16 Update in Intensive Care and Emergency Medicine

Edited by J.L.Vincent

M. Lamy L.G. Thijs (Eds.)

Mediators of Sepsis

With 80 Figures and 41 Tables

Springer-Verlag
Berlin Heidelberg New York
London Paris Tokyo
Hong Kong Barcelona
Budapest

Series Editor

Prof. Dr. Jean Louis Vincent
Clinical Director, Department of Intensive Care, Erasme Hospital
Free University of Brussels, Route de Lennik 808
1070 Brussels, Belgium

Volume Editors

Prof. Dr. Maurice Lamy
Department of Anesthesiology, Centre Hospitalier
Universitaire de Liège, B-35
Domaine Universitaire du Sart Tilman, 4000 Liège, Belgium

Prof. Dr. Lambert G.Thijs
Department of Intensive Care, Free University Hospital
De Boelelaan 1117, 1007 MS Amsterdam, The Netherlands

ISBN 3-540-55841-1 Springer-Verlag Berlin Heidelberg New York
ISBN 0-387-55841-1 Springer-Verlag New York Berlin Heidelberg

Typesetting: HST, Heidelberg. Printing: Zechnersche Buchdruckerei, Speyer
Bookbinding: J. Schäffer, Grünstadt

19/3130-5 4 3 2 1 0 - Printed on acid-free paper

Contents

Mediators and Pathophysiology of Sepsis

List of Contributors

Baumgartner, J.D.
Division of Infectious Diseases, Department of Internal Medicine, CHU Vaudois, 1011 Lausane, Switzerland

Berlot, G.
Anesthesia & Intensive Care Department, Ospedale di Cattinara, University of Trieste, Trieste 34141, Italy

Bernard, C.
Department of Anesthesiology and Intensive Care, Lariboisière University Hospital, 2 Rue Ambroise Paré, 75010 Paris, France

Beutler, B.
Research Laboratories, Howard Hugues Medical Institute, 5353 Harry Hines Boulevard, Dallas TX 75235-9050,USA

Biemond, B.J.
Department of Internal Medicine, Academic Medical Center F4-222, Meibergdreef 9, 1105 AZ Amsterdam, The Netherlands

Bone, R.C.
Section of Pulmonary Medicine, Rush-Presbyterian-St Luke's Medical Center, 1753 West Congress Parkway, Chicago IL 60612, USA

Braquet, P.
Institut Henri Beaufour, 17 Avenue Descartes, 92350 Le Plessis Robinson, France

Brigham, K.L.
Center for Lung Research, Vanderbilt University, School of Medicine, Nashville TN 37232-2650, USA

Brunet, F.
Dept of Intensive Care, Hôpital Cochin, 27 Faubourg St Jacques, 75674 Parix Cedex 14, France

Camus, G.
Laboratory of Human Applied Physiology, ISEPK, B21, University of Liège, Sart Tilman, 4000 Liège, Belgium

Canonico, A.E.
Center for Lung Research, Vanderbilt University, School of Medicine, Nashville TN 37232-2650, USA

Cerra, F.B.
Department of Surgery, University of Minnesota Hospital, 406 Harvard Street South East, Minneapolis MN 55455, USA

Cohen, J.
Infectious Diseases Unit, Hammersmith Hospital, Du Cane Road, London W12 ONN, United Kingdom

Colman, R.W.
Thrombosis Research Center, Temple University School of Medicine, 3400 North Broad Street, Philadelphia PA 19140, USA

Conary, J.T.
Center for Lung Research, Vanderbilt University, School of Medicine, Nashville TN 37232-2650, USA

Dellinger, R.P.
Intensive Care Unit, Baylor College of Medicine, Ben Taub Hospital, 1504 Ben Taub Loop, Houston TX 10017, USA

Dhainaut, J.F.
Dept of Intensive Care,Hôpital Cochin, 27 Faubourg St Jacques, 75674 Paris Cedex 14, France

Dinarello, C.A.
Department of Medicine, Tufts University School of Medicine, 750 Washington Street, Boston MA 02111, USA

Fisher, C.J.
Department of Medicine, University Hospital of Cleveland, 2074 Abington Road, Cleveland OH 44106, USA

Girardin, E.
Department of Pediatrics, Hôpital des Enfants, 1211 Genève 4, Switzerland

Gurll, N.J.
Department of Surgery, University of Iowa Hospitals and Clinics, Iowa City IA 52242, USA

Hack, C.E.
Netherlands Red Cross Blood Transfusion Service, University of Amsterdam, De Boelelaan 1117, 1007 MB Amsterdam, The Netherlands

Hechtman, H.B.
Department of Surgery, Brigham and Woman's Hospital, 75 Francis Street, Boston MA 02115, USA

Hill, J.
Department of Surgery, Brigham and Woman's Hospital, 75 Francis Street, Boston MA 02115, USA

Holaday, J.W.
Medicis Pharmaceutical Corp., 100 East 42nd Street, New York NY 10017, USA

Hosford, D.
Institut Henri Beaufour, 17 Avenue Descartes, 92350 Le Plessis Robinson, France

Kehlet, H.
Department of Surgical Gastroenterology, Hvidovre University Hospital, 2650 Hvidovre, Denmark

Koltai, M.
Institut Henri Beaufour, 17 Avenue Descartes, 92350 Le Plessis Robinson, France

Lamy, M.
Department of Anesthesiology, CHU B35, University of Liège, Sart Tilman, 4000 Liège, Belgium

Levi, M.
Department of Internal Medicine, Academic Medical Center F4-222, Meibergdreef 9, 1105 AZ Amsterdam, The Netherlands

Lindsay, T.F.
Department of Surgery, Brigham and Women's Hospital, 75 Francis Street, Boston MA 02115, USA

Lowry, S.F.
Laboratory of Surgical Metabolism, Cornell University Medical College F-2016, 525 East 68th Street, New York NY 10021, USA

Marra, M.N.
Department of Medicine, University Hospital of Cleveland, 2074 Abington Road, Cleveland OH 44106, USA

Marshall, J.C.
Department of Surgery, Toronto General Hospital, 200 Elizabeth Street, Toronto Ontario M5G 2C4, Canada

Marzi, I.
Department of Surgery, Bad Homburg Hospital, 6380-Bad Homburg, Germany

Michie, H.R.
Department of Surgery, John Radcliff Hospital, Headleyway, Oxford OX3 9DU, United Kingdom

Migliori, S.
Department of Surgery, University of Minnesota Hospital, 406 Harvard Street South East, Minneapolis MN 55455, USA

Mira, J.P.
Department of Intensive Care, Hôpital Cochin, 27 Faubourg St Jacques, 75674 Paris Cedex 14, France

Moldawer, L.L.
Laboratory of Surgical Metabolism, Cornell University Medical College, F-2016, 525 East 68th Street, New York NY 10021, USA

Opal, S.M.
Department of Medicine, Memorial Hospital, 111 Brewster Street Pawtucket, Rhode Island 02860, USA

Parratt, J.R.
Department of Physiology and Pharmacology, University of Strathclyde, 204 George Street, Glasgow G1 1XW, United Kingdom

Payen, D.
Department of Anesthesiology and Intensive Care, Lariboisière University Hospital, 2 Rue Ambroise Paré, 75010 Paris, France

Pincemail, J.
Laboratory of Biochemistry and Radiobiology, Institute of Chemistry B6, University of Liège, Sart Tilman, 4000 Liège, Belgium

Redl, H.
Department of Experimental Traumatology, Ludwig Boltzmann Institute, Donauschingenstrasse 13, 1200 Vienna, Austria

Schlag, G.
Department of Experimental Traumatology, Ludwig Boltzmann Institute, Donauschingenstrasse 13, 1200 Vienna, Austria

Stoclet, J.C.
Laboratoire de Pharmacologie Cellulaire et Moléculaire, Université Louis Pasteur, Strasbourg, France

Straube, R.C.
Department of Infectious Diseases, Clinical Research, Centocor Inc., Malvern PA19355, USA

Suffredini, A.F.
Department of Critical Care, National Institute of Health, Building 10 Room 7-D-43, Bethesda MD 20892, USA

Tedgui, A.
Department of Anesthesiology and Intensive Care, Lariboisière University Hospital, 2 Rue Ambroise Paré, 75010 Paris, France

Thijs, L.G.
Department of Medical Intensive Care, Free University Hospital, De Boelelaan 1117, 1007 MB Amsterdam, The Netherlands

van Deventer, S.J.H.
Departement of International Medicine, Academic Medical Center F4-222, Meibergdreef 9, 1105 AZ Amsterdam, The Netherlands

VanZee, K.J.
Laboratory of Surgical Metabolism, Cornell University Medical College, F-2016, 525 East 68th Street, New York NY 10021, USA

Vincent, J.L.
Department of Intensive Care, Erasme University Hospital, Route de Lennik 808, 1070 Brussels, Belgium

Zimmerman, J.J.
Department of Pediatrics, Children's Hospital, H4/470, 600 Highland Avenue, Madison WI 53792-4108, USA

Abbreviations

ACTH	Adrenocorticotrophic hormone
ARDS	Adult respiratory distress syndrome
BALF	Bronchoalveolar lavage fluid
BPI	Bactericidal permeability increasing protein
CAT	Chloramphenicol acetyltransferase
CSF	Cerebrospinal fluid
EC	Endothelial cell
DIC	Disseminated intravascular coagulation
DMSO	Dimethylsulfoxide
EDRF	Endothelium-derived relaxing factor
ELAM	Endothelial-leukocyte adhesion molecule
FFA	Free fatty acid
GALT	Gut associated lymphoid tissues
GI	Gastrointestinal
GMCSF	Granulocyte-monocyte colony stimulating factor
ICAM	Intercellular adhesion molecule
IL	Interleukin
IL-1ra	Interleukin-1 receptor antagonist
LBP	Lipopolysaccharide binding protein
LPS	Lipopolysaccharide
MAb	Monoclonal antibody
MDF	Myocardial depressant factor
MDS	Myocardial depressant substance
MODS	Multiple organ dysfunction syndrome
MOF	Multiple organ failure
MPO	Myleoperoxidase
NO	Nitric oxide
PAF	Platelet activating factor
PAP	Pulmonary artery pressure
PGE_2	Prostaglandin E_2
PMN	Polymorphonuclear neutrophils
SIRS	Systemic inflammatory response syndrome

SOD	Superoxide dismutase
TBARS	Thiobarbituric acid reactive species
Tx	Thromboxane
TNF	Tumor necrosis factor
tPA	Tissue plasminogen activator
TPN	Total parenteral nutrition
VLDL	Very low density lipoprotein
WBC	White blood cells

Mediators and Pathophysiology of Sepsis

Sepsis and Multiple Organ Failure: Consensus and Controversy

R. C. Bone

Introduction

Sepsis and its related sequelae, including sepsis, shock and multiple organ failure (MOF), are currently the subject of much discussion and some controversy. They are an important source of hospital morbidity and mortality; and a subject that all physicians should be familiar with-yet the pathogenesis of these diseases is still not fully understood. Research into their causes is progressing and new methods of diagnosis and treatment are being developed. In developing the protocols for clinical trials, and too, for basic research into the condition, investigators have run into an important problem: the terms used to describe the conditions have been imprecise or poorly defined. It is important that researchers be able to communicate with each other about their work, and that the knowledge gained through their work is disseminated efficiently and accurately to physicians. It is just as important that the physician dispensing health care to patients be able to accurately describe their condition. Thus, for people involved in medically diagnosing and treating sepsis and for those involved in researching sepsis, the terminology used to define various conditions that relate to sepsis is an important issue.

The importance of precise language is difficult to overstate. For instance, the results of one study cannot legitimately be compared to those of other studies that test the same hypothesis if different definitions were used in the two studies [1–3]. Part of the reason for these inconsistent definitions has arisen when terms are defined differently by the various clinical subspecialties, or sometimes even by individuals within a given field. Also contributing to the controversy is the fact that sepsis and its related conditions are not discrete, well-defined entities but, rather, may be more accurately defined as a gradation of dysfunction. This gradation can be seen as a continuum of illness severity that ranges from the nearly inconsequential to the fatal. It seems that everyone has a vague notion of what the related terms bacteremia, sepsis, septicemia, sepsis syndrome, septic shock and MOF mean, but too often, these words are used interchangeably in speech and in the professional literature, resulting in poor communication and lost meaning.

The importance of accurate definitions may be underscored by the incidence of sepsis. While the actual numbers cannot be known, some 70.000 to 300.000 cases of sepsis are estimated to occur each year in the United States alone [4, 5]. Others have estimated that as many as 80.000 Americans die each year from sepsis and its complications [6]. It is therefore imperative that we have the ability to accurately understand, assess, and communicate precise features of a patient's status. Early recognition and treatment is crucial, given the tendency of sepsis to increase in severity once started; when the complication of sepsis occurs, clinical progression may be rapid and the outcome unfavorable.

Also making the occurrence and treatment of sepsis important to clinicians is the fact that many innovations used in clinical practice may actually have increased its occurrence [5]. These include aggressive oncologic chemotherapy, corticosteroid or immunosuppressive therapy for organ transplantation or inflammatory diseases, the increased survival of patients predisposed to sepsis, and the more frequent use of invasive medical procedures [5, 7]. Even the simplest invasive procedure carries with it the risk of infection as the body surface is opened or abraded, from which sepsis can start. It is ironic that, in our attempts to provide better care, we are making patients more susceptible to the potentially fatal complication of sepsis.

Definitions

Because of the seriousness of sepsis, a number of position papers and rebuttals were published over the last year or two on the subject of its definitions [8–11]. The participants in these discussions, however, could not reach an agreement. Since the need for consensus had become a critical issue, the American Collage of Chest Physicians and the Society of Critical Care Medicine held a consensus conference in an attempt to agree upon a series of terms by which sepsis could be discussed. The following list of terms summarizes the results of that conference.

Infection: Infection is defined as an inflammatory response to the presence of microorganisms or their invasion of normally sterile host tissue.

Bacteremia: Bacteremia is defined as the presence of viable bacteria in the blood. Terms such as viremia, fungemia, parasitemia, and others may also be used when they are present in the blood.

Septicemia: This term has long been used to broadly describe the presence of microorganisms in the blood. The consensus conference decided that it is an ambiguous and imprecise term; its usage should be avoided.

Sepsis: Sepsis is the systemic response to infection. Its manifestations are the same as those for SIRS (see below) but are always associated with the presence of an infectious process. When due to the presence of bacteria, SIRS is synonymous with sepsis.

Severe Sepsis: Severe sepsis is a distinct stage on the continuum of clinical and pathophysiological changes that are associated with sepsis and its sequelae. This term is defined as sepsis with organ dysfunction, abnormal hypoperfusion (that may be characterized by such symptoms as lactic acidosis, oliguria, or acutely altered mental status), or sepsis-induced hypotension.

Sepsis-Induced Hypotension: A systolic blood pressure of less than 90 mm Hg or its reduction by more than 40 mm Hg from baseline in the absence of other causes for such a reduction, constitutes the definition for this term.

Septic Shock: Septic shock is a subset of severe sepsis and consists of a sepsis-induced hypotension that persists, despite adequate fluid resuscitation. Hypoperfusion abnormalities or organ dysfunction are also manifest in septic shock.

Systemic Inflammatory Response Syndrome (SIRS): This term describes a systemic inflammatory response that may or may not result from infection.

Table 1. Definitions

Infection - Microbial phenomenon characterized by an inflammatory response to the presence of microorganisms or the invasion of normally sterile host tissue by those organisms.

Bacteremia - The presence of viable bacteria in the blood.

Systemic inflammatory response syndrome (SIRS) - The systemic inflammatory response to a variety of severe clinical insults (see text). The response is manifested by two or more of the following conditions:

Temperature > 38° C or < 36° C.
Heart rate > 90 beats per minute.
Respiratory rate > 20 breaths per minute or $PaCO_2$ < 32mm Hg.
White blood cell count > 12.000 cells/ml, < 4.000 cells/ml, or > 10% immature (band) forms.

Sepsis - The systemic response to infection. This systemic response is manifested by two or more of the following conditions as a result of infection:

Temperature > 38° C or <36° C.
Heart rate > 90 beats per minute.
Respiratory rate > 20 breaths per minute or $PaCO_2$ < 32mm Hg.
White blood cell count > 12.000 cells/ml, < 4.000 cells/ml, or > 10% immature (band) forms.

Severe sepsis - Sepsis associated with organ dysfunction, hypoperfusion, or hypotension. Hypoperfusion and perfusion abnormalitiers may include, but are not limited to lactic acidosis, oliguria, or an acute alteration in mental status.

Septic shock - Sepsis with hypotension despite adequate fluid resuscitation along with the presence of perfusion abnormalities which may include, but are not limited to, lactic acidosis, oliguria, or an acute alteration in mental status. Patients who are on inotropic or vasopressor agents may not be hypotensive at the time that perfusion abnormalities are measured.

Hypotension - A systolic blood pressure < 90 mm Hg or a reduction of > 40 mm Hg from baseline in the absence of other causes for hypotension.

Multiple organ dysfunction syndrome (MODS): Presence of altered organ function in an actuely ill patient such that homeostasis cannot be maintained without intervention.

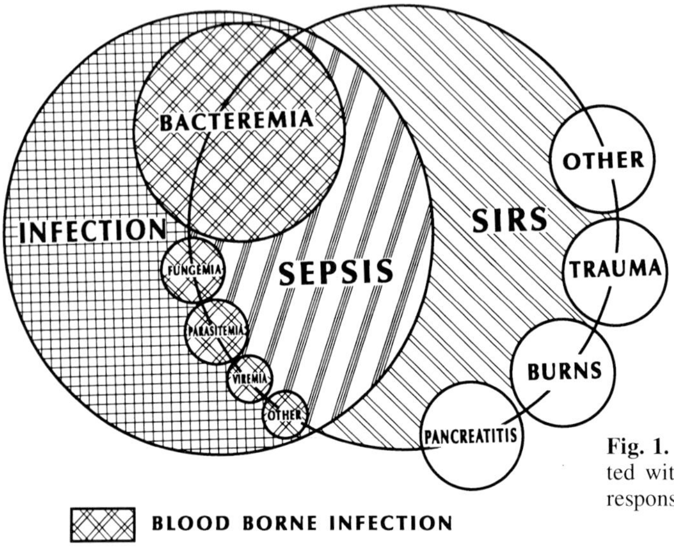

Fig. 1. Conditions associated with the inflammatory response syndrome (SIRS)

This term summarizes our current understanding of the pathophysiology of the disease and encompasses a number of conditions that, previously, may have been considered as separate entities. SIRS is defined as occurring when two or more of the clinical manifestations, outlined in Table 1, are present.

Multiple Organ Dysfunction Syndrome (MODS): This term further defines another point on the continuum of physiological derangements that occur in SIRS. In MODS, organ dysfunction caused by SIRS induced damage reaches the point at which homeostasis cannot be maintained without supportive measures. MODS can either take the form of primary MODS, which arises from a specific insult, such as aspiration injury to the lung resulting culminating in a localized inflammatory response and resulting damage, and secondary MODS, which develops consequent to a host immune response rather than a direct response to an insult. MODS is found at the end of the SIRS/sepsis continuum where fatality is highest.

The essential concept which underlies the more serious of the above conditions is a systemic inflammatory response (Fig. 1). As defined above, this response can be initiated by a variety of events. It has long been assumed that the mortality and morbidity associated with sepsis were due to the presence of bacteria in the blood. However, it is now known that the infection itself is not the cause of the problem but, rather, it is the body's own response to various conditions that causes the damage seen in sepsis. This response is essentially a systemic inflammatory response that can affect various organ systems in the body and is brought about by the action of the body's endogenous molecular mediators. While these molecular entities may be assumed to be adaptive in normal settings, during sepsis their activity becomes injurious. It seems that an „all out" response may occur to circulating endotoxin, resulting in an exaggerated release of the mediators of sepsis. It may be important to note that gram-negative sepsis can result from a very brief bout of endotoxemia-all signs of the bacteria may be gone by the time SIRS manifests itself. It may soon be possible to diagnose SIRS by the presence in the blood of the various mediators of inflammation. Key among these is tumor necrosis factor (TNF), believed to be the first mediator released, largely by endotoxin-activated macrophages, that is followed by a host of other mediator releases. This system is extremely complex and will take much basic research to understand. Each of the mediators may affect the actions of release of other mediators, and there may be mediators involved in this response that have not even been discovered yet.

Identical physiological responses can be produced by gram-positive and gram-negative bacteria; by pathogenic viruses, fungi, and rickettsia; and by non-infectious processes, such as pancreatitis, tissue injury, or even the administration of exogenous TNF or other mediators. Thus, patients with SIRS may have positive or negative blood cultures.

Other terms that have been used in the past include „warm shock“ and „cold shock“. However, while we may better understand the physiology underlying these conditions, their clinical significance is unclear. Warm shock was characterized by the shock symptoms of decreased systemic vascular resistance and increased cardiac output. These are accompanied by leukocyte aggregation, microembolus formation, and endothelial cell injury. The possible later progression to a state of increased vascular resistance, „cold shock“, was rare since most patients maintain decreased systemic vascular resistance even in the late phases of SIRS with shock. Cold shock, with its decreased cardiac output, reflects myocardial depression and the accompanying systemic responses of microvascular insufficiency, inadequate blood flow to tissues, increased lactic acid production, severe organ dysfunction, and even death. However, these terms do not represent solid clinical conditions; patients may manifest symptoms that do not fully match these criteria. Although we can define the physiological changes that occur, it is not understood why they occur. The new definitions of sepsis are broad and inclusive. There is little point to further refining the definitions of such a polymorphic disease entity, particularly when the terms contain little clinical significance.

In 1987, criteria by which sepsis might be defined were studied in a group of prospectively evaluated patients that comprised the placebo treatment group of a double-blind study of methylprednisolone use in patients with SIRS and SIRS with shock [1]. The purpose of that study was to define the parameters of a syndrome that could be distinguished on the basis of readily available, non-invasive clinical criteria at an earlier stage of disease progression than had been previously cited in the literature. By doing so, it was hoped that a point could be defined at which therapeutic interventions might be instituted with the greatest likelihood of preventing the more serious complications of sepsis: septic shock and MOF including the adult respiratory distress syndrome (ARDS), a manifestation of MODS in the lung. The definition of sepsis used in the study allowed the conclusion that 47 % of bacteremic patients went on to develop shock, compared with 30 % of pa-

Table 2. Mortality rate associated with various terms used in SIRS

Term	Mortality rate	Reference
Bacteremia	12-61%*	[6]
Septicemia		
Sepsis	10-20%*	[13]
	50%	[3]
	20-50%	[6]
SIRS	75%	[2]
	25.6%	[4]
SIRS with shock	40-90%	[5]
	27.5-43.2%	[4]
	40-50%	[14]
	10-36%	[15]
Refractory or non-responsive septic shock	77%	[2]
	43%	[4]

*Gram-negative sepsis

tients who were non-bacteremic [4]. Data from the same investigation showed that ARDS developed in 25 % of patients, and that 14-day mortality within the population with ARDS was 22 % [12].

Our own research has shown that the diagnosis of SIRS without septic shock carries with it a mortality rate of approximately 13 %. One would expect that for bacteremia and sepsis, the numbers should be lower, while those for septic shock or refractory septic shock would be much higher. It is not surprising, however, that our review of the literature pointed out remarkable disparity in the mortality statistics in these situations (Table 2). In presenting these mortality data we have, in each instance, used the authors' definitions of the clinical entity under investigation. In doing so, it became obvious that investigators were not always referring to the same disease entity when using any given term. If they had been speaking of the same clinical condition, it is unlikely that we would see the same mortality rates (e.g. 40 %) associated with such clearly disparate clinical conditions as bacteremia on the one hand, and septic shock on the other.

Septic shock has been associated with mortality rates ranging from 10 to 90 % [2–6, 13–15]. At least one study has documented that treatment in the latter stages of SIRS with shock has limited effect on clinical outcome [1]. In a study of corticosteroid usage in septic shock, a 75 % mortality (44 of 59 patients) rate was recorded [2]. An investigation of myocardial depression, which may be responsible for at least some of the symptoms of septic shock, in patients with septic shock demonstrated that the presence of a circulating

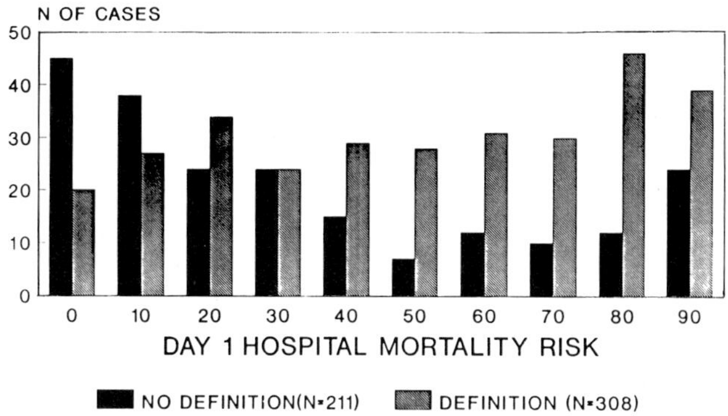

Fig. 2. Risk distributions of 519 ICU admissions for sepsis according to the categorical definition of septic sydrome

myocardial depressant substance (MDS) in the sera was associated with increased mortality (36 %), compared with septic shock patients whose sera were MDS-negative (10 %) [15].

In a study to test the validity of the various definitions [16], hospital mortality risk distribution was calculated on the first day of ICU treatment for 519 patients according to whether or not they met criteria, defined by Bone et al. [17] for septic syndrome. The risk distribution of the 308 (59 %) patients meeting the criteria for this syndrome is not substantially different from the 211 (41 %) patients who did not fulfill the criteria for septic syndrome (Fig. 2).

The result depicted in Fig. 3 shows that when the SIRS definition is applied to the same 519 patients with a primary clinical diagnosis of sepsis, it identified 96.9 % (503 of 519). What this new definition has achieved, therefore, is an increase in the number of patients classified by the definition. Thus, patients excluded by the previous definition (sepsis syndrome) were now included in the SIRS definition. This is important, since the estimated risks of previously excluded patients were equivalent to those who were included.

Other Indicators of SIRS

Arterial blood lactate levels have been used as a measure of the severity of perfusion failure and, hence, of shock [18]. Reduced cardiac output, velocity of blood flow, and measured plasma volume have also been associated with disproportionate increases in arterial blood lactate levels and fatal outcome. However, the use of blood pressure as a monitoring tool can be legitimately criticized since there are no absolute thresholds for indicating disease. Nonetheless, it is readily available in all hospitals and can be uniformly applied. It would probably be of greater use if a reliable baseline measure can be obtained before the more serious complications of SIRS begin.

There have been several attempts to develop scoring systems that define the severity of the inflammatory response; the most commonly used one is the APACHE series of scoring systems. The most recent version, APACHE

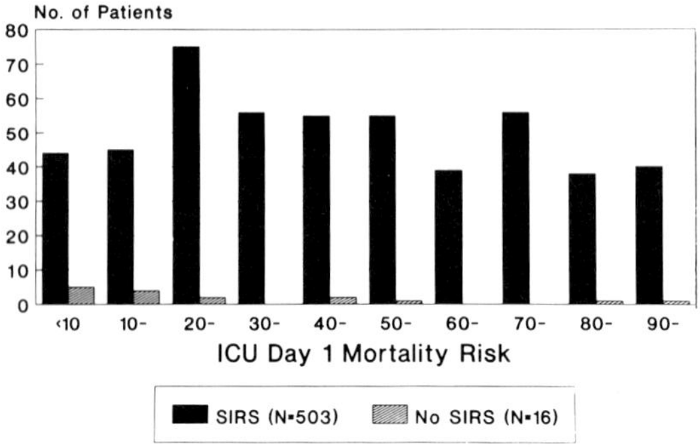

Fig. 3. Risk distributions of 519 ICU admissions for sepsis according to the definition of the systemic inflammatory response syndrome. ■ SIRS (N=503); □ No Sirs (N=169

III, utilizes a database of over 17.000 ICU patients to predict the risk of mortality for individual patients with the systemic inflammatory response. The individual patients are rated by quantifying a number of key physiological and historic variables. The score produced by the APACHE III system can be used by the clinician to predict outcome and as a guide for therapeutic intervention. The use of such scoring systems is also of great importance to researchers investigating the mechanisms of sepsis, allowing consistency of methods and the accurate communication of results. The most important improvement made possible by these new definitions and scoring tests is the consistency of entry criteria for clinical studies; it is important for study subjects to have comparable disease states. The probability estimates obtained through APACHE III scoring can also be used for utilization management, quality assurance comparisons between institutions, and for pre-treatment control of patient risk factors in clinical trials. It must be remembered, however, that these scoring systems are far from perfect; since we do not fully understand the mechanisms that underlie this inflammatory response, it is impossible to pick the key measurable parameters necessary to yield a completely accurate score.

Two other predictive scoring instruments that have been proposed are the Elebute and the surgical sepsis scoring systems. These two systems have been validated in small groups of patients but they have not been shown to have greater predictive power than the APACHE III scoring system [19].

New Treatment Modes

Currently, the only treatments freely available for patients with SIRS and MODS are essentially supportive. Treatment for the symptoms of shock, including volume resuscitation, inotropes, and vasopressors have been a mainstay in the clinicians repertoire. Other treatments have been used when organ failures manifest themselves: mechanical ventilators when the lung is affected, as in ARDS, and dialysis when the kidney is dysfunctional. However, the new treatments made possible by recent advances in biological technology are already being developed and tested. It is in clinical trials of such treatments that the new definitions being advocated here will be particularly important. These new treatments will be directed at the root causes of sepsis rather than the symptoms. For instance, monoclonal antibodies against endotoxin have completed Phase III testing and will soon be on the market for limited use. Another antibody has been developed that binds to TNF although its clinical validation is still in the early phases.

However, there is still much to learn of the pathophysiology of SIRS, and there may be a large number of ways to affect the mediator system underlying the disorder. For instance, it may be possible to block the receptors that bind the various mediators or endotoxin. Since each individual case of SIRS may involve its own unique group of excess mediators, it may be possible, ultimately, for each individual case of sepsis to have its own „cocktail“ of antibodies and receptor blockers to alleviate the condition.

Conclusion

The recently held American College of Chest Physicians-Society for Critical Care Medicine Consensus Conference was intended to help settle issues of terminology [20]. A key problem was revealed with the conference's affirmation that sepsis and its sequelae are best described as a dynamic continuum. Thus, no terminology invoking static terms can be completely satisfactory. However, there are certain clinically relevant periods in the development in sepsis that must be recognized and defined with appropriate terminology. An analysis of multicenter trials of effective agents for sepsis treatment indicates that the early recognition of impending circulatory compromise in patients with sepsis, followed by the institution of prompt and aggressive therapeutic intervention may increase survival [10]. Such recognition requires that clinicians be able to detect both the clinical markers of each of these entities and to discern the sometimes subtle and often rapidly changing signs and symptoms that herald the downward progression of the condition.

The therapeutic uses of monoclonal antibodies to endotoxin and to cytokines, such as TNF, may prove to be the key to controlling the septic conditions. Armed with reasonable and precise definitions to delineate the components of the septic process, we will now be in a better position to compare the various studies covering different treatment modalities. Our increased knowledge of the pathophysiology of sepsis means that we will be able to initiate therapy at an earlier stage in the disease. This may be critical since sepsis appears to be a building process in which mediator release can take the form of an amplifying, cascade-like process. This cascade must be controlled before the sequelae of shock and MOF occur. Only through careful and consistent use of language can we expect to achieve this kind of understanding, and thereby potentially improve clinic outcomes for our patients.

The terms we have been using in the past have come to be more of a hinderance than a help to clinicians and researchers. In particular, considerable confusion arises when imprecise terminology is used in clinical investigations that must be compared. I therefore recommend that the standardized, specific nomenclature used to denote the various phases of the sepsis process that have been proposed by the ACCP-SCCM Consensus Conference be universally accepted and applied.

References

1. Bone RC, Fisher CJ, Clemmer TP, Slotman GJ, Metz CA, Balk RA, and the Methylprednisolone Severe Sepsis Study Group (1987) A controlled clinical trial of highdose methylprednisolone in the treatment of severe sepsis and septic shock. N. Engl J Med 317:353–358
2. Sprung CL, Caralis PV, Marcial EH, et al. (1984) The effects of high-dose corticosteroids in patients with septic shock: A prospective, controlled study. N Engl J Med 311:1137–1143
3. The Veterans Administration Systemic Sepsis Comparative Study Group (1987) Effect of high-dose glucocorticoid therapy on mortality in patients with clinical signs of sepsis. N Engl J Med 317:659–665
4. Bone RC, Fisher CJ, Clemmer TJ, Slotman GJ, Metz CA, Balk RA, and the Methylprednisolone Severe Sepsis Study Group (1989) Sepsis syndrome: A valid clinical entity. Crit Care Med 17:389–393
5. Parker MM, Parrillo JE (1983) Septic shock: Hemodynamics and pathogenesis. JAMA 250:3324–3327
6. Young LS (1990) Gram-negative sepsis. In: Mandell GL, Douglas RG, Bennet JE (eds). Principles and Practice of Infectious Diseases, 3rd edition Churchill Livingston, New York, pp 611–636
7. Shubin H, Weil MH (1976) Bacterial shock. JAMA 235:421
8. Bone RC (1991) Let's agree on terminology: Defintions of sepsis. Crit Care Med 19:973
9. Bone RC (1991) Sepsis, sepsis syndrome, multi-organ failure: A plea for comporable definitions. Ann Intern Med (Editorial) 114:332–333
10. Sprung CL (1991) Definitions of sepsis-Have we reached a consensus? Crit Care Med (Editorial) 19:849–851
11. Canadian Multiple Organ Failure Study Group (1991) „Sepsis"-Clarity of existing terminology-or more confusion? Crit Care Med (Editorial) 19:996–998
12. Bone RC, Fisher CJ, Clemmer TP, Slotman GJ, Metz CA and the Methylprednisolone Severe Sepsis Study Group (1987) Early methylprednisolone treatment for septic syndrome and the adult respiratory distress syndrome. Chest 92:1032–1036
13. Dunn D (1987) Immunotherapeutic advances in the treatment of gram-negative bacterial sepsis. World J Surg 11:233–240
14. Cotran RS, Kumar V, Robbins SL (1989) In: Cotran RS, Kumar V, Robins SL (eds.) Robbins Pathologic Basis of Disease, 4th edition. W. B. Saunders, Philadelphia, pp 114–120
15. Cunnion RE, Parrillo JE (1989) Myocardial dysfunction in sepsis: Recent insights. Chest 95:941–945
16. Knaus WA, Sun X, Nystrom PO, Wagner DP (1992) Evaluation of definition of sepsis. Chest (in press)
17. Bone RC Fisher CJ Jr, Clemmer TP, et al. (1989) Sepsis syndrome: A valid clinical entity. Crit Care Med 17:389–393
18. Rackow EC (1986) Clinical definition of sepsis and septic shock. In: WJ Sibbald, CL Sprung (eds) New Horizons: Perspectives on Sepsis and Septic Shock. Society of Critical Care Medicine, Fullerton, CA, pp 1–10
19. Pilz G, Werden K (1990) Cardiovascular parameters and scoring systems in the evaluation of response to therapy in sepsis and septic shock. Infection. 18:253
20. The ACCP/SCCM Consensus Conference Committee (1992) Definitions for sepsis and organ failure and guidelines for the use of innovative therapies in sepsis. Chest 101:1644–1655

Endotoxin Administration to Humans: A Model of Inflammatory Responses Relevant to Sepsis

A. F. Suffredini

Introduction

Researchers throughout the past century have held an avid interest in the responses elicited in humans by exposure to endotoxin. At the turn of the century, this was based on such divergent themes as the physiological sequelae of fever to the therapeutic effects of bacterial products in patients with malignancies. It is now apparent that these clinical problems shared basic mediators and mechanisms of inflammation that were initiated by exposure to bacterial components including endotoxin. Many of the inflammatory responses elicited by endotoxin share final common pathways with other mediators of inflammation. Further, ample data currently exists which has defined a critical role for endotoxin in the pathogenesis of human gram-negative sepsis, shock and multiple organ failure (MOF) [1, 2]. Thus, with almost one hundred years of *in vitro* and *in vivo* experiments, why should investigators continue to evaluate host responses to endotoxin?

Endotoxin is a novel molecule because it represents an important probe for investigating the humoral and cellular basis of the syndrome of sepsis and septic shock [3]. The administration of endotoxin to humans remains of interest because of the ability to apply new technologies and extend previous concepts of inflammation in a human model of acute inflammatory responses. Further, endotoxin administration to humans provides an opportunity to evaluate the earliest responses that are activated after exposure to an important and common bacterial component. Defining these pathways and their interactions may allow a better understanding of the factors that can be controlled or altered during critical illness.

Limitations of this model of inflammatory responses exist as with any model which attempts to reproduce a clinical syndrome. Contemporary investigators have limited the dose of endotoxin administered to healthy individuals to avoid excessive toxicities. As such, many of the alterations in organ function or circulating mediators observed after endotoxin administration are qualitatively rather than quantitatively similar to that seen in the full syndrome of septic shock. A single dose of intravenous endotoxin administered to an otherwise healthy volunteer cannot be equated to a virulent infection. In clinical sepsis, non-endotoxin bacterial factors may additionally contribute to organ failure, and prior underlying organ damage may potentiate inflammatory injury. Yet even in the context of these limitations, biologically relevant effects pertinent to sepsis and septic shock can often be elicited and manipulated within this model.

Animal studies based on the administration of endotoxin although not restricted by dose have other limitations. Animal species vary considerably in their sensitivity or resistance to endotoxin. The animal species evaluated and the dose of endotoxin required to elicit a specific response influence the clinical relevance of these models [4, 5]. Further, inflammatory responses as well as end-organ responses to endotoxin may vary among animal species [5].

Responses Evaluated using the Human Endotoxin Model

This review is limited to contemporary studies of endotoxin administration to humans performed during the past five years. These have been arbitrarily divided into sections that describe the general systemic effects, alterations in organ function, metabolic, endocrine, hepatic and hematologic effects. Lastly, the effects of endotoxin on humoral and cellular inflammatory responses are reviewed (Table 1).

Endotoxin Preparations used in Human Studies

Investigations performed in the 1940s and 1950s which evaluated the effects of endotoxin often relied upon whole, killed bacterial vaccines [6]. The de-

Table 1. Responses evaluated in contemporary studies of humans following the intravenous administration of endotoxin

Systemic responses	Hematologic alterations
fever	leukocyte flux
Alterations in organ function	Humoral inflammatory responses
cardiovascular	fibrinolysis
pulmonary	hemostasis
gut	kallikrein-kinin generation
renal	complement
blood-ocular barrier	
	Inflammatory cell function
Metabolic responses	neutrophils
oxygen consumption	alveolar macrophages
metabolic substrates	
	Cytokine responses
Endocrine responses	TNFα, IL-1β, IL-6, IL-8, GCSF
hypothalamic-pituitary-adrenal axis	anti-cytokine molecules
stress hormones	neopterin
Liver	
acute phase protein production	

velopment of preparations of purified material greatly assisted the standardization of responses in patients and animals. Preparations used in these earlier studies included endotoxin derived with varying degrees of purity from *Salmonella typhosa, Pseudomonas* species (Piromen) or *Salmonella abortus* equii (Lipexal or Pyrexal). The latter bacterial endotoxin preparation has continued to be used in recent studies of human endotoxin administration [7, 8].

Many investigators have used an endotoxin preparation developed by the Office of Biologics of the U.S. Food and Drug Administration to aid in the standardization of bioassays and research with endotoxin. Reference Standard Endotoxin (*Escherichia coli* 0 113:H 10:K negative, Lot EC-5) is a homogeneous preparation that has been well characterized [9]. This facilitates comparisons of studies performed in humans at different institutions. The usual intravenous dose of reference endotoxin given to normal volunteers ranges from 2 to 4 ng/kg (1 ng is approximately 10 endotoxin units).

General Constitutional and Systemic Responses

With the administration of 2 to 4 ng/kg of reference endotoxin, a monophasic rise in core temperature occurs [10, 14]. The increase in the core temperature is initiated at one hour with the onset of chills and rigors. Accompanying symptoms include varying degrees of headache, myalgias, arthralgias and nausea. During the prodrome to the fever (1 to 2 h post-endotoxin), the subjects appear sallow, peripherally vasoconstricted and have general malaise. Following 4 ng/kg of reference endotoxin, the core temperature rises to a peak of 38.5 to 40 °C at 3 h, and defervescence begins after this period returning to normal by 8 to 12 h post-endotoxin. The symptoms usually abate by 3 to 4 h post-endotoxin and by 6 to 8 h have almost entirely resolved. Both the magnitude of the fever and the constitutional symptoms are dose-dependent. The minimal pyrogenic dose of reference endotoxin is 0.1–0.5 ng/kg [10]. Although significant decreases in systemic blood pressures do not usually occur with the 4 ng/kg dose, subjects can develop orthostatic changes in blood pressure when placed in a upright position during the initial several hours after the infusion of endotoxin.

Endotoxin is cleared rapidly from the circulation after intravenous administration. Low levels of circulating endotoxin were detected 5 to 15 min after the administration of 2 ng/kg IV (endotoxin concentration range 5–13 pg/ml) [12]. In order to assess whether an extravascular source of endotoxin develops during the inflammatory response to endotoxin, we measured endotoxin concentrations at 15 min and 4 h following administration of 4 ng/kg endotoxin and found none (unpublished observations).

The fever and symptoms due to endotoxin can be ablated with prior administration of cyclooxygenase inhibitors such as ibuprofen [13, 14]. In contrast, the phosphodiesterase inhibitor pentoxifylline (given intravenously or orally) is ineffective in ameliorating any of the symptoms or fever associated with acute endotoxemia [7, 14]. The use of cyclooxygenase inhibitors has been used in Phase I therapeutic trials to maximize the tolerated dose of endotoxin given to patients with malignancies [8].

Alterations in Organ Function

Cardiovascular Responses

Investigations performed as early as 1929 noted that administration of typhoid vaccine to healthy humans resulted in an increase in cardiac output, heart rate and oxygen consumption [15]. Bradley et al. [16] evaluated cardiovascular responses in normal and hypertensive subjects after the administration of a pyrogen (typhoid vaccine or contaminated inulin). Cardiac output, renal blood flow and heart rate increased, and peripheral resistance fell [16]. Moser et al. [17] performed detailed studies in subjects given intravenous gram-negative endotoxin (Pyrexal, 0.45 μg). The core temperature peaked at 3 h and was accompanied by an increased cardiac output, heart rate and decreased total systemic resistance [17]. Thus, endotoxin in pyrogenic doses was associated with a hyperdynamic cardiovascular response.

Little information was available however describing cardiac performance during the acute stages of endotoxemia. We evaluated normal subjects using thermodilution pulmonary artery catheters and radionuclide cineangiograms to characterize left ventricular performance during the initial stages of endotoxemia [11]. After the initial cardiac response was evaluated during the first 3 h, normal saline (mean 2.2 liters) was infused in graded increments in order to evaluate ventricular performance at different preloads. 3 hours after endotoxin administration and prior to the volume infusion, the cardiac index and heart rate increased by 53 % and 36 %, respectively, and the mean arterial pressure and systemic vascular resistance index fell by 18 % and 46 %, respectively [11]. After volume loading, the left ventricular ejection fraction fell by 1 % but increased by 14 % in control subjects given saline alone without endotoxin [11]. The left ventricular ejection fraction is relatively independent of preload and varies inversely with afterload and heart rate. The failure of the left ventricular ejection fraction to rise under similar preload and afterload conditions as the controls suggested that endotoxin administration resulted in an intrinsic abnormality of ventricular function [11].

In addition to the ejection fraction, three other measures were used to assess systolic function. The stroke volume and stroke work indices normalized to the end diastolic volume index, and the load independent measure of peak systolic pressure to end systolic volume index. The values of these ratios were compared before and after saline infusion and were significantly different than the control groups response to fluid administration [11]. These changes were independent of changes in left ventricular volume or vascular resistance, and were similar to the changes of depressed ventricular function observed in human septic shock [2]. These data demonstrate that endotoxin administration to normal humans results in a hyperdynamic cardiovascular response with elevated cardiac index and heart rate and decreased systemic vascular resistance index. Further, an intrinsic decrease in left ventricular performance was initiated by intravenous endotoxin characterized by a depressed left ventricular ejection response and depressed systolic function in response to volume administration [11].

Fever is known to have a complex effect on myocardial performance [18]. Bradley et al. [16] noted that the hyperdynamic cardiovascular response was unchanged with the administration of an antipyretic (amidopyrine, a pyrazolon derivative with anti-inflammatory properties similar to salicylates) prior to the administration of a pyrogen. We evaluated normal subjects in an identical fashion to the above study of cardiovascular performance and randomized subjects to receive endotoxin alone or endotoxin following prior administration of oral ibuprofen in a dose sufficient to ameliorate the fever and the constitutional symptoms [19]. Even in the absence of fever, there was no significant diminution of the hyperdynamic cardiovascular response nor any improvement in the previously described alterations in ventricular performance.

Oxygen delivery and consumption increase by almost 50 % after the administration of endotoxin, and little or no significant increase occurs in the oxygen extraction ratio before or after fluid loading [20]. The initial response of oxygen transport variables in humans to endotoxin administration is a normal capacity of tissues to extract and utilize oxygen. The matching of oxygen consumption and delivery during these initial stages of endotoxemia is not impaired [20]. The absence of fever did not significantly attenuate the increase in oxygen consumption and delivery after endotoxin [19]. Thus, the changes in systemic hemodynamics, ventricular performance, and oxygen transport which follow intravenous endotoxin administration to normal humans are not dependent on fever alone and result from endotoxin itself or endogenous inflammatory mediators.

Detailed studies of extremity and splanchnic blood flow have been obtained in normal subjects following endotoxin (2 ng/kg reference endotoxin) using radial artery and femoral and hepatic vein catheters [21]. Indocyanine green dye infusions were used to estimate splanchnic blood flow, and extremity blood flow was measured using electrocapacitance plethysmography. The estimated splanchnic blood flow increased within the first hour after endotoxin, peaking at 3 h (91 % above baseline values). No significant changes occurred in lower extremity blood flow during the study period [21].

Pulmonary Responses

Minimal changes in lung function following endotoxin were suggested by early studies of endotoxemia. With the onset of symptoms and fever, the respiratory rate increased, the $PaCO_2$ decreased and no changes occurred in PaO_2 [17]. In this latter study, the majority of the central pressures were low or normal and no fluid administration was given to the subjects. We noted that the administration of normal saline sufficient to raise the pulmonary wedge pressure to a high normal range (mean 18 mm Hg) resulted in a widening of the alveolar – arterial gradient and a modest but significant fall in PaO_2 [20]. While these changes in PaO_2 were not clinically significant, similar alterations did not occur in normal subjects given saline alone. These findings suggest that fluid administration may result in changes in ventilation/perfusion matching due to increased lung permeability or to alterations in airway resistance.

In contrast to several animal models where intravenous administration of non-lethal doses of endotoxin results in an acute rise in the pulmonary artery pressure [22], no increase in mean pulmonary artery pressure was found in our subjects given endotoxin [11]. This may relate in part to the total dose given. Additionally, species differences in pulmonary vascular reactivity occur and may be due in part to the presence of resident pulmonary intravascular macrophages [23].

Following endotoxin administration, peripheral blood granulocyte counts characteristically fall to a nadir at 1 h (< 1500 granulocytes x $10^3/mm^3$) which is followed by a leukocytosis with peak counts at 6 h greater than 9.000 granulocytes x $10^3/mm^3$ [14]. Animal models of lung injury based on the administration of endotoxin have shown that neutrophils migrate into the lung parenchyma within hours of the administration of endotoxin [22]. Neutrophils can be recovered in bronchoalveolar lavage fluid of sheep within 3 h of the administration of endotoxin [24].

In order to assess whether neutrophils migrated into the alveolar space after intravenous endotoxin administration, we performed bronchoalveolar lavage at an early time point following the leukopenia (1.5–3 h), during the leukocytosis (5 to 6 h) [20], or at 24 h after endotoxin administration (unpublished observations). Ventilation scans with inhaled Tc99m-diethylenetriamine pentacetate (DTPA, a small marker molecule MW 492) were used to assess alterations in alveolar-epithelial permeability (prior to 3 h) or later time points (5–6 h) after the administration of endotoxin. Despite wide changes in the peripheral leukocyte counts ranging from acute leukopenia to leukocytosis, no increase in the total or percent of alveolar neutrophils were detected in any of the subjects evaluated with bronchoalveolar lavage at any time point [20]. No significant increase was found in bronchoalveolar lavage proteins (e.g. IgG/albumin) indicating that alveolar permeability to larger protein molecules is not increased. In contrast, the rate of clearance of inhaled Tc99m-DTPA increased significantly suggesting that an increase in alveolar-epithelial permeability to small molecules occurred after the administration of endotoxin [20].

Thus, a dose of 4 ng/kg of reference endotoxin resulted in wide changes in leukocyte counts and the generation of a variety of inflammatory mediators (see below). Yet the lung appears to be well insulated from the inflammatory events occurring acutely in the circulation. Permeability to small molecules (e.g. DTPA) is increased, and with the administration of fluids, a widening of the alveolar-arterial gradient and modest decrease in the PaO_2 occur within hours after the administration of endotoxin [20].

Gut Function

Endotoxin-induced alterations in gut permeability have been evaluated in normal subjects by administering oral lactulose and mannitol (low-molecular weight (<350) markers which are not metabolized) prior to endotoxin administration [25]. Changes in intestinal permeability were assessed by measuring 12 h urinary excretion of these markers in paired studies. Following endotoxin administration, the absorption and excretion of lactulose and mannitol increased significantly and were maximal 3 to 6 h after endotoxin administration [25]. These data demonstrate that the permeability of the normal intestinal tract changes within hours after administration of intravenous endotoxin. In critical illness, these changes in gut function may be accentuated and contribute to bacteria or endotoxin translocation which may prolong or potentiate organ dysfunction during sepsis or septic shock.

Renal Function

Renal blood flow was measured in normals and patients with hypertension following the administration of a pyrogen [16]. Renal plasma flow was measured with p-amino-hippurate clearance and glomerular filtration rate with inulin or mannitol clearances. Renal blood flow increased within hours of the administration of the pyrogen and these changes occurred even when the febrile response was blocked with an anti-pyretic [16].

In recent studies of metabolic responses following endotoxin, changes in creatinine and urinary urea nitrogen excretion did not differ from controls subjects (26).

Blood-Ocular Permeability

Parenteral administration of endotoxin elicits an ocular response in rabbits and rats that is similar to acute anterior uveitis in humans with increase in anterior chamber cells, protein and permeability of fluorescein dye. The integrity of the blood-aqueous barrier was evaluated in normal subjects after the administration of endotoxin by measuring the appearance of fluorescein in the anterior chamber [27]. No significant changes in the blood-aqueous barrier occurred, suggesting that there is a significant species-specific difference in the ocular response to endotoxin. The capillary permeability of the iris and ciliary body are not altered despite a wide variety of acute systemic inflammatory responses [27].

Metabolic Alterations

Several investigators have measured oxygen consumption following endotoxin administration using expired gas analysis or the indirect Fick principle [17, 19, 21, 26]. Total body oxygen consumption rises significantly within 2 h and remains elevated at 6 h after the administration of endotoxin [21, 26]. Splanchnic oxygen extraction increased by 64 % within 2 h and fell to baseline values at 6 [21]. A disproportionate increase in splanchnic oxygen consumption compared to total body oxygen consumption was seen at 2 h after endotoxin (34 % to 43 %), and this response mimics a similar pattern seen in clinical sepsis [21]. Extremity oxygen remained unchanged until 6 h where it fell below baseline [21].

The administration of endotoxin is associated with increased energy expenditure as reflected by an increase in the metabolic rate and an increase in oxygen consumption [21, 26]. Additionally, the metabolic substrates change in the circulation during this acute response. Mild hyperglycemia has been noted at 2 to 4 h after endotoxin [21, 26]. This is associated with an increase in extremity glucose uptake and increase in net glucose output from the splanchnic bed [21]. While arterial lactates levels do not change, an increase in splanchnic lactate uptake occurs by 2 h and persists for at least 6 h [21]. This is accompanied by a constant efflux of lactate from the extremity which occurs at 4 to 6 h [21]. Arterial hypoaminoacidemia occurs within 2 h and is most prominent for the essential amino-acids as well as glutamine and alanine [21]. This is accompanied by significant increases in splanchnic amino-acid uptake for up to 6 h [21]. Arterial free fatty acids increase and are associated with a net efflux from extremities [21]. These studies demonstrate that the whole body and splanchnic metabolic responses initiated within hours of intravenous endotoxin administration are similar to those observed during sepsis and to critical illness [21, 26].

Endocrine Alterations

Patients with acute critical illness exhibit characteristic host responses to the underlying stress, tissue damage and/or infection. These responses include the elaboration of stress hormones cortisol, glucagon, and catecholamines which are important in the maintenance of homeostasis after injury or stress. The reactivity of the hypothalamic-pituitary-adrenal axis to endotoxin has been well recognized [6, 10]. Endotoxin administration disrupts the usual diurnal variation in cortisol and growth hormone release. Following endotoxin, adrenocorticotrophic hormone (ACTH), cortisol, growth hormone and plasma catecholamines rise acutely by 2 h with peak levels at 3 to 4 h. By 6 h, these hormones have returned to or are approaching baseline values [10, 13, 21, 26]. These acute changes in stress hormones are attenuated by the administration of ibuprofen [13, 26]. Secretion of β-endorphin, an opioid peptide, is linked to ACTH and cortisol release. Serum levels of β-endorphin appear in an identical pattern to that of ACTH and cortisol following endotoxin [28]. No changes in insulin or glucagon levels occur [21].

Other features of the neuroendocrine response to endotoxin have been evaluated. Arginine vasopressin and corticotropin-releasing hormone are hypothalamic hormones that are important in the control of ACTH release [29]. Following endotoxin administration, arginine vasopressin rises and falls simultaneously with ACTH and cortisol [29]. This acute response can be inhibited by the prior administration of ibuprofen suggesting that cyclooxygenase products are proximal mediators of this stress response [29]. No changes in corticotropin-releasing hormone were detected in the peripheral blood samples after endotoxin [29].

An endogenous opioid hormone, αMSH, is important in the control of fever and inflammation. It has been detected in peripheral blood samples within hours following endotoxin-induced fever of greater than 2.6 °C [30]. With less dramatic increases in core temperature, no circulating αMSH was detected in the blood [30].

Liver Acute Phase Protein Responses

Iron metabolism undergoes acute changes following endotoxin administration. Serum iron levels fall as early as 8 h after endotoxin administration and remained depressed at 24 h post-endotoxin [26, 31]. The administration of ibuprofen prior to the endotoxin does not alter this responses [26]. Serum ferritin rises acutely by 4 h and remains elevated at 24 h post-endotoxin [31]. C-reactive protein and serum amyloid A protein are acute phase proteins released by the liver in response to inflammatory stimuli. C-reactive protein levels were elevated threefold at 24 h post-endotoxin and this response was not inhibited when ibuprofen was given prior to the endotoxin [26]. Serum amyloid A protein rises more than 3-fold by 5 h after endotoxin and remains more than 25-fold above baseline at 24 h post-endotoxin [10].

Hematologic Effects

As described above, wide changes in peripheral leukocyte counts occur after the administration of endotoxin. A dose dependent leukopenia occurs characteristically at 1 h with nadir counts of less than 2000 leukocytes per ml. This is followed by a leukocytosis with counts rising to greater than 12000 leukocytes per ml by 8 h. The leukocytosis is associated with the appearance of immature neutrophils or band forms in the blood (approximately 15 % of peripheral counts). Monocytopenia occurs during the first 2 h due to a fall in lymphocytes and monocytes, and persists for almost 24 h after endotoxin. Circulating platelet counts fall transiently by 15 to 20 % [6, 10].

Humoral Inflammatory Responses

Fibrinolytic Proteins

The vascular endothelium is an important target organ for the action of endotoxin directly or through the action of secondary mediators such as IL-1 or TNF. The control of fibrin generated during inflammation is dependent on the balance of thrombogenic factors and protective mechanisms which control thrombus formation and fibrinolysis. Fibrin deposition and microthrombi are found in multiple organs during sepsis and septic shock, and thus the regulation of the fibrinolytic response appears to be a critical factor in the development of MOF.

We evaluated fibrinolytic proteins and their inhibitors after endotoxin administration (4 ng/kg) and found that within 1 h post-endotoxin, the fibrinolytic system is activated (Fig. 1) [32]. Tissue plasminogen activator (tPA) functional activity rose within 1 h and was maximum at 2 h. This was accompanied by the development of complexes that form between the activated fibrinolytic enzyme plasmin and its major inhibitor, α2-plasmin inhibitor. tPA functional activity fell to undetectable levels at 3 h in association with a rise in plasminogen-activator inhibitor-1 which rose more slowly than tPA and was maximum by 5 h [32]. The endothelial cell products, tPA and plasminogen-activator inhibitor-1 release after endotoxin administration are not linked in *vitro,* and presumably their sequential release *in vivo* is due to the action of secondary mediators (e.g. IL-1, TNF). Von Willebrand factor antigen, another marker of endothelial cell stimulation and integral for platelet

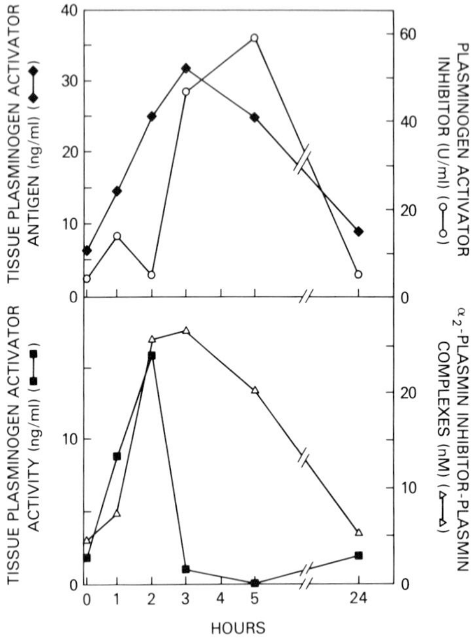

Fig. 1. The fibrinolytic response in a normal subject following 4 ng/kg of intravenous endotoxin. At 2 h post-endotoxin, tissue plasminogen activator activity rises accompanied by a rise in the α2-plasmin inhibitor-plasmin complexes and tPA antigen levels. At 3 h, the plasminogen-activator inhibitor level rises and tPA activity falls to baseline values. At 3 h, tPA antigen and α2-plasmin inhibitor-plasmin complexes begin to fall in parallel, reaching baseline values at 24 h. (From [32]with permission)

adhesion, rose fourfold 3 h after endotoxin and remained elevated at 24 h [32]. Thus, within 1 h following endotoxin administration, the fibrinolytic system is activated by the release of tPA in the blood. By 3 h however, a procoagulant state exists that is characterized by an increase in plasminogen activator inhibitor and greatly diminished tPA activity. Whether this early activation of the fibrinolytic system during endotoxemia prevents the initiation of microvascular thrombosis is unknown [32].

Coagulation Proteins

Levels of prothrombin F_{1+2} fragments, an indicator of activation of the common pathway of coagulation, were elevated as early as 2 h after 2 ng/kg of reference endotoxin, and increased by fourfold at 4 h [12]. Thrombin-antithrombin III complexes similarly increased at 2 h rising 2.4-fold from baseline and returning to baseline by 6 h [12]. These changes indicative of thrombin generation however did not precede the activation of the fibrinolytic pathway but occurred simultaneously with the detection of tPA levels [12]. Thus, the stimulus for early tPA release remains uncertain.

Kallikrein-Kinin System (Contact Activation System)

The contact system is composed of three serine protease zymogen factors XII, XI, and prekallikrein, and a bradykinin precursor high molecular weight kininogen. Kallikrein generation initiates and amplifies several important host defense responses [33]. These include activation of complement, initiation of the coagulation cascade, plasminogen activation, as well as neutrophil stimulation including chemotaxis, superoxide production and elastase release. Additionally, kallikrein is critical in the generation of bradykinin, a potent vasodilator. Factor XIIa-C1-inhibitor, kallikrein-C1-inhibitor, and modified inactive C1-inhibitor were evaluated after endotoxin administration (2 ng/kg), and none of these markers of contact activation were elevated [12]. Using different assays and a higher dose of reference endotoxin (4 ng/kg), we noted that the contact system is activated within 2 h of endotoxin administration [34]. Functional prekallikrein and Factor XI levels fell at 2 to 5 h and this was accompanied by a fivefold rise in $\alpha 2$ macroglobulin-kallikrein complexes by 5 h. Thus, the kallikrein-kinin system is activated within hours after endotoxin administration, and kallikrein and bradykinin may contribute to the observed changes in host inflammatory and hemodynamic responses.

Complement

Complement can be activated by endotoxin *in vitro* by the classic and properdin pathways [35]. Two studies however have not detected changes in complement activation components following intravenous endotoxin administration [12, 36]. Complement anaphylatoxins, C3a desArg, C4a desArg and C5a desArg are not increased after a 2 ng/kg dose of reference endotoxin [12, 36]. Neutrophils exposed to C5a *in vivo* will have deficient chemotaxis *in vitro* because of down regulation of C5a surface receptors [36]. Neutrophil chemotaxis to C5a *in vitro* is not decreased after intravenous endotoxin administration, confirming that no C5a was generated *in vivo* [36].

Effects on Inflammatory Cells and their Products

Tissue damage initiated by neutrophils results from the release of enzymes and reactive oxygen species. Neutrophil release of elastase as reflected by elastase-α_1-antitrypsin complexes occurs by 2 to 3 h [32, 37]. These complexes remain elevated at 24 h post-endotoxin. Neutrophil activation as reflected by the expression of complement opsonin C3 surface receptors (C3b, iC3b) occurs by 3 h [36]. Neutrophil C3b receptors remain expressed at 24 h while iC3b return to baseline levels at 24 h after endotoxin [36]. Neutrophil chemotaxis to formyl-methionyl-leucine-phenylalanine (FMLP) and phagocytosis of opsonized *S. aureus* is not altered by the *in vivo* administration of endotoxin [36].

Neutrophils have different states of reactivity to stimulation depending in part on the stimulus dose a cell is exposed to [38]. Priming of inflammatory cells will potentiate or enhance their subsequent inflammatory responses. The process of priming occurs by exposing leukocytes to small amounts of a stimulus (e.g. endotoxin, C5a, PAF, in a dose an order of magnitude smaller than that required to stimulate the cell directly. Upon exposure to a second agent or stimulus, an enhanced functional response occurs [38]. Through priming, small amounts of endotoxin can contribute to organ dysfunction in animals [39].

We investigated whether intravenous endotoxin would prime human neutrophils for enhanced production of superoxide anion [40]. Additionally, we evaluated the effects of treatment with oral ibuprofen or pentoxifylline prior to endotoxin administration on these responses [40]. Neutrophils obtained *in vivo* at baseline, 15 min or 4 h post-endotoxin were secondarily stimulated with FMLP *in vitro*, and then superoxide production was quantitated using a ferricytochrome C assay. Maximum production of superoxide rose almost threefold at 4 h. No change from baseline superoxide production was apparent at 15 min. The prior administration of ibuprofen or pentoxifylline did not block this priming effect. Thus, intravenous endotoxin primes human neutrophils for an enhanced respiratory burst and production of superoxide anion. The time course of neutrophil priming suggests that the priming occurs *in vivo* as a result of secondary mediators rather than endotoxin itself [40].

Alveolar macrophages obtained after endotoxin administration exhibit a similar priming effect. We obtained alveolar macrophages from normal volunteers by bronchoalveolar lavage several days before and on the day of endotoxin administration [41]. Cells obtained on the control day spontaneously produce only small amounts of IL-1, TNF and PGE_2 in culture. Alveolar macrophages obtained after intravenous endotoxin is given do not have an increased spontaneous release of these mediators. However upon secondary stimulation with endotoxin *in vitro,* an enhanced release of IL-1, TNF and PGE_2 is seen. Thus, endotoxin administration primes alveolar macrophages for an enhanced production of these proinflammatory mediators [41].

Phospholipase A_2 (PLA_2) is critical in the initiation of the arachidonic acid cascade. As an extracellular enzyme it can also be detected in the circulation and increased levels have been associated with organ failure during sepsis [42]. Phospholipase A_2 levels rose at 3 h, peaked at 24 h and began to return to baseline by 48 h post-endotoxin. The magnitude of the PLA_2 response correlated with the maximum TNF response [42].

Histamine is thought to play a major role in vasodilatation and permeability changes during acute inflammatory responses. Histamine levels however do not rise after endotoxin is administered [28]. This is similar to septic shock and suggests that circulating histamine is not a major mediator during these acute inflammatory responses [43].

Cytokine Responses

Peptide regulatory molecules or cytokines play an integral role in the acute inflammatory response initiated by endotoxin. Following exposure to intravenous endotoxin, several acute phase cytokines are released in a characteristic pattern. Many of these cytokines have overlapping proinflammatory activity. Because of this redundancy of function, associations of a single cytokine with a specific inflammatory function can often only be inferred by observations made *in vivo.* The use of specific inhibitors or anti-cytokine molecules will assist in clarifying their specific role in the inflammatory responses.

TNF α has a primary role in mediating many of the effects of endotoxin. TNF detection in peripheral blood occurs as early as 1 h post-endotoxin with peak levels at 90 min to 2 h. This is followed by a rapid disappearance from the circulation with levels approaching baseline by 3 h [13, 44]. Similar patterns are observed when either bioassays or immunoassays are used to detect TNF in the blood [14]. The magnitude of the TNF elevations observed often approaches levels seen in patients with sepsis and septic shock [14]. During this acute TNF response, hepatic venous TNF levels are 2,5-fold higher than simultaneous measurements in radial artery blood samples suggesting that the splanchnic bed is a major site of TNF production [21].

The magnitude of these responses can be altered by pretreatment with cyclooxygenase inhibitors (e.g. ibuprofen). Cyclooxygenase products serve as part of the inhibitory feedback loop that limits monocyte-macrophage TNF production. Pretreatment with ibuprofen prior to endotoxin administration results in an augmented release of TNF at 90 min which is up to fourfold higher than subjects given endotoxin alone [14, 37].

Pentoxifylline, a phosphodiesterase inhibitor, has been shown *in vitro* to inhibit TNF release. When normal volunteers were given 500 mg of pentoxifylline intravenously prior to endotoxin *(S. abortus equil* 100 ng, IV), the acute rise in TNF at 1 and 2 h post-endotoxin was blocked [7]. None of the endotoxin-associated symptoms were improved nor did pentoxifylline blunt the acute rise in IL-6. Oral pentoxifylline did not, however, block TNF release after reference endotoxin was given to normal volunteers [14]. Differences in study design including higher blood levels achieved with intravenous pentoxifylline, different endotoxin preparations, paired doses of endotoxin used in the former study, and higher TNF levels observed with reference endotoxin may account for these different results.

Intestinal mucosal atrophy induced by total parenteral nutrition and prolonged bowel rest has been hypothesized to enhance translocation of endotoxin as well as altering gastrointestinal flora [45]. These changes may result in an enhanced response to injury or inflammatory stimuli. Cytokine responses were evaluated in normal volunteers who were fed enterally or given total parenteral nutrition (TPN) for 7 days prior to the administration of endotoxin [45]. Subjects given total parenteral nutrition were found to have a 2 to 3-fold enhanced release of hepatic vein and radial artery TNF compared to enterally fed controls [45]. Peak levels of epinephrine and glucagaon, and 24 h C-reactive protein was higher in the parenterally fed subjects [45]. Thus, the counter-regulatory hormone and splanchnic cytokine responses were enhanced after TPN and bowel rest suggesting an enhanced responsiveness of the reticuloendothelial system. This was presumably related to changes in intestinal mucosal function which resulted from bowel rest but not malnutrition [45].

Detection of IL-1 after endotoxin has been more elusive than other acute phase cytokines and several groups have been unable to demonstrate significant changes in circulating IL-1 after endotoxin administration [12-14, 21, 37]. Low levels of IL-1 bioactivity have been described at 2–4 h after 2 ng/kg of intravenous endotoxin [44]. Using a radioimmunoassay on chloroform-extracted plasma, IL-1β was found to rise maximally by 2 h and returned to baseline by 4 h [46]. No IL-1α was found in this or other studies [21, 46].

IL-6 is an important proinflammatory cytokine that shares many actions with IL-1 and TNF including pyrogenicity. It has major actions on acute hepatic protein synthesis and serves as an important immunomodulator. Following endotoxin, IL-6 rises with maximum levels by 2 h after endotoxin and returns to baseline by 5 to 6 h [47]. Ibuprofen given prior to endotoxin enhances the IL-6 responses. This may occur as a direct response to cyclooxygenase inhibition or as a counterregulatory cytokine response to the enhanced TNF release [14, 37].

IL-8 serves as a potent stimulator of neutrophil function. Neutrophils exposed to IL-8 result in increased neutrophil chemotaxis, degranulation and expression of cell surface markers [14]. We measured the release of IL-8 and found that it rises acutely at 90 min with maximum levels at 2 to 3 h post-endotoxin [14]. The maximum levels occur after an earlier rise in TNF activity and parallel a rise in IL-6 activity. Administration of ibuprofen prior to giving endotoxin resulted in an enhanced release of IL-8. This may represent a similar mechanism to that described for enhanced TNF response after cyclooxygenase inhibition [14].

Granulocyte colony stimulating factor (GCSF) is an important growth factor for marrow progenitor cells, and additionally is a potent activator of neutrophils. Following endotoxin, GCSF rises initially by 2 h and was maximal by 6 h post-endotoxin. At 24 h, levels have returned to baseline [48]. A summary of the acute changes in TNF, IL-6, IL-8, and GCSF serum values following intravenous endotoxin is shown in Fig. 2.

Thymocyte co-stimulatory activity rises after the administration of endotoxin and reflects the actions of one or more of the following cytokines: IL-1, IL-2, IL-4, IL-6, IL-7 [28]. Presumably, this increase in thymocyte co-stimulatory activity after intravenous endotoxin is related in part to IL-1 and IL-6 elevations as specific assays have not detected increases in circulating IL-2 post-endotoxin [28]. Lymphotoxin or TNFβ and γ-interferon are also undetectable after the administration of endotoxin [13, 44].

It is apparent that many of the potent actions of cytokines are self-limited. Several naturally occurring inhibitors of IL-1 and TNFα have been described in the urine of febrile patients and patients with malignancies [49, 50]. Endotoxin administration to healthy subjects can induce the release of serum factors that inhibit the action of IL-1 and TNFα *in vitro* [51]. The peak levels of activity occur in parallel with the peak TNF levels and with fever and may be in part due to shed TNF receptors [51]. The IL-1 inhibitory activity of this earlier study may be identical to the recently described IL-1 receptor antagonist which is released simultaneously with IL-1 after endotoxin administration to normal volunteers [52]. The role of these inhibitors in modifying the inflammatory responses due to IL-1 and TNF remain to be clarified.

Neopterin is released from activated macrophages after stimulation by γ-interferon or endotoxin and serum levels are elevated in several inflammatory diseases including septic shock. We measured levels of this neopterin

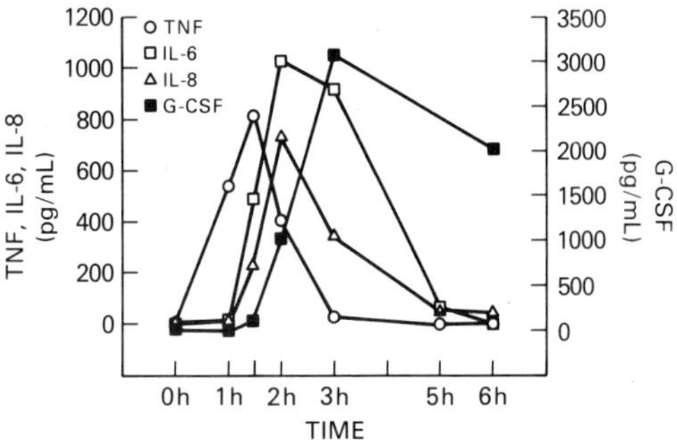

Fig. 2. Mean values (pg/ml) of immunoreactive TNF, IL-6, IL-8 and GCSF following intravenous administration of 4 ng/kg of reference endotoxin to normal humans. (Data derived in part from reference [14] which is reproduced with permission).

following endotoxin and no changes were found within the first 6 h post-endotoxin. Levels at 24 h however were elevated two to fourfold and remained elevated at 48 h [53]. Neopterin levels correlated strongly with total TNF and IL-6 release [54]. Thus neopterin, a marker of cellular immune activation has a delayed but sustained rise after endotoxin administration, and well after the acute phase responses have subsided [53].

Conclusion

The administration of intravenous endotoxin to humans represents a useful model of acute inflammatory events that are likely to occur during the initial stages of gram-negative infections. Within hours of the administration of a small dose of endotoxin, changes occur in systemic hemodynamics, ventricular function, pulmonary gas exchange, and lung and gut permeability which are qualitatively similar to those observed in sepsis.

A wide variety of inflammatory mediators are released often in conjunction with counter-regulatory responses which appear to limit the effects of these mediators. These include activation of the fibrinolytic system and kallikrein-kinin generation. Several proinflammatory cytokines are released including IL-1β, TNFα, IL-6, IL-8 and GCSF. IL-1β and TNFα are accompanied by the release of their respective antagonists or inhibitors. Phagocytic leukocytes are primed for enhanced inflammatory responses after endotoxin administration. Many of these inflammatory responses can be modulated in part by the administration of cylooxygenase and phosphodiesterase inhibitors. Further studies with administration of specific antiinflammatory agents (e.g. anti-cytokine molecules) will assist in extending the understanding of these inflammatory events and their relevance to acute critical illness.

References

1. Danner RL, Elin RJ, Hosseini JM, Wesley RA, Reilly JM, Parrillo JE (1991) Endotoxemia in human septic shock. Chest 99:169–175
2. Parrillo JE, Parker MM, Natanson C, et al.(1990) Septic shock in humans: Advances in the understanding of pathogenesis, cardiovascular dysfunction, and therapy. Ann Intern Med 113:227–242
3. Raetz CRH, Ulevitch RJ, Wright SD, Sibley CH, Ding A, Nathan CF (1991) Gram-negative endotoxin: An extraordinary lipid with profound effects on eukaryotic signal transduction. FASEB J 5:2652–2660
4. Gilbert R (1960) Mechanisms of the hemodynamic effects of endotoxin. Physiol Rev 40: 245–279
5. Berry LJ (1985) Introduction. In: Berry LJ (ed) Cellular biology of endotoxin, Handbook of Endotoxin, Vol 3. Elsevier, Amsterdam, pp XVII–XXI
6. Wolff SM (1973) Biological effects of bacterial endotoxin in man. J Infect Dis 128:259–264
7. Zabel P, Schönharting MM, Wolter DT, Schade UF (1989) Oxpentifylline in endotoxaemia. Lancet 2:1474–1477
8. Engelhardt R, Mackensen A, Galanos C, Andreesen R (1990) Biological response to intravenously administered endotoxin in patients with advanced cancer. J Biol Response Mod 9: 480–491

9. Hochstein HD, Mills DF, Outschoorn AS, Rastogi SC (1983) The processing and collaborative assay of reference endotoxin. J Biol Stand 11:251–260
10. Elin RJ, Wolff SM, McAdam KPWJ, et al (1981) Properties of reference *Escherichla coli* endotoxin and its phthalylated derivative in humans. J Infect Dis 144:329–336
11. Suffredini AF, Fromm RE, Parker MM, et al. (1989) The response of normal humans to the administration of endotoxin. N Engl J Med 321:280–287
12. van Deventer SJH, Büller HR, ten Cate JW, Aarden LA, Hack CE, Sturk A (1990) Experimental endotoxemia in humans: Analysis of cytokine release and coagulation, fibrinolytic, and complement pathways. Blood 76:2520–2526
13. Michie HR, Manogue KR, Spriggs DR, et al.(1988) Detection of circulating tumor necrosis factor after endotoxin administration. N Engl J Med 23:1481–1486
14. Martich GD, Danner RL, Ceska M, Suffredini AF (1991) Detection of interleukin-8 and tumor necrosis factor in normal humans following intravenous endotoxin: The effect of anti-inflammatory agents. J Exp Med 173:1021–1024
15. Grollman A (1929) Variations in the cardiac output of man. V: The cardiac output of man during the malaise and pyrexia following the injection of typhoid vaccine. J Clin Invest 8: 25–32
16. Bradley SE, Chasis H, Goldring W, Smith H (1945) Hemodynamic alterations in normotensive and hypertensive subjects during the pyrogenic reaction. J Clin Invest 24:749–758
17. Moser KM, Perry RB, Luchsinger PC (1963) Cardiopulmonary consequences of pyrogen-induced hyperexia in man. J Clin Invest 42:626–634
18. Greisman SE (1991) Cardiovascular alterations during fever. In: Mackowiak P (ed) Fever: Basic mechanisms and management. Raven Press, New York, pp 143–165
19. Martich GD, Parker MM, Cunnion RE, Suffredini AF (1992) Effects of ibuprofen and pentoxifylline on the cardiovascular response of normal humans to endotoxin. J Appl Physiol (in press)
20. Suffredini AF, Shelhamer JH, Neumann RD, Brenner M, Baltaro RJ, Parrillo JE (1992) Pulmonary and oxygen transport effects of intravenously administered endotoxin in normal humans. Am Rev Respir Dis (in press)
21. Fong Y, Marano MA, Moldawer LL, et al.(1990) The acute splanchnic and peripheral tissue metabolic response to endotoxin in humans. J Clin Invest 85:1896–1904
22. Brigham KL, Meyrick B (1986) Endotoxin and lung injury. Am Rev Respir Dis 133:913–927
23. Miyamato K, Schultz E, Heath T, Mitchell MD, Albertine KH, Staub NC (1988) Pulmonary intravascular macrophages and hemodynamic effects of liposomes in sheep. J Appl Physiol 64:1143–1152
24. Kindt GC, Gadek JE, Weiland JE (1991) Initial recruitment of neutrophils to alveolar structures in acute lung injury. J Appl Physiol 70:1575–1585
25. O'Dwyer ST, Michie HR, Ziegler TR, Revhaug A, Smith RJ, Wilmore DW (1988) A single dose of endotoxin increases intestinal permeability in healthy humans. Arch Surg 123:1459–1464
26. Revhaug A, Michie HR, Manson JMcK, et al.(1988) Inhibition of cyclooxygenase attenuates the metabolic response to endotoxin in humans. Arch Surg 123:162–170
27. Herman DC, Suffredini AF, Parrillo JE, Palestine AG (1991) Ocular permeability after systemic administration of endotoxin to humans. Curr Eye Res 10:121–126
28. Casale TB, Ballas ZK, Kaliner MA, Keahey TM (1990) The effects of intravenous endotoxin on various host-effector molecules. J Allergy Clin Immunol 85:45–51
29. Michie HR, Majzoub JA, O'Dwyer ST, Revhaug A, Wilmore DW (1990) Both cyclooxygenase-dependent and cyclooxygenase-independent pathways mediate the neuroendocrine response in humans. Surgery 108:254–261
30. Catania A, Suffredini AF, Lipton JM (1991) Alpha-MSH response to endotoxin in normal human subjects. FASEB J 5:A1392
31. Elin RJ, Wolff SM, Finch CA (1977) Effect of induced fever on serum iron and ferritin concentration in man. Blood 49:147–153
32. Suffredini AF, Harpel PC, Parrillo JE (1989) The promotion and subsequent inhibition of plasminogen following intravenous endotoxin administration to normal humans. N Engl J Med 320:1165–1172
33. Colman RW (1984) Surface-mediated defense reactions: The plasma contact activation system. J Clin Invest 73:1249–1253

34. De La Cadena RA, Suffredini AF, Kaufman N, Parrillo JE, Colman RW (1990) Activation of the kallikrein-kinin system after endotoxin administration to normal human volunteers. Clin Res 38:346A
35. Morrison DC, Kline LF (1977) Activation of the classical and properdin pathways of complement by bacterial lipopolysaccharides (LPS). J Immuhol 118:362–368
36. Moore FD, Moss NA, Revhaug A, Wilmore DW, Mannick JA, Rodrick ML (1987) A single dose of endotoxin activates neutrophils without activating complement. Surgery 102:200–205
37. Spinas GA, Bloesch D, Keller U, Zimmerli W, Cammisuli S (1991) Pretreatment with ibuprofen augments circulating tumor necrosis factor-α, interleukin-6, and elastase during acute endotoxemia. J Infect Dis 163: 89–95
38. Cochrane CG (1987) The enhancement of inflammatory injury. Am Rev Respir Dis 136:1–2
39. Worthen GS, Haslett C, Rees AJ, et al. (1987) Neutrophil-mediated pulmonary vascular injury: Synergistic effect of trace amounts of lipopolysaccharide and neutrophil stimuli on vascular permeability and neutrophil sequestration in the lung. Am Rev Respir Dis 136:19–28
40. Martich GD, Danner RL, Van Dervort AL, Patterson E, Suffredini AF (1990) Priming of neutrophils after intravenous endotoxin administration to normal humans: Effects of oral pentoxifylline or ibuprofen. Clin Res 38:306A
41. Smith PD, Suffredini AF, Lamerson CL, et al. (1988) Endotoxin administration to normal humans causes increased alveolar permeability and priming of alveolar macrophages to produce enhanced superoxide and IL-1 production. Clin Res 36: 374A
42. Pruzanski W, Stefanski E, Wilmore DW, et al. (1990) Sequential activation of TNF phospholipase A2 axis following IV endotoxin challenge in human volunteers. FASEB J 4:A2147
43. Jacobs R. Kaliner M, Shelhamer JH, Parrillo JE (1989) Blood histamine concentrations are not elevated in humans with septic shock. Crit Care Med 17:30–35
44. Hesse DG, Tracey KJ, Fong Y, et al. (1988) Cytokine appearance in human endotoxemia and primate bacteremia. Surg Gynecol Obstet 166:147–153
45. Fong Y, Marano MA, Barber A, et al.(1989) Total parenteral nutrition and bowel rest modify the metabolic response to endotoxin in humans. Ann Surg 210:449–456
46. Cannon JG, Tompkins RG, Gelfand JA, et al. (1990) Circulating interleukin-1 and tumor necrosis factor in septic shock and experimental endotoxin fever. J Infect Dis 161:79–84
47. Fong Y, Moldawer LL, Marano M, et al. (1989) Endotoxemia elicits increased circulating β2-IFN/IL-6 in man. J Immunol 142:2321–2324
48. Mackensen A, Galanos C, Engelhardt R (1991) Treatment of cancer patients with endotoxin induces release of endogenous cytokines. Pathobiology 59:264–267
49. Seckinger P, Williamson K, Balavoine JF, et al. (1987) A urine inhibitor of interleukin-1 activity affects both interleukin-1α and 1β but not tumor necrosis factor α. J Immunol 139: 1541–1545
50. Engelmann H, Novick D, Wallach D (1990) Two tumor necrosis factor-binding proteins purified from human urine: Evidence for immunological cross-reactivity with cell surface tumor necrosis factor receptors. J Biol Chem 265:1531–1536
51. Spinas GA, Bloesch D, Kaufmann MT, Keller U, Dayer JM (1990) Induction of plasma inhibitors of interleukin-1 and TNF-α activity by endotoxin administration to normal humans. Am J Physiol 259:993–997
52. Granowitz EV, Santos AA, Poutsiaka DD, et al. (1991) Production of interleukin-l-receptor antagonist during experimental endotoxaemia. Lancet 2:1423–1424
53. Bloom J, Suffredini AF, Parrillo JE, Palestine A (1990) Serum neopterin levels after intravenous endotoxin administration to normal humans. Immunobiology 181:317–323
54. Martich GD, Boujoukos AJ, Reda DG, Suffredini AF (1991) Relation of serum neopterin to the hemodynamic and cytokine response following intravenous endotoxin administration to normal humans. Crit Care Med 19:S14

Mediators of Lung Injury Following Ischemia and Reperfusion

J. Hill, T. F. Lindsay, and H. B. Hechtman

Introduction

Multisystem organ failure (MOF) continues to complicate the clinical course of many patients with trauma and sepsis. It has been long appreciated that the lung is a particularly sensitive target organ following remote trauma. In 1938, VH Moon [1] described pulmonary congestion and edema in „wet autopsies“ of soldiers who had died of septic shock following traumatic injuries. Lung injury and edema are now well recognized complications following ischemia and reperfusion of tissues remote from the lung, including the lower torso during abdominal aortic aneurysm repair and reperfusion of the ischemic intestine or liver [2–4]. In addition, lung injury may result from lung trauma itself following such insults as pulmonary artery occlusion, acid aspiration, pneumothorax, atelectasis and contusion [5, 6].

In the 1950's, Francis D. Moore of the Brigham and Womens Hospital, Boston, MA. [7] in documenting lung injury following trauma proposed that infected or damaged tissue elaborated circulating factors he called – „woundagons“ – that signal the host to initiate the inflammatory, cardiovascular and pulmonary responses that characterize critical illness. The importance of systemic mediators is particularly apparent following intestinal ischemia. Thus, experimental occlusion of the superior mesenteric artery is often fatal even before the intestine loses its viability. Reperfusion of the ischemic intestine leads to an exacerbation of the local injury, circulatory collapse and accelerated death. Whilst both loss of fluid in the bowel and peritoneal cavity as well as systemic organ injury contribute to death in an untreated individual, death will occur despite fluid resuscitation and maintenance of a normal blood volume. Indeed, two of the first three patients who underwent superior mesenteric artery embolectomy died of pulmonary edema 48 h after surgery. At post mortem examination, the bowel was macroscopically normal [8].

Although pulmonary edema seen in routine clinical practice is most often due to cardiac failure and increased hydrostatic pressure in the pulmonary microvasculature, the pulmonary edema that follows ischemia and reperfusion is secondary to altered permeability of the lung microvascular endothelial barrier. This permeability is mediated by circulating humoral factors and cells. Reperfusion of any organ or tissue leads to the release of agents that have accumulated during ischemia or are synthesized or activated during reperfusion. On reperfusion, oxygen availability leads to eicosanoid and oxygen free radical synthesis. Further, complement is activated, and cytokines and platelet activating factor (PAF) synthesized. All are capable of altering microvascular endothelial function and therefore have a potential role in mediating ischemia and reperfusion induced lung injury.

Eicosanoids

Ischemia is a stimulus for production and release during reperfusion of the eicosanoids thromboxane (Tx) A_2 and leukotriene (LT) B_4. On removal of a hindlimb tourniquet, Tx production occurs within minutes of reperfusion and plasma levels return toward normal within 30 min. [2]. The early site of synthesis of this eicosanoid is unknown, but ischemic tissue itself is likely an important source. Thereafter, circulating neutrophils become dominant and finally lung parenchyma has been shown to play a key synthetic role. In humans and dogs, platelets are not activated by limb ischemia. Further, Tx production is prevented in neutropenic animals indicating that platelets are not an important Tx source. That the lung itself contributes to thromboxane synthesis following limb ischemia and reperfusion can be seen firstly by the observation that systemic arterial TxB_2 levels (the stable hydrolysis product of TxA_2) during surgery for abdominal aortic aneurysm are higher than TxB_2 levels in pulmonary arterial blood, and secondly that TxB_2 levels in pulmonary lymph are higher than levels in plasma [2, 9].

TxA_2 is a potent vasoconstrictor that is responsible for the transient elevation in pulmonary arterial pressure seen following lower torso ischemia. Inhibition of Tx production in sheep or dogs with a Tx-synthetase inhibitor or use of a Tx-receptor antagonist prevents this pulmonary hypertension [9]. Tx also mediates a rise in pulmonary artery pressure during aortic clamping and reperfusion in abdominal aortic aneurysm surgery [2]. Tx is synthesized during aortic clamping because collaterals permit simultaneous ischemia and reperfusion of the lower torso. This is in distinction from tourniquet application to the hindlimb.

In isolated guinea pig lungs, Tx synthesis results from tumor necrosis factor (TNF) infusion and leads to a neutrophil dependent increase in pulmonary capillary pressure and endothelial permeability. Inhibiton of thromboxane synthesis in this *in vitro* setting prevents the increase in pulmonary capillary pressure but not endothelial permeability [10]. Following hindlimb ischemia, synthetic Tx inhibition or lavage of Tx synthesis inhibitors prevents both neutrophil sequestration and lung permeability. These data indicate that thromboxane plays an important role in mediating pathological changes in pulmonary vascular pressure and permeability.

A direct effect of Tx is on the microvascular endothelium, leading to a decrease in barrier function by disassembling acting microfilaments which regulate the cell cytoskeleton. *In vitro* observations show that the interendothelial junctions become widened with a resultant increased permeability. The major *in vivo* Tx effect is more apt to be as a chemoactivator and chemoattractant for neutrophils leading to their increased adhesion to endothelium and release of injurious oxidative products and proteases.

Inhibition of Tx synthesis also prevents increased lung microvascular permeability following systemic complement activation, acid aspiration and lung microembolization, but not endotoxemia. It is likely that different mediators predominate in the pulmonary injury in various inflammatory settings. Following skeletal muscle ischemia, Tx appears to be an early and important mediator of increased lung microvascular permeability.

LTB_4 levels are also elevated following limb ischemia or coronary occlusion. LTB_4 is a powerful chemoattractant. In addition, it increases neutrophil adhesion to endothelium by activating an adhesion molecule: the CD18 integrin. This same adhesion molecule mediates diapedesis through endothelium. Other prominent LTB_4 effects on the neutrophil include increased superoxide production, protease release and Tx production. The primacy of LTB_4 or Tx has not been established. Either agent can induce synthesis of the other. The lipoxygenase inhibitor diethylcarbamazine prevents a rise in LTB_4 and TxA_2 levels, limits the pulmonary leukosequestration and increased microvascular permeability following hindlimb ischemia [11]. Tx inhibition will also limit LTB_4 synthesis and pulmonary injury. When lavaged into the human lung, LTB_4 promotes neutrophil diapedesis but does not lead to an increase in bronchoalveolar lavage fluid protein concentration and when injected intravenously, does not induce macromolecular flux across the pulmonary microvascular endothelium. Increased LTB_4 levels have been documented in patients with adult respiratory distress syndrome (ARDS), but its precise role in mediating this condition is uncertain.

Cytokines

Evidence indicates that both TNF and interleukin-1 (IL-1) are involved in the pathogenesis of ARDS and MOF. TNF and IL-1 are synthesized in nearly all organs containing phagocytes and blood mononuclear cells, in response to a large number of stimuli. These include endotoxin, C5a, LTB_4, inteferon-γ, interleukin-4 and viral antigens. In addition, TNF and IL-1 can stimulate the synthesis of each other. Endotoxin is a particularly potent stimulus for both cytokines. Low doses induce elevated TNF levels within minutes in experimental animals [12] and human volunteers [13]. In these settings, levels of TNF peak after 90 to 120 min and then return to below detectable levels after about 4 h.

Following an injection of endotoxin, most of the TNF synthesized by a cell is released into the circulation, but some does remain cell bound and may mediate paracrine biological activities. As blood mononuclear cells contain a nascent pool of mRNA for TNF, its biosynthesis proceeds within minutes after cellular activation. In addition to tissue phagocytes and monocytes, polymorphonuclear leukocytes have recently been shown capable of synthesizing small quantities of TNF [14]. Non-phagocytic cells such as endothelial and smooth muscle cells can also produce IL-1 [15]. IL-1 lacks a distinct cleavage sequence, and thus a considerable amount of IL-1 remains cell associated. Membrane bound IL-1, first described in 1985, is biologically active and is thought to account for a significant part of its activity [16]. Thus, IL-1 in contrast to the other cytokines may act mainly as a cell associated mediator. Its presence in the circulation apart from monocytes may indicate overwhelming infection. Thus, IL-Iβ but not IL-lα has been detected in the circulation of patients with meningococcal meningitis and septic purpura. On the other hand, neither IL-lα or lL-Iβ were assayable in the circulation of human volunteers given low doses of intravenous endotoxin whereas elevated levels of TNFα and IL-6 were readily detected [13]. Baboons and rabbits challenged with lethal doses of endotoxin do have elevated levels of IL-1β in the circulation.

TNF is readily produced *in vitro* by pulmonary macrophages, liver Kuppfer cells, peritoneal macrophages and endothelial cells. TNF derived from these tissue macrophages may exert important local paracrine actions. In such cases, local tissue levels may be of greater importance than circulating levels of TNF in mediating organ failure. Elevated concentrations of TNF have been reported in the bronchoalveolar lavage of patients with ARDS.

An infusion of TNF or IL-1 causes a lung injury characterized by increased permeability and neutrophil sequestration. The mechanism of action of these cytokines is thought to involve an activation of both neutrophils and lung endothelium. Thus, TNF causes neutrophil degranulation and superoxide production [17]. TNF also induces a rapid functional upregulation of the neutrophil adhesion receptor, the CD11b/CD18 complex, which promotes adhesion of neutrophils to endothelium [18]. Further, stimulation of the endothelium by either TNF or IL-1 induces over the course of hours the synthesis and expression of antigens on the surface of endothelial cells. The intercellular adhesion molecule (ICAM) which is the ligand for CD11b/CD18 is upregulated maximally after 24 h, endothelial leukocyte adhesion molecule 1 (ELAM-1) which is the ligand for LAM-1 [19] is upregulated over the course of 2-4 h and both result in a gradual increase in neutrophil adherence over several hours. In addition, endothelial cells exposed to TNF synthesize IL-1, and once exposed to TNF or IL-1 become more susceptible to lysis by activated neutrophils. TNF and IL-1 also induce endothelial procoagulant activity so that endothelium becomes thrombogenic. This may then lead to capillary thrombosis and inadequate tissue perfusion. This intravascular coagulation may be compounded because of the ability of the cytokines to inhibit plasminogen activator as well as limit its synthesis, thereby preventing fibrinolysis. Finally, there is alteration of the thrombomodulin/protein C anticoagulation pathway.

Several reports support the thesis that cytokine related increases in permeability are mediated by neutrophils. Thus the increased lung permeability caused by an experimental infusion of TNF can be prevented by neutrophil depletion [10]. When injected into skin, peritoneum or lung, IL-1 induces emigration of neutrophils and an associated increased microvascular permeability [20,23]. That neutrophil depletion prevents the increased permeability following an injection of IL-1 into the skin suggests their causal relationship to this event [21]. Studies of rats undergoing hindlimb and hepatic ischemia and reperfusion are known to undergo the sequence: TNF-α release, neutrophil sequestration in the lungs and lung permeability. TNF inhibition in these settings significantly reduces both neutrophil sequestration and lung permeability [4, 24]. One recent study however did not confirm these findings. The authors found that TNF-α inhibition following intestinal ischemia did not reduce lung neutrophil sequestration although increased lung permeability was prevented [3].

TNF and IL-1 act synergistically in inducing shock [25, 26] prostaglandin synthesis, and neutrophil chemotaxis [20]. Either TNF or IL-1 inhibitors when used independently have been shown to prevent lung injury, shock and death following endotoxin or *E.coli* administration [12, 27-29].

Two human IL-1 receptor antagonist proteins have recently been purified and cloned. Both block IL-1 binding to its receptor and seem to be identical in effect. The recombinant IL-1 receptor antagonist proteins bind completely to the IL-1 receptor and block the action of IL-1 while exhibiting no detectable agonist activity and not affecting TNF binding to its receptor. *In vitro*, the IL-1 receptor antagonist protein prevents IL-1 induced neutrophil-endothelial adhesion in a concentration dependent manner [30]. The following *in vivo* effects of an IL-1 infusion or local injection are prevented by the IL-1 receptor antagonist protein; hypotension, emigration of neutrophils into the peritoneal cavity or skin, acute phase protein release and glucocorticoid release into blood [22, 31]. IL-1 receptor antagonist proteins effect an 80 % reduction in neutrophil emigration into the peritoneal cavity, and 40 % reduction of neutrophil infiltration into lung alveoli following lipopolysaccharide (LPS) administration to these sites [22]. Finally, an IL-1 receptor antagonist has been found to significantly reduce neutrophil sequestration and infarct size in dogs subjected to myocardial ischemia and reperfusion [32].

TNF and IL-1 are the most important inflammatory mediators. IL-6 also has weak inflammatory activity. It is an endogenous pyrogen and induces acute-phase responses. Evidence for a role of IL-6 in mediating lung disease is lacking.

In order to test the roles of TNF-α, IL-1 and neutrophils in mediating lung injury following intestinal ischemia, rats were subjected to 1 h of superior mesenteric ischemia followed by 3 h reperfusion. TNF was inhibited with a polyclonal antibody and IL-1 was inhibited with a recombinant receptor antagonist (IRAP). Results showed that there was rapid TNF production and release into the circulation followed by gradual clearance. IL-1 could not be detected in the circulation despite evidence of its activity, perhaps because its circulating levels were too low or because it was synthesized locally in the lungs and remained cell bound. The lungs entrapped PMNs and there was evidence of a progressive increase in lung permeability. Inhibition of either

TNF or IL-1 reduced lung leukosequestration and prevented the increased lung permeability. The sequestration of neutrophils over the 3 h period of monitored reperfusion is in keeping with activation of the pulmonary microvascular endothelium to generate adhesion molecules. The data in this study provide further evidence that TNF and IL-1 are important mediators of remote tissue injury following ischemia and reperfusion. Secondly, these cytokines demonstrate an extraordinary synergism in action shown by the ability to obtain equivalent protective effects by inhibition of either TNF or IL-1.

Platelet Activating Factor (PAF)

PAF is a phospholipid synthesized by neutrophils, macrophages and endothelial cells. All or most of the PAF generated at these sites remains cell associated. It has been proposed that PAF acts as a second messenger. Thus, when neutrophils or macrophages are stimulated with a calcium ionophore or formyl-methionyl-leucyl-phenylalanine (fMLP), PAF is generated. The same stimuli also induce prostacyclin, LTB_4 and superoxide release from these white blood cells. However, PAF generation was found to either precede or be coincident with eicosanoid and superoxide release from the cell. Indeed, selective PAF antagonists prevented the eicosanoid and superoxide generation. In the same study, endothelial cells stimulated with ionophore generated cell associated PAF while prostacyclin was released. PAF antagonists prevented the prostacyclin release [33].

Endothelium exposed to IL-1 synthesizes PAF and expresses adhesion molecules on its surface which increase neutrophil adhesion. If the endothelial cell associated PAF was removed, or a PAF antagonist was introduced, no reduction of neutrophil adhesion was observed [34]. In a model of acute lung injury induced by exposure of LPS primed neutrophils to N-formyl peptide, a PAF antagonist prevented the increased lung permeability, but did not affect the increased neutrophil sequestration [35]. Thus, rather than influencing neutrophil-endothelial adhesion, PAF may mediate cellular events such as eicosanoid and superoxide generation that follow adhesion.

An infusion of PAF induces systemic hypotension and a generalized increase in microvascular permeability. There is associated MOF affecting the lungs, gastrointestinal tract, heart and kidneys. PAF is a powerful chemoactivator. It increases neutrophil adhesion to endothelium and adhesion dependent superoxide production within minutes. Reperfusion following 2 h of superior mesenteric artery occlusion in dogs is associated with systemic hypotension, pulmonary permeability and elevated levels of PAF. Treatment with a PAF antagonist prevented this arterial hypotension, but its ability to prevent the lung injury was not studied [36]. However, in the majority of *in vivo* settings where PAF antagonists have demonstrated benefit, elevated circulating PAF levels have not been detected. It is unlikely to be an important circulating mediator because it is predominantly cell associated.

Complement

Complement plays a role in host defense against infection and is involved in the inflammatory tissue damage seen in classic animal models of immune complex deposition such as the Arthus phenomenon, and in patients with autoimmune disease. Complement activation generates the anaphylotoxins C3a, C4a and C5a from C3, C4 and C5, respectively. C5a in particular is a potent mediator of inflammation. These peptides function as hormone-like messenger molecules and bind to specific cell-surface receptors with high affinity. Cells binding to these peptides are polymorphonuclear leukocytes, macrophages, mast cells, basophils and smooth muscle cells. The cellular responses to complement stimulation are release of arachidonic acid metabolites, PAF, histamine, serotonin and oxygen free radicals. In addition, the binding of C5a to the surface of a neutrophil produces other profound changes including degranulation, chemokinesis, and enhanced adherence of neutrophils to each other. Complement activation by cobra venom factor leads to deposition of C3 on endothelium with increased neutrophil adhesion. This occurs within minutes, is independent of protein synthesis and lasts for up to 8 h [37]. Complement activation also causes direct cell damage when the membrane attack complex C5b-9 is inserted into the cell membrane. This forms a cylinder like structure with resultant loss of membrane integrity, the cell cannot maintain its osmotic equilibrium leading to swelling and bursting.

The first indication that complement may play a role in the pathogenesis of ischemia and reperfusion injury was the finding that myocardial ischemia activated complement. A second study confirmed these findings, and in addition, found mitochondrial fragments in cardiac lymph that activated the classical and alternate pathway of complement. Subsequent studies using cobra venom factor to activate and subsequently deplete C3 and C5 demonstrated a reduction in myocardial necrosis after coronary artery occlusion [38].

The causal relationship of complement activation to remote lung injury is not clear. Arguments favoring the involvement of complement are that its intravascular activation with cobra venom factor or zymosan results in acute lung injury and lung leukosequestration. Further, lung injury during hemodialysis and cardiopulmonary bypass [39] leads to an elevation of the complement product C3a desArg. Thirdly, elevated levels of C5a predict the onset of ARDS [40]. Finally, endotoxin and pancreatitis, both risk factors for ARDS, activate intravascular complement.

However, not all workers have confirmed these findings. Weinberg et al. [41] found that complement activation had no predictive value for the onset or progression of ARDS, and Duchateau et al. [42] found variable complement activation in several other predisposing conditions for ARDS. It is possible that some of the confusion is due to indirect complement effects. Thus, in addition to inducing lung injury, systemic complement activation with zymosan induces characteristic hemodynamic changes of hyperdynamic sepsis with hepatic and renal hypoperfusion. The lung injury may be due to this septic like state. C5a also induces transcription of both TNF and IL-1, known mediators of sepsis and organ injury.

There are five regulatory proteins of the complement system, two are in plasma, factor H and C4-binding protein, and three are membrane bound, complement receptor 1(CR1), decay-accelerating factor and membrane co-factor protein. These proteins have structural and functional similarities and are grouped together as the family that regulate complement activation. All the proteins suppress complement activation by reversibly binding to the C3b or C4b (or both) subunits of the bi and trimolecular complexes that are the convertases of the two complement pathways [43]. Binding to these complexes causes either displacement of the catalytic subunits of the convertases Bb and C2a, proteolytic inactivation of C3b and C4b by factor 1 or both [43].

CR1 is a molecule with a long extracellular region, a transmembrane segment and a cytoplasmic domain. In the circulatory system of man, 90 % of CR1 is on erythrocytes. CR1 serves as a cofactor for factor I-mediated cleavage of C3b to iC3b and can limit the amount of damage caused by the complement cascade. Thus, CR1 by favoring conversion, of C3b to iC3b, prevents activation of C5. In addition, iC3b cannot bind factor B, which blocks further complement activation by the amplification loop of the alternate pathway. CR1 also inhibits the activity of C4b, thereby limiting the sequential activation and amplification aspect of the classical pathway. A soluble form of CR1 has recently been engineered from human erythrocytes which lacks the cytoplasmic and transmembrane domains of CR1. This human soluble complement receptor type 1 (sCR1) retains the C3b and C4b binding functions and factor I-cofactor activities of membrane associated CR1 [43].

Complement inhibition with sCR1 has been reported to decrease the size of infarcted myocardium following myocardial ischemia and reperfusion [43]. sCRI was demonstrated to reduce endothelial binding of C3 and C5b-9, and neutrophil accumulation at the site of injury was significantly reduced. These observations with sCR1 confirmed the role of complement in mediating myocardial ischemia and reperfusion that had been suggested by experiments using cobra venom factor.

To test whether ischemia and reperfusion induced remote lung injuries are complement dependent, rats were subjected to 1 h of intestinal ischemia or 4 h of hindlimb ischemia. After this time, injury to the lung was quantitated as was neutrophil sequestration. Reperfusion of ischemic intestine or hindlimb and saline treatment led to a remote lung injury manifested by albumin leak and increased neutrophil sequestration. Animals treated with sCR1 demonstrated depression of complement lytic capacity indicating that a biologically active concentration of inhibitor was present. Following either intestinal or hindlimb ischemia, sCR1 induced complement inhibition and abrogated the pulmonary albumin leak in a dose dependent fashion. These data show that the pulmonary injury is complement-dependent. Interestingly, sCR1 did not prevent lung neutrophil accumulation. This indicates that non-complement dependent neutrophil or endothelial adhesion receptors lead to the remote leukosequestration, and secondly that lung neutrophil accumulations were insufficient to alter permeability.

Oxygen Free Radicals

Oxygen radicals are able to damage the entire array of biomolecules found in tissues, including nucleic acids, membrane lipids, structural and transport proteins, enzymes and receptors [44]. Superoxide ($O_2^{\cdot-}$) is formed during the metabolic processing of many substances of biological importance, including epinephrine, thiols, hemoglobin and products of cyclooxygenase and lipoxygenase. The enzyme, superoxide dismutase (SOD), which is present intra and extracellularly, has an important role in scavenging these free radicals, preventing them from causing damage. There are at least 3 SOD isoenzymes in man; CuZn SOD in the cell cytosol, Mn-SOD in the mitochondrial matrix, and extracellular SOD. Neutrophils via NADPH and endothelial cells, and other tissue via xanthine oxidase are capable of producing large amounts of superoxide. Oxygen free radicals may be beneficial by permitting bacterial killing by neutrophils, but they are also capable of causing inappropriate tissue damage [44].

Hydrogen peroxide can be produced directly by xanthine oxidase, or indirectly through the spontaneous dismutation of $O_2^{\cdot-}$. The spontaneous dismutation of $O_2^{\cdot-}$ proceeds rapidly in aqueous solution, so the production of $O_2^{\cdot-}$ is always accompanied by H_2O_2. $O_2^{\cdot-}$ and H_2O_2 reacts in the presence of certain transition metals such as iron or copper, in the Haber-Weiss reaction, to produce the highly reactive hydroxyl radical ($OH^{\cdot}$).

Evidence for the involvement of free radicals in ischemia and reperfusion injury is based mainly on the protective effects of agents that limit the production of these cytotoxic oxidants or effectively scavenge the radicals after they have been produced. Free radical inhibition with superoxide dismutase, catalase, dimethylsulfoxide and dimethylthiourea attenuates post-ischemic tissue injury in many organs including lungs, heart, intestine and muscle. Free radical inhibition also ameliorates the lung injury following experimental lower torso ischemia and abdominal aortic aneurysm repair [45]. Oxygen radical scavengers also prevent neutrophil infiltration into the ischemic and reperfused tissue which has led to the hypothesis that oxygen free radicals act primarily as neutrophil chemoattractants [46].

Oxygen free radical scavengers have not proven to be of benefit in other settings of lung injury. Thus endotoxin is thought to lead to complement fragment C5a release and activation of polymorphonuclear leukocytes with oxygen radical generation. Although increased oxygen free radical production can be measured following endotoxin administration, the lung injury and hemodynamic changes associated with endotoxemia are unaffected by treatment with superoxide dismutase, catalase or dimethylthiourea. Two recent studies in man using a human recombinant superoxide dismutase to treat myocardial or renal ischemia and reperfusion injury following angioplasty or transplantation have not demonstrated a benefit [47, 48].

Difficulty in assigning clear roles to oxygen free radicals arises because the antagonists are not specific. For example, superoxide dismutase, dimethylthiourea and dimethylsulfoxide all inhibit Tx and probably other eicosanoid synthesis in addition to scavenging free radicals. In many pathological states, oxygen free radical scavengers are at best only partially effective and despite the enormous amount of data that has been collected, the precise relationship between oxygen free radical generation and tissue injury remains unclear.

Neutrophils

During the 1960's and 1970's, observations documented that during inflammation neutrophils actively secreted products which injured cells [44, 49]. These products include oxygen metabolites and proteases such as elastase and collagenase. Other pertinent observations regarding the importance of neutrophils were the findings that the increased permeability resulting from an injection of LTB_4, C5a or fMLP into the skin was prevented by prior neutrophil depletion [50].

Weiss [44] demonstrated that neutrophils stimulated with phorbol myristate acetate damaged endothelial cells by secreting H_2O_2 since the injury could be prevented with catalase, an agent that scavenged H_2O_2. It was also found that the endothelial damage was mediated by neutrophil elastase [49]. The mechanism of neutrophil injury is by the formation of a protected microenvironment. The fundamental strategy of this microenvironment is to form close union between the neutrophil and its target in order to allow prompt contact of H_2O_2 at high concentration. Evidence to support this concept is based on the following findings. Neutrophils lyse substrate protein only when in close contact. Phorbol myristate acetate induces lung injury when neutrophils are in direct contact with endothelium. Neutrophils stimulation by fMLP [49], C5a or endotoxin leads to their adhesion to endothelial cells, an event necessary for injury to occur (Fig. 1.) Adhesion is mediated by molecules expressed on the surface of both cell types. When close contact or a protected microenvironment has been established, oxygen radicals and proteases are released. Any plasma protease inhibitors gaining access to this restricted space are antagonized by the neutrophil secretory products H_2O_2 and myeloperoxidase, both of which have been shown to inhibit the main plasma protease inhibitor alpha-1 antitrypsin. Not only does myeloperoxidase protect proteases from inactivation, it can also lead to their activation [44]. Oxygen radicals and proteases appear to act synergistically to cause tissue damage. Thus, microvascular pemeability increased in the lungs can be induced by perfusion of both elastase and H_2O_2, but not by either agent alone. The lung injury following reperfusion of the ischemic lower torso which is known to be neutrophil dependent [11], can be prevented by in-

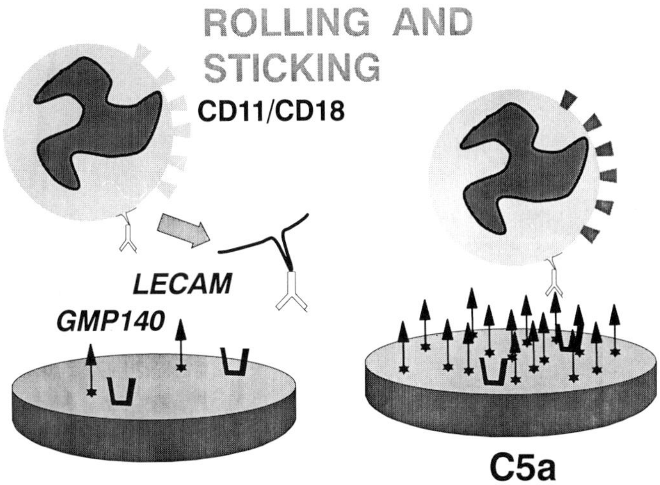

Fig. 1. Initial neutrophil-endothelial interaction is via the selectin family of adhesion molecules. Neutrophil L-selectin (LECAM) couples with endothelial P-selectin (GMP-140) which is rapidly expressed (minutes) in response to an abluminal chemoactivator such as C5a or LTB_4. This initial adhesion occurs at normal flow and shear states and is manifest as rolling and occasional sticking. If large amounts of chemoactivators are released into the blood vessel lumen they will cause L-selectin to be shed. There will be no rolling and sticking and later development of firm adhesion will be impaired.

hibition of either free radicals or proteases [51]. Neutrophil depletion has been shown to ameliorate hepatic and intestinal ischemia and reperfusion injury [52, 53]. Further, neutrophils have also been implicated in the remote lung injury following intestinal ischemia. Schmeling et al. [54] demonstrated increased lung permeability and neutrophil sequestration after 2 h of ischemia and 2 h reperfusion [54].

Neutrophil-endothelial adhesion is carefully controlled by adhesion molecules on both the neutrophil and endothelium. Adhesion molecules on the neutrophil belong to the integrin and selectin families. The development of monoclonal antibodies to these adhesion receptors has enabled the collection of precise data on the role of neutrophils in experimental lung injury.

Integrin Family Adhesion Receptors

Members of the integrin family include CD11/CD18 which are expressed on all leukocytes. The common β-chain, CD18, is linked to one of three α-subunits, CD11a (LFA-1), CD11b (Mac-1, Mo1, CR3) or CD11c (Gp150). CD11a/CD18 is expressed on all leukocytes. However CD11b/CD18 and CD11c/CD18 expression is limited to granulocytes and large granular lymphocytes. It is the CD11a/CD18 and CD11b/CD18 subunits that are primarily involved in mediating the adherence of neutrophils to endothelium [49, 55, 56].

Stimulation of neutrophils with the chemotactic factors C5a, PAF, Tx, LTB_4 or TNF increases neutrophil adhesion to endothelium within minutes by a mechanism which is independent of protein synthesis [18, 55, 57]. The adhesion is usually transient, lasting only 15–20 min [55], but is sufficient to induce a neutropenia within 1 min of intravenous administration of C5a. It is equally dependent on CD11a and CD11b and completely dependent on CD18 as shown by using selective antibodies to the various subunits [18, 55, 57, 58].

Neutrophils in solution stimulated by TNF or PAF produce increased amounts of H_2O_2. The same stimuli applied to neutrophils adherent to endothelium or to tissue matrix proteins yield massive increases in H_2O_2 production [17, 57]. Adhesion and H_2O_2 production were inhibited by monoclonal antibodies (mAbs) to CD18 [17, 57]. In a series of experiments performed by Shappel et al. [57] neutrophils were stimulated with various chemotactic factors and attempts were made to modulate adhesion and adhesion dependent H_2O_2 production using several antibodies to the integrin adhesion receptors. In general, H_2O_2 production was inhibited together with adhesion. However, when canine neutrophils were stimulated with PAF to induce adherence to keyhole limpet hemocyanin coated glass, antibodies to CD11b prevented H_2O_2 production, but not adhesion. This demonstrated that these two events could be dissociated. The CD11b/CD18 integrin has also been shown to mediate neutrophil degranulation [59]. Thus, chemotactic stimulation of neutrophils or activation with endotoxin or TNF increases their adhesion to endothelium by CD11a/CD18 and CD11b/CD18 dependent mechanisms. This chemotactically stimulated adhesion increases neutrophil superoxide production and granule release by CD11b/CD18 dependent mechanisms.

Increased cell surface expression (upregulation) of CD11b/CD18 was noted to be temporarily associated with changes in adherence. This led to the thesis that increased surface expression caused increased adherence. However, treatment of neutrophils with human (rh) granulocyte macrophage-colony stimulating factor produced an increased surface expression of CD11b/CD18, but did not cause an increased adhesion of the neutrophils to cultured endothelial monolayers (60]. A dissociation between quantitative cell surface expression of CD18 and diapedesis of neutrophils following ischemia has recently been demonstrated [61]. It is also true that increased neutrophil adhesion can occur without increased surface expression of CD11b/CD18. These findings suggest that increased cell surface expression is neither necessary nor sufficient for increased adherence to endothelium. It is most likely that a conformational change in CD11b/CD18 leads to activation of the receptors and increased adhesion of neutrophils to endothelium.

Stimulation of endothelium with the cytokines TNF or IL-1 also increases neutrophil adhesion to endothelium (Fig. 2). This mechanism however, involves alteration of adhesion proteins on the endothelium. Following incuba-

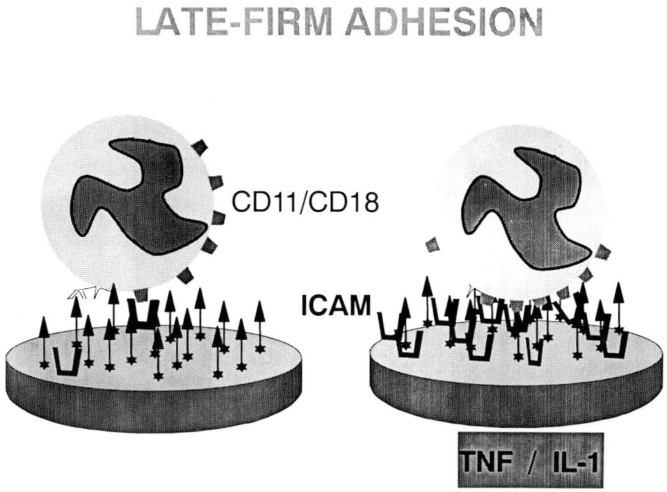

Fig. 2. Firm adhesion develops when the leukocyte integrin CD1l/CD18 couple with ICAM. The endothelial ligand is produced over the course of hours in response to unlikely cytokine stimulation without initial selectin adhesion, late firm adhesion is unlikely to develop, except in regions of low shear such as the lungs. This perhaps explains why the lungs are initial targets in ARDS. In this setting, circulating chemoactivators remove selectins.

tion of human umbilical vein endothelium for 4 h with IL-1, neutrophil adhesion was greatly increased. CD18 antibodies reduced this adhesion by 78 %, CD11a antibodies by 40 % and CD11b antibodies by 34 %, suggesting that adhesion was mediated equally by CD11a and CD11b [58]. Smith et al. [56] confirmed that neutrophil adherence to cytokine stimulated endothelium was CD11a/CD18 dependent, but using four different antibodies to the CD11b integrin, was unable to prevent adhesion. Both these *in vitro* studies were performed under static conditions. They demonstrate a role for CD11a, but are contradictory regarding the role of CD11b. Under venous flow conditions, neutrophil adhesion to endothelium incubated with IL-1 was not inhibited by CD18 antibodies. Further, the neutrophils from patients with leukocyte adhesion deficiency (LAD) (deficiency of CD18) also adhered to endothelium under these conditions. However, with flow, transendothelial migration of neutrophils was inhibited by more than 80 % [62].

Important concepts emerging from the above studies are first that adhesion is necessary for neutrophils to diapedese, release H_2O_2 and degranulate. Secondly, antibodies against the integrins may inhibit neutrophil function (H_2O_2 release) independent of adhesion. Thirdly, the mechanism of adhesion is dependent on flow conditions.

In Vivo Studies Using Antibodies to Integrin Adhesion Molecules

The potential for treatment of patients with shock or trauma using monoclonal antibodies to neutrophil adhesion proteins was first suggested in animal studies of hemorrhagic hypotension. Animals treated with CD18 monoclonal antibodies required smaller volumes of resuscitation fluid to maintain blood pressure and hematocrit. There was attenuation of gastric, but not pulmonary injury [63]. Several studies have shown a benefit in using CD18 monoclonal antibodies to treat experimental lung injury induced by ischemia and reperfusion of the lung itself, *Pseudomonas aeruginosa* infusion, or lower torso ischemia and reperfusion [5, 64, 65]. Neutrophil emigration in the lung has been found to be both CD18-dependent and CD18-independent [66]. CD18 monoclonal antibody 60.3 prevented neutrophil accumulation into the lungs induced by phorbol myristate acetate, *E. coli* organisms or *E. coli* endotoxin but had no significant effect on neutrophil accumulation induced by acid aspiration or *Salmonella pneumoniae.*

We have recently used two different monoclonal antibodies to neutrophil adhesion molecules to investigate lung injury following intestinal ischemia. Superior mesenteric artery occlusion in the rabbit for 1 h followed by 3 h of reperfusion induced severe hypotension, leukopenia and a remote lung injury characterized by increased permeability and lung leukosequestration. Treatment with a monoclonal antibody to the neutrophil CD18 integrin (mAb R15.7) did not moderate the systemic hypotension, but prevented the increased lung permeability and reduced lung sequestration of neutrophils by 70 %. These data indicate that in this model, increased lung permeability is fully, and neutrophil adhesion is partly CD18 dependent. In keeping with the decreased neutrophil sequestration, the CD18 mAb also prevented leukopenia. A corroborative study in pigs of *Pseudomonas aeruginosa* induced shock and lung injury, showed that a CD18 mAb did not ameliorate the hemodynamic effects, but prevented the development of lung injury and leukopenia [65].

One hour of superior mesenteric artery occlusion and 3 h of reperfusion in the rat also induced increased lung permeability and leukosequestration. A CD11b monoclonal antibody (R17) prevented the development of lung permeabililty but did not significantly reduce sequestration of neutrophils. Further, the antibody did not appear to alter white blood cell kinetics since there was no leukocytosis or lung leukosequestration when R17 was administered to sham animals. As lung endothelium is exposed to high circulating levels of TNF during intestinal ischemia and reperfusion, we speculate that the CD11b/CD18 independent lung leukosequestration in our study is related to the other integrin CD11a/CD18 as well as selectin mediated adhesion. The latter postulate is necessary since the CD18 mAb did not completely prevent leukosequestration. The beneficial effects of CD11b mAbs thus relate more to inhibition of neutrophil function than sequestration. An alternate explanation of the inability of the CD11b mAb to alter sequestration is that neutrophil activation has led to increased PMN stiffening secondary to actin polymerization and non-specific trapping in the pulmonary microcirculation. That this is unlikely is indicated by the ability of a CD18 mAb to reduce leukosequestration. The findings in the present study that a Mac-1 monoclonal antibody prevented permeability edema in the lungs but not neutrophil entrapment is an example of the dissociation between lung injury and sequestration of neutrophils. This is in concert with the report of lung injury induced by LPS primed neutrophils stimulated with fMLP, where treatment with a platelet activating factor antagonist prevented increased lung permeability but not leukosequestration [35].

Since adhesion molecules are important in promoting neutrophil diapedesis through the microvasculature at sites of infection, „anti-adhesion“ therapy may increase susceptibility to infection. Certainly the genetic disease LAD results in severe problems with infections. In the short term, inhibition of integrin function may be well tolerated. Thus, mortality from acute intra-abdominal abscesses in rabbits was not increased following two doses of CD18 [67]. However, knowledge of the effects of neutrophil integrin antibodies on the overall function of the immune system is still poor. A CD11b directed mAb has a potential advantage over that of mAb against CD18 in that it does not effect lymphocyte binding and may therefore not induce the same degree of susceptibility to infection.

Endothelium

An increase in the permeability of lung microvascular endothelium characterizes ischemia and reperfusion induced lung injury. The endothelium is not a passive bystander in this process of injury. It expresses adhesion receptors which act as ligands for neutrophil adhesion molecules. The endothelium also synthesizes other mediators including free radicals, eicosanoids, PAF, and IL-1, that may contribute to the inflammatory process. The key endothelial adhesion molecules that are involved in acute inflammatory lung disease are intercellular adhesion molecule (ICAM) and endothelial leukocyte adhesion molecule (ELAM-1, or E-selectin).

Three intercellular adhesion molecules have been identified: ICAM-1, ICAM-2 and ICAM-3. All are members of the immunoglobulin superfamily. ICAM-1 is constitutively expressed on endothelium. Its expression is increased by a protein synthesis dependent mechanism when endothelium is exposed to TNF, IL-1, LPS or interferon-γ [68]. Interleukin-1 induced upregulation is seen 30 min after incubation, increases steadily and reaches a peak after 24 h [58]. Increased surface expression of ICAM-1 results in increased neutrophil adhesion [58]. Antibodies to ICAM-1 inhibit neutrophil adhesion to cytokine stimulated endothelium [69]. Endothelial ICAM-1 is a ligand for neutrophil CD11a/CD18 (Fig. 2) [56, 69]. ICAM-1 is also thought be an endothelial ligand for neutrophil CD11b/CD18 [56, 69]. Thus ICAM-1 is involved in CD11a and CD11b mediated neutrophil adherence to endothelium and is upregulated after cytokine stimulation.

Following pulmonary artery occlusion for 24 h, reperfusion leads to increased lung permeability and increased neutrophil sequestration. Antibodies to ICAM-1 prevent both events. Increased expression of ICAM-1 was demonstrated on pulmonary endothelium following the reperfusion period [70]. Similarly, the lung permeability increase that follows atelectasis was prevented with monoclonal antibodies to either CD18 or ICAM-1 (unpublished observations). The lung injury induced by PMA stimulation of neutrophils also dependent on ICAM-1 and CD18.

The selectin family, also called lectin-cell adhesion molecules (LEC-CAMS) is composed of three members: E-selectin (ELAM-1), L-selectin also called MEL-14 or LAM 1 and P-selectin also known as CD62, GMP-140, PADGEM. All three selectins help regulate leukocyte binding to endothelium at inflammatory sites. They are expressed only on cells within the vasculature (endothelial cells, lymphocytes, neutrophils, monocytes and platelets). E-selectin mediates neutrophil binding to cytokine stimulated endothelium. It is not expressed constitutively, but is induced rapidly by IL-1, TNF and LPS [68, 71] at sites of inflammation [72]. Following stimulation, E-selectin is maximally expressed at 4 h and declines to near baseline by 24 h. When E-selectin is maximally expressed, mAbs to this antigen reduce neutrophil adherence by only 47 %. On the other hand, a significant portion of neutrophil adherence is not inhibited by CD18 mAb. CD18 is not a ligand for E-selectin. These observations are consistent with neutrophil binding to both E-selectin as well as ICAM-1 [58]. The combination of CD18 and E-selectin antibodies reduced adhesion by 94 %, demonstrating CD18 dependent and CD18 independent mechanisms of neutrophil adhesion to endothelium. L-selectin (LAM-1, MEL-14) and sialyl Lewis x have both been identified as neutrophil receptors of E-selectin [73, 74]. Sialyl Lewis x is widely distributed on the neutrophil surface, but is concentrated on microvillus projections on the L-selectin molecule. This high concentration of sialyl Lewis x results in selective adhesion of L-selectin with E-selectin [74]. E-and L-selectin interactions are thought to mediate the initial neutrophil-endothelial adhesion. This occurs under conditions of flow and high shear. This initial sticking and rolling of neutrophils is then followed by CD18/ICAM mediated firm adhesion. The latter bond is required for neutrophil degranulation, superoxide production and diapedesis.

Recently, a monoclonal antibody to E-selectin has been shown to prevent lung injury and neutrophil sequestration induced by immune complex alveolitis [75]. The benefits of E- or L-selectin mAbs have not yet been tested in other settings of lung injury. As the selectins appear to mediate initial neutrophil-endothelial adhesion, it is possible that they will be effective in preventing experimental lung disease that is CD18/ICAM-1 dependent. However, under conditions of low shear, neutrophil-endothelial adhesion becomes increasingly CD18 dependent [62]. Thus, the proportions of LAM-1 and CD18 dependent adhesion in the lung may vary with changes in shear forces that accompany lung injury. It is also possible that entry of chemoattractants into the circulation will change operations of L-selectins.

Contact of these agents with neutrophils would then be largely determined by CD18/ICAM binding which occurs in organs such as the lungs with low shear forces.

Conclusion

A number of inflammatory mediators generated in response to ischemia and reperfusion have now been elucidated. These include the eicosanoids, particularly thromboxane A_2, leukotriene B_4, platelet activating factor, the cytokines, complement, oxygen free radicals, neutrophil and endothelial activation factors such as adhesion receptors and the neutrophil products superoxide and elastase. There exists a complex interrelationship between these agents. The current development of specific antagonists to a number of these mediators promises several new classes of therapeutic tools for the therapy of respiratory failure.

References

1. Moon VH (1938) Inflammation. In: Shock and related capillary phenomena (Chapt. V), Oxford University Press, New York. pp 64–81
2. Paterson IS, Klausner JM, Goldman G, et al. (1989) Pulmonary edema after aneurysm surgery is modified by mannitol. Ann Surg 210:796–801
3. Caty MG, Guice KS, Oldham KT, Remick DG, Kunkel SI (1990) Evidence for tumor necrosis factor-induced pulmonary microvascular injury after intestinal ischemia reperfusion injury. Ann Surg 212:694–700
4. Colletti LM, Remick DG, Burtch GD, Kunkel SL, Streiter RM, Campbell DA (1990) Role of tumour necrosis factor alpha in the pathophysiologic alterations after hepatic ischemia/reperfusion injury in the rat. J Clin Invest 85:1936–1943
5. Horgan MJ, Wright SD, Malik AB (1990) Antibody against leukocyte integrin (CD18) prevents reperfusion-induced lung vascular injury. Am J Physiol 259:315–319
6. Goldman G, Welbourn R, Lindsay T, Hill J, Shepro D, Hechtman HB (1991) Neutrophil adhesion receptors mediate remote aspiration injury. FASEB J A:6503
7. Moore FD (1959) In: Metabolic care of the surgical patient, WB Saunders Co, Philadelphia, PA, pp 97.
8. Klass AA (1953) Acute mesenteric arterial occlusion: Restoration of blood flow by embolectomy. J Int Coll Surg 20:687–694
9. Klausner JM, Paterson IS, Goldman G, Valeri CR, Shepro D, Hechtman HB (1989) Thromboxane A_2 mediates increased pulmonary microvascular permeability following limb ischemia. Circ Res 64:1178–1189.
10. Hocking DC, Phillips PG, Ferro TJ, Johnson A (1990) Mechanisms of pulmonary edema induced by tumor necrosis factor-α. Circ Res 67:68–76
11. Klausner JM, Paterson IS, Valeri CR, Shepro D, Hechtman HB (1988) Limb ischemia-induced increase in permeability is mediated by leukocytes and leukotrienes. Ann Surg 208:755–760
12. Wakabayashi G, Gelfand JA, Burke JF, Thompson RC, Dinarello CA (1991) A specific receptor antagonist for interleukin 1 prevents Escherichia coli-induced shock in rabbits. FASEB J 5:338–343
13. Michie HR, Manogue KR, Spriggs DR, et al.(1988) Detection of circulating tumor necrosis factor after endotoxin administration. N Eng J Med 318:1481–1486

14. Dubravec DB, Spriggs DR, Mannick JA, Rodrick ML (1990) Circulating human peripheral blood granulocytes synthesize and secrete tumor necrosis factor α. Proc Natl Acad Sci USA 87:6758–6761
15. Dinarello CA (1991) Interleukin-1 and Interleukin-1 antagonism. Blood 77:1627–1652
16. Kurt-Jones EA, Beller DI, Mizel SB (1985) Identification of a membrane-associated interleukin-1 in macrophages. Proc Natl Acad Sci USA 82:1204–1208
17. Nathan C, Srimal S, Farber C, et al(1989) Cytokine-induced respiratory burst of human neutrophils: Dependence on extracellular matrix proteins and CD18/CD18 integrins. J cell Biol 109:1341–1349
18. Gamble JR, Harlan JM, Klebanoff SJ, Vadas MA (1985) Stimulation of the adherence of neutrophils to umbilical vein endothelium by human recombinant tumor necrosis factor. Proc Natl Acad Sci USA 82:8667–8671
19. Smith CW, Kishimoto TK, Abassi O, et al. (1991) Chemotactic factors regulate lectin adhesion molecule 1 (LECAM-1)-dependent neutrophil adhesion to cytokine-stimulated endothelial cells in vitro. J Clin Invest 87:609–618
20. Movat HZ, Burrowes CE, Cybulsky MI, Dinarello CA (1987) Acute inflammation and a Schwartzman-like reaction induced by interleukin-1 and tumor necrosis factor. Synergistic action of the cytokines in the induction of inflammation and microvascular injury. Am J Pathol 129:463–476
21. Abe Y, Sekiya S, Yamashita T, Sendo F (1990) Vascular hyperpermeability induced by tumor necrosis factor and its augmentation by IL-1 and IFN-γ is inhibited by selective depletion of neutrophils with a monoclonal antibody. J Immunol 145:2902–2907
22. Ulich TR, Yin S, del Castillo J, Eisenberg SP, Thompson RC (1991) The intratracheal administration of endotoxin and cytokines. The interleukin-1 receptor antagonist inhibits endotoxin-and IL-1-induced acute inflammation. Am J Pathol 138:521–524
23. Goldblum SE, Jay M, Yoneda K, Cohen DA, McClain CJ, Gillespie MN (1987) Monokine-induced acute lung injury in rabbits. J Appl Physiol 63:2093–2100
24. Welbourn R, Goldman G, Riordan MO (1991) Role for tumor necrosis is factor as a mediator of lung injury following lower torso ischemia. Am J Physiol 70:2645–2650
25. Okusawa S, Gelfand JA, Ikejima T, Connolly RJ, Dinarello CA (1988) Interleukin-1 induces a shock-like state in rabbits. Synergism with tumor necrosis factor and the effect of cyclooxygenase inhibition. J Clin Invest 81:1162–1172,
26. Waage A, Espevik T (1988) Interleukin 1 potentiates the lethal effects of tumor necrosis factor-α/cachectin in mice. J Exp Med 167:1987–1992
27. Beutler B, Milsark IW, Cerami AC, et al. (1985) Passive immunization against cachectin/tumor necrosis factor protects mice from lethal effect of endotoxin. Science 229:869–871
28. Tracey KJ, Fong Y, Hesse DG, et al (1987) Anti-cachetin/TNF monoclonal antibodies prevent septic shock during lethal bacteraemia. Nature 330:662–664
29. Ohlsson K, Björk P, Bergenfeldt M, Hageman R, Thompson RC (1990) Interleukin- 1 receptor antagonist reduces mortality from endotoxin shock. Nature 348:550–552
30. Carter DB, MR Deibel, CJ Dunn, et al. (1990) Purification, cloning, expression and biological characterization of an interleukin-1 receptor antagonist protein. Nature 344:633–638
31. McIntyre KW, Stepan GJ, Kolinsky KD, et al. (1991) Inhibition of interleukin-1 binding and bioactivity in vitro, and modulation of acute inflammation in vivo by IL-1 receptor antagonist and anti-IL-1 receptor monoclonal antibody. J Exp Med 173:931–939
32. Karolle BL, Weiss SJ, Huber AR, Lim MJ, Buda AJ (1991) The recombinant receptor antagonist to interleukin-1 reduces myocardial neutrophil accumulation and tissue injury following ischemia and reperfusion. Circulation 84:A336
33. Stewart AG, Dubbin PN, Harris T, Dusting GJ (1990) Platelet-activating factor may act as a second messenger in the release of ecosanoids and superoxide anions from leukocytes and endothelial cells. Proc Natl Acad Sci USA 87:3215–3219
34. Kuijpers VW, Hakkert BC, Hoogerwerf M, Leeuwenberg JF, Roos D (1991) Role of endothelial leukocyte adhesion molecule-1 and platelet activating factor in neutrophil adherence to IL-1 -prestimulated endothelial cells. Endothelial leukocyte adhesion molecule-1 mediated CD18 activation. J Immunol 147:1369–1376

35. Anderson BO, Poggetti RS, Shanley PF, et al. (1991) Primed neutrophils injure rat lung through a platelet-activating factor-dependent mechanism. J Surg Res 50:510–514
36. Mozes T, Braquet P, Filep J (1989) Platelet-activating factor: An endogenous mediator of mesenteric ischemia-reperfusion-induced shock. Am J Physiol 257:872–877
37. Marks RM, Todd RF III, Ward PA (1989) Rapid induction of neutrophil-endothelial adhesion by endothelial complement fixation. Nature 339:314–317
38. Crawford MH, Grover FL, Kolb WP, et al. (1988) Complement and neutrophil activation in the pathogenesis of ischemic myocardial injury. Circulation 78:1449–1458
39. Moore FD Jr, Wamer KG, Assousa S, Valeri CR, Khuri SF (1988) The effects of complement activation during cardiopulmonary bypass. Attenuation by hypothermia, heparin and hemodilution. Ann Surg 208:95–103
40. Hammerschmidt DE, Weaver LJ, Hudson LD, Craddock PR, Jacob HS (1980) Association of complement activation and elevated plasma C5a with adult respiratory distress syndrome: Pathophysiologic relevance and possible prognostic value. Lancet 1:947–949,
41. Weinberg P, Matthay M, Webster R, Roskos K, Goldstein I, Murray J (1984) Biologically active products of complement and acute lung injury in patients with the sepsis syndrome. Am Rev Resp Dis 130:791–796
42. Duchateau J, Haas M, Schreyen H, Radoux L, Sprangers I, Noel F (1984) Complement activation in patients at risk of developing the adult respiratory distress syndrome. Am Rev Resp Dis 130:1058–1064
43. Weisman HF, Bartow T, Leppo MK et al. (1991) Soluble human complement receptor type 1: In vivo inhibitor of complement suppressing post-ischemic myocardial inflammation and necrosis. Science 249:146–151
44. Weiss SJ (1989) Tissue destruction by neutrophils. N Engl J Med 320:365–376,
45. Klausner JM, Paterson IS, Kobzik L, Valeri CR, Shepro D, Hechtman HB (1989) Oxygen free radicals mediate ischemia-induced lung injury. Surgery 104:192–199
46. Petrone WF, English DK, Wong K, McCord JM (1980) Free radicals and inflammation superoxide-dependent activation of neutrophil chemotactic factor in plasma. Proc Natl Acad Sci USA 77:1159–1163
47. Wems S, Brinker J, Gruber J, et al.(1989) A randomized, double-blind trial of recombinant human superoxide dismutase (SOD) in patients undergoing PTCA for acute MI. Circulation 80 (Suppl): 113
48. Schneeberger H, Illner WD, Abendroth D, et al. (1989) First clinical experiences with superoxide dismutase in kidney transplantation: Results of a double blind randomized study. Transplantation Proceedings 21:1245–1246
49. Harlan JM (1985) Leukocyte-Endothelial interactions. Blood 65:513–525
50. Wedmore CV, Williams TJ (1981) Control of vascular permeability by polymorphnuclear leukocytes in inflammation. Nature 289:646–650
51. Welbourn CRB, Goldman G, Paterson IS, Valeri CR, Shepro D, Hechtman HB (1991) Neutrophil elastase and oxygen radicals: Synergism in lung injury after hindlimb ischemia. Am J Physiol 260:1852–1856
52. Jaeschke H, Farhood A, Wayne-Smith C (1990) Neutrophils contribute to ischemia/reperfusion injury in rat liver in vivo. FASEB J 4:3355–3359
53. Hernandez LA, Grisham MB, Twohig B, Arfors KE, Harlan JM, Granger DN (1987) Role of neutrophils in ischemia/reperfusion-induced microvascular injury. Am J Physiol 253:699–703
54. Schmeling DJ, Caty MG, Oldham KT, Guice KS, Hinshaw DB (1989) Evidence for a neutrophil related acute lung injury following intestinal ischemia-reperfusion injury. Surgery 106:195–203
55. Lo SK, Van Seventer GA, Levin SM, Wright SD (1989) Two leukocyte receptors (CD11a/CD18 and CD11b/CD18) mediate transient adhesion to endothelium by binding to different ligands. J Immunol 143:3325–3329-
56. Smith CW, Marlin SD, Rothlein R, Toman C, Anderson DA (1989) Cooperative interactions of LFA-1 and Mac-1 with intercellular adhesion molecule-1 in facilitating adherence and transendothelial migration of human neutrophils in vitro. J Clin Invest 83:2008–2017
57. Shappell SB, Toman C, Anderson DC, Taylor AA, Entman ML, Wayne Smith C (1990) Mac-1 (CD11b/CD18) mediates adherence-dependence hydrogen peroxide production by human and canine neutrophils. J Immunol 144:2702–2711

58. Luscinskas FW, Brock AF, Arnaout MA, Gimbrone NM (1989) Endothelial-leukocyte adhesion molecule-l-dependent and leukocyte (CD11/CD18)-independent mechanisms contribute to polymorphonuclear leukocyte adhesion to cytokine-activated human vascular endothelium. J Immunol 142:2257–2263
59. Schleiffenbaum B, Moser R, Patarroyo M, Fehr J (1989)Me cell surface glycoprotein Mac-1 (CD11b/CD18) mediates neutrophil adhesion and modulates degranulation independently of its cell surface expression. J Immunol 142:3527–3545
60. Lopez AF, Williamson DJ, Gamble JR, et al. (1986) A recombinant human granulocyte-macrophage colony-stimulation factor (rhGM-CSF) stimulates *in vitro* mature human neutrophil and eosinophil function, surface receptor expression and survival. J Clin Invest 78:1220–1228f
61. Welbourn R, Goldman G, Kobzik L, Valeri CR, Shepro D, Hechtman HB (1990) Neutrophil adherence receptors (CD18) in ischemia: Dissociation between quantitative cell surface expression and diapedesis mediated by leukotriene B4. J Immunol 145:1906–1911
62. Lawrence MB, Smith CW, Eskin SG, McIntire LV (1990) Effect of venous shear stress on CD18-mediated neutrophil adhesion to cultured endothelium. Blood 75:227–237
63. Vedder NB, Winn RK, Rice CL, Chi EY, Arfors KE, Harlan JM (1988) A monoclonal antibody to the adherence-promoting leukocyte glycoprotein, CD18, reduces organ injury and improves survival from haemorrhagic shock and resuscitation in rabbits. J Clin Invest 81:939–944
64. Welboum R, Goldman G, Valeri CR, Shepro D, Hechtman HB (1992) Lung injury following hindlimb ischemia is mediated by neutrophil CD18 adherence receptors. Circ Res (In press)
65. Walsh CJ, Carey PD, Cook DJ, Bechard DE, Fowler AA, Sugarman HJ (1991) Anti CD18 antibody attenuates neutropenia and alveolar capillary-membrane injury during gram-negative sepsis. Surgery 110:205–212
66. Doerschuk CM, Winn RK, Coxson HO, Harlan JM (1990) CD18-dependent and independent mechanisms of neutrophil emigration in the pulmonary and systemic microcirculation of rabbits. J Immunol 144:2327–2333
67. Mileski W, Winn R, Harlan J, Rice C (1989) Inhibition of neutrophil adhesion in sepsis. Surg Forum 40:107–108
68. Pober JS, Gimbrone MA, Lapierre LA, et al. (1986) Overlapping patterns of activation of human endothelial cells by interleukin-1, tumor necrosis factor, and immune interferon. J Immunol 137:1893–1896
69. Smith CW, Rothlein R, Hughes B, Mariscalco M, Schmalsteig F, Anderson DC (1988) Recognition of an endothelial determinant for CD 18-dependent human neutrophil adherence and transendothelial migration. J Clin Invest 82:1746–1756,
70. Horgan MJ, Ge M, Gu J, Rothlein R, Malik AB (1991) Protective effect of monoclonal antibody RR1 directed against intercellular adhesion molecule ICAM-1 in reperfusion lung injury. Am Rev Resp Dis 143:A578
71. Bevilacqua MP, Pober JS, Wheeler ME, Cotran RS, Gimbrone MA Jr (1 985) Interleukin-1 acts on cultured human vascular endothelial cells to increase the adhesion of polymorphonuclear leukocytes, monocytes and related leukocyte cell lines. J Clin Invest 76:2003–2011
72. Munro JM, Pober JS, Cotran RS (1989) Tumor necrosis factor and interferon-gamma induce distinct patterns of endothelial activation and associated leukocyte accumulation in skin of Papio anubis. Am J Path 135:121–133
73. Philips ML, Nudelman E, Gaeta FC, et al. (1991) ELAM-1 mediates cell adhesion by recognition of a carbohydrate ligand, sialyl-le$_x$. Science 250:1130–1135
74. Picker LJ, Wamock RA, Bums AR, Doerschuk CM, Berg EL, Butcher EC (1991) The neutrophil selectin LECAM-1 presents carbohydrate ligands to the vascular selectins ELAM-1 and GMP- 140. Cell 66:921–933
75. Mulligan MS, Varani J, Dame MK, et al. (1991) Role of endothelial-leukocyte adhesion molecule 1 (ELAM-1) in neutrophil-mediated lung injury in rats. J Clin Invest 88:1396–1406

Cytokines in Shock: 1992

B. Beutler

Introduction

We have recently learned many lessons regarding the role of hematopoietically derived cells, and the marcophage in particular, in the etiology of gram-negative septic shock. Perhaps the most important lesson, and the lesson which still invites the most avid experimentation, was that taught by the C3H/HeJ mouse. These animals carry a genetic defect, localized to the 4th chromosome [1], which deprives them of the ability to respond to lipopolysaccharide (LPS). As a result, the mice can sustain the injection of enormous quantities of LPS; the dose-lethality curve for this strain is shifted "downfield" by a factor of 100 or more [2]. Indeed, it is not clear that the animals ever succumb to the injection of highly purified LPS preparations.

Michalek et al. [3] demonstrated that hematopoietic stem cells obtained from normal, histocompatible donor animals render C3H/HeJ mice susceptible to the lethal effect of LPS when used to reconstitute their stem cell population following lethal irradiation. Then, too, C3H/HeJ marrow administered to lethally irradiated responder mice, leads to the production of chimeric animals that fail to respond to LPS. Thus, a decade ago, it became obvious that LPS works its lethal effect through an indirect mechanism, involving mediators of hematopoietic origin. This is not the whole story of LPS action. However, it is a crucial one, for two reasons. It emphasizes the fact that all of LPS signal transduction is channeled through the product of a single gene, known as the *Lps* gene [1]. Second, it reveals that LPS is, by itself, relatively harmless, and that endogenous mediators make it the violent poison that it appears to be.

Cytokines Released in Response to LPS Mediate the Biological Actions of LPS

The Central Role of Tumor Necrosis Factor (TNF) as a Mediator of Endotoxic Shock

Endotoxin induces a wide array of changes when it is administered to experimental animals [4,5]. Among these, its ability to cause interstitial pnemonitis (adult respiratory distress syndrome; ARDS), acute renal tubular necrosis, coagulopathy, and hypoglycemia contributes most markedly to its overall lethal effect. More subtle changes have also been recorded. Endotoxin causes hypertriglyceridemia which, while not harmful in itself, is a biochemical indicator of the molecular processes that endotoxin can set in motion [6]. If an animal happens to have a tumor, it has been observed that LPS may be disproportionately destructive to the tumor mass [7,8]. The phenomenon of hemorrhagic necrosis of tumors generated much excitement earlier in this century, insofar as pathogenic bacteria and their products were thought to comprise a potential means of chemotherapy [9-13].

Hypertriglyceridemia and tumor necrosis are superficially unrelated to one another. However, both occur in the context of septic shock or endotoxemia. As it developed, both phenomena are attributable to the release of a single cytokine mediator which was identified, on the one hand, as "tumor necrosis factor" (TNF) and on the other hand, as "cachectin". The term TNF will be used to designate the mediator for the remainder of this chapter, since this abbreviation has come in very widespread use.

The role played by TNF as a central mediator of endotoxic shock was determined through a series of investigations involving both human and animal subjects. Its assignment, as such, rests upon the following observations:

1. In animals of diverse species [14-17], and in humans [18], TNF is produced by mononuclear phagocytes over a time course that precedes the onset of the toxic effects of LPS, and in amounts that would likely prove to be very toxic.
2. Agents which sensitize to the lethal effect of LPS often act to increase the biosynthesis of TNF (as in the case of facultative intercellular pathogens like *Bacillus Calmette-Guerin, Corynebacterium parvum,* and *Mycobacterium lepraemurium*)[8,19-21], or increase sensitivity to the toxic effects of TNF (as in the case of lead acetate or D-galactosamine) [22,23].
3. TNF is a highly toxic molecule, which is capable of reproducing much of the tissue injury and metabolic derangement witnessed in the setting of endotoxic shock [24]. Notably, TNF causes injury to the lungs, gastrointestinal tract, kidney, and other vital organs; it produces a profound metabolic acidosis, and transient shifts in plasma glucose concentration (an initial phase of hypertriglyceridemia followed by a late phase of hypertriglyceridemia), hypotension, and coagulopathy.
4. Passive immunization against TNF has been shown to elicit substantial protection against the lethal effect of LPS [25]. This observation has been made in several species, using both monoclonal [26] and polyclonal [25,27] reagents, and most recently, using a soluble form of the TNF receptor. The effect of passive immunization is only manifested if antibody is given in advance of LPS administration, consistent with the rapid production and clearance of TNF that occur subsequent to endotoxin challenge [17].
5. In humans, septic shock is associated with high levels of circulating TNF, and these levels may be inversely correlated with survival [28].

TNF is presumed to cause injury associated with endotoxic shock through several mechanisms. However, the most important of its effect include its ability to activate neutrophils [29-33] and vascular endothelial cells [29,34-40], leading to margination of the former, coagulopathy, and organ damage.

It has been noted that passive immunization against TNF prevents LPS induced activation of IL-1 synthesis and IL-6 synthesis *in vivo* [41]. Thus, while production of these other cytokines may be directly induced by LPS *in vitro* , their production *in vivo* apparently depends upon prior biosynthesis of TNF. In this sense, although each of these mediators undoubtedly participates in the development of the septic syndrome, TNF may be considered as the primary mediator. Its kinetics of synthesis are such that peak levels are observed before peak levels of IL-1, IL-6, or interferon-γ [41]. More recently, administration of the IL-1 receptor antagonist, a form of IL-1 which engages the IL-1 receptor but fails to elicit a response in any of the biological assays thus far studied [42-44], protects animals against infusion of LPS or gram-negative organisms. It might thus be inferred that the IL-1 produced in response to TNF contributes to the pathogenesis of gram-negative septic shock. Interestingly, however, although IL-1 has been shown to provoke hypotension and a hyperdynamic cardiovascular state in rabbits, it has never been shown to be directly lethal to animals, as has been the case with TNF. The effects of IL-1 may therefore be seen as less global than the effects of TNF (e.g. TNF may provoke the release of a "shower" cytokines, each of which is somewhat toxic, and which act together to reproduce the findings in sepsis). Blockade of any of the individual participant in the cascade, by antibody or inhibitor, may have a protective effect with respect to the development of shock.

Interferon-γ is known to synergize with TNF in many biological assays [45-55]. Its ability to sensitize animals to the lethal effect of TNF has also been described [56]. Indeed, interferon-γ, produced in response to a gram-negative bacterial infection like salmonellosis, may lead to such enhanced sensitivity to TNF that an infected mouse may be killed by infusion of nanogram quantities of the cytokine. Given that such amounts of TNF are untraceable *in vivo* within a few minutes following their injection [17], one might suppose that quantities of TNF that cannot be detected by assay of serum samples may work profound effects on the host in the presence of appropriate sensitizing agents. Thus, it is not implausible to suggest that TNF may, at undetectable concentrations, cause wasting in animals with various sensitizing tumors.

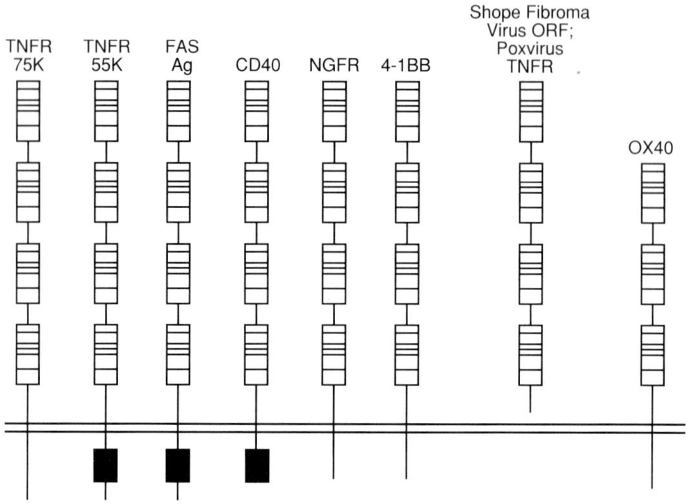

Fig. 1. The TNF receptor family. Defined by repeated cysteine-rich motifs, the TNF receptor now includes nine members, as illustrated above. Bars within boxes represent intrachain disulfide bonds. The double line represents the plasma membrane. The dark boxes indicate regions of homology between the 55 TNF receptor, the FAS antigen, and CD40 antigen which are tought to mediate apoptosis. ORF = open reading frame; TNFR = TNF receptor; NGFR = nerve growth factor receptor

Mechanisms of TNF Action

How does TNF cause shock and tissue injury ? Undoubtedly, as noted above, it does not do so alone. Not only does it stimulate the production of other cytokines, but the production of terminal mediators of shock (e.g. leukotrienes , platelet activating factor (PAF), and other molecules of low molecular weight that are capable of causing tissue injury). The complexity of the response to TNF mirrors the complexity of the response to the inducing agent (e.g. LPS) itself. However, a focal point for the understanding of TNF action has emerged with the molecular cloning of cDNAs and genes encoding the two known TNF receptors. In fact, it has become clear that the TNF receptors are but two members of an extended receptor "family" (Fig. 1) [57].

Each TNF receptor consists of a single glycosylated polypeptide chain with a single membrane spanning domain, separating the extracellular (binding) domain from the cytoplasmic (signaling) domain. One of the molecules is 55 kD in size, whereas the other is 75 kD in size. The difference in size results mostly from differences in glycosylation of the two species. Both types of receptors are found on most cells and tissues, although the density of the 75 kD receptor is relatively greater on cells of lymphoid origin, and the density of the 55 kD receptor is relatively greater on cells of epithelial origin.

There is no significant homology between the cytoplasmic domains of the 55 kD and 75 kD receptors on comparison of their amino-acid sequences. This would suggest that quite different signals are transduced by each molecule. A general sense of function has by now been obtained, in that the 55 kD molecule is known to be responsible for the cytolysis and cytotoxicity, and perhaps most of the other known effects of TNF, whereas the 75 kD molecule stimulates lymphoproliferation.

The extracellular domains of the two TNF receptors are homologous to one another, exhibiting approximately 25% sequence identity at the amino-acid level. Despite this relatively modest level of structural similarity, each receptor is capable of engaging both of TNF-α (cachectin) and TNF-β (lymphotoxin), which themselves have only 28% homology at the amino-acid level [58]. Somewhat surprisingly, in view of the evident flexibility of the TNF receptor interaction, human TNF does not bind to the mouse TNF 75 kD receptor. Thus, human TNF is not able to stimulate the proliferation of mouse T cells. This finding has important implications related to the toxicity of TNF, and the role played by each receptor in the pathogenesis of shock.

Four cysteine-rich internal repeats characterize the extracellular domain of the TNF receptors. It is this motif that defines the TNF receptor family. Not all of the repeats are required for binding to the TNF trimer. Deletion of the innermost repeat is tolerated; deletion of the most N-terminal repeat destroys the binding activity of the receptor [59].

The TNF molecule is trimeric in structure [60]. Each trimer contains three receptor binding sites, and X-ray diffraction studies of co-crystals composed of receptor and TNF trimer have begun to reveal the interaction between these proteins in exacting detail. The TNF receptor is engaged by the trimer at intersubunit surfaces. Thus, a monomer of TNF, even if it were soluble, could not be expected to bind the receptor. A TNF dimer could be expected to bind a single receptor monomer. And a TNF trimer (the predominant form of TNF in solution) may be expected to bind three receptor monomers, holding them tightly together.

TNF is now known to elicit a biological response by crosslinking three receptor monomers on the cell surface. A TNF-like effect can therefore be elicited by other agents that are capable of crosslinking the receptor (e.g. anti-receptor antibodies) [61]. Interestingly, although the TNF trimer must bind to a cell membrane containing a mixture of 55 kD and 75 kD receptors, the interaction is exclusionary: it appears that only three of the smaller receptor type, or three of the larger receptor type molecules will ordinarily engage a single trimer. Mixed hexamers do not occur, or occur very infrequently.

The nature of the signal elicited following receptor crosslinking is still very poorly understood. Neither receptor has a cytoplasmic domain suggestive of kinase activity. It has been suggested that G proteins couple the response to TNF in endothelial cells [62], although similar evidence has not accrued to implicate G proteins in other tissues or cell types. The cytolytic response to TNF seems to be mediated by a discrete collection of amino-acids located within the cytoplasmic domain of the 55 kD molecule.

The earliest effect of TNF that has been linked to biological responses, including the induction of other genes, is the activation of NF-κB [57]. This presumably occurs via modification of the cytoplasmic inhibitor of NF-κB, i.e. IκB. As noted below, NF-κB stimulates transcription of the TNF gene itself in cells that produce TNF, and as such, TNF may induce its own synthesis in some systems. Activation of NF-κB presumably involves a kinase cascade, but the details of the process are not clear. NF-κB activation may also occur in response to oxidative stress, though again, the proximal molecules that sense oxidants are unclear. It has been claimed, that TNF constitutes a form of oxidative stress on cells [63], and that antioxidants such as N-acetylcysteine interrupt cell killing by TNF. The importance of this signaling mechanism is currently being investigated.

Several proteins seem to interrupt the cytolytic action of TNF. These include the major heat shock protein (Hsp-70) (Jäättelä M., personal communication), manganous superoxide dismutase (MnSOD) [64], and plasminogen activator inhibitor (PAI-2) [65]. Such findings seem to imply a multifactorial mechanism in cell killing by TNF. Hsp are known to assist in the refolding of denatured proteins, and perhaps act as intracellular protein carriers as well. MnSOD may protect cells against oxidative damage. PAI-2 most probably guards against proteolysis within the cytosol just as it does outside the cell. However, the importance of these proteins in non-cytolytic events has yet to be studied.

The TNF Receptor Family: Belated Recognition of New Cytokines

Once the TNF receptor cDNAs were cloned, it became apparent that several other proteins belonged to the same structural group, defined chiefly by a repeating cysteine-rich extracellular domain motif [57]. Among these was the receptor for nerve growth factor (NGF). NGF is a dimeric protein, and may, like TNF, trigger a biological response by causing receptor aggregation on the cell surface; however, this remains a matter of speculation. In addition, CD40, a membrane antigen of previously unknown function, was found to bear homology to the TNF receptor. The ligand of CD40 has recently been identified, and its cDNA cloned. Termed CD40L, this protein bears 28% homology to TNF-α, and thus, is no more structurally distant than TNF-β. It might properly be termed "TNF-γ"; however, it must be pointed out that the protein does not engage either of the two known TNF receptors, and unlike TNF-α and TNF-β, does not trigger biological responses that define TNF. Its role in the pathogenesis of shock, inflammation, and cachexia remains to be established.

The identification of the TNF receptor was carried out in parallel with the identification of another protein, termed the FAS antigen, which was recognized as the target of monoclonal antibodies that were isolated for their ability to cause apoptosis, the programed death of target cells [66]. Since TNF kills cells by an apoptotic process, it was believed for some time that the

FAS antigen and the TNF receptor might be identical to one another. However, when each of the cDNAs was cloned, it became apparent that FAS was homologous to, but distinct from, the 55 kD TNF receptor [67,68]. The FAS antigen, like the TNF receptors, exhibited cysteine-rich repeats in its extracellular domain. It also exhibits homology to the 55 kD receptor (but not the 75 kD receptor) on the cytoplasmic side: a conserved "box" of amino-acids is observed on comparison of the two sequences, and it is presumably this region that is critical for signaling leading to cytolysis. FAS does not engage TNF-α or TNF-β, and its natural ligand remains undiscovered, though the subject of intense investigation. It would seem likely that the ligand, when isolated, may indeed prove to mediate certain effects similar to those mediated by TNF.

Very recently, it emerged that a mouse mutation known as *Lpr*, which leads to lymphadenopathy and a lupus-like syndrome when expressed in homozygous form, represents a defect of the locus encoding FAS [69]. Mice homozygous for the classical *Lpr* mutation fails to express the FAS mRNA, although the exact nature of the mutation (i.e. a promoter mutation, or a mutation affecting splicing) remains to be established. A second mutation of the same locus leads to the formation of an inactive protein, and yields much the same phenotype.

These exciting findings raise many questions about the phenotype that would be produced if the TNF 55 kD receptor were ablated *in vivo*, not to mention the phenotype that would result from ablation of either or both of the TNF genes. As might be expected, a "knockout" of each of the genes involved, through homologous recombination techniques, is being attempted in many laboratories throughout the world.

Mutant Forms of TNF Exhibit Lower Toxicity In Vivo

The fact that human TNF is less toxic to mice than is mouse TNF, and the fact that human TNF fails to bind to the mouse TNF 75 kD receptor stimulated a reasoned search for mutations that might alter binding to the 75 kD receptor in humans. The surface residues on the TNF trimer that are required in interaction with both receptors have been well mapped [70]. Through substitution experiments, it was determined that mutations at residue 32 of the mature TNF trimer forbid interaction of human TNF with the human or mouse 75 kD TNF receptor without substantially altering interaction with 55 kD receptor [71].

The mutant form of TNF thus retains its full cytotoxic potential. Yet it is substantially less toxic to living animals than the unmodified counterpart. Such a mutein may offer a valuable means of treating neoplastic disease, given that the therapeutic index of such a molecule may be far higher than the native form of TNF. Moreover, the fact that a molecule that fails to bind the 75 kD receptor exhibits far lower toxicity to animals suggests that the 75 kD receptor, acting alone or in conjuction with the 55 kD receptor, provides signals critical for the development of shock.

The Tissue Origins of TNF and Other Cytokines

The lethal mediator of endotoxic shock must, of necessity, be hematopoietically derived [3]. That is not to say, that all of the TNF produced *in vivo*, nor all of any cytokine, need derive from cells of hematopoietic origin. In fact, it is increasingly clear that most cytokines, including TNF, are produced by extrahematopoietic cells, and that certain extrahematopoietic cells like macrophages, have the capacity to respond to endotoxin.

IL-1, for example, has been shown to be produced by keratinocytes [72-74], microglia [75], astrocytes [76], and endothelial cells [37,77], to name a few sources. Similarly, IL-6 is produced by cells of diverse origin. Although TNF was long believed to be produced principally by macrophages in response to LPS, and by T cells and B cells in response to other stimuli, it now appears that it also is produced by many other cells [76,78-84].

The identification of tissue sources of TNF and other cytokines in endotoxic states has been problematic. TNF synthesis is largely controlled at a translational level, as noted above. Therefore, TNF mRNA is detectable in the tissues of healthy individuals [85,86] and does not necessarily imply the production of TNF protein. The protein itself is efficiently secreted, at least from macrophages (Beutler, unpublished data) and therefore, is difficult to detect by immunocytochemical analysis. Moreover, once produced, TNF is rapidly consumed through interaction with its ubiquitous cell surface receptor [17]. Much of the TNF produced may act at short range, and may never gain access to the circulation.

These problems were recently addressed through the design of a reporter "minigene" that mimics the function of the authentic TNF gene. When introduced into the murine genome, this reporter transgene causes the synthesis of the enzyme chloramphenicol acetyltransferase (CAT) within cells which normally produce TNF. CAT, a bacterial enzyme, has no counterpart in mammalian cells under the conditions of assay used. It remains within the cytosol of the cells that synthesize it, is highly stable, and may be detected with great sensitivity. Thus, it serves as an ideal marker of TNF synthesis.

Transgenic mice bearing the CAT reporter express CAT activity only in the thymus prior to injection of LPS, reflecting the constitutive synthesis of TNF within this organ [87,88]. Following injection of LPS, CAT activity is expressed in the kidney, spleen, lung, uterus, falopian, tube pancreas, and heart of transgenic animals, suggesting that these tissues comprise the principal sources of TNF *in vivo* [89]. Somewhat surprisingly, the liver fails to produce CAT, despite its rich content of Kuppfer cells. In parallel studies, mice were injected with LPS, their organs were removed, and the production of TNF by various tissues was examined *in vitro*. The results essentially confirmed the observations made using the reporter transgene, although it was necessary to trypsinize the heart to obtain myocardial cell preparations, to isolate islets from the pancreas (which are responsible for the TNF produced by this organ), and to isolate renal glomeruli (which are the chief source of TNF within the kidney).

The fact that several of the organs that produce TNF are "target organs" in septic shock raises questions as to the role of circulating TNF in this disease. It is, on the one hand, possible that circulating TNF causes much of the damage in endotoxic shock. On the other hand, it may be that much of the injury that occurs results from local production of the protein, and its subsequent action at short range.

The transgenic approach to localization of cytokine synthesis has yet to be applied to other mediators, although it would potentially be useful in locating the sources of IL-1 synthesis, and the synthesis of interferon-γ. Ultimately, such reporters might be used to assess the production of various cytokines *in vivo* in various disease states, including authentic infectious diseases of mice.

Regulation of Cytokine Synthesis

The production of cytokines is controlled at more than one level, and different stimuli eventuate biosynthesis through different signaling pathways. In the first place, it must be presumed that the cytokine genes are permanently inactivated in many cell types, perhaps as a result of development processes. Thus, the respective genes are "available" for transcription in a limited subset of tissues. The tissue distribution of cytokine gene expression is probably influenced by this circumstance more than by any other.

Promoters of many cytokine genes contain putative binding sites for the transcription factor NF-κB, through phosphorylation of the cytosolic inhibitor IκB would seem to be a common feature of cell activation. At the same time, some degree of selectivity is exercised, since not all cytokines are elaborated in response to an inflammatory signal.

Transcriptional activation of cytokine biosynthesis is clearly not the entire story. Most cytokine mRNA molecules display a conserved UA-rich element within the 3'-untranslated region (UTR), which has been associated both with instability of the mRNA [90], and with translational inhibition [91]. The degree of instability, and still more, the degree of translational inhibition, appear to be governed by the state of the cell activation [92,93]. Thus, post-transcriptional regulation of cytokine genes may heavily influence the rate of protein synthesis.

The role of 3'-UTR sequence elements upon mRNA stability and translation has been most thoroughly studied in the case of the TNF gene, although certain generalizations have now been extended to the interferon-β gene as well. It has been shown, through the use of reporter constructs, that the TNF 3'-UTR strongly suppresses translation in resting macrophages, but is only weakly suppressive in LPS-activated macrophages [92]. Thus, based upon the presence of 3'-UTR sequences alone, greater than 200-fold induction is observed. This degree of induction is the most powerful yet reported at a translational level in mammalian systems. When the inducing effect of the TNF promoter is combined with the inducing effect of the 3'-UTR by incorporating both elements into a reporter construct, as much as 4.000-fold induction has been observed [94]. This finding supports the conclusion that the two elements function independently of one another, in order to allow the massive induction of the TNF gene that is witnessed at the protein level.

Inhibition of Cytokine Synthesis

As noted above, the pathway leading to initiation of TNF biosynthesis within macrophages is likely to be highly "branched". Such is the nature of most signaling pathways within cells. Reflecting this fact, it appears that there are several means of blocking cytokine synthesis within cells, at least when synthesis is initiated by contact with LPS (Fig. 2).

Glucocorticoid agonists are well known to protect experimental animals against the lethal effect of an LPS challenge. Their effect is entirely preemptive; if administered after LPS, they are virtually without effect. Thus, it is not surprising that they are of little or no use in clinical settings, wherein contact with the stimulus has occurred prior to the onset of therapy. Moreo-

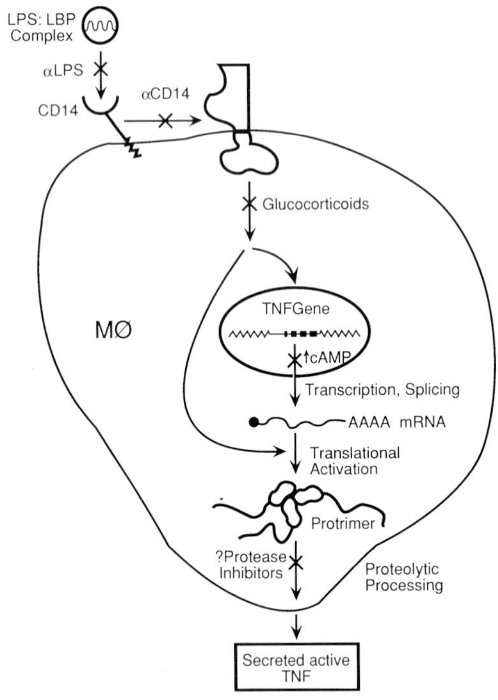

Fig. 2. Steps in activation of the biosynthesis and specific inhibition by pharmacologic agents. αLPS and αCD14 refer to antibodies against LPS and CD14, respectively

ver, they may actually hamper recovery from an authentic infection by virtue of their myriad effects on host immunity. However, the effect of glucocorticoids on cytokine synthesis in instructive, since it suggests that it is possible to interrupt signaling by LPS at a very early stage, perhaps at the level of the LPS "receptor" itself.

So much is clear from the fact that glucocorticoids block both transcription of the TNF gene and translation of the TNF mRNA [95]. Thus, both of the major limbs of the signaling pathway are affected. The pre-emptive nature of the glucocorticoid effect is evident at the cellular level, insofar as pretreatment of macrophages with dexamethasone blocks TNF biosynthesis, whereas treatment after induction by LPS is essentially without effect [95]. It would seem likely that glucocorticoids stimulate the production of inhibitors that impede LPS signaling, but are powerless to arrest activation once it is in progress.

A second class of agents which prevent TNF biosynthesis, and perhaps the biosynthesis of other cytokines as well, includes phosphodiesterase inhibitors and cyclic AMP (cAMP) analogues. It would appear that any agent that elevates intracellular cAMP concentration blocks TNF production. However, the mechanism of action of these agents differs from that of the glucocorticoids, in that it is strictly pretranslational. Pentoxifylline, for example, downregulates the expression of the TNF gene at a transcriptional level, and has no effect on the expression of reporter genes bearing the TNF 3'-UTR, which is essential in the regulation of TNF mRNA translation [96].

The combination of glucocorticoids and phosphordiesterase inhibitors is more effective in the prevention of TNF synthesis than either agent alone, both *in vivo* and *in vitro* [97]. While some phosphodiesterase inhibitors (e.g. theophylline and pentoxiphylline) are too toxic to administer in quantities sufficient to block TNF biosynthesis *in vivo*, others (e.g.amrinone) are not, and impact upon survival following endotoxin challenge, perhaps through a combination of effects.

Intervention after the Release of Cytokines

Undoubtedly, cytokines can cause much harm to the host, although equally, it is clear that they fulfill important physiological functions. It would seem worthwhile to block cytokine release under selected conditions; however, it is also to be expected that some degree of immunocompromise might result from such maneuvers, as certain micro-organisms have been shown to be more highly lethal in animals treated with antibodies against cytokines; for example, mice in a state of TNF "blockade" are more susceptible to the lethal effect of *Listeria* organisms [98], malarial parasites [99], and mycobacteria [100]. A central paradox of shock, however, is that while techniques of antimicrobial therapy have become relatively advanced, the incidence of a lethal outcome in sepsis has changed but little. It is to be hoped that inhibition of cytokine synthesis and action, accomplished under the cover of chemotherapeutic agents, might improve this situation.

Both monoclonal and polyclonal antibodies against TNF, IL-1, and other cytokines have long been available, and are capable of effectively neutralizing the activity of these proteins. They have shown encouraging results when used in animal studies [25,26]. Combinations of antibodies against several cytokines have not yet been explored as a treatment modality in shock; it would seem probable that at some point, virtually complete protection might be achieved.

Because of their inherent immunogenicity, anti-cytokine antibodies are less than ideal for use in human subjects. The use of natural and/or synthetic inhibitors of cytokine action may circumvent this problem.

A natural inhibitor of IL-1 (the IL-1 receptor antagonist IL-1ra) is found in the plasma of LPS-treated animals [42,43], and may partially mitigate the actions of IL-2. The antagonist bears considerable sequence homology to IL-1α and IL-1β, and shares the IL-1 receptors occupied by the latter ligands, but, so far as is presently known, elicits no agonist response [44]. High doses of IL-1ra have been shown to protect rabbits against the lethal effects of LPS [101].

Recently, the TNF receptor extracellular domain has been spliced to the IgG heavy chain in order to generate bivalent TNF ligands that neutralize cytokine activity [102]. This soluble version of the TNF receptor, exhibits remarkably high affinity for TNF, should prove to be nearly non-antigenic, and is known to be quite stable *in vivo* [102]. Similar chimeric receptors have been used to inhibit interferon-γ, IL-1, and perhaps other cytokines. Since they are easy to produce through a variety of expression systems, they offer the hope that a "cocktail" of cytokine inhibitors might one day be used to block the toxic effects of cytokines as required in certain clinical situations.

Conclusions: The Future

As briefly discussed above, the details of signaling pathways activated by LPS are very sketchy. Undoubtly, the most critical element within the signaling pathway, and perhaps the first element of the pathway, is the protein encoded by the *Lps* gene. An attempt to clone this gene is underway in several laboratories. The potential reward of achieving this is very great: it is tantalizing to consider that a single selective antagonist of the *Lps* gene product might render a human temporarily refractory to *Lps*, even as unresponsive as the C3H/HeJ mouse. Yet such an agent might prove to be devoid of the long-term immunosuppressive consequences characteristic of glucocorticoid hormones. At a larger level, many questions about shock, and the overall response to LPS remain to be answered. Why does a pathway for response exist at all ? And why are humans uniquely susceptible to LPS, whereas subhuman primates are highly resistant ? The answer to these questions may tell us a great deal about the immune system as a whole.

References

1. Watson J, Kelly K, Largen M, Taylor BA (1978) The genetic mapping of a defective LPS response gene in C3H/HeJ mice. J Immunol 120:422–424
2. Sultzer BM (1968) Genetic control of leucocyte responses to endotoxin. Nature 219:1253–1254
3. Michalek SM, Moore RN, McGhee JR, Rosenstreich DL, Mergenhagen SE (1980) The primary role of lymphoreticular cells in the mediation of host responses to bacterial endotoxin. J Inf Dis 141:55–63
4. Morrison DC, Ryan JL (1979) Bacterial endotoxins and host immune responses. Adv Immunol 28:293–450
5. Morrison DC, Ulevitch RJ (1978) The effects of bacterial endotoxins on host mediation systems. Am J Pathol 93:526–617
6. Kawakami M, Cerami A (1981) Studies of endotoxin-induced decrease in lipoprotein lipase activity. J Exp Med 154:631–639
7. O'Malley WE, Achinstein B, Shear MJ (1962) Action of bacterial polysaccharide on tumors. II. Damage of sarcoma 37 by serum of mice treated with Serratia marcescens polysaccharide, and induced tolerance. J Natl Canc Inst 29:1169–1175
8. Carswell EA, Old LJ, Kassel RL, Green S, Fiore N, Williamson B (1975) An endotoxin-induced serum factor that causes necrosis of tumors. Proc Natl Acad Sci 72:3666–3670
9. Coley WB (1893) The treatment of malignant tumors by repeated inoculations of erysipelas; with a report of ten original cases. Am J Med Sci 105:487–511
10. Coley WB (1894) Treatment of inoperable malignant tumors with toxins of erysipelas and the Bacillus prodigiosus. Trans Am Surg Assoc 12:183–212
11. Coley WB (1896) The therapeutic value of the mixed toxins of the streptococcus of erysipelas in the treatment of inoperable malignant tumors, with a report of 100 cases. Am J Med Sci 112:251–281
12. Coley WB (1896) Further observations upon the treatment of malignant tumors with the mixed toxins of erysipelas and Bacillus prodigiosus with a report of 160 cases. Bull Johns Hopkins Hosp 65:157–162
13. Coley WB (1906) Late results of the treatment of inoperable sarcoma by the mixed toxins of erysipelas and Bacillus prodigiosus. Am J Med Sci 131:375-430
14. Mannel DN, Moore RN, Mergenhagen SE (1980) Marcophages as a source of tumoricidal activity (tumor-necrotizing factor). Inf Immun 30:523–530
15. Ruff MR, Gifford GE (1981) Rabbit tumor necrosis factor: Mechanism of action. Inf Immun 31:380–385
16. Mannel DN, Meltzer MS, Mergenhagen SE (1980) Generation and characterization of a lipopolysaccharide-induced and serum-derived cytotoxic factor for tumor cells. Inf Immun 28:204–211
17. Beutler B, Milsark IW, Cerami A (1985) Cachectin/tumor necrosis factor: Production, destribution, and metabolic fate in vivo. J Immunol 135:3972–3977
18. Michie HR, Manogue KR, Spriggs DR, et al. (1988) Detection of circulating tumor necrosis factor after endotoxin administration. N Engl J Med 318:1481–1486
19. Haranaka K, Satomi N, Sakurai A, Haranaka R (1984) Role of first stimulating agents in the production of tumor necrosis factor. Canc Immunol Immunother 18:87–90
20. Green S, Dobrjansky A, Chiasson MA, Carswell E, Schwartz MK, Old LJ (1977) Corynebacterium parvum as the priming in the production of tumor necrosis factor in the mouse. J Natl Canc Inst 59:1519–1522
21. Ha DK, Gardner ID, Lawton JW (1983) Characterization of marcophage function in Mycobacterium lepraemurium-infected mice: Sensitivity of mice to endotoxin and release of mediators and lysosomal enzymes after the endotoxin treatment. Parasite Immunol 5:513–526
22. Galanos C, Freudenberg MA, Reutter W (1979) Galactosamine-induced sensitization to the lethal effects of endotoxin. Pro Natl Acad Sci 76:5939–5943
23. Lehmann V, Freudenberg MA, Galanos C (1987) Lethal toxicity of lipopolysaccharide and tumor necrosis factor in normal and d-galactosamine-treated mice. J Exp Med 165:657–663

24. Tracey KJ, Beutler B, Lowry SF,ct al. (1986) Shock and tissue injury induced by recombinant human cachectin. Science 234:470–474
25. Beutler B, Milsark IW, Cerami A (1985) Passive immunization against cachectin/tumor necrosis factor (TNF) protects mice from the lethal effect of endotoxin. Science 229:869–871
26. Tracey KJ, Fong Y, Hesse DG, et al. (1987) Anti-cachectin/TNF monoclonal antibodies prevent septic shock during lethal bacteraemia. Nature 330:662–666
27. Mathison JC, Wolfson E, Ulevitch RJ (1988) Participation of tumor necrosis factor in the mediation of gram-negative bacterial lipopolysaccharide-induced injury in rabbits. J Clin Invest 81:1925–1937
28. Waage A, Halstensen A, Espevik T (1987) Association between tumor necrosis factor in serum and fatal outcome in patients with meningococcal disease. Lancet 1:355–357
29. Gamble JR, Harlan JM, Klebanoff SJ, Lopez AF, Vadas Ma (1985) Stimulation of the adherence of neutrophils to umbilicial vein endothelium by human recombinant tumor necrosis factor . Proc Natl Acad Sci 82:8667–8671
30. Shalaby MR, Aggarwal BB, Rinderknecht E, Svedersky LP, Finkle BS, Palladino MAJr (1985) Activation of human polymorphonuclear neutrophil functions by interferon-gamma and tumor necrosis factors. J Immunol 135:2069–2073
31. Klebanoff SJ, Vadas MA, Harlan JM, et al. (1986) Stimulation of neutrophils by tumor necrosis factor . J Immunol 136: 4220-4225
32. Tsujimoto M, Yokota S, Vilcek J, Weissmann G (1986) Tumor necrosis factor provokes superoxide anion generation from neutrophils. Biochem Biophys Res Commun137:1094–1100
33. Gamble JR, Smith WB, Vadas MA (1992) TNF modulation of endothelial and neutrophil adhesion . In: Beutler B (ed) Tumor necrosis factors: The molecules and their emerging role in medicine. Raven Press, New York, NY, pp 65-86
34. Bevilacqua MP, Pober JS, Majeau GR, Fiers W, Cotran RS, Gimbrone MA Jr (1986) Recombinant tumor necrosis factor induces procoagulant activity in cultured human vascular endothelium: Characterization and comparison with the actions of interleukin. 1. Proc Natl Acad Sci 83:4533–4537
35. Collins T, Lapierre LA, Fiers W, Strominger JL, Pober JS (1986) Recombinant human tumor necrosis factor increases mRNA levels and surface expression of HLA-A,B antigens in vascular endothelial cells and dermal fibroblasts *in vitro*. Proc Natl Acad Sci 83:446–460
36. Libby P, Ordovas JM, Auger KR, Robbins AH, Birinyi LK, Dinarello CA (1986) Endotoxin and tumor necrosis factor induce interleukin-1 gene expression in adult human vascular endothelial cells. Am J Pathol 124:179–185
37. Nawroth P, Bank I, Handley D, Cassimeris J, Chess L, Stern D (1986) Tumor necrosis factor/cachectin interacts with endothelial cell receptors to induce release of interleukin 1.J Exp Med 163:1363–1375
38. Pober JS, Gimbrone MA Jr, Lapierre LA, et al. (1986) Overlapping patterns of activation of human endothelial cells by interleukin 1, tumor necrosis factor, and immune interferon. J Immunol 127:1893–1896
39. Pober JS, Bevilacqua MP, Mendrick DL, Lapierre LA, Fiers W, Gimbrone MA Jr (1986) Two distinct monokines, interleukin 1 and tumor necrosis factor, each independently induce biosynthesis and transient expression of the same antigen on the surface of cultured human vascular endothelial cells. J Immunol 136:1680–1687
40. Pohlman TH, Stanness KA, Beatty PG, Ochs HD, Harlan JM (1986) An endothelial cell surface factor(s) induced *in vitro* by lipopolysaccharide, interleukin-1, and tumor necrosis factor-α increases neurtophil adherence by a CDw18-dependent mechanism. J Immunol 136:4548–4553
41. Fong Y, Tracey KJ, Moldawer LL, et al. (1989) Antibodies to cachectin/tumor necrosis factor reduce interleukin 1β and interleukin 6 appearance during lethal bacteremia. J Exp Med 170:1627–1633
42. Eisenberg SP, Evans RJ, Arend WP, et al. (1990) Primary structure and functional expression from complementary DNA of a human interleukin-1 receptor antagonist. Nature 343:341–346
43. Hammun CH, Wilcox CJ, Arend WP, et al. (1990) Interleukin-1 receptor antagonist activity of a human interleukin-1 inhibitor. Nature 343:336–340

44. Dinarello CA, Thompson RC (1991) Blocking IL-1: Interleukin 1 receptor antagonist *in vivo* and *in vitro.* Immunol Today 12:404–409
45. Broxmeyer HE, Williams DE, Lu L, et al. (1986) The suppressive influence of human tumor necrosis factors on bone marrow hematopoietic progenitor cells from normal donors and patients with leukemia: Synergism of tumor necrosis factor and interferon-γ. J Immunol 136:4487–4495
46. Sone S, Lopez-Berestein G, Fidler IJ (1986) Potentiation of direct antitumor cytotoxicity and production of tumor cytolytic factors in human blood monocytes by human recombinant interferon-γ and muramyl dipeptide derivatives. Canc Immunol Immunother 21:93–99
47. Tsujimoto M, Feinman R, Vilcek J (1986) Differential effects of type I IFN and IFN-γ on the binding of tumor necrosis factor to receptors in two human cell lines. J Immunol 137:2272–2276
48. Esparza I, Mannel D, Ruppel A, Falk W, Krammer PH (1987) Interferon-γ (IFN-γ) and lymphotoxin (LT) or tumor necrosis factor (TNF) synergize to activate macrophages for tumoricidal and schistosomulicidal functions. Lymphokine Res (Abs) 6:1715
49. Tribble H, Schneider M, Bowersox O, Talmadge JE (1987) Combination immunotherapy with RH TNF and RM IFN G: Increased therapy and toxicity. Fed Proc (Abs) 46:561
50. Agah R, Malloy B, Sherrod A, Mazumder A (1988) Successful therapy of natural killer-resistant pulmonary metastases by the synergism of γ-interferon with tumor necrosis factor and interleukin-2 in mice. Cancer Res 48:2245–2248
51. Chapekar MS, Glazer RI (1988) The synergistic cytocidal effect produced by immune interferon and tumor necrosis factor in HT-29 cells in associated with inhibition of rRNA processing and (2', 5') oligo (A) activation of RNase L. Biochem Biophy Res Comm 151:1180–1187
52. Bonavida B, Jewett A (1989) Activation of human peripheral blood-derived monocytes by OK-432 (Strecptococcus pyogenes): Augmented cytotoxicity and secretion of TNF and synergy with rIFN-γ. Cell Immunol 123:373–383
53. Barker JNWN, Sarma V, Mitra RS, Dixit VM, Nickoloff BJ (1990) Marked synergism between tumor necrosis factor-α and interferon-γ in regulation of keratinocyte-derived adhesion molecules and chemotactic factors. J Clin Invest 83:605–608
54. Beresini MH, Sugarman BJ, Shepard HM, Epstein LB (1990) Synergistic induction of polypeptides by tumor necrosis factor and interferon-γ in cells sensitive or resistant to tumor necrosis factor: Assessment by computer based analysis of two-dimensional gels using the PDQUEST system. Electrophoresis 11:232–241
55. Kumaratilake LM, Ferrante A, Bates EJ, Kowanko IC (1990) Augmentation of the human monocyte/macrophage chemiluminescence response during short-term exposure to interferon-γ and tumor necrosis factor-α. Clin Exp Immunol 80:257–262
56. Matsuura M, Galanos C (1990) Induction of hypersensivitiy to endotoxin and tumor necrosis factor by sublethal infection with *Salmonella typhimurium.* Infect Immun 58:935–937
57. Pfitzenmaier K, Himmler A, Schutze S, Scheurich P, Kronke M (1992) TNF receptors and TNF signal transduction. In: Beutler B (ed) Tumor necrosis factors: The molecules and their emerging role in medicine. Raven Press, New York, pp 439–472
58. Pennica D, Nedwin GE, Hayflick JS, et al. (1984) Human tumor necrosis factor: Precursor structure, expression and homology to lymphotoxin. Nature 312:724–729
59. Marsters SA, Frutkin AD, Simpson NJ, Fendly BM, Ashkenazi A (1992) Identification of cysteine-rich domains of the type 1 tumor necrosis factor receptor involved in ligand binding. J Biol Chem 267:5747–5750
60. Eck MJ, Sprang SR (1989) The structure of tumor necrosis factor-α at 2.6A resolution: Implications for receptor binding. J Biol Chem 264:17595–17605
61. Engelmann H, Holtmann H, Brakebusch C, et al. (1990) Antibodies to a soluble form of a tumor necrosis factor (TNF) receptor have TNF-like activity. J Biol Chem 265:14497–14504
62. Brett J, Gerlach H, Nawroth P, Steinberg S, Godman S, Stern D (1989) Tumor necrosis factor/cachectin increases permeability of endothelial cell monolayers by a mechanism involving regulatory G proteins. J Exp Med 169:1977–1991
63. Roederer M, Staal FJT, Raju PA, Ela SW, Herzenberg LA (1990) Cytokine-stimulated human immunodeficiency virus replication is inhibited by N-acetyl-L-cysteine. Proc Natl Acad Sci USA 87:4884–4888

64. Wong GHW, Elwell JH, Oberley LW, Goeddel DV (1989) Manganous superoxide dismutase is essential for cellular resistance to cytotoxicity of tumor necrosis factor. Cell 58:923–931
65. Baglioni C (1992) Mechanisms of cytotoxicity, cytolysis, and growth stimulation by TNF. In: Beutler (ed) Tumor necrosis factors: The molecules and their emerging role in medicine. Raven Press, New York, pp 425–472
66. Yonehara S, Ishii A, Yonehara M (1989) A cell-killing monoclonal antibody (anti-Fas) to a cell surface antigen co-down-regulated with the receptor of tumor necrosis factor. J Exp Med 169:1747–1756
67. Itoh N, Yonehara S, Ishii A, et al. (1991) The polypeptide encoded by the cDNA for human cell surface antigen Fas can mediate apoptosis. Cell 66:233–243
68. Watanabe-Fukunaga R, Brannan CI, Itoh N, et al. (1992) The cDNA structure, expression, and chromosomal assignment of the mouse Fas antigen. J Immunol 148:1274–1279
69. Watanabe-Fukunaga R, Brannan CI, Copeland NG, Jenkins NA, Nagata S (1992) Lymphoproliferation disorder in mice explained by defects in Fas antigen that mediates apoptosis. Nature 356:314–317
70. Sprang SR, Eck MJ (1992) The 3-D Structure of TNF: In Beutler B (ed) Tumor necrosis factors: The molecules and their emerging role in medicine. Raven Press, New York, pp 11-32
71. Van Ostade X, Vandenabeele P, Everaerdt B, et al. (1992) Human TNF mutants with reduced binding to the TNF-R75. Eur Cyto Net (Abs.) 3:137–137
72. Dente L, Ciliberto G, Cortese R (1985) Structure of the human α-1-acid glycoprotein gene: Sequence homology with other human acute phase protein genes. Nucleic Acids Res 13:3941–3952
73. Sauder DN (1984) Epidermal cytokines: Properties of epidermal cell thymocyte-activating factor (ETAF). Lymphokine Res 3:145–151
74. Kupper TS, Ballard DW, Chua AO, et al. (1986) Human keratinocytes contain mRNA indistinguishable from monocyte interleukin 1α and β mRNA. J Exp Med 164:2095–2100
75. Giulian D, Baker TJ, Shih LN, Lachman LB (1986) Interleukin-1 of the central nervous system is produced by ameboid microglia. J Exp Med 164:594–604
76. Chung IY, Benveniste EN (1990) Tumor necrosis factor-α production by astrocytes: Induction by lipopolyaccharide, IFN-γ, and IL-1β. J Immunol 144:2999–3007
77. Poubelle PE, Grassi J, Pradelles P, Marceau F (1990) Pharmacological modulation of interleukin 1 production by cultured endothelial cells from human umbilical veins. Immunopharmacology 19:121–130
78. Spriggs DR, Imamura K, Rodriguez C, Sariban E, Kufe DW (1988) Tumor necrosis factor expression in human epithelial tumor cell lines. J Clin Invest 81:455–460
79. Hsu P-L, Hsu S-M (1989) Production of tumor necrosis factor-α and lymphotoxin by cells of Hodgkin's neoplastic cell lines HDLM-1 and KM-H2. Am J Pathol 135:735–745
80. Gowen M, Chapman K, Littlewood A, Hughes D, Evans D, Russell G (1990) Production of tumor necrosis factor by human osteoblasts is modulated by other cytokines, but not by osteotropic hormones. Endocrinology 126:1250–1255
81. Ohno I, Tanno Y, Yamauchi K, Takishima T (1990) Gene expression and production of tumor necrosis factor by a rat basophilic leukaemia cell line (RBL-2H3) with IgE receptor triggering. Immunology 70:88–93
82. Ohno I, Tanno Y, Yamauchi K, Takishima T (1990) Production of tumor necrosis factor by mastocytoma P815 cells. Immunology 69:312–315
83. Zolti M, Meirom R, Shemesh M, Wollach D, Mashiach S, Shore L, Rafael ZB (1990) Granulosa cells are a source and target organ for tumor necrosis factor-α. FEBS Lett 261:253–255
84. Jaattela M, Kuusela P, Saksela E (1988) Demonstration of tumor necrosis factor in human amniotic fluids and supernatants of placental and decidual tissues. Lab Invest 58:48–52
85. Tovey MG, Content J, Gresser I, et al. (1988) Genes for IFN-β-2 (IL-6), tumor necrosis factor, and IL-1 are expressed at high levels in the organs of normal individuals. J Immunol 141:3106–3110
86. Ulich TR, Guo K, Castillo JD (1989) Endotoxin-induced cytokine gene expression in vivo. I. Expression of tumor necrosis factor mRNA in visceral organs under physiologic conditions and during endotoxemia. Am J Pathol 134:11–14

87. Kossodo S, Giroir B, Brown T, Pointaire P, Grau G, Beutler B (1991) Constitutive expression of cachectin/TNF in the thymus: Fulfillment of an essential developmental function. Clinical Res (Abs) 39:250A
88. Giroir BP, Brown T, Beutler B (1992) Constitutive synthesis of tumor necrosis factor in the thymus. Proc Natl Acad Sci (In Press)
89. Giroir BP, Johnson JH, Brown T, Allen GL, BeutlerB (1992) The tissue distribution of TNF biosynthesis during endotoxemia. J Clin Invest (In Press)
90. Shaw G, Kamen R (1986) A conserved AU sequence from the 3' untranslated region of GM-CSF mRNA mediates selective mRNA degradation. Cell 46:659–667
91. Kruys V, Marinx O, Shaw G, Deschamps J, Huez G (1989) Translational blockade imposed by cytokine-derived UA-rich sequences. Science 245:852–855
92. Han J, Brown T, Beutler B (1990) Endotoxin-responsive sequences control cachectin/TNF biosynthesis at the translational level. J Exp Med 171:465–475
93. Han J, Beutler B (1990) The essential role of the UA-rich sequence in endotoxin-induced cachectin/TNF synthesis. Eur Cyto Net 1:71–75
94. Beutler B, Brown T (1991) A CAT reporter construct allows ultrasensitive estimation of TNF synthesis, and suggests that the TNF gene has been silenced in non-macrophage cell lines. J Clin Invest 87:1336–1344
95. Beutler B, Krochin N, Milsark IW, Luedke C, Cerami A (1986) Control of cachectin (tumor necrosis factor) synthesis: Mechanisms of endotoxin resistance. Science 232:977–980
96. Han J, Thompson P, Beutler B (1990) Dexamethasone and pentoxifylline inhibit endotoxin-induced cachectin/TNF synthesis at separate points in the signaling pathway. J Exp Med 172:391–394
97. Giroir BP, Beutler B (1992) Effect of amrinone on tumor necrosis factor production in endotoxic shock. Circulatory Shock 36:200–207
98. Havell EA (1989) Evidence that tumor necrosis factor has an important role in antibacterial resistance. J Immunol 143:2894–2899
99. Grau GE, Fajardo LF, Piguet PF, Allet B, Lambert PH, Vassalli P (1987) Tumor necrosis factor (cachectin) as an essential mediator in murine cerebral malaria. Science 237:1210–1212
100. Kindler V, Sappino AP, Grau GE, Piguet PF, Vassalli P (1989) The inducing role of tumor necrosis factor in the development of bacterial granulomas during BCG infection. Cell 56:731–740
101. Ohlsson K, Bjork P, Bergenfeldt M, Hageman R, Thompson RC (1990) Interleukin-1 receptor antagonist reduces mortality from endotoxin shock. Nature 348:550–552
102. Peppel K, Crawford D, Beutler B (1991) A tumor necrosis factor (TNF) receptor-IgG heavy chain chimeric protein as a bivalent antagonist of TNF activity. J Exp Med 174:1483–1489

TNFα and Soluble TNF Receptors in Meningococcemia

E. Girardin

Introduction

In septic shock, most of the damage does not come from the invading pathogen but from the host reaction to it. A large variety of humoral mediators were implicated in endotoxemia associated pathology. Two main lines of evidence indicate that TNFα is a key mediator. First, the injection of recombinant human TNFα can by itself induce pathological changes of shock [1-6]. Second, the administration of neutralizing anti-TNF antibodies prevents these changes [7-10].

High circulating TNFα levels were indeed found after experimental injection of endotoxin in human [6]. The importance of TNFα in the etiopathology of septic shock in man was supported by numerous reports of high TNFα circulating concentrations in septic conditions [11-15]. In these studies, the circulating amount of TNFα correlated with the clinical outcome.

Apart from the situation where overproductions of TNFα contributes to the mortality and morbidity of diseases, TNFα exerts beneficial effects in numerous situations. It is an important mediator of inflammation participating to intercellular communication in normal or diseased tissue. It was found to be protective in some animal infectious models: *Legionella pneumophila* [16], *Salmonella* [17] and *Listeria monocytogenes* [18,19].

Because of this duality of action, it is of crucial importance to understand the mechanisms which control TNFα either at the level of production or at the level of biological activity. Recently, the importance of natural TNFα inhibitors in modulating the biological response of TNFα has been stressed.

TNF Binding Proteins

TNFα inhibitory activities have been found in urine of febrile patients [20]. Purification to homogeneity of this inhibitory material revealed a protein with a novel amino-acid sequence [21-23]. The inhibitory protein reversed completely the cytotoxicity of TNFα on TNF-susceptible cell lines but affected to a lesser extent the cytotoxicity of TNFβ, a closely related protein to TNFα. This specificity was confirmed by the absence of inhibition of IL-1β and IL-1α biological activities [21]. A direct specific binding of the inhibitory protein to TNFα and, to a lesser extent, to TNFβ was found [24]. No binding was observed with IL-1 or interferon γ.

With a different method of purification, the inhibitory material resolved into two active components: the TNF binding protein I (TBPI) which is similar to the one previously discussed, and the TNF binding protein II (TBPII) which differs from TBPI by the lack of immunological cross-reactivity and different NH_2-terminal amino-acid sequences [25,26].

TNF Receptors

In the past few years, several groups have identified cell surface receptors for TNF in a variety of cells and cell lines.

Two distinct TNF receptor molecules were identified which differ in molecular mass, in ligand binding affinity, immunoreactivity and proteolytic fingerprints [27,28]. Monoclonal antibodies raised against these TNF receptor fractions confirmed the existence of two distinct receptors. No immunological cross-reactivity was observed between these anti-TNF-receptor antibodies. In western blot and immunoprecipitation analysis, they recognized proteins of molecular mass of about 75 KD and 55 KD. Altogether, these studies indicated that two immunologically distinct TNF receptors were expressed to varying degrees in the different cell types. These receptors were termed TNF receptor I (TNF-RI) with a molecular mass of 55 KD and TNF receptor II (TNF-RII) with a molecular mass of 75 KD [22,29-33].

The cyclic DNA encoding human TNF-RI [29] and TNF-RII [30,34) have been then isolated. The predicted structure of the two receptors showed an intracellular domain, a transmembrane protein and an extracellular domain. The extracellular regions of the two receptors display sequence similarities. In contrast, the intracellular regions of TNF-RI and TNF-RII are entirely unrelated [34]. This difference in structure may indicate that TNF-RI and TNF-RII may transmit a signal for distinct cellular functions [35].

The proteolytic cleavage of the two TNF receptor molecules resulted in two soluble fragments which represent part of the extracellular domain of the receptors. A stricking homology was found between TBPI, TBPII and the extracellular domain of TNF-RI and TNF-RII, respectively. This finding was based on amino-acid sequence identity and immunological cross-reactivity with polyclonal and monoclonal antibodies [26,28,36-38]. These data lead to the concept of an extracellular domain of TNF-RI and TNF-RII having inhibitory properties against TNFα.

TNFα in Meningococcemia

Severe infectious purpura has a high mortality rate despite antibiotic treatment and improvement in intensive care therapy. This syndrome is most frequently due to *Neisseria meningitidis,* and occasionally to *Haemophilus influenzae.* Most of the relevant manifestations of meningococcemia are thought to be induced by endotoxin of gram-negative bacteria as circulating endotoxin concentrations were shown to correlate with the development of multiple organ failure and death [39,40]. Clinical and biological risk factors have been described for the identification of children with meningococcal sepsis who have a high probability of lethal outcome [41-43]. It is then particularly interesting to study the profile of TNFα production in this desease.

In 1987, an association between serum TNFα concentrations and outcome was found in patients with meningococcal disease [44]. In this study, TNFα levels were measured by bioassay in patients with bacteriologically or serologically proved meningococcal disease.

Seventy nine patients were included, only 2 of them being less than 10 years old. Twenty six patients had meningitis without septicemia or shock. Forty two patients had septicemia, 12 of them being in shock without cell reaction in the CSF, a group known to be at high risk for death. TNFα was detected in 10 patients out of the 11 who died, and in 8 patients out of the 68 who survived. In another study, TNFα circulating concentrations were measured in a group of children with severe infectious purpura [45]. Since this initial report, other children have been included and the data presented here are for the whole group of patients. 73 children with a clinical diagnosis of sepsis with purpuric lesions were enrolled if they were in shock or if they had 3 or more of the following biochemial abnormalities known to be biological risk factors for a lethal outcome: a blood leukocytes count below 10 x 10^9/1, a blood platelet count below 100 x 10^9/1, a fibrinogen level below 1.5 g/1, a serum carbon dioxide level under 15 mmol/1, and a cerebrospinal fluid cell count under 0.1 x 10^9/1. TNFα were assayed with competitive inhibition radio immunoassay. The mean age of the patients was 4 years 4 months. The mean time between the onset of the disease and the TNFα determinations was 7 ± 6 hours. TNFα serum levels correlated with the number of risk factors present on admission and with the mortality of the disease. In these patients, low levels of fibrinogen were highly correlated with poor outcome. A negative correlation was found between fibrinogen levels and TNFα concentrations suggesting a relation between TNFα production and the severity of disseminated intravascular coagulation. When patients were

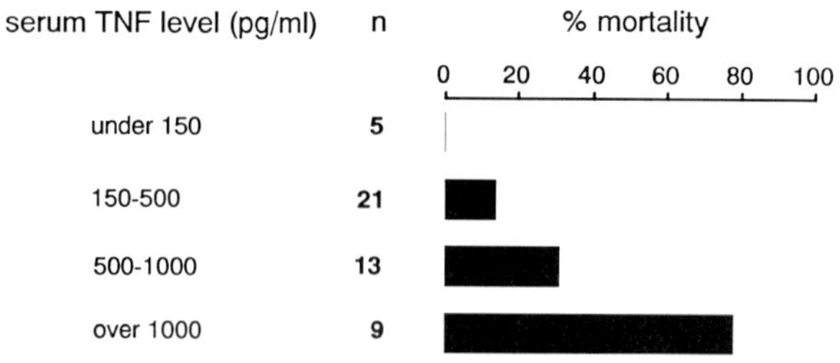

Fig. 1. Correlation between mortality and serum levels of TNFα on admission.

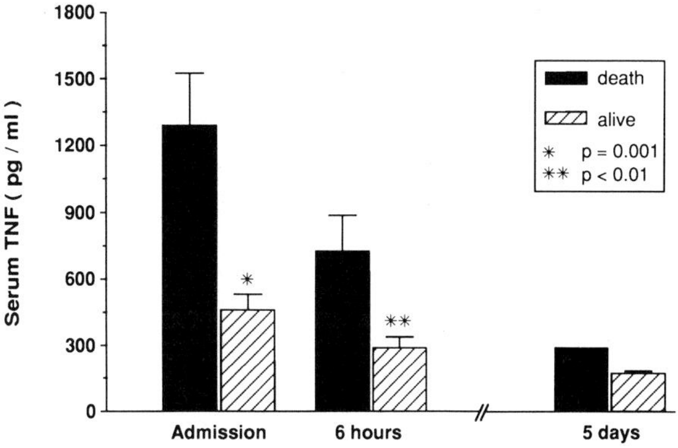

Fig. 2. Evolution of TNFα serum concentrations analyzed according to the outcome. After 6 h, the TNF levels decrease approximatively by half in both groups. At this time, the concentrations remain significantly higher in the group of patients with poor outcome.

divided according to their serum TNFα levels found on admission, the percentage of mortality was directly related to the TNFα concentrations (Fig. 1). In these patients, serum TNFα were studied after 6 h and 5 days of evolution (Fig. 2). TNFα concentrations decreased by half during the first 6 h, both in survivors and in patients with a poor outcome. The intervals between the onset of the disease and the first cytokine determinations were short, indicating that the peak concentrations of TNFα occurred at the very beginning of the disease. Altogether, these data are consistent with the implication of TNFα in the pathogenesis of severe infectious purpura. Other circulating cytokines were measured in high quantity in the serum of patients with meningococcal disease. IL-6 levels were higher in patients with lethal outcome [46,47]. A correlation between TNFα and the logarithm of IL-6 serum concentrations was found at the beginning of the disease and after 6 h [47]. This relation and the time interval between the release of TNFα and IL-6 in meningococcemia [46] are compatible with a release of IL-6 induced by TNFα [48,49]. IL-1 [45,46] and interferon γ [45] were exclusively detected in serum of patients who had high TNFα levels, severe disease and poor outcome. Thus in severe meningococcemia, TNFα is not the only circulatory cytokine detected in response to the endotoxin. One can speculate that IL-1 and interferon γ participate to the overproduction of TNFα by upregulating the response of macrophages to endotoxin in the most severe cases.

Soluble TNF Receptors in Meningococcemia

The two receptor fragments TNF-RI and TNF-RII can be detected in biological fluids by enzyme-linked immunological binding assay. Their profiles in different clinical conditions are currently investigated. In cancer patients, serum levels on TNF-RI and TNF-RII were increased and correlated with the staging of solid malignant tumors [50]. In children with severe meningococcemia, the receptor serum concentrations were measured on admission at the hospital and after 6 h of evolution. High circulating amounts of TNF-RI and TNF-RII were found: 29.9 pg/ml for TNF-RI, and 76 pg/ml for TNF-RII [51]. Normal values in our laboratory are 2.2 pg/ml for TNF-RI, and 0.8 pg/ml for TNF-RII. When the serum circulating IL-6 levels, the TNFα and the TNF receptor concentrations were analyzed according to the outcome, the two cytokines and the TNF receptors I and II concentrations were significantly higher in the group of deceased patients than in the group of surviving patients (Table 1). Considering the inhibitory effects of the two receptors, we wondered whether the ratio of TNFα over TNF receptors would be a better indicator of mortality. Indeed, the ratio was higher in the deceased patients; however, its reliability in prognosing fatal outcome was similar to that of TNF receptor alone. On admission at the hospital, a significant correlation was observed between circulating levels of TNFα and both TNF receptor I ($p < 0.001$) and II ($p = 0.012$). In Fig. 3, patients are represented by their number of risk factors on admission at the hospital, with circles showing deceased patients. The relation was analyzed using a locally weighted smoothing model [52] which revealed two distinct linear relationships. For TNFα concentrations below 500 pg/ml, the relation was steep with small changes in TNFα leading to important increases in TNFα receptors levels. The relations flattened for TNFα concentrations higher than 500 pg/ml. Patients who had the highest number of biological risk factors and those with the highest mortality rate are localized on the flat portion of the relation. As the extracellular domain of TNF receptors have inhibitory properties against TNFα, the relative proportion between ligand and ligand inhibitors may be of great importance in the pathophysiology of the development of the shock. These data show that an imbalance between ligand and ligand inhibitors occurred at the beginning of the disease as, when TNFα exceeded 500 pg/ml, the concentrations of the receptors did not increase proportionally.

Table 1. Relation between clinical and biological data obtained on admission at the hospital and outcome

Variables	Nr.	Survival	Death
TNF-α (pg/ml)	35	486 ± 80	1466 ± 285
IL-6 (ng/ml)	34	22,4 ± 5.4	216.3 ± 84.2
TNF-RI (ng/ml)	31	26.3 ± 2.1	35.4 ± 3.0
TNF-RII (ng/ml)	26	67.8 ± 7.2	93.3 ± 8.1
TNFα/TNF-RI ratio	31	0.018 ± 0.003	0.040 ± 0.008
TNFα/TNF-RII ratio	28	0.08 ± 0.001	0.016 ± 0.003

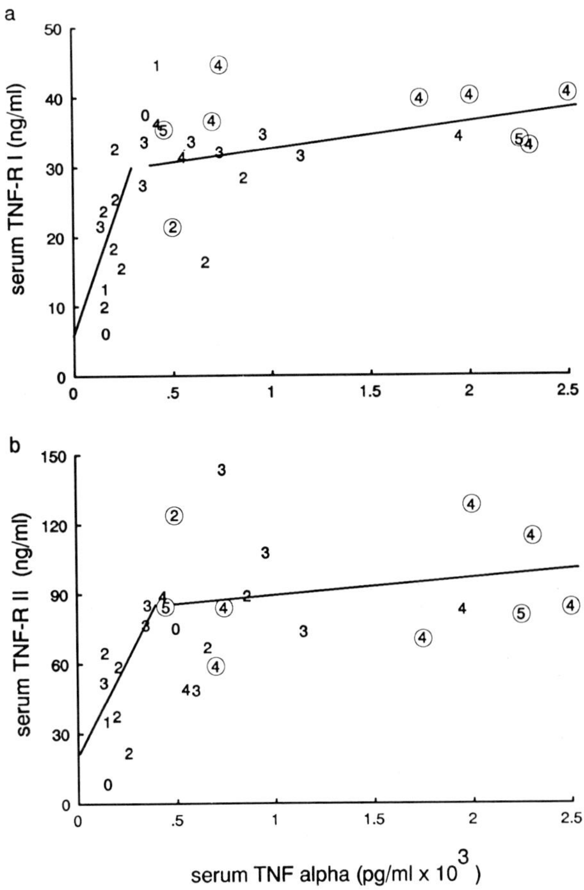

Fig. 3. Correlation between TNFα and TNF-RI or TNF-RII. Patients are shown in the correlation by the number of their biological risk factors on admission at the hospital. Circles represent deceased patients. All the deaths occurred between 10 and 48 h after admission. (From [51] with permission).

After 6 h, we observed a disparity of the evolution of TNFα and its receptors which could be related to a difference in the kinetics between the ligand and its inhibitor. A decrease of 28% in TNFα concentrations was observed in non-surviving patients as well as in those who recovered. In contrast, concentrations of TNF-RI remained stable during the first 6 h of evolution for the two groups of patients. The evolution of TNF-RII was also different. A drop of 35% was observed in the patients who recovered, but an increase of 6% was seen in the non-surviving patients. This difference in evolution of the two receptors may be indicative of a distinct regulation of receptor expression or of differences in the cleavage mechanisms of the extracellular portion of the receptors [36].

Altogether these data demonstrated that TNF-RI and TNF-RII are produced in high amounts in severe meningococcal sepsis, a condition where circulating concentrations of TNFα are elevated. The kinetic of the receptor and of the ligand was different. On admission at the hospital, a plateau was observed in the relation between the ligand and the inhibitors. One can speculate that this imbalance between TNF and TNF receptors may determine the clinical outcome. Recently, the recombinant human TNF receptor fragments have been found to be bioreactive and protective against lethality in a model of D-galactosamine-sensitized mice injected with endotoxin [53]. If the hypothesis of imbalance between ligand and ligand inhibitors is confirmed, administration of exogenous TNF-R may be beneficial in blocking excess of TNFα.

Conclusion

High TNFα circulating levels were reported in meningococcemia both when TNFα was measured by bioassay and by immunoassay. Naturally occurring TNFα inhibitors were also found to be increased during meningococcemia. The concept of unbound TNF and of TNF/TNF receptor complexes will contribute to a better understanding of the TNF-induced illnesses.

References

1. Tracey KJ, Fong Y, Hesse DG, et al. (1988) Cachectin (tumor necrosis factor, TNF-alpha) participates in the metabolic derangements induced by gram-negative bacteremia. Surg Forum 39:8–10
2. Tracey KJ, Lowry SF, Fahey TJ, et al. (1987) Cachectin/tumor necrosis factor induces lethal shock and stress hormone responses in the dog. Surg Gynecol Obstet 164:415–422
3. Remick DG, Kunkel RG, Larrick JW, Kunkel SL (1987) Acute in vivo effects of human recombinant tumor necrosis factor. Lab Invest 56:583–590
4. Kettelhut IC, Fiers W, Goldberg AL (1987) The toxic effects of tumor necrosis factor in vivo and their prevention by cyclooxygenase inhibitors. Proc Natl Acad Sci USA 84:4273–4277
5. Warren RS, Starnes HF Jr, Gabrilove JL, Oettgen HF, Brennan MF (1987) The acute metabolic effects of tumor necrosis factor administration in humans. Arch Surg 122:1396–1400
6. Michie HR, Manogue KR, Spriggs DR, et al. (1988) Detection of circulating tumor necrosis factor after endotoxin administration. N Engl J Med 318:1481–1486
7. Beutler B, Milsark IW, Cerami AC (1985) Passive immunization against cachectin/tumor necrosis factor protects mice from lethal effect of endotoxin. Science 229:869–871
8. Hinshaw LB, Tekamp-Olson P, Chang ACK, et al. (1990) Survival of primates in LD 100 septic shock following therapy with antibody to tumor necrosis factor (TNFalpha). Circ Shock 30:279–292
9. Tracey KJ, Fong Y, Hesse DG, et al. (1987) Anti-cachectin/TNF monoclonal antibodies prevent septic shock during lethal bacteraemia. Nature 330:662–664

10. Silva AT, Bayston KF, Cohen J (1990) Prophylactic and therapeutic effects of a monoclonal antibody to tumor necrosis factor-alpha in experimental gram-negative shock. J Infect Dis 162:421–427
11. Offner F, Philippe J, Vogelaers D, et al. (1990) Serum tumor necrosis factor levels in patients with infectious disease and septic shock. J Lab Clin Med 116: 100–105
12. Cannon JG, Tompkins RG, Gelfand JA, et al. (1990) Circulating interleukin-1 and tumor necrosis factor in septic shock and experimental endotoxin fever. J Infect Dis 161:79–84
13. Marks JD, Marks CB, Luce JM, et al. (1990) Plasma tumor necrosis factor in patients with septic shock. Mortality rate, incidence of adult respiratory distress syndrome, and effects of methylprednisolone administration. Am Rev Respir Dis 141:94–97
14. Debets JMH, Kampmeijer R, Van der Linden MPMH, Buurman WA, Van der Linden CJ (1989) Plasma tumor necrosis factor and mortality in critically ill septic patients. Crit Care Med 17:489–494
15. Calandra T, Baumgartner JD, Grau GE, et al. and the Swiss-Dutch J5 study group (1990) Prognostic values of tumor necrosis factor/cachectin, interleukin-1, alpha-interferon and gamma-interferon in the serum of patients with septic shock. J Infect Dis 161: 982–987
16. Blanchard DK, Djeu JY, Klein TW, Friedman H, Stewart WE (1988) Protective effects of tumor necrosis factor in experimental legionella pneumophila infections of mice via activation of PMN function. J Leukoc Biol 43:429–435
17. Nakano Y, Onozuka K, Erada Y, Shinomiya H, Nakano M (1990) Protective effect of recombinant tumor necrosis factor-alpha in murine salmonellosis. J Immunol 144:1935–1941
18. Nakane A, Minagawa T, Kato K (1988) Endogenous tumor necrosis factor (cachectin) is essential to host resistance against Listeria monocytogenes infection. Infect Immun 56:2563–2569
19. Desiderio JV, Kiener PA, Lin PF, Warr GA (1989) Protection of mice against Listeria monocytogenes infection by recombinant human tumor necrosis factor alpha. Infect Immun 57:1615–1617
20. Seckinger P, Isaaz S, Dayer JM (1988) A human inhibitor of tumor necrosis factor alpha. J Exp Med 167:1511–1516
21. Seckinger P, Isaaz S, Dayer JM (1989) Purification and biologic characterization of a specific tumor necrosis factor-alpha inhibitor. J Biol Chem 264:11966–11973
22. Schall TJ, Lewis M, Koller KJ, et al. (1990) Molecular cloning and expression of a receptor for human tumor necrosis factor. Cell 61:361–370
23. Lantz M, Gullberg U, Nilsson E, Olsson I (1990) Characterization in vitro of a human tumor necrosis factor-binding protein - A soluble form of a tumor necrosis factor receptor. J Clin Invest 86:1396–1402
24. Engelmann H, Aderka D, Rubinstein M, Rotman D, Wallach D (1989) A tumor necrosis factor-binding protein purified to homogeneity from human urine protects cells from tumor necrosis factor toxicity. J Biol Chem 264:11974–11980
25. Engelmann H, Novick D, Wallach D (1990) Two tumor necrosis factor-binding proteins purified from human urine - Evidence for immunological cross-reactivity with cell surface tumor necrosis factor receptors. J Biol Chem 265:1531–1536
26. Seckinger P, Zhang JH, Hauptmann B, Dayer JM (1990) Characterization of a tumor necrosis factor-alpha inhibitor - Evidence of immunological cross-reactivity with the TNF receptor. Proc Natl Acad Sci USA 87:5188–5192
27. Aggarwal BB, Eessalu TE, Hass PE (1985) Characterization of receptors for human tumor necrosis and their regulation by gamma-interferon. Nature 318:665–667
28. Hohmann HP, Remy R, Brockhaus M, van Loon APGM (1989) Two different cell types have different major receptors for human tumor necrosis factor (TNF-a). J Biol Chem 264:14927–14934
29. Loetscher H, Pan YCE, Lahm HW, et al. (1990) Molecular cloning and expression of the human 55 KD tumor necrosis factor receptor. Cell 61:351–359
30. Smith CA, Davis T, Anderson D, et al. (1990) Receptor for tumor necrosis factor defines an unusual family of cellular and viral proteins. Science 248:1019–1023

31. Gatanaga T, Hwang CD, Kohr W, et al. (1990) Purification and characterization of an inhibitor (soluble tumor necrosis factor receptor) for tumor necrosis factor and lymphotoxin obtained from the serum ultrafiltrates of human cancer patients. Proc Natl Acad Sci USA 87:8781–8784
32. Gray PW, Barrett K, Chantry D, Turner M, Feldmann M (1990) Cloning of human tumor necrosis factor receptor cDNA and expression of recombinant soluble TNF-binding protein. Proc Natl Acad Sci USA 87:7380–7384
33. Kohno T, Brewer MT, Baker SL, et al. (1990) A second tumor necrosis factor receptor gene product can shed a naturally occurring tumor necrosis factor inhibitor. Proc Natl Acad Sci USA 87:8331–8335
34. Dembic Z, Loetscher H, Gubler U, et al. (1990) Two human TNF receptors have similar extracellular, but distinct intracellular, domain sequences. Cytokine 2:231–237
35. Loetscher H, Steinmetz M, Lesslauer W (1991) Tumor necrosis factor: Receptors and inhibitors. Cancer Cells 3: 221-226
36. Brockhaus M, Schoenfeld HJ, Schlaeger EJ, Hunziker W, Lesslauer W, Loetscher H (1990) Identification of 2 types of tumor necrosis factor receptors on human cell lines by monoclonal antibodies. Proc Natl Acad Sci USA 87:3127–3131
37. Hohmann HP, Remy R, Poschl B, Vanloon AP (1990) Tumor necrosis factor-alpha and factor-beta bind to the same 2 types of tumor necrosis factor receptors and maximally activate the transcription factor nf-kappa-b at low receptor occupancy and within minutes after receptor binding. J Biol Chem 265:15183–15188
38. Nophar Y, Kemper O, Brakebusch C, et al. (1990) Soluble forms of tumor necrosis factor receptors (TNF-RS) - the cDNA for the type-I TNF-R, cloned using amino-acid sequence data of its soluble form, encodes both the cell surface and a soluble form of the receptor. EMBO J 9:3269–3278
39. Braendtzaeg P, Kierulf P, Gaustad P, et al. (1989) Plasma endotoxin as a predictor of multiple organ failure and death in systemic meningococcal disease. J Infect Dis 159:195–204
40. Davis CE, Arnold K (1974) Role of meningococcal endotoxin in meningococcal purpura. J Exp Med 140:159–171
41. Stiehm ER, Damrosch DS (1966) Factors in the prognosis of meningococcal infection: Review of 63 cases with emphasis on recognition and management of the severely ill patient. J Pediatr 68:458–467
42. Kahn A, Blum D (1978) Factors for poor prognosis in fulminating meningococcemia: Conclusions from observation of 67 childhood cases. Clin Pediatr 17:680–687
43. Leclerc F, Hue V, Martinot A, Delepoulle F (1991) Scoring systems for accurate prognosis of patients with meningococcal infections. Am J Dis Child 145:1090–1091
44. Waage A, Halstensen A, Espevik T (1987) Association between tumor necrosis factor in serum and fatal outcome in patients with meningococcal disease. Lancet 1:355–357
45. Girardin E, Grau GE, Dayer JM, Roux-Lombard P, J5 study group, Lambert PH (1988) Tumor necrosis factor and interleukin-1 in the serum of children with severe infectious purpura. N Engl J Med 319:397–400
46. Waage A, Braendtzaeg P, Halstensen A, Kierulf P, Espevik T (1989) The complex pattern of cytokines in serum from patients with meningococcal septic shock. Association between interleukin 6, interleukin 1, and fatal outcome. J Exp Med 169:333–338
47. Girardin E, Baumgartner JD, Beaufils F, an al. and the J5 study group (1992) Treatment of severe infectious purpura in children with human plasma from donors immunized with Escherichia coli J5: A prospective, double blind study. J Infect Dis 165:695–701
48. Fong Y, Moldawer LL, Marano M, et al. (1990) Endotoxemia elicits increased circulating beta$_2$-IFN/IL-6 in man. J Immunol 142:2321–2324
49. Brouckaert P, Spriggs DR, Demetri G, Kufe DW, Fiers W (1989) Circulating interleukin 6 during a continuous infusion of tumor necrosis factor and interferon gamma. J Exp Med 169:2257–2262
50. Aderka D, Engelmann H, Hornik V, et al. (1991) Increased serum levels of soluble receptors for tumor necrosis factor in cancer patients. Cancer Res 51:5602–5607

51. Girardin E, Roux-Lombard P, Grau GE, Suter P, Gallati M, J5 study group, Dayer JM (1992) Imbalance between tumor necrosis factor alpha and soluble TNF receptor levels in severe meningococcemia. Immunology (in press)
52. Cleveland WS (1979) Robust locally weighted regression and smoothing scatterplots. J Am Statist Assoc 74:829–836
53. Lesslauer W, Tabuchi H, Gentz R, et al. (1991) Recombinant soluble tumor necrosis factor receptor proteins protect mice from lipopolysaccharide-induced lethality. Eur J Immunol 21:2883–2886

Role of the Complement Cascade in Severe Sepsis

L.G. Thijs and C.E. Hack

Introduction

Activation of the complement system has been implicated as one of the possible mechanisms involved in the extremely complex pathophysiology of septic shock. Bacteria and their products like endotoxin can activate this system even in the absence of antibodies [1]. Complement activation results in the generation of several peptides which have strong biological properties and are called anaphylatoxins [2]. Hypotension, leukopenia and increased pulmonary permeability are features of systemic complement activation which are also observed in human septic shock. In this chapter, we will review the available evidence for the role of activation of the complement system in severe sepsis, and some of its sequelae.

The Complement System

The complement system consists of at least 18 factors comprising about 4% of the total amount of plasma proteins. The complement system can be activated in two ways: by the classical pathway and by an alternative pathway (Fig. 1).

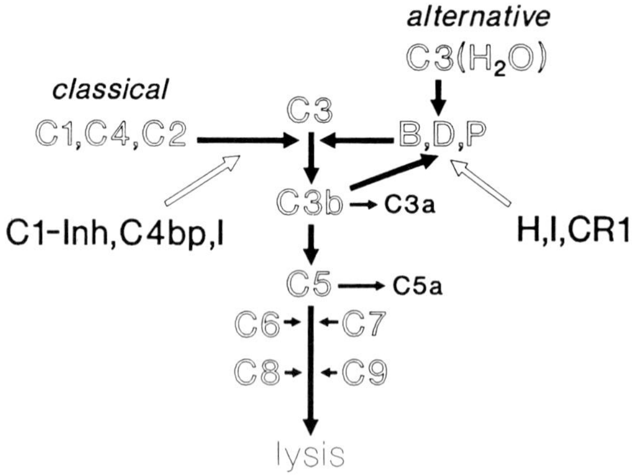

Fig. 1. Schematic representation of the two pathways of complement activation. For abbreviations see text.

Classical Pathway

This pathway is activated mainly by antigen-antibody complexes containing IgG (except IgG4) or IgM, but also by aggregated IgG, some microorganisms and polyanions. The components of the complement system circulate as inactive precursors until they are activated sequently. In many steps, this process involves limited proteolytic cleavage with formation of two fragments of unequal size. The larger fragment continues the sequence of complement reactions while the smaller fragment often contributes to the inflammatory response. Activation starts with recognition of the antibodies by C1, which consists of 3 components (C1q, C1r, C1s), held together by calcium and the subsequent binding of C1q to the Fc fragment of the antibody in the immune complex on the cell surface. Binding of C1q results in the activation of subunit C1r which in turn leads to activation of C1s (C1s = C1 esterase). C1s cleaves C4 into C4a and C4b. The latter larger fragment forms (in the presence of Mg^{++}) a complex with C2, which in turn is split by C1s into C2a and C2b. C2a leaves the complex that now consists of C4b2b, the classical C3-convertase which activates C3. Several naturally circulating inhibitors of this pathway are known: C1 esterase inhibitor (binds to C1r and C1s). C4 binding protein (may dissociate C4b2b complex) and factor I which further degrades C4b bound to C4 binding protein.

Alternative Pathway

A number of factors (B, D and P) are involved in another pathway which leads to activation of C3. Under physiological conditions, a continuous interaction takes place between factors B, D, P and C3. Factor B binds in the presence of Mg^{++} to C3. This C3 is different from native C3 in that sense that its thio-ester is hydrolyzed. This hydrolyzed form of C3 is continuously formed from native C3 at low rate. Factor D subsequently cleaves B into Bb and Ba resulting in a C3Bb complex, the C3-convertase of the alternative pathway. This complex is stabilized by factor P. C3-convertase cleaves C3 into C3a and C3b. Once C3b is formed (this can also be generated via the classical pathway), a process of amplification is startet: C3b reacts with factor B (C3bB complex) which is transformed by factor D into C3bBb, a protein complex with C3-convertase activity, and stabilized by factor P. In the fluid phase, factor I together with factor H can inactivate this complex by degrading C3b. Thus, the inhibitors I and H prevent a continuous activation of the alternative pathway in a normal organism, an as a result activation of amplification is limited under normal conditions. So-called activators of the alternative pathway fix some C3b formed by the continuous but low-grade activation and amplification of the alternative pathway. However, by hampering factors H and I to exert their inhibitory functions on the C3b fixed, they allow a strong amplification which then proceeds to activation of C5 and further complement factors. Among the alternative pathway activators are:

lipopolysaccharides (LPS) from bacterial cell walls, immune complexes (IgG, IgA, IgM), virus particles, yeast, cobra venom factor, and others.

The Final Steps of Complement Activation

C3b formed via the classical pathway binds to the C4b2b complex resulting in the C4b2b3b complex (C5-convertase). In a similar way C3b produced via the alternative route (and by amplification) binds to the C3bBb complex resulting in another C5-convertase: C3b(n)Bb complex. Both convertases cleave C5 into a smaller fragment C5a and a larger fragment C5b. The latter one reacts with C6 and C7 to form C5b67. This stabilized complex can dissociate from the cell membrane and attack other cells. With the help of C8 and several C9 molecules, C5b6789 is formed (terminal complement complex, TCC) which makes "holes" in the cell membrane resulting in lysis of the cell.

Several complement factors such as C3 are degraded. After cleavage of C3 into C3a and C3b, C3b may bind covalently to cells and immune complexes (labile), and also to C3b-receptors (stabile) which are present on granulocytes, monocytes, macrophages and B-lymphocytes. Subsequently, C3b is cleaved by factor I (together with factor H) to form C3bi which is further cleaved into C3c (large fragment) and C3dg (small fragment) by proteolytic enzymes.

Biological Effects of Complement Activation

Activation of the complement system induces a variety of biochemical processes that contribute to host defense against microorganisms.

Factors Bound to Activators: An important function of the activated complement system is to kill cells by lysis (C5b, C6, C7, C8, C9). Activation may be brought about by these cells as such, but also by activators such as immune complexes in their neighbourhood (innocent bystander). During complement activation, a number of factors (C3b, C3d, C3bi, C4b) may fix to the activator (opsonization) via which the latter becomes subsequently bound to receptors on phagocytes that are specific for these complement factors (immune adherence). In this process, the activator will ultimately be removed by phagocytosis.

Small Peptides Split Off during Activation: The most important group is formed by the anaphylatoxins C3a, C4a and C5a (Table 1). These peptides increase vascular permeability and induce smooth muscle contraction. Both C3a and C5a can interact with mast cells and basophilic granulocytes, and induce degranulation and release of histamine and other vascular (vasodilating) mediators. Anaphylatoxins like C3a in particular may directly activate platelets with subsequent release of vasoactive mediators. The release of pla-

Table 1. Biological effects of anaphylatoxins (C5a)

1. chemotactic for neutrophils and monocytes
2. aggregation and degranulation of neutophils
3. stimulation of generation of:
   O_2 free radicals
   leukotrienes (LTB4)
   prostaglandins
   proteases (e.g. elastase)
   PAF
   lysozomal enzymes
4. stimulation of monocytes: *TNF, IL-1, IL-6*
5. degranulation of mast cells: *histamine*
6. expression of tissue factor
7. increase vascular permeability
8. hypotension (peripheral vasodilation?
   pulmonary vasoconstriction?)

telet activating factor (PAF) is among others induced by C5a. Activated complement components also mobilize leukocytes from the bone marrow (C3e), and promote adherence and aggregation of granulocytes to the vascular endothelium (C5a). Also, C5a attracts phagocytic leukocytes (granulocytes, monocytes) and macrophages to the site of microbial invasion (chemotaxis) and stimulates killing mechanisms of the phagocyte, such as the generation of oxygen free radicals and the release of enzymes from lysosomal granules [3]. Activated complement components stimulate the generation of products of the arachidonic cascade. Recently, it has been demonstrated that natural C3a and C5a can induce IL-1 and TNF production by human monocytes in a dose-dependent fashion [4,5], and enhance release of these cytokines induced by endotoxin [5]. Also recombinant C5a acts synergistically with endotoxin in this respect [5]. Natural and recombinant C5a are also potent inducers of the synthesis and release of IL-6 [6]. Anaphylatoxins are apparently potent stimulators of mononuclear secretion of various cytokines that are involved in the pathogenesis of septic shock. TNF is on the other hand able to increase complement receptor expression on human neutrophils [7]. Moreover, complement activation products such as C5a and the terminal complement complex (TCC) promote coagulation by inducing expression of tissue factor [8,9].

Complement Activation in Human Sepsis

The complement system can be activated by bacteria in the presence and even in the absence of antibodies. Therefore, and because of the biological effects of complement activation (see above), the system has long been suspected to be involved in the pathogenesis of sepsis. In one of the first published series on the role of complement in sepsis, C3 levels were measured in blood of patients with gram-negative bacteremia at the onset of fever [10]. Bacteremic patients essentially had the same mean C3 levels as a control group of non-infected patients, but with a considerably wider range. However, patients suffering from shock and those dying had markedly decreased C3 levels. These studies were extended to include measurements of additional complement factors, again at the onset of fever, in another group of patients with gram-negative bacteremia [11]. Patients who developed shock, had significantly lower levels of factors B and P and C3, C5, C6 and C9 when compared with those with uncomplicated bacteremia. No difference in mean levels of C1, C2 and C4 were found between the two groups. This study suggested a preferential activation of the alternative pathway in patients who progressed into shock. Similar findings were published by others [12]. Subsequently, several series have been published in which patients were studied in established or late septic shock, and these included measurement of levels of a variable number of complement factors [13-16]. In essence, these studies confirmed that the levels of most complement factors were lowered in septic shock and this was considered as evidence for increased consumption of these factors.

In one study, C3 levels in patients admitted for hemorrhagic shock or multisystem trauma were completely unaffected when severe sepsis with or without shock supervened [17]. Complement activation is a very dynamic process, and plasma levels of native factors reflect both synthesis (acute phase reaction) and consumption, while hemodilution (by volume loading as part of the treatment) and leakage to the extravascular space due to capillary damage lower plasma levels. Measurement of native factors may, therefore, not be such a sensitive index of complement activation. Later studies have confirmed that complement activation occurs in sepsis by demonstrating that the levels of activated products of complement are increased. Elevated levels of C3 activation products [18], C3a-desarg [19-27], C4a-desarg [19,25,27], C5a-desarg [19-21,25,26], C5a-like activity [28,29], and TCC [18,25,30,31] have been found in septic patients.

Most studies have been performed in gram-negative sepsis (10,11,15,16,32]. In those studies in which both gram-negative and gram-positive septic patients were evaluated, in general no differences between these groups were observed with respect to the levels of (lowered) native [13,14] or (elevated) activated complement [20,27], although in one study slightly higher levels of C5a-like activity were found in gram-negative sepsis [29]. Patients clinically judged as suffering from septic shock but without positive blood cultures have similar [20] or lower [29] levels of activated complement factors than patients with positive blood cultures.

There has been some debate whether activation takes place through the classical [13,32], the alternative [11,16] or both pathways [12,14,15] in patients with septic shock. It has been suggested that this disagreement could be attributed to differences in the time elapsed between the onset of shock and the time of measurement [14]. Complement activation through the alter-

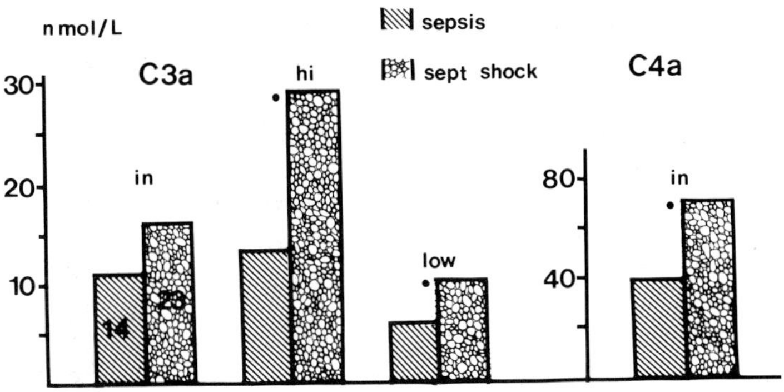

Fig. 2 Levels of C3a and C4a in 37 patients with sepsis (n=14) and septic shock (n=23); in = initial values on admission; hi = highest value during course of disease; low = lowest value. ˙= $p < 0.05$. Upper limit of normal value for C3a = 5 nmol/l; for C4a = 21 nmol/1

native pathway seems to be an early event in sepsis and can take place before hemodynamic alterations are observed [12-14]. It is suggested that activation of the classical pathway would occur later [13,14]. Therefore, both pathways seem to be activated, albeit in varying proportions in the various stages of septic shock. In a recent study measuring C4d and Bb, and Ba levels, it was concluded that the majority of patients had activation of both pathways [31].

Earlier studies in which native complement factors were measured, the lowest values were found in patients who ultimately died [10,12,14,33]. These levels may therefore have prognostic significance, although Leon et al. [13] did not find differences between survivors and nonsurvivors. In this series, initial low values of complement factors returned to normal in survivors. Serial studies may thus be better related to outcome than single measurements.

In our studies, we demonstrated that C3a-desarg levels are almost uniformly elevated in patients with sepsis [27]. Levels of this activated complement factor fluctuated significantly during the day and during the course of disease. Levels of C4a-desarg closely paralleled the levels of C3a-desarg indicating that in these patients activation had mainly followed the classical pathway. Initial, highest and lowest levels of C3a-desarg observed during the disease period were all significantly higher in patients with shock compared to normotensive septic patients (Fig. 2). Also, these levels were significantly higher in nonsurvivors than in survivors (Fig. 3). Mortality increased with increasing C3a-desarg levels which therefore have prognostic value. We found a significant inverse correlation between C3a-desarg and C4a-desarg levels on the one hand, and leukocyte and platelet count on the other (Fig. 4). This may indicate that complement activation is involved in aggregation of these elements in the microcirculation.

Excessive activation of the complement system can be induced by excessive amounts of activator but probably also by insufficient activity of natural

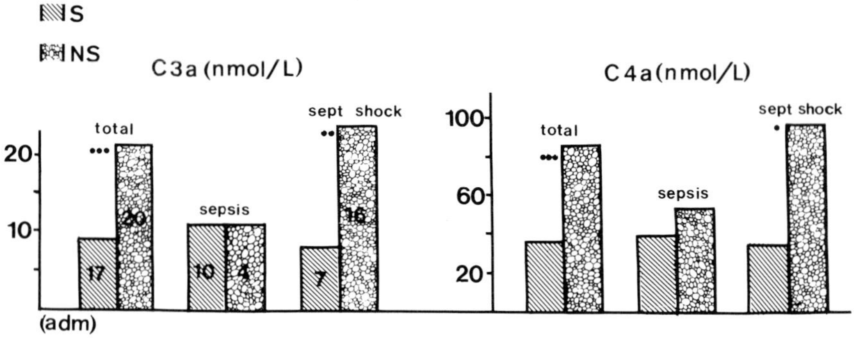

Fig. 3 Initial mean levels of C3a and C4a on admission (adm) in patients with sepsis (n=14) and septic shock (n=23). S = survivors, NS = nonsurvivors, · = p <0.05, ·· = p <0.01, ··· = p <0.005

inhibitors. Factor H and factor I are natural inhibitors of the alternative pathway. Levels of these factors have been found lower in patients in shock and nonsurviving patients, than in those with uncomplicated sepsis [15].

Activation of the classical pathway is regulated by C1-esterase inhibitor (C1-Inh), a protein that belongs to the superfamily of serine protease inhibitors. C1-Inh is not only the main inhibitor of activated C1, but also that of the contact system proteases factor XIIa and kallikrein. Thus, C1-Inh is the main inhibitor of two plasma cascade systems that share the property of generating very potent vasoactive peptides (anaphylatoxins and bradykinin). Intravascular activation of complement and contact system is potentially harmful. Presumably for this reason, plasma levels of C1-Inh increase during acute phase reactions. During uncomplicated sepsis, plasma levels of C1-Inh indeed rise [33] but are often found lowered in patients in (fatal) shock [15,33]. Recently, we analyzed the state of C1-Inh in sepsis [34]. We found that in most patients, and in particular those with lethal complications, functional levels of this inhibitor were normal or even decreased in spite of

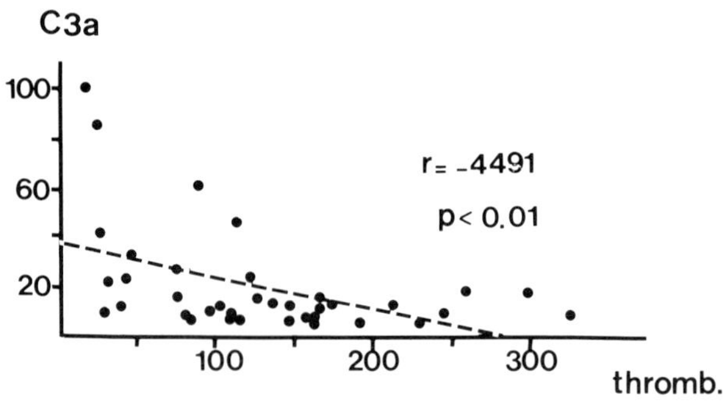

Fig. 4 Relationship between C3a plasma levels and platelet counts in 37 individual patients with sepsis and septic shock.

its acute phase properties. In addition, antigenic levels were higher than functional levels indicating the presence of non-functional C1-Inh. This may be due to binding of C1-Inh to C1-esterase, factor XIIa or kallikrein, or to inactivation of C1-Inh by proteolysis. Complexes of factor XIIa-C1-Inh, C1-C1-Inh, and kallikrein-C1-Inh were however elevated in only a minority of the patients [35]. In contrast, levels of proteolytically inactivated C1-Inh (iC1-Inh) were markedly elevated in the majority of patients [34]. Levels of iC1-Inh were significantly higher in patients in shock than in normotensive patients and also higher in nonsurvivors than in survivors. Calculation of the contribution of iC1-Inh and the various inhibitor complexes to the total amount of nonfunctional C1-Inh revealed that iC1-Inh was by far the most important. The cause of this proteolytical degradation is not known, but among the possibilities are elastase released by activated neutrophils or a strong activation of the contact system.

All evidence discussed above indicates a greater turnover of both classical and alternative pathways during septic shock periods than during periods without shock, and that episodes which end fatally have more intense activation of these pathways than episodes which are survived. This could mean that complement derived products play an important pathogenic role in septic shock. Moreover, plasma levels of the functionally active regulatory proteins may be important in dictating the turnover of the complement system in septic shock. Alternatively, these findings may simply reflect increased utilization of both complement components and control proteins during shock and fatally ending episodes in an attempt to detoxify circulating endotoxins [15].

Complement Activation and Shock

Several observations indicate that complement activation may be involved in the pathogenesis of the circulatory disturbances of septic shock. The shock syndrome develops in about 40% of patients with sepsis and this largely contributes to the mortality of sepsis. Levels of native complement factors are almost uniformly lowest in septic patients with (fatal) shock [10-13,32,33]. Also, concentrations of activated complement factors C3a-desarg [21,27], C3a activity [18], C4a-desarg [27], C5a-desarg [20], and TCC [18] are usually higher in patients in shock than in septic patients without clinical signs of shock. This may suggest a relationship between excessive complement activation and the development of shock, but both may also simply reflect the seriousness of the septic insult.

Several studies have shown that endotoxin is a powerful complement activator in the animal model [36-40]. Also *in vitro* incubation of *E. coli* in fresh serum produces a dose related formation of C3a and C5a [26] and TCC [30]. Recently, it has been shown that also gram-positive microorganisms can induce complement activation and produce similar effects as *E. coli* in the animal model [41]. In these models hypotension is a uniform feature and

Table 2. Complement activation induced hypotension in sepsis

Evidence
- C5a induces hypotension in various models
- Decomplimentation abolishes the hypotensive response to endotoxin
- anti-C5a antibodies attenuate hypotension in sepsis

Possible mechanisms
- periphal vasodilation (prostacyclin?)
- splanchnic pooling with decline of venous return
- pulmonary vasoconstriction (thromboxane A_2?)
- direct effects on the heart

it has been suggested that activated complement factors may contribute to its development [40] (Table 2).

The anaphylatoxin C5a has hypotensive effects in various animal models [40,42-44] and decomplementation abolishes the hypotensive response to endotoxin [38].

It has been shown that low doses of TNF and endotoxin act synergistically on complement activation and that the acute development of shock and tissue injury in response to low doses of TNF with endotoxin depends on an intact complement system [45]. Several mechanisms have been proposed for this hypotensive reaction to C5a. Peripheral vasodilation might be such a mechanism, as C5a may act on the peripheral resistance vessels by inducing (local) production of prostacyclin [46-48], and a causal relationship between prostacyclin formation and arterial hypotension has been suggested [48]. Intravenous administration of zymosan in the rat produces a hyperdynamic circulation with a low vascular resistance and a high cardiac output with a decrease in total hemolytic complement (CH50) [49]. At high doses of zymosan, however, cardiac output declines, systemic vascular resistance increases and blood pressure drops. The high correlation between zymosan dose and degree of complement activation suggests a causal relationship between complement activation and the observed hemodynamic changes. The pattern of these hemodynamic alterations is remarkably similar to that observed in human septic shock. In patients with septic shock, a significant inverse correlation between initial plasma C5a-like activity and both systemic vascular resistance and mean arterial blood pressure has been found [29]. No statistically significant correlation was observed with either cardiac output or left ventricular ejection fraction. In our study in septic patients no significant correlation was found between C3a-desarg levels and systemic vascular resistance for the group as a whole [27]. However, in individual patients in whom more than six data points were available, such an inverse correlation was also found [50]. In another study, C3a-desarg concentration inversely correlated with mean arterial pressure in patients with septic shock in whom also prostacyclin levels were significantly elevated [21]. These observations suggest that complement activation may produce or contribute to peripheral vascular alterations in human septic shock and this may be related to formation of prostaglandins.

Another mechanism which may explain complement-induced hypotension is portal venous pooling followed by a decrease in venous return and cardiac output [43], but this might be a typical response in the dog.

Also pulmonary vasoconstriction is reported to occur after anaphylatoxin administration or complement activation [43] and this phenomenon may contribute to arterial hypotension. In rats, C5a induces systemic arterial hypotension coinciding with an increase in central venous pressure, a decline in cardiac output, neutropenia, and with an unchanged systemic vascular resistance, but with redistribution of total blood flow [44]. This hypotensive response is paralleled by an increase in plasma 6ketoPGF1a and TBX2 levels and is abolished by a cyclooxygenase inhibitor (without altering C5a-induced neutropenia), and reduced by an H2-receptor blocker. Thromboxane synthetase inhibition does not prevent C5a-induced hypotension, but lowers central venous pressure and systemic vascular resistance. One might speculate that the neutrophil is the prime target for C5a as receptors specific for C5a have been identified on its surface, and that activation of this cell contributes to the hemodynamic responses observed with C5a. However, neutropenia as such does not prevent C5a-induced neutropenia whereas C5a-induced hypotension is markedly attenuated [40]. Thus, C5a-induced hypotension seems to be a neutrophil-independet reaction. It is suggested that hypotension is mediated through cyclooxygenase products and to some degree by histamine and that is appears to be (in this model) a secundary effect of pulmonary vasoconstriction probably mediated by thromboxane A2 [44].

Also direct effects of anaphylatoxins on the heart may contribute to hypotension. In a rabbit model, intracoronary administration of C3a causes tachycardia, impairment of atrioventricular conduction, left ventricular contractile failure, coronary vasoconstriction and histamine release [51]. Histamine, leukotrienes and prostaglandins may mediate these various cardiac effects of C3a [51].

In primates, administration of a polyclonal antibody to C5a is able to only partially attenuate the hypotensive response to live E. coli infusion [52]. In a rat endotoxin model, similar effects have been observed with F(ab') 2 fragments of a polyclonal anti-C5a antibody [40]. Both studies show that neutralization of C5a not completely prevents hypotension in sepsis, suggesting that other mechanisms are also involved. However, it should be noted that the efficacy of antibodies to neutralize C5a activity in vivo may not be optimal, and therefore, some C5a induced effects may not have been blocked in both studies. In addition, in neither study the anti-C5a antibodies affected neutropenia suggesting that neutropenia in sepsis is not dependent on complement activation. In an extensive review on the biological effects of endotoxin in several animal models, Fine [39] concluded that the early transient and relatively benign hypotensive response is related to complement activation, whereas the later prolonged and potentially fatal hypotension is probably not.

Complement Activation and ARDS

The adult respiratory distress syndrome (ARDS) is a common complication of septic shock and still carries an extremely high mortality. The incidence of ARDS following a severe septic insult varies between 18 and 38% [20,53,54]. Several observations in the literature suggest that compliment activation is involved in the pathogenesis of this sydrome. In particular C5a can mediate neutrophil adhesion, aggregation, activation, and subsequent pulmonary endothelial damage [55-58]. This sequence of events i.e. margination and sequestration of neutrophils in the lung where they release toxic substances leading to endothelial cell injury, may be the primary pathogenetic mechanism for the development of ARDS in septic shock. Among these toxic products are oxygen free radicals and proteases (e.g. elastase, trypsin, chymotrypsin and cathepsin G). Recent studies have shown that neutrophil-mediated injury of endothelial cells involves interactions of oxygen products and proteases [59].

The hypothesis that complement activation and neutrophil sequestration and activation in the pulmonary vasculature with subsequent pulmonary vascular injury is the underlying mechanism responsible for acute lung injury, originally stems from observations during hemodialysis [60]. During hemodialysis, activation of the complement system was demonstrated and this was associated with transient neutropenia and pulmonary dysfunction. It was shown that plasma passed over dialysis cellophane activated complement via the alternative pathway and that after reinfusion of activated, autologous plasma neutrophils became trapped in the microvasculature [60]. In addition, infusion in rabbits of autologous, cellophane-incubated plasma produced acute neutropenia and significant hypoxemia, with on histologic examination gross intravascular leukostasis with interstitial edema in the lung [60]. In sheep, this maneuvre was accompanied by a marked increase in pulmonary lymph flow. This syndrome could be prevented by pre-inactivation of complement and by prior induction of leukopenia. Also, enhanced clearance of neutrophils in the pulmonary vascular bed was demonstrated [60]. These observations linked complement activation, pulmonary leukostasis and injury, acute leukopenia and pulmonary dysfunction. Subsequently, a number of experimental studies in animals have provided evidence for the role of complement in the pathogenesis of acute lung injury and ARDS which will be discussed later. Clinical studies in ARDS have shown that the early phase of acute lung injury is associated with the sequestration of large numbers of neutrophils in the lung. Transient leukopenia is sometimes also a feature of early septic shock and it has been suggested that a fall in leukocytes in the peripheral circulation heralds the onset of the development of ARDS [61]. In

Table 3. Complement activation and ARDS

- Zymosan (or CVF)* - induced complement activation causes neutropenia, hypoxemia, aggregation of neutrophils in the lung with edema, and increased pulmonary lymph flow
- C5a causes similar abnormalities
- Complement-deficient animals show less pulmonary injury during sepsis
- Antibodies to C5a attenuate pulmonary injury in sepsis
- Inconsistent correlation between levels of activated complement factors and development of human ARDS

*CVF = cobra venom factor

Table 3, the evidence for a role of complement activation in the development of ARDS is briefly summarized. This will be discussed in the following paragraphs.

Animal Studies

Infusion of endotoxin in the animal experiment has been used as a model of ARDS. In these experiments, the development of acute lung injury is preceded by neutrophil sequestration in the pulmonary vasculature as demonstrated in histologic sections [62-64]. This is followed by increased lung microvascular permeability and enhanced pulmonary lymph flow [62,63,65]. These changes are also associated with generalized neutropenia and can be abrogated by neutrophil depletion [62,63,65]. Thus, there is a significant body of evidence to support the premise that neutrophil sequestration in the microvasculature of the lung is an early event in endotoxemia that seems to be critical to the development of microvascular injury.

Since endotoxin is able to activate both the alternative and the classical pathways [1,39], it has been postulated that complement activation might be an important mediator of these processes. Several investigators have indeed shown that complement activation as such can induce intravascular neutrophil sequestration and have suggested that this results in damage to the microvasculature in the lung. Zymosan-induced complement-activated plasma (alternative pathway) is able to cause early neutropenia, progressive hypoxemia, respiratory alkalosis and tachypnea in a rabbit model [66-68]. In sheep, zymosan-incubated plasma produces similar abnormalities together with a marked increase in pulmonary lymph flow [60]. Microscopy of the lungs reveals aggregation and plugging of neutrophils in small vessels and capillaries of the lung. Electronmicroscopy shows degranulation and disintegration of neutrophils, interstitial edema and endothelial cell injury [66,68]. When the animals were rendered neutropenic, these changes did not occur [66]. The combination of hypoxia and systemic complement activation appears to aggravate this microvascular injury with the occurrence of protein rich alveolar edema and hemorrhage in the lung [68]. Similarly, intravascular activation of the complement system with cobra venom factor in rats causes acute lung injury as quantified by the increase in lung vascular permeability [69]. Also in this model, damage to the endothelial cell lining of lung alveolar capillaries and plugging of neutrophils that are in direct contact with the vascular basement membrane is observed. Lung injury can dramatically be attenuated by either prior depletion of neutrophils or by intravenous catalase or superoxide dismutase, supporting that complement-mediated neutrophil aggregation with subsequent production of oxygen free radicals is an important event in acute lung injury [69]. Infusion of a single activated complement factor C5a can also produce increased permeability in the lung [70]. Studies using intravital microscopy have confirmed that neutrophil aggregation and leukoembolization occur in the microcirculation upon administration of C5a or zymosan-activated plasma [71]. Moreover, this phenomenon was accompanied by extravasation of plasma proteins in a pattern suggestive of endothelial damage. These studies have clearly shown that complement activation in several models can mimic abnormalities as present in ARDS.

What evidence do we have that pulmonary injury caused by sepsis or endotoxemia is mediated by complement activation? In a study comparing the effects of caecal ligation and puncture-induced peritonitis in both C5-sufficient and C5-deficient mice, morphometric studies demonstrated a significant increase in intracapillary granulocrit and air-blood barrier thickness in C5-sufficient mice associated with a decline in PaO_2, abnormalities that were not present in septic C5-deficient mice [72]. In an elegant study, Hosea et al. [70] demonstrated that complement-depleted and C5-deficient animals, unlike normal and C4-deficient animals, did not localize injected bacteria (ingested by neutrophils) to the lungs. This finding again suggests that C5a, a strong chemotactic factor, is critical in this process and is required for pulmonary edema formation. Further support for this hypothesis comes from studies in which the effects of a polyclonal antibody to C5a-desarg on the development of ARDS in septic primates was evaluated [52]. In this model, infusion of live *E. coli* resulted in severe sepsis with a decline in systemic vascular resistance and blood pressure and development of ARDS. Anti-C5a antibodies could prevent hypoxemia and the increase in extravascular lungwater and markedly attenuated therefore signs of ARDS. Moreover, the peak levels of C5a were significantly less in the anti-C5a treated animals, but C5 depletion was not prevented demonstrating that activation of the parent C5 molecules was not prevented [73].

Intravenous endotoxin administration in a rabbit model caused a marked dose dependent sequestration of radioactive labeled neutrophils in the pulmonary vasculature as detected by external quantitative scintigraphy and ultrastructural autoradiography of the lungs [74]. Pretreatment *ex vivo* of neutrophils with endotoxin also caused a dose-dependent pulmonary sequestration of these pretreated labeled neutrophils, but no generalized neutropenia. There was no evidence of complement activation on the surface of pretreated neutrophils suggesting that initiation of pulmonary sequestration by low dose endotoxin is a complement-independet effect on the neutrophil rather than on the endothelium [74]. Thus, endotoxin may directly promote neutrophil sequestration. Indeed, some studies have suggested that complement activation *per se* is unable to fully simulate the effects of endotoxin [64,67,75,76]

Although the adherence of neutrophils to endothelium is likely to be the first step in neutrophil-mediated injury, the sequestration of neutrophils within the pulmonary vasculature itself appears insufficient to cause injury [67,75]. Small doses of endotoxin enhances injury to cultured endothelial cells mediated by stimulated neutrophils [77] and endotoxin may directly promote neutrophil sequestration in the lung [74]. Trace amounts of endotoxin in combination with either a synthetic chemotactic peptide or chemotactic fragments of C5 were able to markedly increase pulmonary permeability, which did not occur with either of these compounds alone [76]. Neutrophil depletion completely abolished this phenomenon. Also, ultrastructural studies revealed enhanced neutrophil sequestration and alterations in endothelial cells when combinations were administered [76]. Thus, endothelial cell injury seems to increase by the combination of small amounts of endotoxin and neutrophil chemotactic factors.

In conclusion, there is much evidence in experimental models that complement activation with a predominant role for C5a, is involved in the pathogenesis of ARDS, but also that additional factors and/or mechanisms are necessary to fully express its effects.

Human Studies

In one of the first studies using a neutrophil aggregation technique to estimate C5a (plasma C5a-like activity), a strong and highly significant correlation was found between the presence of C5a-like activity and the development of ARDS [28]. It was suggested that detection of an elevated C5a level could be a useful predictor of ARDS. Subsequent studies however have shown variable results. Using a similar technique, Duchateau et al. [78] found in (mainly nonseptic) patients at risk for ARDS evidence for early complement activation as detected by high C5a-like activity (and C3d/C3 ratios). However, this activation correlated poorly with the actual development of ARDS. They suggested that additional factors may contribute to the evolution to a full-blown ARDS. Interestingly, it was shown that initial pulmonary clearance of C5a-like activity was followed by release of C5a-like activity from the pulmonary circulation [78].

Total hemolytic complement (CH50) is usually lowered during sepsis, but this is not different between patients who will or will not develop ARDS or between patients with and without ARDS [25].

Initial C3a-desarg levels have been found to be significantly higher in patients who developed or manifested signs of ARDS than in uncomplicated patients [24,79-81]. A weak but statistically significant correlation has been observed between the level of C3a-desarg and pulmonary alveolo-capillary permeability [24]. However in most studies, no statistically significant differences have been found in initial levels of C3a-desarg and C5a-desarg between patients who develop this syndrome and those who have an uneventful course [20,22,25-27,29,30]. In addition, no correlation has been found between levels of these anaphylatoxins and the initial severity of lung injury, nor did they predict development or worsening of associated acute lung injury [20]. There are, however, some observations which suggest that persistently elevated or rising levels of C3a-desarg are associated with the development of ARDS [26,30]. Others have not found differences between septic patients with and without ARDS or changes in C3a-desarg or C5a-desarg levels when a clinical diagnosis of ARDS was made during the course of disease [25]. In our own study of patients with sepsis and septic shock, initial as well as highest or lowest levels of C3a-desarg during the whole observation period, were not different between patients with and without ARDS [27]. Possibly, local complement activation is more important for the development of ARDS. For example, measurement of the concentration of C3a-desarg in BAL fluid appeared to be a more sensitive parameter than plasma levels in patients with ARDS [23].

It has been suggested that persistence of elevated C4a-desarg is associated with multiorgan system failure [19]. However, in a large prospective study, levels of this complement activation product were not different in septic patients with and without ARDS, nor did the levels change at the time of a clinical diagnosis of ARDS [25]. Also, measurement of Ba, Bb, C4d, iC3b and C3d failed to distinguish the patients at risk from the patients with ARDS [31]. Measurement of anaphylatoxin levels may, however, underestimate the extent of complement activation as both C3a and C5a are rapidly cleared from the circulation by complement receptors on the surface of phagocytic cells including neutrophils. This is illustrated by the study of Solomkin et al. [79] who demonstrated that in patients at risk for ARDS neutrophils showed signs of prior exposure to C5a without demonstrable elevated C5a levels in the peripheral blood. In contrast, the fluid phase terminal complement complex (sC5b-9, TCC) is a more stable complement activation byproduct and its presence in plasma indicates that the complement cascade has been activated to completion [82]. Therefore, TCC levels may be a more consistent marker of complement activation than fragments of C3 and C5 [25] although this has been questioned [31].

Langlois and Gawryl [25] found that TCC levels were the only marker of complement activation that was higher in patients with ARDS than in non-ARDS septic patients. Moreover, in all septic patients who developed ARDS the TCC levels increased significantly two days prior to the clinical diagnosis of ARDS, while these levels remained constant in patients in whom no acute lung injury developed. Thus, this complex could be a useful predictive marker of ARDS. In another study, a correlation was found between persistence of elevated TCC levels and the development of ARDS [30]. However, Parsons and Giclas [31] did not find a difference in TCC levels between patients at risk for ARDS and ARDS patients. These authors also did not observe a consistent pattern in plasma levels of this complex when ARDS actually developed.

In summary, the majority of reports indicate that measurement of activation products of the complement system does not provide a clinically reliable predictor for the development and severity of ARDS. A possible exception could be the determination of terminal complement complexes but this needs further study.

In a study in patients with acute illness including abdominal sepsis, C5a-desarg levels were not elevated. However, neutrophil migratory responses to FMLP (N-formyl-methionyl-leucyl-phenylalanine) and/or C5a were deactivated in those patients who developed ARDS [24,79). Neutrophils from these patients showed a fall in beta-glucuronidase and lysozyme levels. Both findings are consistent with prior exposure to C5a *in vivo*. C5a-exposure *in vitro* was not able to reproduce migratory dysfunction and lysozyme loss of neutrophils, suggesting that *in vivo* other stimuli are necessary to produce these effects [79]. Several studies have documented the occurrence of ARDS in severely neutropenic patients arguing for a heterogenous pathogenesis for this syndrome [83-85]. Complement activation may, therefore, be a necessary but not sufficient pathogenetic mechanism in the evolution of ARDS. Other additional factors necessary to produce significant acute lung injury could be hypoxia [68], cytokines, prostaglandins [75,80], and (trace amounts of) endotoxin [74,76] and other mediators. The role of cytokines is extensively discussed elsewhere in this book. Small concentrations of endotoxin enhance C5a-stimulated release of superoxide anions [86] and elastase [87] from neutrophils. It seems, therefore, that endotoxin can prime neutrophils for subsequent stimulation by C5a [74,76]. Even trace amounts of endotoxin in conjunction with intravascular complement fragments or other neutrophil stimuli can increase neutrophil sequestration in the capillaries and enhance a neutrophil-dependent increase in pulmonary vascular permeability [76]. Mean endotoxin levels were significantly higher (and were persistently present) in patients with ARDS or in those who subsequently developed ARDS than in patients at risk [81]. In this study, the combination of activated complement factors and endotoxin levels in plasma better discriminated between patient with full-blown ARDS and patients at risk than did the presence of activated complement factors (C3a, C5a) alone. Therefore, the combination of endotoxin and complement fragments may be one mechanism involved in the development of ARDS [81].

Conclusion

There is no doubt that the complement system is activated in human sepsis and septic shock. The strong biological properties of some activated complement factors, basically designed to localize and eliminate causative microorganisms, may, when produced in excessive amounts, turn against the body itself. However, complement activation is just one mechanism amongst many others including an array of mediators such as TNF, IL-1, IL-6, IL-8, arachidonic acid metabolites, platelet activating factor, involved in the pathophysiology of sepsis. Besides, these various mediators show important interactions. Complement activation for example may stimulate release of TNF, IL-1 and IL-6 production, histamine, serotonine, arachidonic acid products, and oxygen free radicals by interactions with neutrophils, monocytes and platelets. Many of these complex interactions have not been fully elucidated. Complement activation *in vivo* provides one of the triggers for cytokine production. It is therefore not surprising that, at this moment, it is impossible to appreciate the precise contribution of complement activation to the pathophysiology of human septic shock. Some experimental and clinical data have been presented which suggest a role for complement activation, in particular in the early phase of sepsis. These data, however, also clearly indicate that other additional mechanisms are necessary to produce the clinical syndrome of sepsis and its major complications, shock and ARDS, as part of multiorgan system failure.

References

1. Morrison DC, Kline LF (1977) Activation of the classical and properdin pathways of complement by bacterial lipopolysaccharides (LPS). I Immunol 118:362–368
2. Vogt W (1986) Anaphylatoxins: Possible roles in disease. Complement 3:177–188
3. Yancey KB (1988) Biological properties of human C5a: Selected in vitro and in vivo studies. Clin Exp Immunol 71:207–210
4. Okusawa S, Yancey KB, Van der Meer JWM, et al. (1988) C5a stimulates secretion of tumor necrosis factor from human mononuclear cells in vitro. J Exp Med 168:443–448
5. Cavaillon JM, Fitting C, Haeffner-Cavaillon N (1990) Recombinant C5a enhances interleukin-1 and tumor necrosis factor release by lipopolysaccharide-stimulated monocytes and macrophages. Eur J Immunol 20:253–257
6. Scholz W, McClurg MR, Cardenas GJ, et al. (1990) C5a-mediated release of interleukin-6 by human monocytes. Clin Immunol Immunopathol 57:297–307
7. Berger M, Wetzler EM, Wallis RS (1988) Tumor necrosis factor is the major monocyte product that increases complement receptor expression on mature human neutrophils. Blood 71:151–158
8. Bjork J, Hugli TE, Smedegard G (1985) Microvascular effects of anaphylatoxins C3a and C5a. J Immunol 134:1115–1119
9. Hamilton KK, Hattori R, Esmon CT, Sims PJ (1990) Complement proteins C5b-9 induce vesiculation of the endothelial plasma membrane and expose catalytic surface of assembly of the prothrombinase enzyme complex. J Biol Chem 265:3809–3814
10. McCabe WR (1973) Serum complement levels in bacteremia due to gram-negative organisms. N Engl J Med 288:21–23
11. Fearon DT, Ruddy S, Schur PH, McCabe WR (1975) Activation of the properdin pathway of complement in patients with gram-negative bacteremia. N Engl J Med 292:937–940
12. Füst G, Petras G, Ujhelyi E (1976) Activation of the complement system during infections due to gram-negative bacteria. Clin Immunol Immunopathol 5:293–302
13. León C, Rodrigo MJ, Tomasa A, et al. (1982) Complement activation in septic shock due to gram-negative and gram-positive bacteria. Crit Care Med 10:308–310
14. Sprung CL, Schultz DR, Marcial E, et al. (1986) Complement activation in septic shock patients. Crit Care Med 14:525–528

15. Whaley K, Yee Khong T, McCartney AG, et al. (1979) Complement activation and its control in gram-negative endotoxin shock. J Clin Lab Immunol 2:117–124
16. Witte J, Jochum M, Scherer R, Schramm W, Hochstrasser K, Fritz H (1982) Disturbances of selected plasma proteins in hyperdynamic septic shock. Intensive Care Med 8:215–222
17. Shatney CH, Benner C (1985) Sequential serum complement (C3) and immunoglobulin levels in shock/trauma patients developing acute fulminant systemic sepsis. Circ Shock 16:9–17
18. Brandtzaeg P, Mollnes TE, Kierulf P (1989) Complement activation and endotoxin levels in systemic meningococcal disease. J Infect Dis 160:58–65
19. Heideman M, Hugli TE (1984) Anaphylatoxin generation in multisystem organ failure. J Trauma 24:1038–1043
20. Weinberg PF, Matthay MA, Webster RO, Roskos KV, Goldstein IM, Murray JF (1984) Biologically active products of complement and acute lung injury in patients with the sepsis syndrome. Am Rev Respir Dis 130:791–796
21. Slotman GJ, Burchard KW, Williams JJ, D'Arezzo A, Yellin SA (1986) Interaction of prostaglandins, activated complement, and granulocytes in clinical sepsis and hypotension. Surgery 99:744–751
22. Ketai LH, Grum CM (1986) C3a and adult respiratory distress syndrome after massive transfusion. Crit Care Med 14:1001–1003
23. Hällgren R, Samuelsson T. Modig J (1987) Complement activation and increased alveolar-capillary permeability after major surgery and in adult respiratory distress syndrome. Crit Care Med 15:189–193
24. Tennenberg SD, Jacobs MP, Solomkin JS (1987) Complement-mediated neutrophil activation in sepsis - and trauma - related adult respiratory distress syndrome. Arch Surg 122:26–32
25. Langlois PF, Gawryl MS (1988) Accentuated formation of the terminal C5b-9 complement complex in patient plasma precedes development of the adult respiratory distress syndrome. Am Rev Respir Dis 138:368–375
26. Bengtson A, Heideman M (1988) Anaphylatoxin formation in sepsis. Arch Surg 123:645–649
27. Hack CE, Nuijens JH, Felt-Bersma RJF, et al. (1989) Elevated plasma levels of the anaphylatoxins C3a and C4a are associated with a fatal outcome in sepsis. Am J Med 86:20–26
28. Hammerschmidt DE, Weaver LJ, Hudson LD, Craddock PR, Jacob HS (1980) Association of complement activation and elevated plasma-C5a with adult respiratory distress syndrome. Lancet 1:947–949
29. Ognibene FP, Parker MM, Burch-Whitman C, et al. (1988) Neutrophil aggregating activity and septic shock in humans: Neutrophil aggregation by C5a-like material occurs more frequently than complement component depletion and correlates with depression of systemic vascular resistance. J Crit Care 3:103–111
30. Heideman, M, Norder-Hansson B, Bengtson A, Mollnes TE (1988) Terminal complement complexes and anaphylatoxins in septic and ischemic patients. Arch Surg 123:188–192
31. Parsons PE, Giclas PC (1990) The terminal complement complex (sC5b-9) is not specifically associated with the development of the adult respiratory distress syndrome. Am Rev Respir Dis 141:98–103
32. George C, Carlet J, Sobel A, et al. (1980) Circulating immune complexes in patients with gram-negative septic shock. Intensive Care Med 6:123–127
33. Kalter ES, Daha MR, ten Cate JW, Verhoef J, Bouma BN (1985) Activation and inhibition of Hageman factor-dependent pathways and the complement system in uncomplicated bacteremia or bacterial shock. J Infect Dis 151:1019–1027
34. Nuijens JH, Eerenberg-Belmer AJM, Huijbregts CCM, et al. (1989) Proteolytic inactivation of plasma C1 inhibitor in sepsis. J Clin Invest 84:443–450
35. Nuijens JH, Huijbregts CCM, Eerenberg-Belmer AJM, et al. (1988) Quantification of plasma factor XIIa-C1-inhibitor and kallikrein-C1-inhibitor complexes in sepsis. Blood 72:1841–1848
36. Heideman M, Kaijser B, Gelin LE (1979) Complement activation early in endotoxin shock. J Surg Res 26:74–78

37. Gilbert VE, Braude AI (1962) Reduction of serum complement in rabbits after injection of endotoxin. J Exp Med 116:477–490
38. Garner R, Chater BV, Brown DL (1974) The role of complement in endotoxin shock and disseminated intravascular coagulation: Experimental observations in the dog. Brit J Haematol 28:393–401
39. Fine DP (1985) Role of complement in endotoxin shock. In: Hinshaw LB (ed) Handbook of endotoxin, Vol 2, Elsevier Scientific Publishers, pp 129–144
40. Smedegard G, Cui L, Hugli TE (1989) Endotoxin-induced shock in the rat. A role for C5a. Am J Pathol 135:489–497
41. Wakabayashi G, Gelfand JA, Jung WK, Connolly RJ, Burke JF, Dinarello CA (1991) Staphylococcus epidermidis induces complement activation, tumor necrosis factor and interleukin-1, a shock-like state and tissue injury in rabbits without endotoxemia. J Clin Invest 87:1925–1935
42. Bodammer G, Vogt W (1967) Actions of anaphylatoxin on circulation and respiration in the guinea pig. Int Arch Allergy 32:417–428
43. Pavel K, Piper PJ, Smedegard G (1979) Anaphylatoxin-induced shock and two patterns of anaphylactic shock: Hemodynamics and mediators. Acta Physiol Scand 105:393–403
44. Lundberg C, Marceau F, Hugli TE (1987) C5a-induced hemodynamic and hematologic changes in the rabbit. Role of cyclooxygenase products and polymorphonuclear leukocytes. Am J Pathol 128:471–483
45. Hsueh W, Sun X, Rioja LN, Gonzales-Crussi F (1990) The role of the complement system in shock and tissue injury induced by tumour necrosis factor and endotoxin. Immunology 70:309–314
46. Rampart M, Bull H, Herman AG (1983) Activated complement and anaphylatoxins increase the in vitro production of prostacyclin by rabbit aorta endothelium. Arch Pharmacol 322:158–165
47. Hugli TE, Marceau F (1985) Effects of the C5a anaphylatoxin and its relationship to cyclooxygenase metabolites in rabbit vascular strips. Br J Pharmacol 84:725–733
48. Bult M, Herman, AG, Laekeman GM, Rampart M (1985) Formation of prostanoids during intravascular complement activation in rabbits. Br J Pharmacol 84:329–336
49. Schirmer WJ, Schirmer JM, Naff GB, Fry DE (1988) Systemic complement activation produces hemodynamic changes characteristic of sepsis. Arch Surg 123:316–321
50. Thijs LG, Hack CE, Nuijens JH, Groeneveld ABJ (1989) Peripheral circulation in septic shock. In: Schlag G, Redl H (eds) Second Vienna Shock Forum, Alan R Liss Inc., pp 163–174
51. Hachfeld del Balzo U, Levi R, Polley MJ (1985) Cardiac dysfunction caused by purified human C3a anaphylatoxin. Proc Natl Acad Sci 82:886–890
52. Stevens JH, O'Hanley P, Shapiro JM, et al. (1986) Effects of anti-C5a antibodies on the adult respiratory distress syndrome in septic primates. J Clin Invest 77:1812–1816
53. Kaplan RL, Sahn SA, Petty TL (1979) Incidence and outcome of the respiratory distress sydrome in gram-negative sepsis. Arch Intern Med 139:867–886
54. Pepe PE, Potkin RT, Holtman Reus D, Hudson LD, Carrico CJ (1982) Clinical predictors of the adult respiratory distress syndrome. Am J Surg 144:124–130
55. Craddock PR, Hammershmidt D, White JG, Dalmasso AP, Jacob HS (1977) Complement (C5a)-induced granulocyte aggregation in vitro. A possible mechanism of complement-mediated leukostasis and leukopenia. J Clin Invest 60:260–264
56. Sacks T, Moldrow PR, Craddock PR, Bowers TK, Jacob HS (1978) Oxygen radicals mediate endothelial cell damage by complement-stimulated granulocytes. J Clin Invest 61:1161–1167
57. Tate RM, Repine JE (1983) Neutrophils and the adult respiratory distress syndrome: State of the art. Am Rev Respir Dis 128:802–806
58. Tonnesen MG, Smedley LA, Henson PM (1984) Neutrophil-endothelial cell interactions: Modulation of neutrophil adhesiveness induced by complement fragments C5a and C5a-desArg and formyl-methionyl-leucyl phenylalanine in vitro. J Clin Invest 74:1581–1592
59. Varani J, Ginsburg I, Schuger L, et al. (1989) Endothelial cell killing by neutrophils. Synergistic interaction of oxygen products and proteases. Am J Pathol 135:435–438

60. Craddock PR, Fehr J, Brigham KL, Kronenberg RS, Jacob HS (1977) Complement and leukocyte-mediated pulmonary dysfunction in hemodialysis. N Engl J Med 296:769–774
61. Thommasen HV, Russel JA, Boyko WJ, Hogg JC (1984) Transient leucopenia associated with adult respiratory distress syndrome. Lancet 1:809–812
62. Brigham KL, Woolverton WC, Blake LH, Staub NC (1974) Increased sheep lung permeability caused by Pseudomonas bacteria. J Clin Invest 54: 792–804
63. Brigham KL, Bowers R, Haynes L (1979) Increased sheep lung vascular permeability caused by E. coli endotoxin. Circ Res 45:292–297
64. Myrick BO, Brigham KL (1983) Acute effects of Escherichia coli endotoxin on the pulmonary microcirculation of anesthetized sheep. Structure-function relationships. Lab Invest 48:458–470
65. Heflin AG, Brigham KL (1981) Prevention by granulocyte depletion of increased vascular permeability of sheep lung following endotoxemia. J Clin Invest 68:1253–1260
66. Hohn DC, Meyers AJ, Cherini ST, Beckmann A, Markinson RE, Churg AM (1980) Production of acute pulmonary injury by leukocytes and activated complement. Surgery 88:48–58
67. Webster RO, Larsen GL, Mitchell BC, Goins AJ, Henson PM (1982) Absence of inflammatory lung injury in rabbits challenged intravascularly with complement-derived chemotactic factors. Am Rev Respir Dis 125:335–340
68. Nuytinck JKS, Goris RJA, Weerts JGE, Schillings PHM, Schuurmans-Stekhoven JH (1986) Acute generalized microvascular injury by activated complement and hypoxia: The basis of the adult respiratory distress syndrome and multiple organ failure? Br J Exp Path 67:537–548
69. Till GO, Johnson KJ, Kunkel R, Ward PA (1982) Intravascular activation of complement and acute lung injury. J Clin Invest 69:1126–1135
70. Hosea S, Brown E, Hammer C, Frank M (1980) Role of complement activation in a model of adult respiratory distress syndrome. J Clin Invest 66:375–382
71. Hammerschmidt DE, Harris PD, Wayland JH, Craddock PR, Jacob HS (1981) Complement-induced granulocyte aggregation in vivo. Am J Pathol 102:146–150
72. Olson LM, Moss GS, Baukus O, Das Gupta TK (1985) The role of C5 in septic lung injury. Ann Surg 202:771–776
73. Hangen DH, Stevens JH, Satoh PS, Hall EW, O'Hanley PT, Raffin TA (1989) Complement levels in septic primates treated with anti-C5a antibodies. J Surg Res 46:195–199
74. Haslett C, Worthen GS, Giclas PC, Morrison DC, Henson JE, Henson PM (1987) The pulmonary vascular sequestration of neutrophils in endotoxemia is initiated by an effect of endotoxin on the neutrophil in the rabbit. Am Rev Respir Dis 136:9–18
75. Henson PM, Larsen GL, Webster RO, et al. (1982) Pulmonary vascular alteration and injury induced by complement fragments: Synergistic effect of complement activation, neutrophil sequestration, and prostaglandins. Ann NY Acad Sci 384:287–300
76. Worthen GS, Haslett C, Rees AJ, Gumbay RS, Henson JE, Henson PM (1987) Neutrophil-mediated pulmonary vascular injury. Synergistic effect of trace amounts of lipopolysaccharide and neutrophil stimuli on vascular permeability and neutrophil sequestration in the lung. Am Rev Respir Dis 136:19–28
77. Smedly LA, Tonnesen MG, Sandhaus RA, et al. (1986) Neutrophil-mediated injury to endothelial cells: Enhancement by endotoxin and essential role of neutrophil elastase. J Clin Invest 77:1233–1242
78. Duchateau J, Haas M, Schreyen H, et al. (1984) Complement activation in patients at risk of developing the adult respiratory distress syndrome. Am Rev Respir Dis 130:1058–1064
79. Solomkin JS, Cotta LA, Satoh PS, Hurst JM, Nelson RD (1985) Complement activation and clearance in acute illness and injury: Evidence for C5a as a cell-directed mediator of the adult respiratory distress syndrome in man. Surgery 97:668–678
80. Slotman GJ, Burchard KW, Yellin SA, Williams JJ (1986) Prostaglandin and complement interaction in clinical acute respiratory failure. Arch Surg 121:271–274
81. Parsons PE, Wortehn GS, Moore EE, Tate RM, Henson PM (1989) The association of circulating endotoxin with the development of the adult respiratory distress syndrome. Am Rev Respir Dis 140:294–301

82. Muller-Eberhard H (1986) The membrane attack complex of complement. Ann Rev Immunol 4:503–528
83. Ognibene FP, Martin SE, Parker MM, et al. (1986) Adult respiratory distress syndrome in patients with severe neutropenia. N Engl J Med 315:547–551
84. Laufe MD, Simon RH, Flint A, et al. (1986) Adult respiratory distress syndrome in neutropenic patients. Am J Med 80:1022–1026
85. Maunder RJ, Hackman RC, Riff E, et al. (1986) Occurrence of the adult respiratory distress syndrome in neutropenic patients. Am Rev Respir Dis 133:313–316
86. Guthrie LA, McPhail LC, Henson PM, Johanston RB (1984) Priming of neutrophils for enhanced release of oxygen metabolites by bacterial lipopolysaccharide. J Exp Med 160:1656–1671
87. Fittshen CF, Sandhaus RA, Worthen GS, Henson PM (1988) Bacterial lipopolysaccharide enhances chemoattractant induced elastase secretion by human neutrophils. J Leukocyte Biol 43:547–556

The Role of the Kallikrein-Kinin System in Septic Shock

R.W. Colman

Introduction

Gram-negative septicemia is a major cause of morbidity in hospitalized patients, with an incidence of about 250.000 documented cases in the United States, or about one case in one thousand individuals. If positive blood cultures are associated with significant hypotension, the mortality ranges from 40-60% [1], and septic shock is one of the major causes of death in the intensive care unit. Because the cardiac output is normal or increased in septicemic hypotension [2], the primary cause of the decreased mean arterial blood pressure must be the decreased peripheral resistance due to vasodilation. Among the candidate mediators, one must consider tumor necrosis factor [3], interleukin-1 [4], prostacyclin [5], and complement fragments such as the anaphylatoxins [6]. Because bradykinin, liberated from kininogen by plasma kallikrein, is one of the most potent vasodilators [7], it may play a major role in the shock associated with gram-negative bacteremia. Thus, the contact system is an appropriate candidate as a source of mediators to account for the hypotension accompanying gram-negative bacteremia. This chapter presents the evidence from patient observation and animal models for the participation of the kallikrein-kinin system in hypotensive septicemia.

Proteins of the Contact System

Four proteins, coagulation factor XII (FXII), prekallikrein (PK), factor XI (FXI), and high molecular weight kininogen (HK), are required for the activation, and three, C1-inhibitor (C1-INH), α_2-macroglobulin (α_2M), and α_1-antitrypsin (α_1-AT), for the inhibition of the surface-medidated pathways. The zymogens, FXII, PK, and FXI, are converted, by limited proteolysis, into the active serine proteases. HK is a non-enzymatic procofactor for these interconversions, and C1-INH is the major inhibitor of activated kallikrein and activated FXII, α_2M of kallikrein and α_1-AT of factor XIa. These proteases interact at the biochemical interfaces of intrinsic coagulation with other plasma proteolytic pathways. These enzymes are required in the initiation, amplification, and propagation of surface-mediated defense reactions by activating C1, factor VII, prorenin, and plasminogen directly, as well as by stimulating neutrophils and by releasing bradykinin. Thus, the molecular events of the contact phase of coagulation, activation, and inhibition affect a number of important plasma biochemical systems and may play an important role in hypotensive septicemia.

Factor XII

FXII is a single-chain β-globulin with a molecular weight of 76.000 and an isoelectric point of 6.1 to 6.5. In plasma, FXII circulates as an inactive zymogen with an estimated concentration of 29 μg/ml. Its complete amino-acid sequence of 596 residues has been determined [8]. Upon contact with model negatively charged surfaces such as glass, kaolin, and dextran sulfate, FXII is autoactivated (solid-phase activation) [9]. Biologic components, which include articular cartilage, skin, fatty acids, and endotoxin, also promote solid-phase activation of FXII. Cerebroside sulfates, a biological component of all cell membranes [10], certain glycosaminoglycans, and components of mucosal mast cell are very potent activators of FXII. Enzymatic activation of FXII (fluid-phase activation) gives rise to successively smaller molecules, each with the same active site. Two proteolytic products of activated FXII have been well characterized. FXIIa is formed by cleavage of the bond connecting Arg^{353}-Val^{354}, generating a two-chain molecule composed of a heavy chain (353 residues) and a light chain (243 residues) held together by a disulfide bond. The heavy chain of FXIIa contains homologous structural regions similar to those found in tissue-type plasminogen activator [8] of unknown function except for the "finger" region which contains the surface binding site [11]. FXII fragment (Mr 30.000) is produced by cleavage of the bonds between Arg^{334}-Asn^{335}, Arg^{343}-$Leu^{344,}$ and Arg^{353}-$Val^{354,}$ resulting in two polypeptide chains (9 and 243 residues in size), held together by a disulfide bond.

Factor XI

Factor XI, a fast γ-globulin with an isoelectric point of 8.9 to 9.1, is a two-chain hemodimer with an estimated molecular weight of 160 kDa by non-reduced SDS-PAGE [12]. On reduced SDS-PAGE, the molecule consists of two apparently identical 80 kDa subunits held together by disulfide bonds. FXI circulates in plasma (2 μg to 7 μg/ml) as a complex with the contact phase procofactor HK [13]. Once adsorbed to an anionic surface through HK (after the HK is converted to its active form HKa [14]), FXI is activated by FXIIa [12], by cleavage of the peptide bond Arg^{369}-Ile^{370} on each chain. The resulting serine protease is composed of two light chains containing the active sites and two heavy chains bridged by disulfide bonds [15]. In turn, activated FXIa catalyzes the activation of FIX by the cleavage of internal Arg-Ala and Arg-Val bonds with the release of a small glycopeptide with a molecular weight of 11 kDa. From the sequence of a cDNA insert coding for

FXI, the primary structure has been elucidated [15]. Four tandem repeats designated as "apple" domains [16] are present in the heavy chain of FXIa. Distinct and separate binding sites for the cofactor HK and for the substrate FIX are present on each of the heavy chains of FXIa.

Prekallikrein

Plasma prekallikrein is a fast γ-globulin with an isoelectric point between 8.5 and 9.0 [17], and it circulates in blood with an estimated concentration of 35 to 50 μg/ml. Approximately 75% circulates bound to HK [18], and the remainder as free PK. By SDS-PAGE, plasma PK consists of two components of Mr 85.000 and 88.000, which differ in the degree of glycosylation. Plasma PK is synthesized in the liver [19]. Analysis of the cDNA for PK has allowed determination of the amino-acid sequence [20] which shows a 50% homology with factor XI. The conversion of PK to kallikrein occurs either on a surface, which is catalyzed by FXIIa or by factor XII fragment in the fluid phase [21]. The surface-mediated activation of PK is similar to the activation of factor XI (see previous paragraph). A single bond (Arg^{371}-Ile^{372}) is split, generating a heavy chain of 371 amino-acids which contains four tandem repeats of 91 amino-acids similar to the "apple" domains of factor XI [22]. The light chain contains the catalytic triad His, Asp, and Ser. The heavy chain is required for complexing with HK [23]. The HK binding domain of PK resides on the C-terminal, 231 amino-acids of the heavy chain (amino-acids 141-371) [24]. In addition, studies using a monoclonal antibody to PK heavy chain indicate that there is also a site on this C-terminal portion of the heavy chain for the interaction with activated factor XII that is separate and distinct from the HK binding site.

The light chain of kallikrein is the site for reactions with protease inhibitors. In plasma, kallikrein is rapidly inactivated by α2-macroglobulin and C1-INH. C1-INH forms a 1/1 stoichiometric complex with kallikrein [25] resulting in complete loss of proteolytic and amidolytic activity. Alpha-2-macroglobulin inhibits the kinin-forming activity of kallikrein, but only partially inhibits its esterolytic activity and its amidolytic activity [26] by forming a covalent complex with kallikrein.

High Molecular Weight Kininogen

Two forms of kininogen exist in human plasma. The high molecular weight kininogen (HK) displays an apparent molecular weight of 120.000 on reduced SDS-PAGE [27]. The low molecular weight kininogen (LK) has a molecular weight of 68.000 daltons on SDS-PAGE. HK is an α-globulin with an isoelectric point of 4.3 and a plasma concentration of 70-90 μg/ml [27]. LK is a β-globulin with an isoelectric point of 4.7 and a plasma concentration of approximately 160 μg/ml [28]. HK and LK have an identical amino-terminal heavy chain, the bradykinin moiety, but each has a unique carboxyl-terminal light chain. Both HK and LK are coded for by the same single copy gene [29]. Differential splicing of the primary transcript from kininogen yields two mRNAs. The major function of the heavy chain of LK and HK is to inhibit proteases with cysteine at their active sites including the calcium-activated cysteine proteases (calpains) [30]. The HK light chain is that portion of the HK molecule that possesses the HK coagulant activity [31], i.e. the ability to bind to anionic surfaces [32] and the ability to associate with the zymogens PK and FXI [33]. The region responsible for surface binding has been hypothesized to be in the histidine-glycine rich region, and recent studies [34] have shown that critical amino-acids (residues 459-475) within the histidine-glycine rich region are responsible for binding an artificial negatively charged surface.

Plasma kallikrein cleaves HK in a three-step sequential manner [35]. The first two cleavages yield bradykinin (non-apeptide) and an intermediate kinin-free protein. The third cleavage results in a stable kinin-free protein composed of two disulfide-linked 64.000 dalton and 45.000 dalton chains and liberates a small 7 kDa peptide. This cleaved form of human HK appears to bind to a greater extent to an activating surface [14]. Thus, in plasma, HK exists as a procofactor that can be activated to HKa by cleavage with kallikrein [14]. FXIa appears to cleave HK at a different sequence of bonds initially, and prolonged exposure of HK to FXIa results in complete proteolysis of the HK light chain into small molecular weight peptides with a loss of coagulant cofactor activity [36].

Regulation of the System

The regulators of activation of this system are naturally occurring plasma protease inhibitors, C1-INH, α2-macroglobulin, and α1-antitrypsin. C1-INH is the major inhibitor of this system and contributes more than 90% of the inhibitory activity in plasma toward both FXIIa [37] and FXIIf [38]. When plasma is activated by kaolin at 37° C, C1-INH accounts for 75% of the inhibition of kallikrein with α2-macroglobulin responsible for 25% [39]. The rate of inhibition of kallikrein, activated FXIIa or FXIIf in plasma is relatively rapid, but FXIa is inactivated approximately 10 times more slowly. The predominant inhibitor of FXIa, α1-antitrypsin, accounts for two-thirds of the inhibitory activity of plasma toward FXIa [40]. Inhibition of the contact activation enzymes differs from that of the serine proteases in the later stages of the coagulation cascade, which are predominantly regulated by antithrombin III. Not only is antithrombin III a poor inhibitor of FXIIa, FXIa and kallikrein, but heparin, which markedly accelerates inactivation of FXa and thrombin by antithrombin III, exhibits minimal enhancement of the inactivation of the contact enzymes [41].

Relationship of the Contact System to Blood Pressure Regulation

Kallikrein cleavage of HK results in the release of bradykinin, one of the most potent vasodilators known [7]. One of the plasma inactivators of bradykinin, kininase II [42], has been shown to be identical to angiotensin-converting enzyme. The net effect of this enzyme is to tend to raise blood pressure by destroying bradykinin (a vasodilator) and producing angiotensin II (a vasoconstrictor).

Interaction of the Complement and Contact Systems

C1-INH, the major plasma protease inhibitor of FXIIa, FXIIf, and kallikrein, is also the major inhibitor of the activated first component of complement C1r and C1s [43]. FXIIf can activate the classic pathway of complement by interacting with macromolecular C1 [44]. C1 activation by FXIIf is enzymatic, and is due to direct activation of the C1r subcomponent of C1 and to a lesser degree to C1s [44].

Laboratory Detection of Contact System Activation

From the biochemical reactions of the enzymes, cofactors and inhibitors, one can predict the changes in plasma (Table 1).

Following activation, factor XII and prekallikrein are converted to active enzymes that rapidly react with C1-INH to form complexes of factor XIIa-C1-INH and kallikrein-C1-INH. The result is depletion of the functional FXIIa and Kal. However, if the complexes have not been cleared from the circulation, the detectable levels of prekallikrein and factor XII antigens should appear normal. Functional C1-INH also declines, but, as measured by antigen, it remains constant or may even increase, suggesting that it behaves as a weak acute phase reactant [41]. As functional C1-INH is cleaved to an

Table 1. Assays of contact system in hypotensive septicemia

Factor	↓	Factor XII	↔	XIIa - C1-INH
Prekallikrein	↓	Prekallikrein	↔	K-C1-INH ↑ α_2M-Kal ↑
C1-INH	↓	C1–INH	↔ or ↑	
HK	↓	HK	↓	Bradykinin ↑
FXI	↑	Factor XI	?	FXIa - α_1AT ↑

Abbrev: HK: high molecular weight kininogen; XIIa: factor XIIa; C1-INH: C1 inhibitor; K: kallikrein; ↓: decreased; ↔: unchanged; ↑:increased inactive form, α2M becomes a more important inhibitor and α2M-Kal complexes form. HK is a substrate that liberates bradykinin when attacked by plasma kallikrein. The rise in bradykinin is only transient because 95% is cleared during one passage through the lungs. The functional coagulant activity as well as the detectable antigen of HK decrease in parallel. This is most likely due to destruction by factor XIa [36], which is known to cleave and inactivate HK. Paradoxically, for unknown reasons, functional factor XI increases. Factor XIa-α1-antitrypsin complexes have been found to be low in disseminated intravascular coagulation (DIC) [45].

Studies of the Kallikrein-Kinin System in Clinical Sepsis

In our early investigations of patients with gram-negative sepsis, we were limited to functional studies of factor XII, prekallikrein and C1-INH. In the first, we studied 54 individuals. Four groups were distinguished: normal, hypotensive due to blood loss, normotensive with bacteremia, and hypotensive bacteremia [46]. Those individuals who were hypotensive due to blood loss did not differ from normal in functional levels of factor XII, prekallikrein and C1-INH. Those with septicemia alone showed some decrease, but it was not significant statistically. Only the hypotensive septicemia groups showed significantly decreased levels of contact factors, indicating activation of the kallikrein-kinin system. Another 23 patients with clinical and laboratory criteria for DIC [47] associated with septicemia or viremia with endothelial injury, experienced a decrease of functional factor XII, prekallikrein and C1-INH consistent with factor XII activation. In contrast, in patients with neoplasia where tumor or monocyte tissue factor may be the initiating agent, no significant changes occurred in the kallikrein-kinin system [48]. In a third group of patients with postoperative septicemia [49], decreased prekallikrein activity and elevated bradykinin were associated with positive blood cultures and hypotension.

We next introduced the use of immunological assays of contact system proteins in investigating an experimental infection of humans with typhoid fever during a vaccine trial [50]. In a typical patient with typhoid fever, prekallikrein inhibitor activity decreased concomitant with the fall in platelets, appearance of a positive blood culture, and fever. All patients with typhoid fever showed a decrease in functional prekallikrein and C1-INH but the corresponding antigens remain unaffected. We hypothesized that this could be explained by the occurrence of kallikrein-C1-INH complexes circulating *in vivo*. We detected this complex using crossed immunoelectrophoresis during the febrile episode. This complex not only expressed kallikrein antigen but also C1-INH antigen, and demonstrated a more anodal migration than prekallikrein. This was the first demonstration of circulating kallikrein-C1-INH complexes.

The adult respiratory distress syndrome (ARDS) is a clinical complex of non-cardiogenic pulmonary edema with refractory hypoxemia and decreased pulmonary compliance. ARDS may occur following a variety of insults, and results from an abnormally permeable alveolar-capillary membrane. Activation of proteins of the contact system may play a significant role in the pathogenesis of this disorder by stimulating neutrophils to synthesize and release substances that can cause endothelial and epithelial injury and enhance the inflammatory response. Many cases are due to sepsis. Schapira et al. [51] demonstrated prekallikrein activation in ARDS. In a recent study, we introduced the measurement of HK activity and antigen [52]. Patients with ARDS have significantly reduced plasma levels of factor XII and PK. We found that HK was also decreased, and documented increased levels of C1-INH antigen with decreased levels of C1-INH activity. The measurement of plasma HK in patients with septic shock may therefore have prognostic value. In young victims of traumatic injuries complicated by sepsis, a good correlation exists between HK levels and survival [1]. A profound drop in HK levels usually is associated with a lethal outcome in hospitalized patients with septic shock, while HK levels rise toward normal in those patients who survive. In contrast, PK decrease seems to be sensitive but less closely related to survival. Decreased levels of prekallikrein have been documented not only in bacteremia but in septicemia due to viruses, fungi, and Rickettsia [53, 54]. Patients with Rocky Mountain spotted fever have decreased PK levels with increased kallikrein-C1-INH complexes [55, 56]. However, in most cases of septic shock, kallikrein-C1-INH complexes did not increase [57]. We therefore developed a "sandwich" ELISA for α_2M-Kal complexes [58] and found that in septicemic hypotension, α_2M-Kal complexes were elevated but not in septicemia alone. Prekallikrein activity was decreased and prekallikrein antigen was normal [41, 52].

In a more controlled study, *E. coli* endotoxin was infused into normal volunteers, and PK and FXI decreased in addition to an increase in plasma levels of α_2M-Kal complexes [59]. These changes were relatively small in magnitude, probably relative to the low concentrations of endotoxin infused.

All of these human studies document that the contact system is markedly activated during septicemic hypotension and moderately activated during endotoxin infusion. However, to prove that the activation is related to either the shock or DIC, animal studies are required. Infusion of endotoxin into Rhesus monkeys [60] caused hypotension, and elevated bradykinin levels were measured. Unfortunately, it is now known that the methods for collecting the plasma for bradykinin measurements did not exclude *in vitro* activation. Mason et al. [46] infused endotoxin into mice and rats and documented a decrease in prekallikrein and kallikrein inhibitor levels. Weisser et al. [61] demonstrated that the pattern of the acute response to endotoxin or bacterial infection in pigs resembled that in man. Further, they documented a decrease in prekallikrein during endotoxin infusion. Accordingly, we selected a septic pig model for a study of a potent protease inhibitor in gram-negative septicemia [15].

Our studies of the inactivation and the formation of enzyme-inhibitor complexes of each contact system enzyme by each plasma protease inhibitor indicate that each inhibitor functions relatively slowly compared to the rapid inhibition of elastase by α_1-antitrypsin (α_1-AT). For therapeutic purposes, a much more rapid reaction was needed. A variant of α_1-antitrypsin, designated α_1-antitrypsin-Pittsburgh (α_1-ATP), identified as a point mutation involving the replacement of methionine at position 358 in the cleavage site of the molecule by arginine, occurred in a single patient where it functioned as a potent thrombin inhibitor [62] and caused uncontrollable bleeding. Because the enzymes of the contact phase of plasma proteolysis (factor XIa, activated factor XII and kallikrein) primarily cleave bonds containing arginine in the P1 position, we hypothesized and demonstrated that α_1-ATP might function as an efficient inhibitor of these enzymes [63]. When purified factor XIa was incubated with pure α_1-ATP at plasma concentrations, the data indicated that the second-order rate constant, k", for the inactivation of factor XIa by α_1-antitrypsin-Pittsburgh, was 1600-fold higher than normal α_1AT, and 630-fold greater than antithrombin III toward inactivation of factor XIa. When purified kallikrein was incubated with ATP, the rapid inactivation by α_1-ATP was 10.000-fold greater than normal AT III, a weak inactivator, under the same conditions, and 160-fold greater than antithrombin III, which has moderate inhibitor activity toward kallikrein. Therefore, α_1ATP is also a potent inhibitor of plasma kallikrein. The k" for inactivation of factor XIIf by α_1-ATP was found to be $1.6 \times 10^4\ M^{-1}s^{-1}$. This rate of reaction is very striking, since normal α_1-AT does not detectably inactivate factor XIIf. Furthermore, α_1-ATP was calculated to be 150-fold more potent than antithrombin III in the inactivation of factor XIIf [64].

Because, in gram-negative septicemia, the activation of contact proteases, consumption of plasma protease inhibitors, and concomitant hypotension occur, we hypothesized that infusion of α_1-ATP might increase the survival rate by blocking this pathway. Because α_1-ATP also blocks thrombin action, it

Table 2. Effect of pretreatment with rAT-P on plasma proteins in pigs during sepsis[a]

	Bacteria + dextrose ± saline (Group I)	Bacteria + r-ATP (Group II)
ATIII[b]	69.9 ± 24.3	91.8 ± 19.7
Prekallikrein	84.0 ± 23.5	90.2 ± 6.8
Factor XI[b]	82.4 ± 31.5	104.7 ± 10.9
Fibrinogen[b]	81.1 ± 34.2	100.7 ± 2.5
FDP (μg/ml)[bc]	7.4	2.13

Results are expressed as the mean ± SD of the percent of initial value (prior to bacterial infusion. [a]Values were determined 1 h after bacterial infusion. [b]$P<0.05$. [c]FDP expressed as geometric mean. Normal range is 1.2-4.9 μg/ml. (From [65] with permission)

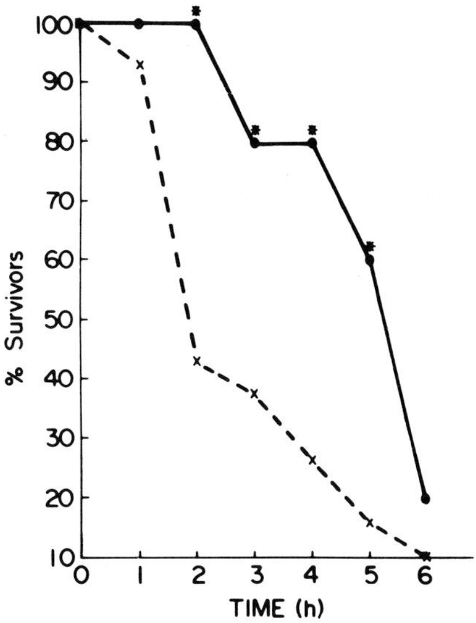

Fig. 1. Comparison of survival rates of septic treated and untreated pigs. The survival rate of Group I (untreated septic pigs, n = 14) and Group II (r-ATP treated septic pigs, n = 5) were evaluated for statistical significance. Group I x---x; Group II. .---. *P.<0.05 (From [65] with permission)

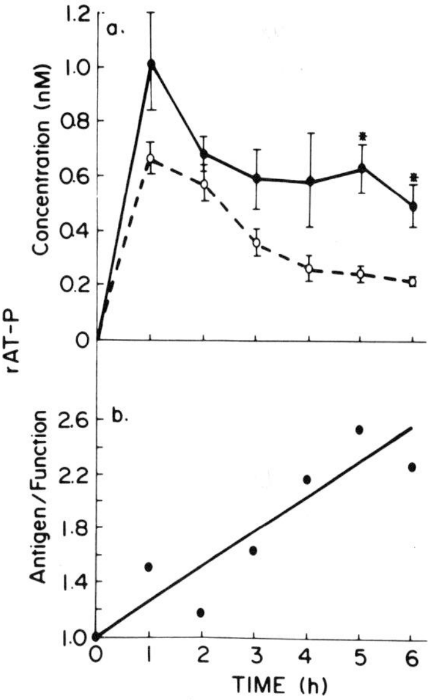

Fig. 2. Top. Comparison or r-ATP function and antigen *in vivo*. Antigenic (•) and functional (o) levels of r-ATP were determined in the plasma of septic pigs after the initial 100-mg infusion as well as during the continuous infusion of the inhibitor. The data represent the mean SEM ± Bottom. The ratio of antigenic (total r-ATP protein) and function r-ATP were plotted versus time (From [65] with permission)

might also prevent the development of DIC, which is a common manifestation of this disease. The experimental model consisted of two groups of pigs [65]. Group I was composed of 14 animals infused with *Pseudomonas aeruginosa* and saline, while Group II was composed of 5 animals infused with *Pseudomonas* (2×10^8 CFU) and recombinant α_1-ATP (r-α_1ATP) produced in yeast. To control for variation in response to a set concentration of bacteria,

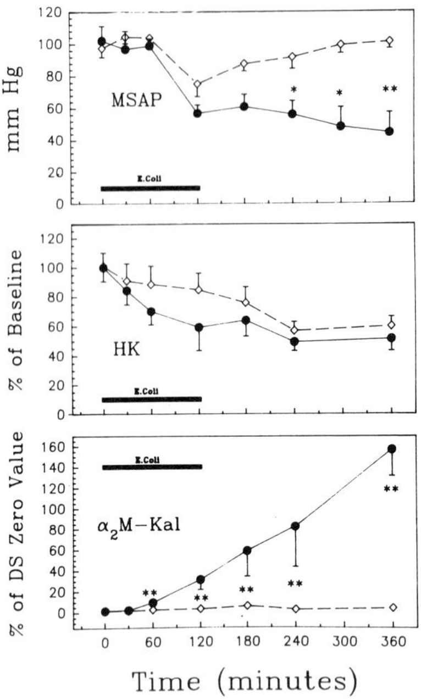

Fig. 3. Mean systemic arterial pressure (MSAP), and levels of high molecular weight kininogen (HK) and α2M-Kal complexes of lethal (•) and nonlethal (o) group. The differences between lethal and nonlethal groups, determined by Mann-Whitney U test, are significant (*p<0.025) and highly significant (**p<0.01) (From [66] with permission)

each animal was infused with sufficient bacteria to maintain the pulmonary artery pressure (PAP) at twice baseline as well as comparable sytemic artery pressure between the two groups at the same time. Thus, no effect of the inhibitor on the blood pressure could be assessed. Assay of plasma proteolytic systems at 1 h revealed significant differences between the group treated with r-α_1ATP and the untreated septic control group (Table 2). The untreated septic animals (Group 1) had significantly lower values of ATIII, factor XI and fibrinogen, and significantly higher levels of FDP. Thus, the untreated group failed to show the coagulation and contact system changes. Survival in group 2 was significantly increased during 2-5 h but not at 6 h (Fig. 1). We found that by 5 h the antigenic level was 60% of the original 1 μM obtained, but the functional levels were only 0.25 μM due to complex formation of the r-α_1ATP with the endogenously activated proteases (Fig. 2). Although these results indicated that the mutant inhibitor afforded protection in experimental gram-negative septicemia, because r-α_1ATP acts on thrombin, plasma, kallikrein, factor XIIa and factor XIa, its mechanism of action is unclear.

We therefore decided to utilize an established experimental baboon model of bacteremia which allowed the use of both diagnostic and therapeutic immunological tools, because monoclonal and polyclonal antibodies to the contact system crossreacted with the homologous proteins in baboon plasma. Two concentrations of *E. coli* were used to produce lethal and non-lethal hypotension (Fig. 3). The lethal group (n = 5) developed irreversible hypotension which significantly correlated with the decline in functional levels of

HK and an increase in α_2M-Kal complexes [66]. The non-lethal group (n=9) experienced reversible hypotension, a less striking decline in HK, and only slight elevation in α_2M-Kal. No significant changes were found in levels of factor XII, prekallikrein and factor XI in either group. A significant change in the contact system, which reflects the fatal outcome, is the rise in α_2M-Kal. This study suggests that irreversible hypotension correlates with prolonged activation of the contact system. To further investigate this relationship, we studied whether the infusion of a monoclonal antibody (MAb) to factor XII, which could neutralize its coagulant activity, could modulate the pathophysiological response and the biochemical changes in the contact system [67]. When the MAb was infused prior to a lethal concentration of *E. coli,* the factor XII activity fell to 40% of its value when the MAb was present at 1.5 mM. The contact system was inhibited as judged by the prevention of the decrease in functional HK and the increase in α_2M-Kal complexes seen in the untreated group. Moreover, the irreversible phase of the hypotension was prevented, although the initial rapid fall in blood pressure still occurred, and the survival of the antibody-treated group was prolonged. Interestingly, the DIC which occurs in the lethal untreated group, marked by a fall in fibrinogen, factor V and platelet count and a rise in fibrinogen degradation products, was not affected by the antibody. We conclude that the hypotension is probably mediated, at least in part, by the contact system but that the DIC is initiated by other pathways, probably the tissue factor pathway.

Conclusion

Biochemical observations during clinical sepsis using functional and immunological measurements of enzymes, cofactors and inhibitors of the kallikrein-kinin system indicate that activation of these proteases occur during hypotensive gram-negative septicemia and ARDS. Using animal models of septicemia, we demonstrated that protease inhibitors or neutralizing monoclonal antibodies to proteins of the contact system inhibit or prevent the formation of kallikrein and the decrease in kininogen. In addition, the irreversible phase of hypotension can be prevented and survival prolonged. Thus, bradykinin is one of the important mediators of hypotension. In contrast, the contact system plays little role in the associated DIC.

Acknowledgments. This review was supported by a Specialized Center of Research in Thrombosis, HL45486.

References

1. Hirsch EF, Nakajima T, Oshima G, Erdos EG, Herman CM (1974) Kinin system responses in sepsis after trauma in man. J Surg Res 17:147–153
2. Suffredini AF, Fromm RE, Parker MM, et al. (1989) The cardiovascular response of normal humans to the administration of endotoxin. N Engl J Med 321:280–287
3. Beutler B, Cerami A (1987) Cachectin: More than a tumor necrosis factor. N Engl J Med 316:379–385
4. Wakabayashi G, Gelfand JA, Burke JF, Thompson RC, Dinarello CA (1991) A specific receptor antagonist for interleukin 1 prevents Escherichia coli-induced shock in rabbits. FASEB J 5:338–343
5. Carmona RH, Tsao TC, Trunkey DD (1984) The role of prostacyclin and thromboxane in sepsis and septic shock. Arch Surg 119:189–192
6. Hack CE, Nuijens JH, Felt-Bersma RJ, et al. (1989) Elevated plasma levels of the anaphylatoxins C3a and C4a are associated with a fatal outcome in sepsis. Am J Med 86:20-26
7. Jacobsen S (1966) Substrates for plasma kinin-forming enzymes in human, dog and rabbit plasmas. Br J Pharmacol 26:403–411
8. Cool DE, Edgell CJ, Louie GV, Zoller MJ, Brayer GD, MacGillivray RT (1985) Characterization of human blood coagulation factor XII cDNA: Prediction of the primary structure of factor XII and the tertiary structure of beta-factor XIIa. J Biol Chem 260:13666–13676
9. Silverberg M, Dunn JT, Garen L, kaplan AP (1980) Autoactivation of human Hageman factor: Demonstration using a synthetic substrate. J Biol Chem 225:7281–7286
10. Tans G, Rosing J, Griffin JH (1983) Sulfatide-dependent autoactivation of human blood coagulation factor XII (Hageman Factor). J Biol Chem 258:8215–8222
11. Pixley RA, Stumpo LG, Birkmeyer K, Silver L, Colman RW (1987) A monoclonal antibody recognizing an icosapeptide sequence in the heavy chain of human factor XII inhibits surface catalyzed activation. J Biol Chem 262:10140–10145
12. Kurachi K, Davie EW (1977) Activation of human factor XI (plasma thromboplastin antecedent) by factor XIIa (activated Hageman Factor). Biochemistry 16:5831–5839
13. Thompson RE, Mandle R Jr, Kaplan AP (1977) Association of factor XI and high molecular weight kininogen in human plasma. J Clin Invest 60:1376–1380
14. Scott CF, Silver LD, Schapira M, Colman RW (1984) Cleavage of human high molecular weight kininogen markedly enhances its coagulant activity: Evidence that this molecule exists as a procofactor. J Clin Invest 73:954–962
15. Fujikawa K, Chung DW, Hendrickson LE, Davie EW (1986) Amino-acid sequence of human factor XI, a blood coagulation factor with four tandem repeats that are highly homologous with plasma prekallikrein. Biochemistry 25:2417–2424
16. McMullen BA, Fujikawa, K, Davie EW (1991) Location of the disulfide bonds in human coagulation factor XI: The presence of tandem apple domains. Biochemistry 30:2056–2060
17. McConnell DJ, Mason B (1970) The isolation of human plasma prekallikrein. Br J Pharmacol 38:490-502
18. Mandle RJ, Colman RW, Kaplan AP (1976) Identification of prekallikrein and high molecular weight kininogen as a complex in human plasma. Proc natl Acad Sci USA 73: 4179–4183
19. Wong P, Colman RW, Talamo RC, Babior BM (1972) Kallikrein-bradykinin system in chronic alcoholic liver disease. Ann Intern Med 77:205–209
20. Chung DW, Fujikawa K, McMullen BA, Davie EW (1986) Human plasma prekallikrein, a zymogen to a serine protease that contains four tandem repeats. Biochemistry 25:2410–2417
21. Wuepper KD, Cochrane CG (1972) Plasma prekallikrein: Isolation, characterization, and mechanism of activation. J Exp med 135:1–20
22. McMullen BA, Fujikawa K, Davie EW (1991) Location of the disulfide bonds in human plasma prekallikrein: The presence of four novel apple domains in the amino terminal portion of the molecule. Biochemistry 30:2050–2056
23. Burger D, Schleuning WD, Schapira M (1986) Human plasma prekallikrein: Immunoaffinity, purification and activation to alpha- and beta-kallikrein. J Biol Chem 261:324–327

24. Page JD, Colman RW (1991) Localization of distinct functional domains on prekallikrein for interaction with both high molecular weight kininogen and activated factor XII in a 28 kDa fragment (amino-acids 141-371). J Biol Chem 266:8143–8148
25. Gigli I, Mason JW, Colman RW, Austen KF (1970) Interaction of plasma kallikrein with C1-inhibitor. J Immunol 104:574–581
26. Schapira M, Scott CF, Colmann RW (1981) Protection of human plasma kallikrein from inactivation of C1-inhibitor and other protease inhibitors: The role of high molecular weight kininogen. Biochemistry 20:2738–2743
27. Kerbiriou DM, Griffin JH (1979) Human high molecular weight kininogen: Studies of structure-function relationships and of proteolysis of the molecule occurring during contact activation of plasma. J Biol Chem 245:12020–12027
28. Muller-Esterl W, Vohle-Timmerman M, Boos B, Dittman B (1982) Purification and properties of human low molecular weight kininogen. Biochem Biophys Acta 706:145–152
29. Kitamura N, Kitagawa H, Fukushima D, et al. (1985) Structural organization of the kininogen gene and a model for its evolution. J Biol Chem 260:8610–8617
30. Schmaier AH, Bradford H, Silver ID, et al. (1986) High molecular weight kininogen is an inhibitor of platelet calpain. J Clin Invest 77:1565–1573
31. Thompson RE, Mandle R Jr, Kaplan AP (1978) Characterization of human high molecular weight kininogen: Procoagulant activity associated with the light chain of kinin-free high molecular weight kininogen. J Exp Med 147:488–499
32. Retzios AD, Rosenfeld R, Schiffman S (1987) Effects of chemical modifications on the surface- and protein-binding properties of the light chain of human high molecular weight kininogen. J Biol Chem 262:3074–3081
33. Tait JF, Fujikawa K (1987) Primary structure requirements for the binding of human high molecular weight kininogen to plasma prekallikrein and factor XI. J Biol Chem 262:11651–11656
34. DeLa Cadena RA, Colman RW (1989) Effect of synthetic peptides derived from HMW-kininogen on its surface mediated coagulant activity. Clin Res 37:379a
35. Mori K, Nagasawa S (1981) Studies on human high molecular weight (HMW) kininogen. II. Structural change of HMW kininogen by the action of human plasma kallikrein. J Biochem 89:1465–1473
36. Scott CF, Silver LD, Purdon AD, Colman RW (1985) Cleavage of human high molecular weight kininogen by factor XIa *in* vitro: Effect on structure and function. J Biol Chem 260:10856–10863
37. Pixley RA, Schapira M, Colman RW (1985) The regulation of human factor XIIa by plasma proteinase inhibitors. J Biol Chem 260:1723–1729
38. De Agostini A, Lijnen HR, Pixley RA, Colman RW, Schapira M (1984) Inactivation of factor XII active fragment in normal plasma: Predominant role of C1-inhibitor. J Clin Invest 73:1542–1549
39. Schmaier AH, Gustafson E, Idell S, Colman RW (1984) Plasma prekallikrein assay: Reversible inhibition of C1-inhibitor by chloroform and its use in measuring prekallikrein in different mammalian species. J Lab Clin Med 104:882–892
40. Scott CF, Schapira M, James HL, Cohen AB, Colman RW (1982) Inactivation of factor XIa by plasma protease inhibitors: Predominant role of α1-protease inhibitor and protective effect of high molecular weight kininogen. J Clin Invest 69:844–852
41. Colman RW, Scott CF, Pixley RA, DeLa Cadena RA (1989) Effect of heparin on the inhibition of the contact system enzymes. Ann NY Acad Sci USA 556:95–103
42. Yang HY, Erdos EG (1967) Second kininase in human blood plasma. Nature 215:1402–1403
43. Laurell AB, Johnson U, Martensson U, Sjoholm AG (1978) Formation of complexes composed of C1r, C1s, and C1 inactivator in human serum on activation of C1. Acta Pathol Microbiol Scand 86C:299–306
44. Ghebrehiwet B, Silverberg M, Kaplan AP (1981) Activation of the classical pathway of complement by Hageman factor fragment. J Exp Med 153:665–676
45. Nishikado H, Komiyama Y, Masuda M, Egawa M, Murata K (1986) Factor XIa-α1-antitrypsin complex: Elevation in patients with DIC. Thromb Res 44:489–501
46. Mason JW, Kleeberg U, Dolan P, Colman RW (1970) Plasma kallikrein and Hageman factor in gram-negative bacteremia. Ann Intern Med 73:545–551

47. Colman RW, Robboy SJ, Minna JD (1972) Disseminated intravascular coagulation (DIC): An approach. Am J Med 52:679–689
48. Mason JW, Colman RW (1971) The role of Hageman factor in disseminated intravascular coagulation induced by septicemia, neoplasia or liver disease. Thromb Diath Haemorrh 26:325
49. O'Donnell TF, Clowes GH, Talamo RC, Colman RW (1976) Kinin activation in the blood of patients with sepsis. Surg Gynecol Obstet 143:539–545
50. Colman RW, Edelman R, Scott CF, Gilman RH (1978) Plasma kallikrein activation and inhibition during typhoid fever. J Clin Invest 61:287–296
51. Schapira M, Gardaz JP, Py P, Lew PD, Perrin LH, Suter PM (1985) Prekallikrein activation in the adult respiratory distress syndrome. Bull Eur Physiopathol Respir 21:237–241
52. Carvalho AC, DeMarinis S, Scott CF, Silver LD, Schmaier AH, Colman RW (1988) Activation of the contact system of plasma proteolysis in the adult respiratory distress syndrome. J Lab Clin Med 112:270–277
53. Robinson JA, Kondnycky ML, Loeb HS, Racic MR, Gunnar RM (1975) Endotoxin, prekallikrein, complement and systemic vascular resistance: Sequential measurements in man. Am J Med 59:61–67
54. Saito H, Poon MC, Vicic W, Goldsmith GH Jr, Menitove JE (1978) Human plasma prekallikrein (Fletcher factor) clotting activity and antigen in health and disease. J Lab Clin Med 92:84–95
55. Yamada T, Harber P, Pettit GW, Wing DA, Oster CN (1978) Activation of the kallikrein-kinin system in Rocky Mountain spotted fever. Ann Intern Med 88:764–768
56. Rao AK, Schapira M, Clements ML, et al. (1988) A prospective study of platelets and plasma proteolytic systems during the early stages of Rocky Mountain spotted fever. N Engl J Med 318:1021–1028
57. Nuijens JH, Huijbregts CC, Eerenberg-Belmer AJ, et al. (1988) Quantification of plasma factor XIIa-C1-inhibitor and kallikrein-C1-inhibitor complexes in sepsis. Blood 72:1841–1848
58. Kaufman N, Page JD, Pixley RA, Schein R, Schmaier AH, Colman RW (1991) Alpha-2-macroglobulin-kallikrein complexes detect contact system activation in hereditary angioedema and human sepsis. Blood 77:2660–2667
59. DeLa Cadena RA, Suffredini AF, Kaufman N, Parrillo JE, Colman RW (1990) Activation of the kallikrein-kinin system after endotoxin administration to normal human volunteers. Clin Res 38:346a
60. Nies AS, Forsyth RP, Williams HE, Melmon KL (1968) Contribution of kinin to endotoxin shock in unanesthetized Rhesus monkeys. Circ Res 22:155–164
61. Weisser A, Clowes GH, Colman RW, Talamo RC (1973) Sepsis and endotoxemia in pigs: A comparison of mortality and pathophysiology. In: Haberland GL, Lewis DH (eds) New Aspects of Trasylol Therapy: The Lung in Shock. Schattauer-Verlag, New York, pp 159–174
62. Owen MC, Brennan SO, Lewis JH, Carrell RW (1983) Mutation of antitrypsin to antithrombin: Alpha-1-antitrypsin Pittsburgh (358 Met-Arg) abated bleeding disorder. N Engl J Med 309:694–698
63. Scott CF, Carrell RW, Glaser CB, Kueppers F, Lewis JH, Colman RW (1986) Alpha-1-antitrypsin Pittsburgh: A potent inhibitor of human plasma factor IXa, kallikrein and factor XIIf. J Clin Invest 77:631–634
64. Schapira M, Ramus MA, Jallat S, Carvallo D, Courtney M (1986) Recombinant alpha-1-antitrypsin Pittsburgh (Met358-Arg) is a potent inhibitor of plasma kallikrein and activated factor XII fragment. J Clin Invest 77:635–637
65. Colman RW, Flores DN, DeLa Cadena RA, et al. (1988) Recombinant alpha-1-antitrypsin Pittsburgh attenuates experimental gram-negative septicemia. Am J Pathol 130:418–426
66. Pixley RA, DeLa Cadena R, Page JD, et al. (1992) Activation of the contact system in lethal hypotensive bacteremia in a baboon model. Am J Pathol 140:897–906
67. Pixley RA, DeLa Cadena RA, Kaufman N, et al. (1990) In vivo use of a monoclonal antibody to factor XII (Hageman factor) in a lethal hypotensive septicemic baboon model. Blood 76:433a

The Procoagulant State in Sepsis: Experimental Models and New Modalities for Intervention

B.J. Biemond, M. Levi, and S.J.H. van Deventer

Introduction

Sepsis is a clinical syndrome comprising derangements of inflammatory, hemodynamic, metabolic and coagulation systems. Sepsis is frequently complicated by irreversible shock, diffuse intravascular coagulation and multiple organ failure (MOF), and despite of the availability of improved supportive measures in intensive care units, the mortality due to sepsis remains around 40-60% [1].

Many investigators have been trying to understand the pathogenic mechanisms of the septic syndrome in order to find new modalities for intervention in the processes involved in the development of the septic syndrome.

This chapter will first focus on the mechanisms involved in the development of the procoagulant state during sepsis which often results in diffuse intravascular coagulation and subsequently MOF. Various experimental models in humans and in animals for the study of coagulation activation in sepsis will be reviewed, and some new specific interventional approaches will be discussed.

Procoagulant State During Sepsis

Experimental Models

In order to develop effective therapeutic strategies that target the coagulation system in sepsis, it is important to determine the mechanisms involved in the development of coagulation disorders associated with sepsis. At present, models of experimental sepsis can be divided into *in vitro* and *in vivo* models. The *in vitro* models often consist of cell-culture systems in which for example cultures of human endothelial cells can be exposed to mediators such as endotoxin or tumor necrosis factor (TNF). These simplified systems can provide adequate answers on the significance of molecular processes at the surface of the endothelial cell, but a main problem of these *in vitro* models is the difficulty to translate the results to the *in vivo* situation. One obvious confounding factor is the lack of possible interactions with other mediators, which cannot be taken into account. In *in vitro* systems this is not a theoretical concern, as it has repeatedly been found that inflammatory mediators may have additive or synergistic effects, and that their combined effects may markedly differ from their individual biological activities.

Experimental studies performed in smaller animals such as the rat and the rabbit do not have these disadvantages, but are nevertheless difficult to compare with the human situation. For instance, the dose of endotoxin per kilogram necessary for the induction of a septic syndrome in an animal such as the rat, is many times higher than needed to induce sepsis in humans. Primate animal models, such as baboons or chimpanzees, appear to be more suitable to study the pathogenetic mechanisms involved in the development of the septic syndrome. In baboons (Papio Cyanocephalus cynocephalus), the efficacy of potential therapeutic substances can be studied by assessing their ability to improve the survival of a lethal *Escherichia coli* infusion [2,3]. In such animal models, the effect of the therapeutic intervention on the coagulopathy induced by septicemia can be defined using well-defined endpoints, such as the amount of fibrinogen consumption and fibrin deposition.

To study the more specific mediators and mechanisms involved in the coagulative response to septicemia, it is necessary to measure either peptides liberated from the coagulation factor zymogens during their activation (activation peptides) or complexes between activated coagulation factors and their natural inhibitors. Because activated coagulation factors in plasma have a very short half-life, direct measurements of these factors during coagulation activation is not feasible. In our experience, the chimpanzee proved to be the only animal in which the specific human assays for these activation peptides and protease-complexes can be used [4]. Because the response of the chimpanzee to an infusion of a low dose of endotoxin is practically identical to the human response, the chimpanzee seems to be a very suitable animal model for coagulopathies associated with sepsis [5]. By using monoclonal antibodies against human epitopes and other specific preparations (not yet suitable for the use in humans), this model can give more insight in the pathogenesis and potential therapeutic approaches in endotoxemia.

Infusion of low doses of endotoxin into healthy volunteers appears to be a very useful model to study coagulation activation during endotoxemia in humans. This model can give more insight in the early dynamics and route of coagulation activation during endotoxemia. Finally, clinical studies in septic patients may be helpful, although these studies are difficult to interpret because of the invariably late stages of coagulation activation at presentation, that in many cases have already proceeded to full-blow disseminated intravascular coagulation (DIC).

In conclusion, it appears that, besides clinical studies in septic patients, studies in primates such as baboons or chimpanzees, as well as experimental studies in healthy volunteers, are particulary useful in the investigation of the hemostatic dysbalance in sepsis.

Endotoxin, Cytokines and Coagulation Activation

Experimental and clinical studies have shown that endotoxin, a lipopolysaccharide (LPS) from the outer membrane of gram-negative bacteria, plays a

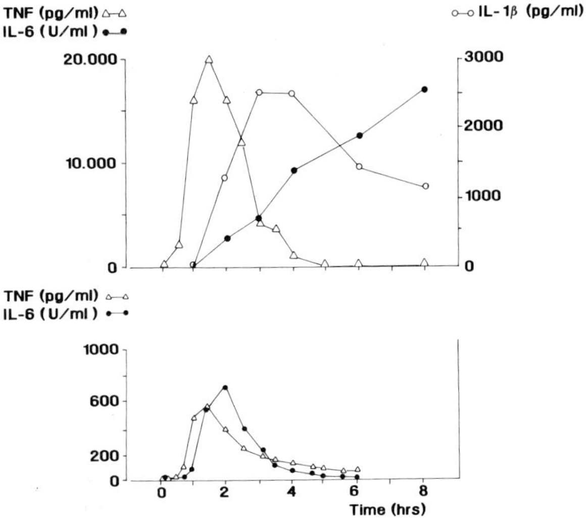

Fig. 1. The appearance in the circulation of TNF, IL-1β and IL-6 after a lethal infusion of E. Coli in baboons (upper panel) and after an intravenous injection of low dose endotoxin in healthy humans (lower panel). In the latter experiment IL-1 activity was not detected in serum

pivotal role in the development of the septic syndrome. Van Deventer et al. [5] observed that the presence of endotoxin in the circulation of febrile patients (endotoxemia) is a more reliable predictor of the development of the clinical syndrome of septicemia than the presence of viable bacteria (bacteremia). Brandtzaeg et al. [6] confirmed this observation and found that the endotoxin level is an important prognostic marker in the clinical outcome of patients with a meningococcal septicemia. Recently, Michie et al. [7] and Van Deventer et al. [8] confirmed that the administration of endotoxin to healthy volunteers induced symptoms of septicemia including fever, tachycardia and decreased mean arterial pressure.

The biological effects of endotoxin appear to be mediated by endogenous proteins (cytokines) which play an important role in the development of the septic syndrome. These cytokines, in particular tumor necrosis factor (TNF), interleukin-1 (IL-1) and interleukin-6 (IL-6), are mainly synthesized and released by monocytes and macrophages, and are the primary mediators in the inflammatory process following endotoxemia. TNF appears as one of the first cytokines in circulation after a challenge with either bacteria or endotoxin [9]. For example, it was shown by Michie et al. [7] and van Deventer et al. [8] that the administration of endotoxin to healthy volunteers induced a rapid release of TNF starting at 30-45 min after the infusion of endotoxin (Fig. 1) and reaching a peak at 60 to 90 min. In models of lethal bacteremia in subhuman primates, the release of TNF is closely followed by a subsequent rise of IL-1. Both cytokines play an important role in the inflammatory response during sepsis and contribute to the activation of leukocytes (in part by induction of IL-8) and the development of endothelial damage. Passive immunization of baboons against TNF resulted in a reduction of the lethality of the septic syndrome induced by the infusion of endotoxin [13]. Infusion of recombinant TNF (r-TNF) in dogs or in human volunteers provoked the occurrence of sepsis-like symptoms such as chills, fever, tachycardia, and an increased leukocyte count [14,16]. Several investigators found IL-6 levels to be markedly elevated in sepsis and to be related to the clinical outcome [10,11]. The temporal difference between the appearance of TNF and IL-6 in the circulation in human volunteers suggests that the release of IL-6 is stimulated by TNF. This hypothesis was confirmed by an observation that monoclonal antibodies directed against TNF almost completely blocked the release of IL-6 following an infusion of a lethal dose of *E. coli* in baboons [12]. In combination, these observations strongly suggest a pivotal role of TNF in the initiation of the septic syndrome.

In many cases, sepsis is complicated by derangements in the hemostatic balance resulting in a procoagulant state. This procoagulant state is a main cause for the development of DIC which results in fibrin deposition in the microvascular system that may be implicated in MOF. Interestingly, it appears that the release of cytokines during endotoxemia induces the procoagulant state by activation of the coagulation system. Activation of the coagulation cascade has been investigated following the infusion of endotoxin in healthy volunteers or chimpanzees or following the infusion of TNF in healthy volunteers or cancer patients [4, 8, 15, 16]. All studies demonstrated factor X activation by measuring the factor X activation peptide (FXP) which is liberated from the zymogen factor X, following activation. Thrombin generation was assessed by measuring F1+2, a fragment liberated from prothrombin during its activation, and by measuring thrombin-antithrombin III complexes and fibrinopeptide A (Fig. 2). Infusion of TNF in healthy volunteers resulted in a sharp rise of FXP at 30-45 min and an increase in F1+2

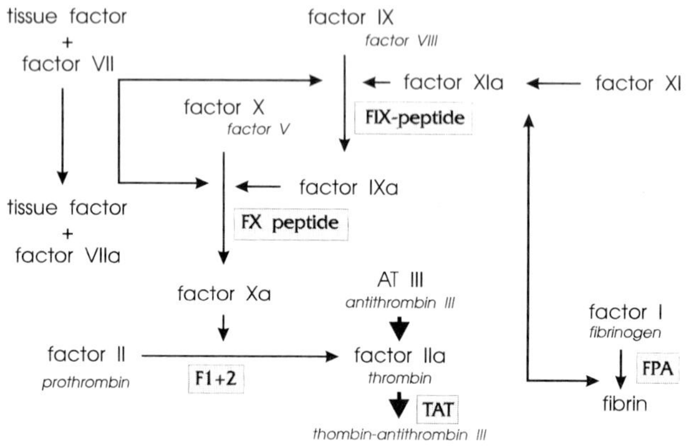

Fig. 2. The location of the different activation peptides (FIX-peptide, FX-peptide, F1+2 and FPA) and thrombin-antithrombin-III-complexes (TAT) in the coagulation cascade. By measuring the activation peptides and activation-complexes coagulation activation can be studied very closely

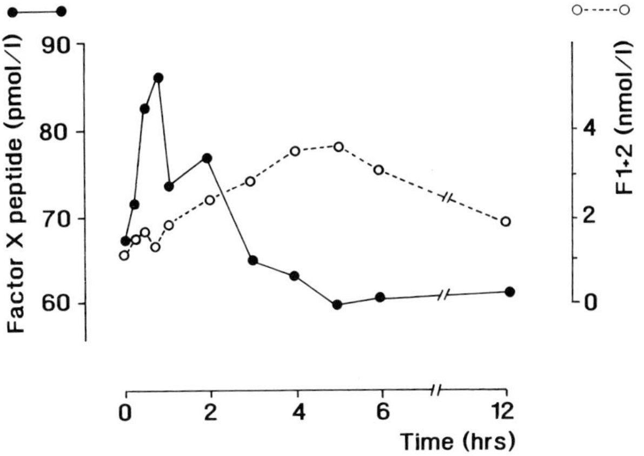

Fig. 3. Mean plasma levels of Factor X activation peptide (FXp) and the prothrombin fragment F1+2 after an intravenous bolus injection of recombinant human TNF in healthy humans

plasma levels at 3-5 h (Fig. 3). These results indicated a rapid activation of the common pathway of the coagulation cascade. Factor X, the first factor of the common pathway, can be activated by either factor IX or by the factor VII-tissue factor complex. Factor IX is thought to be activated by the contact system, comprising the conversion of the zymogens factor XII and prekallikrein to factor XIIa and kallikrein. In patients with sepsis, decreased plasma levels of factor XII and prekallikrein, and increased levels of factor XII-C1 inhibitor complexes and kallikrein-C1 inhibitor complexes have been reported, which are interpreted to indicate contact activation. In contrast, van der Poll et al. [16] and van Deventer et al. [8] showed that the zymogens factor XII and prekallikrein as well as the level of factor XII-C1 inhibitor complexes and kallikrein-C1 inhibitor complexes remained within the normal range after TNF or endotoxin infusion in healthy volunteers indicating that the intrinsic pathway and the contact system are not involved in the initiation of coagulation activation during sepsis. This was further stressed by measuring the level of factor IX activation peptide (FIXP), liberated from the zymogen factor IX following activation, which was not affected by the infusion of TNF. These findings suggested that the initial activation of coagulation by endotoxin or TNF is not induced by the contact system but probably by the extrinsic coagulation pathway or by an alternative route via MAC-1 receptors at the surface of monocytes as suggested by Altieri et al. [17]. The extrinsic pathway is activated by complex formation of tissue factor and factor VIIa resulting in an enhanced conversion of factor X. Indeed, in meningococcal sepsis in children, an increased tissue factor (TF) activation and expression on monocytes has been reported [18]. The release of TNF might be responsible for the activation and expression of TF on monocytes and the subsequent induction of coagulation activation via the extrinsic pathway

[16]. The rapid time-course of the factor X activation following intravenous administration of TNF, however, could also indicate exposure of TF that is expressed at cryptogenic sites, for example at subendothelial sites, to the blood. In contrast to all these studies however de Boer et al. [19] found, following the lethal infusion of *E. coli* in baboons, generation of thrombin as reflected by an increase in circulating levels of thrombin-antithrombin complexes (TAT-complexes), before TNF release could be detected. A possible explanation, suggested by the authors, might be the initial activation of TF by the complement system rather than the cytokine release in this model.

In any case, the discussed observations in endotoxin- or TNF-challenged volunteers suggest an important role for tissue factor in the initial activation of coagulation in sepsis. Besides the coagulation activation induced by TF activation/expression, the procoagulant state is further promoted by the downregulation of protein C and protein S activity. Protein C and protein S are plasma proteins with anticoagulant functions. Protein C is an important inhibitor of factor Va and factor VIIIa and is activated by complex formation of thrombin with an endothelial cell surface protein, thrombomodulin. The anticoagulant capacity of protein C is enhanced by its natural co-factor protein S. The downregulation of thrombomodulin during sepsis, that is likely caused by TNF, results in diminished protein C activity and may enhance the procoagulant state. In plasma, 60 % of the cofactor protein S is complexed to a complement regulatory protein, C4b binding protein (C4bBP). The anticoagulant capacity of protein C is enhanced by the free fraction of protein S. Taylor et al. [20] proposed that increased plasma levels of C4bBP may result in a relative protein S deficiency as a consequence of the acute phase reaction in inflammatory diseases, which would further contribute to a procoagulant state during sepsis. In support of this hypothesis, in a recent study Taylor et al. [20] showed that the infusion of C4bBP in combination with a sublethal dose of *E. coli* into baboons resulted in a lethal response with severe organ damage due to diffuse intravascular coagulation.

Besides the activation of the coagulation cascade, endotoxemia also affects the fibrinolytic system. Suffredini et al. [21] found increased tissue-type plasminogen activator (tPA) activity and plasminogen activator inhibitor (PAI) activity 2 h after the start of the infusion of endotoxin. Van Deventer et al. [8] and van der Poll et al. [22] described an enhanced fibrinolytic activity during the first 2 h following TNF or endotoxin administration to healthy volunteers. In this study, an increase in plasminogen activation activity, mediated by an increase in tissue-type plasminogen activator (tPA) and urokinase plasminogen activator (uPA) resulted in increased plasmin generation as indicated by a rise of plasmin-α_2-antiplasmin complexes (PAP). One hour after the infusion of TNF, an increase of plasminogen activator inhibitor (PAI) resulted in a rapid decline of plasminogen activator activity and as a consequence plasmin generation. Therefore, it appears that the infusion of TNF induced a rapid activation and subsequent inhibition of the fibrinolytic system in healthy humans. Comparing these results with the findings of studies on coagulation activation after TNF or endotoxin administration [8, 16], the authors conclude that at the time of maximal thrombin generation (i.e. 4 h after the infusion of TNF or endotoxin) fibrinolysis was already offset (Fig. 4). This results in a remarkable dysbalance between the procoagulant and fibrinolytic system, resulting in a net procoagulant state 3 h after TNF administration.

Intervention

On the basis of our present understanding of sepsis, treatment aimed at the pathogenic pathways of this syndrome can be applied at two different levels. First, by eradicating the microorganisms responsible for the septicemia by the administration of antibiotics or surgical drainage, and second, by applying novel modalities of intervention that inhibit cascade systems or endogenous mediators of sepsis.

Monoclonal antibodies and monoclonal antibody fragment (Fab's) form an important class of reagents that can be used to block various mediators of sepsis *in vivo*. Monoclonal antibodies have been directed against endotoxin, in order to reduce the deleterious effect triggered by endotoxemia. Ziegler et al. [23] recently showed in a randomized, placebo controlled clinical trial, that the administration of a monoclonal antibody (HA-1A), directed against a lipid A epitope on the *E. coli* rough mutant (J5), reduced mortality in patients with a gram-negative sepsis. Although the HA-1A treatment, particularly in a subgroup of patients in whom endotoxemia was present, significantly reduced mortality, a large number of HA-1A treated patients still died, indicating the need for additional new intervention strategies.

Cytokines, such as TNF, IL-1 and IL-6, appear to be important mediators in the pathogenesis of sepsis and drugs interfering with the production and release of TNF or drugs capable of neutralizing TNF may have beneficial effects on en-

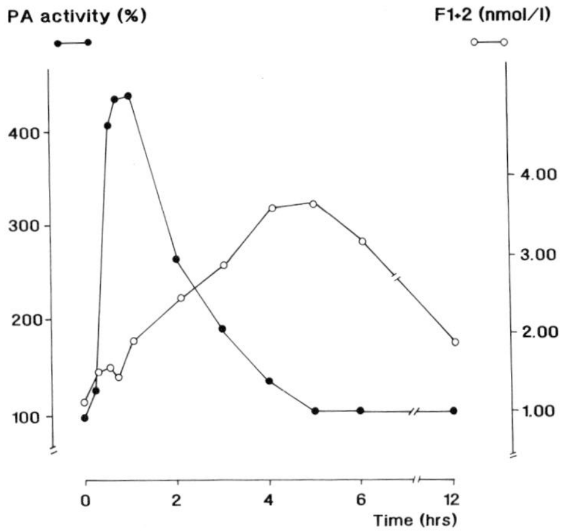

Fig. 4. Comparison of the dynamics of the fibrinolytic and procoagulant responses to intravenous injection of recombinant human TNF: mean plasminogen activator (PA) activity, and mean plasma concentrations of prothrombin fragment F1+2

dotoxic shock. Tracey et al. [24] showed that neutralizing Fab's, directed against TNF, administered 1 h before the infusion of *E. coli* in baboons, protected against shock but did not prevent fatal organ failure. A more complete protection against shock, MOF and death was conferred by administration of the antibodies 2 h in advance of the bacterial challenge. Hinshaw et al. [25], however, were able to protect baboons from the deleterious effects of sepsis by the administration of monoclonal antibodies directed against TNF, which were given 30 min after the infusion of *E. Coli* bacteria.

Pentoxifylline is an effective inhibitor of transcription of the TNF gene in cell cultures stimulated with endotoxin [26]. In a study in pigs with induced faecal peritonitis, pentoxifylline improved the hemodynamic variables and survival [27]. Zabel et al. [28] showed that the administration of pentoxifylline did block the endotoxin-induced synthesis of TNF in human volunteers. We have recently shown that pentoxifylline treatment prevented coagulation activation in a model of endotoxin induced coagulation activation in chimpanzees, as measured by plasma levels of thrombin-antithrombin complexes and specific activation peptides of factor X, prothrombin and fibrinogen [29].

The cytokine IL-1 has been implicated as an important mediator of septic shock. It has been shown to induce tachycardia and hypotension and to act synergistically with TNF causing tissue damage [30]. A recombinant human IL-1 receptor antagonist (IL-1ra) capable of blocking the effect of IL-1 *in vitro* [31, 32], has been used to determine the role of IL-1 in models of septic shock in rabbits [33]. In this model, the endotoxin induced lethality and the toxicity of IL-1 release could be reversed by the administration of IL-1ra at least 2 h after the injection of endotoxin.

Sepsis is associated with coagulation activation and subsequent formation of (micro)-thrombi intravascularly, ultimately leading to MOF. Secondary to consumption of coagulation factors and platelets, bleeding may occur. The present treatment for this derangement consists of suppletion of coagulation factors and platelet transfusion, while some advocate the use of intravenous heparin, although considerable debate exists on the role of heparin therapy in DIC [34]. Recently, animal studies in baboons and chimpanzees and studies in human volunteers and septic patients have indicated several more specific strategies for treatment of coagulation activation in sepsis.

The expression and activation of tissue factor (TF) on monocytes, macrophages and endothelial cells is probably an important factor in the initiation of a procoagulant state during septicemia. In order to counteract the initial coagulation activation, Taylor et al. [35] blocked the expression of TF by infusion of monoclonal antibodies directed against TF. The administration of these antibodies to baboons prevented the coagulopathic and lethal effects of the *E. coli* infusion. Recent experiments by our own group in a model of endotoxin-induced coagulation activation in chimpanzees confirmed the pivotal role of TF in the initiation of coagulation activation in sepsis [36].

The procoagulant state during septicemia is partly promoted by the downregulation and consumption of protein C and antithrombin III, natural inhibitors of the coagulation activation. Both anticoagulants have been administered to septic baboons in order to study the effect of suppletion on coagulopathy and mortality during septicemia. The intravascular infusion of a lethal dose of *E. coli* into baboons is a relevant primate model of septic shock associated with coagulopathy, organ failure and death. Taylor et al. [3] showed that the administration of activated protein C prevented the coagulopathic, hepatotoxic and lethal effect of the infusion of *E. coli* bacteria in baboons. Moreover, by blocking the activation of protein C with selective monoclonal antibodies, the dose of *E. coli* to elicit a fatal septic shock in baboons could be reduced 10 times, indicating a protective effect of activated protein C on the induction of septic shock. The administration of antithrombin III (AT III) did also protect the baboons against the otherwise lethal dose of *E. coli* [37]. The reduced mortality in these studies suggests that the coagulopathic response to *E. coli* might be one of the essential components involved in the high mortality of septic shock in baboons. The application of a selective monoclonal antibody against activated factor X (DEGR-anti Xa) however, at a dose sufficient to inhibit fibrinogen consumption and, as a consequence, fibrin formation during sepsis *in vivo*, did not reduce the lethal effects of *E. coli* infusion in baboons [38].

Many recently introduced modalities of intervention have been studied *in vitro* or in smaller animal models of septic shock. Most of the reagents discussed in this chapter have been studied in primate animal models. Primate animal models seem to be more reliable to study new therapeutic strategies that are not yet suitable for humans than the smaller animal models or *in vitro* experiments. However, one needs to be very careful in translating the observations in primates to the clinical human situation. Nevertheless, it is our hope that these reagents will be studied in clinical trials soon and may result in a more effective management of sepsis and septic shock.

Conclusions

The formation of fibrin thrombin in sepsis is a consequence of activation of the coagulation system and inhibition of the fibrinolytic response. Although the contact system is usually active in septic patients, our studies in human volunteers and subhuman primates indicate that the major route of endotoxin- and TNF-induced coagulation activation is the extrinsic pathway. In endoxin-challenged chimpanzees, thrombin formation can be inhibited by either prevention of the synthesis of TNF, or by monoclonal antibodies specific for tissue factor. The most promising intervention strategies in patients with DIC include immunotherapeutical treatments directed at endotoxin or TNF. More specific tools that may become available for clinical use are monoclonal antibodies that recognize tissue factor (inhibiting the extrinsic route of coagulation activation) and activated protein C (a natural inhibitor of the common route of coagulation activation).

References

1. Harris RL, Musher DM, Bloom K, et al. (1987) Manifestations of sepsis. Arch Intern Med 147:1895
2. Hinshaw LB, Brackett DJ, Archer LT, Beller BK, Wilson MF (1983) Detection of the hyperdynamic state of sepsis in the baboon during lethal E. Coli infusion. J Trauma 23:361–365
3. Taylor FB, Chang Jr. A, Esmon CT, D'Angelo A, Vigano-D'Angelo S, Blick KE (1987) Protein C prevents the coagulopathic and lethal effects of Escherichia Coli infusion in the baboon. J Clin Invest 79:918–925
4. Levi M, Ten Cate H, Bauer KA, et al. (1992) Pentoxifylline inhibits endotoxin-induced activation of coagulation and fibrinolysis in a chimpanzee model of endotoxemia. (In press)
5. Van Deventer SJH, Buller HR, Ten Cate JW, Sturk A, Pauw W (1988) Endoxaemia: An early predictor of septicemia in febrile patients. The Lancet 1:605–609
6. Brandtzaeg P, Kierulf P, Gaustad P, et al. (1989) Plasma endotoxin as a predictor of multiple organ failure and death in systemic meningococcal disease. J Infect Dis 159:195–204
7. Michie HR, Manogue KR, Spriggs DR, et al. (1988) Detection of circulating tumor necrosis factor after endotoxin administration. New Eng J Med 318:1481–1486
8. Van Deventer SJH, Buller HR, Ten Cate JW, Aarden LA, Hack CE, Sturk A (1990) Experimental endotoxemia in humans: Analysis of cytokine release and coagulation, fibrinolytic, and complement pathways. Blood 76:2520–2526
9. Waage A, Halstensen A, Espevik T (1987) Association between tumor necrosis factor in serum and fatal outcome in patients with meningococcal disease. Lancet 1:355–357
10. Hack CE, De Groot ER, Felt-Bersma RJF, et al. (1989) Increased plasma levels of interleukin-6 in sepsis. Blood 74:1704–1710
11. Waage A, Brandtzaeg P, Halstensen A, Kierulf P, Espevik T (1989) The complex pattern of cytokines in serum from patients with meningococcal septic shock. Association between interleukin-6, interleukin-1 and fatal outcome. J Exp Med 169:333–338
12. Fong Y, Tracey KJ, Moldawer LL (1989) Antibodies to cachectin/tumor necrosis factor reduce interleukin 1β and interleukin 6 appearance during lethal bacteremia. J Exp Med 170:1627–1633
13. Beutler B, Milsark IW, Cerami AC (1985) Passive immunization against cachectin/tumor necrosis factor protects mice from lethal effect of endotoxin. Science 229:869–871
14. Natanson C, Eichenholz PW, Danner RL, et al. (1989) Endotoxin and tumor necrosis factor challenges in dogs simulate the cardiovascular profile of human septic shock. J Exp Med 169:823–832
15. Bauer KA, Ten Cate H, Barzegar S, Spriggs DR, Sherman ML, Rosenberg RD (1989) Tumor necrosis factor infusions have a procoagulant effect on the hemostatic mechanism of humans. Blood 74:165–172
16. Van Der Poll T, Buller HR, Ten Cate H, et al. (1990) Activation of coagulation after administration of tumor necrosis factor to normal subjects. New Eng J Med 322:1622–1627
17. Altieri DC, Morrissey JH, Edgington TS (1988) Adhesive receptor Mac-1 coordinates the activation of factor X on stimulated cells of monocytic and myeloid differentiation: An alternative initiation of the coagulation protein cascade. Proc Natl Acad Sci USA 85:7462–7466
18. Osterud B, Flaegstad T (1983) Increased tissue thromboplastin activity in monocytes of patients with meningococcal infection: Related to unfavourable prognosis. Thromb Haemost 49:5–7
19. De Boer JP, Creasey AA, Chang A, et al. (1992) Activation of coagulation and fibrinolysis in baboons following infusion with lethal or sublethal dose of E. Coli. (in press)
20. Taylor FB, Chang A, Ferrel G, et al. (1991) C4b-binding protein exacerbates the host response to Escherichia Coli. Blood 78:357–363
21. Suffredini AF, Harpel PC, Parillo JE (1989) Promotion and subsequent inhibition of plasminogen activator after administration of intraveneous endotoxin to normal subjects. New Eng J Med 320:1165–1172
22. Van Der Poll T, Levi M, Buller HR, et al. (1991) Fibrinolytic response to tumor necrosis factor in healthy subjects. J Exp Med 174:729–732
23. Ziegler EJ, Fisher CJ Jr., Sprung CL et al. (1991) Treatment of gram-negative bacteremia and septic shock with HA-1A human monoclonal antibody against endotoxin. New Eng J Med 324:429–436

24. Tracey KJ, Fong Y, Hesse DG, et al. (1987) Anti-cachectin/TNF monoclonal antibodies prevent septic shock during lethal bacteremia. Nature: 330:662–664
25. Hinshaw LB, TeKamp-Olson P, Chang AC, et al. (1990) Survival of primates in LD100 septic shock following therapy with antibody to tumor necrosis factor (TNF alpha). Circ Shock 30:279–292
26. Strieter RM, Remick DG, Ward PA, et al. (1988) Cellular and molecular regulation of tumor necrosis factor-alfa production by pentoxifylline. Biochem Biophys Res Comm 155:1230–1236
27. Tighe D, Moss R, Hynd J, et al. (1988) Pentoxifylline reverses haemodynamic and histological changes associated with peritonitis in pigs. In: Mandell GL, Novick J Jr., et al. (eds): Pentoxifylline and leukocyte function. Somerville NJ, HRP Inc. pp 184–189
28. Zabel P, Wolter DT, Schonharting MM, Schade UF (1989) Oxpentifylline in endotoxemia. The Lancet 2:1474–1477
29. Levi M, Ten Cate H, Bauer KA, et al. (1991) Dose dependent endotoxin induced cytokine release and coagulation activation in chimpanzees. Thromb Haemostas 65:410 (Abs.)
30. Okusawa S, Gelfand JA, Ikejima T, Connolly RJ, Dinarello CA (1988) Interleukin-1 induces a shock-like state in rabbits. J Clin Invest 81:1162–1172
31. Hannum CH, Wilcox CJ, Arend WP, et al. (1990) Interleukin-1 receptor antagonist activity of a human interleukin-1 inhibitor. Nature 343:336–340
32. Eisenberg SP, Evans RJ, Arend WP, et al. (1990) Primary structure and functional expression from complementary DNA of a human interleukin-1 receptor antagonist. Nature 343:341–346
33. Ohlsson K, Bjork P, Bergenfeldt M, Hageman R, Thompson RC (1990) Interleukin-1 receptor antagonist reduces mortality from endotoxin shock. Nature 348:550–552
34. Mant MJ, Gartner King E. (1979) Severe, acute disseminated intravascular coagulation. A reappraisal of its pathophysiology, clinical significance and therapy based on 47 patients. Am J Med 67:557–563
35. Taylor FB Jr., Chang A, Ruf W, et al. (1991) Lethal E. Coli septic shock is prevented by blokking tissue factor with monoclonal antibody. Circ Shock 33:127–134
36. Levi M, Ten Cate H, Bauer KA, et al. (1990) Endotoxin induced tumor necrosis factor release and coagulation activation in vivo. Blood 76:1698 (Abs.)
37. Taylor FB Jr., Emerson TE Jr., Chang AK, Blick KE (1988) Antithrombin III prevents the lethal effects of E. Coli infusion in baboons. Circ Shock 26:227–235
38. Taylor FB Jr., Chang ACK, Peer GT, et al. (1991) DEGR-Factor Xa blocks disseminated intravascular coagulation initiated by Escherichia coli without preventing shock or organ damage. Blood 78:364–368

Leukocyte-Endothelial Interactions in Trauma and Sepsis

H. Redl, G. Schlag, and I. Marzi

Introduction

The development of organ failure may occur within the first days after trauma (early organ failure) or after one or two weeks (late organ failure) in ICU patients. The reaction that leads to organ damage and organ failure is a generalized inflammatory event [1]. This inflammation may be non-bacterial in the early stage of organ failure, and be aggravated by the influence of bacterial factors during the development of late organ failure. The non-bacterial inflammatory reaction is induced by the initial injury and is usually based on three factors: tissue ischemia/hypoxia, reperfusion events with generation of oxygen radicals; stimulation of phagocytes by complement split products or other humoral inflammatory factors; and the interaction with endothelial cells. This chapter focuses on PMN/endothelial activation with special emphasis on the PMN-endothelial interaction. The results of these events will be discussed in the trauma and the sepsis situation.

Granulocyte Activation

Anaphylatoxins can activate WBC in trauma. Among the different leukocyte populations, granulocytes are the most fast-acting cells of the body's inflammatory response mechanism, and therefore in the focus of endothelial cells (EC)-leukocyte interactions.

Traumatic tissue damage leads to unmasking of different cellular components, which might be the reason for the massive complement activation seen after polytrauma. Similar conclusions have been drawn from experiments where homogenized muscle tissue was infused into experiment animals [2]. Equally, ischemic tissue causes massive complement activation, resulting in elevated levels of the anaphylatoxins C3a and C5a [3]. The important reactions during complement activation are probably the release of C3a, C5a, and the formation of terminal complement complexes, which in turn can activate and damage cells. C3a is most useful for monitoring this complement activation. Initially, high levels of circulating C3a have demonstrated to be related to the subsequent development of organ failure and mortality [4]. C3a levels were also seen to be significantly higher in patients with early organ failure and early mortality after severe polytrauma (Fig. 1).

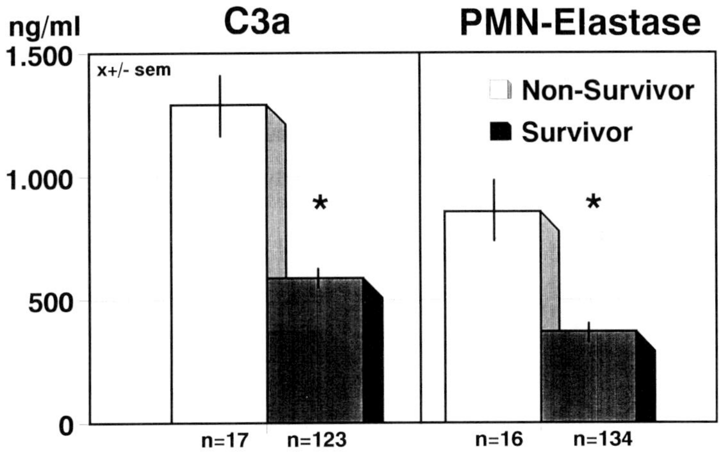

Fig. 1. Non-surviving polytraumatized patients had significantly higher complement and granulocyte activation than survivors as measured by plasma C3a and plasma PMN-elastase levels (Data from a multicenter polytrauma study together with J. Goris, H. Benzer, A. Aasen and W. Sandtner, with permission)

Activated complement components stimulate PMN to perform the respiratory burst reaction with the formation of reactive oxygen species and the release of cytotoxic proteases.

A good example is elastase liberated by PMN, measured as the elastase alpha-1-proteinase inhibitor complex in plasma [5]. There is a positive correlation between trauma severity and elastase plasma levels in patients [6]. Elastase levels were found to be significantly higher in non-surviving polytrauma patients (Fig. 1). There is also a significant correlation between sepsis and PMN-elastase plasma levels and the severity of multi organ failure (MOF) [6], which indicates a link between the activation of granulocytes and the development of organ failure [6,7]. We were able to apply this method in the baboon (IMAC-technique - Merck) [8] and found much higher elastase levels in severe septic than in traumatic baboons (Fig. 2). In the baboon model situation, one of the reasons for the higher activation state of leukocytes might be the *E. coli* related release of endotoxin into the plasma (up to 11 ng/ml), which was not seen in the trauma animals. Similarily, most of the LPS inducible cytokines, except for IL-6, were found in the sepsis but seldom in the trauma situation (IL-6 trauma 11 (3-360) ng/ml, sepsis 4197 (1476 - 5468) ng/ml).

Among the PMN activators also the formation of TNF has been observed in the initial phase of hemorrhage and trauma [9]. This early cytokine formation is either triggered by complement activation products or by ischemia

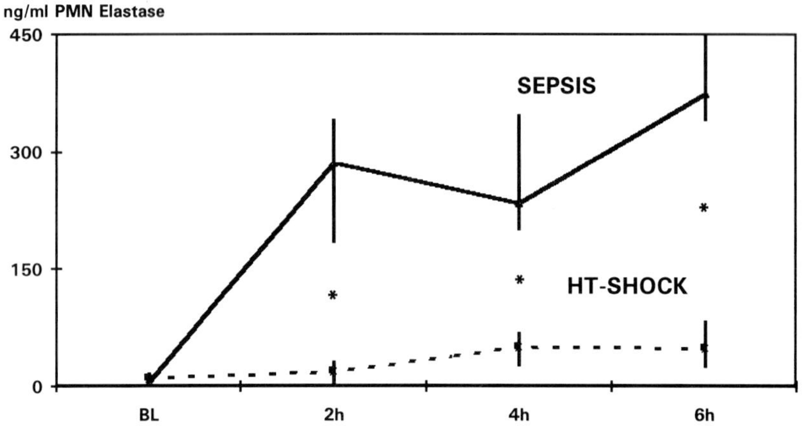

Fig. 2. Baboons with bacteremia (10^{10}CFU/kg (n = 7) were found to have significantly higher granulocyte-specific elastase levels in plasma (= more PMN activation) than baboons subjected to a polytrauma with hemorrhagic shock (n = 9) (From [14,41] with permission)

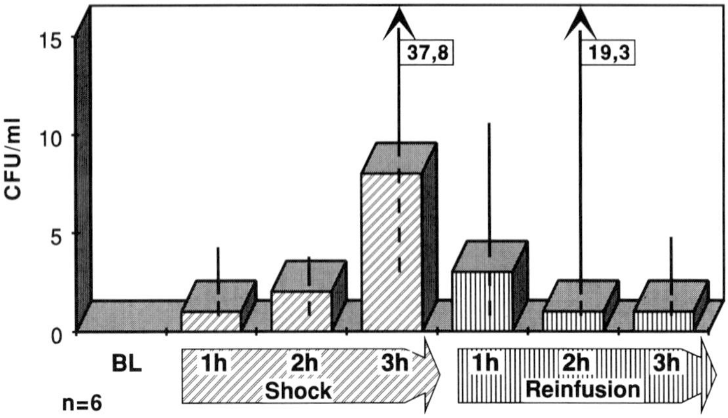

Fig. 3. Bacterial translocation (Colony Forming Units in blood - CFU/ml) in a baboon model of hemorrhagic-traumatic shock (n = 6) (From Schlag et al., in press)

[10]. An additional stimulus could be bacterial toxin liberation during bacterial translocation (Fig. 3) [11]. Via such a bacterial (endotoxin) translocation and in sepsis, activation of PMN occurs via action of humoral products (e.g. C5a), by bacterial products (e.g. chemotactic peptides, LPS, or cytokines (e.g. TNF, IL-8).

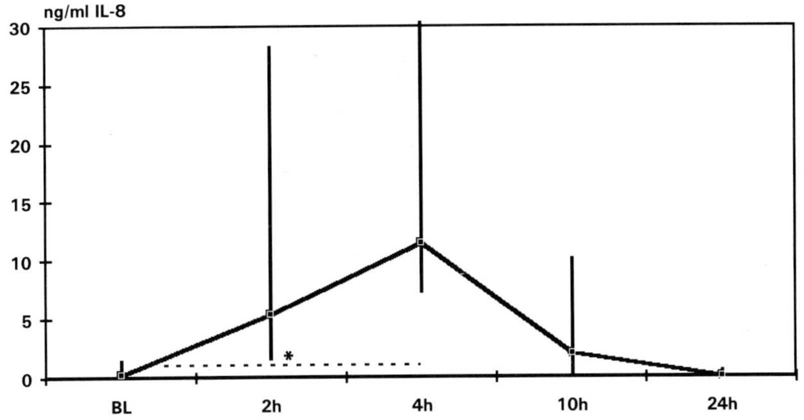

Fig. 4. Neutrophil activating peptide-1 (IL-8) plasma levels significantly increased during baboon septicemia (n = 4) after infusion of 5 x 10^8E.coli/kg over 2 h (*p <0.05

Several studies have clearly indicated the importance of TNF since TNF blockade leads to decreased mortality [12,13]. Aside from TNF, the proinflammatory cytokines IL-1 (see chapter by Dinarello in this volume) and IL-8 are thought to be of central importance for PMN and endothelial activation and in the pathophysiology of sepsis. We have first described the *in vivo* appearance of IL-8 in baboons during lethal *E. coli* bacteremia [14]. IL-8 *in vivo* was also demonstrated in sublethal endotoxemia and after administration of human IL-1 [15]. IL-8 appearance in septicemia was found to follow the kinetics of IL-1 and IL-6 appearance, which peaked much later than TNF (Fig. 4) [14]. IL-6 and IL-1 release is dependent on TNF generation [16]. We investigated whether TNF might be responsible for IL-8 production in baboon septicemia and found that using TNF-antibody resulted in a significant reduction of circulating IL-8 [17]. NAP-1/IL-8 might be considered a potentially important mediator of host response to sepsis, due to its chemoattractant and PMN activation properties. These features indicate that IL-8 could be a major mediator of PMN activation in sepsis and thus of (PMN dependent) organ failure.

The importance of PMN for tissue damage in general and of adhesion (molecule) upregulation during PMN activation is supported by numerous studies with experimentally induced leukopenia which demonstrated that organ damage, e.g. in the lung, could be prevented [18,22]. Neutrophil depletion did not prevent edema formation in the lungs after endotoxin administration if depletion was performed with nitrogen mustard and not with hydroxyurea [23]. In contrast, nitrogen mustard PMN depleted rabbits did not reveal lung injury induced by endotoxin and chemotactic peptide [24].

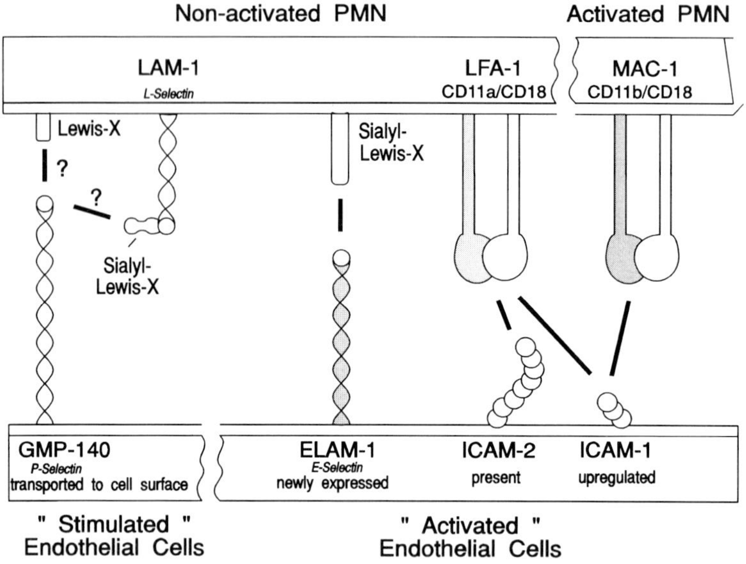

Fig. 5. Possible interactions between granulocytes and endothelial cells responsible for adherence phenomena (From [46] with permission)

PMN activation also induces an upregulation of neutrophil adherence molecules, especially of the CD18 complex, and a loss of LAM-1. The CDw18 complex is part of the supergene integrin family and consists of glycoproteins arranged in one beta-chain (CD18) and three different alpha-chains (CD11a, or CD11b, or CD11c), and can be influenced by several inflammatory mediators [25]. Of special interest is the CD11b (Mac-1) [26], which is both an important complement receptor (CR3) involved in phagocytosis, and one of the ligands of the endothelial adherence molecule ICAM-1, and is thus involved in the endothelial-leukocyte interaction. Beside the CD18 complex of which Mac-1 is upregulated, there are further complementary molecules on the leukocyte surface, which are either constitutive (e.g. Lewis-X, LFA-1), or lost during PMN activation (e.g. LAM-1) (Fig. 5).

In addition to granulocytes, monocytes and lymphocytes also bind (e.g. to the endothelium [27,28]) by means of these adhesive proteins. The relative contribution of each of these molecules to leukoycte/endothelial adhesion varies depending on the cell type and the stimulus used, as shown by Arnaout et al. [29].

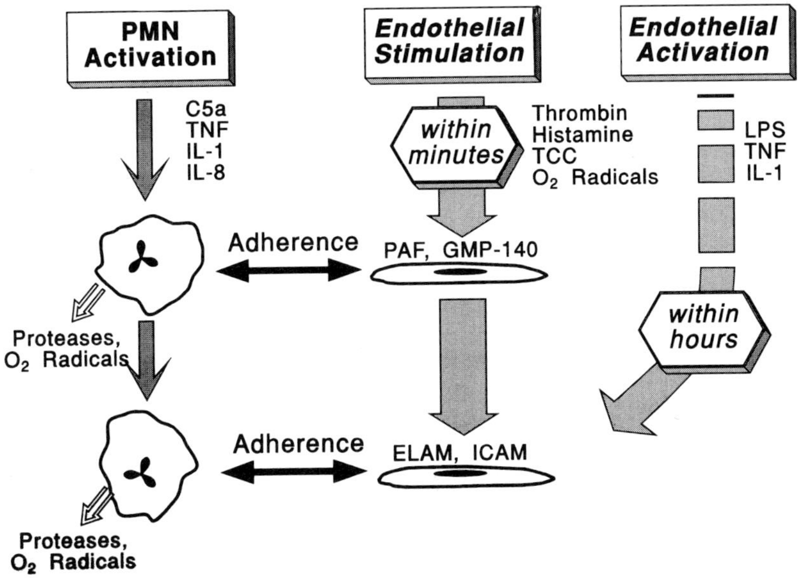

Fig. 6. Fast endothelial stimulation (protein synthesis independent) versus slow endothelial activation (protein synthesis dependent)

Endothelial Effects (Fig. 6)

One of the important tasks of EC is the communication between circulating blood cells and specific cells of the organs, with EC acting as "doorkeepers" in blood cell margination and extravasation. Along with this task, EC are important sites of synthesis of shock mediators. At the same time they are target cells for many substances released during traumatic and septic shock [30].

Endothelial Stimulation

Endothelial cell stimulation (according to the definition of J. Pober) is a fast protein synthesis independent response, which might occur in the early posttraumatic/postshock period in that hydrogen peroxide can induce PAF formation on the endothelial surface [31], which upon contact with neutrophils could lead to neutrophil activation via the PAF receptors. Endothelial stimulation occurs also in response to agonists such as thrombin and histamine [32]. EC stimulation involves the transport of the adherence molecule GMP-140, which is located in Weibel-Palade bodies (WPB), to the surface of EC, which leads to fusion of the WPB with the plasma membrane so that GMP-140 molecules can interact with neutrophils [32].

It is proposed that both GMP-140 together with PAF on the EC and the PAF receptor on the neutrophils together with the Lewis X structure are responsible for early adherence of neutrophils to endothelial cells. This initial contact between EC and PMN seems to be independent of neutrophil activation. Presumably, PMN are only activated through contact with PAF/PAF-R. *In vivo* evidence for this hypothesis has been obtained from splanchnic shock experiments in rats. Leukocyte adherence was noted upon reperfusion as judged by vital microscopy, and was attenuated by SOD, and especially by PAF antagonists in this model (Fig. 7) [33,34].

Endothelial Activation

A distinct sequence of events occurs if the EC are activated by LPS or by cytokines. The *in vitro* properties of the endothelium inducible by LPS and cytokines include cytokine expression, procoagulant activity, immunologic functions and increased adhesiveness for leukocytes due to expression of adherence molecules. These events are within the definition of "endothelial activation" [35]. We could demonstrate that a *(de novo)* expression of adhesion molecules occurs under septic conditions in subprimate animal models by using two antibodies to the ELAM-1 structure (Fig. 8) [8], which seems to be TNF dependent [17].

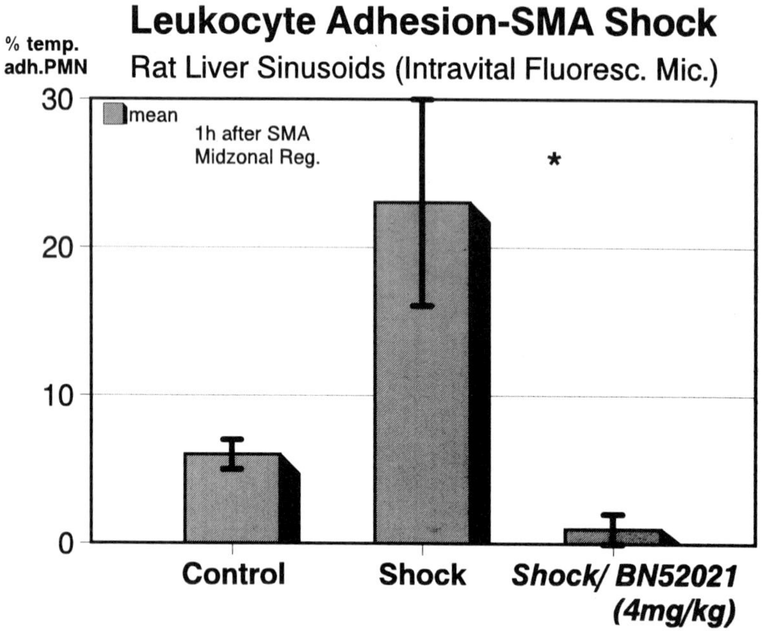

Fig. 7. Leukocyte adhesion in the liver (midzonal region) after superic mensenteric artery (SMA) shock in rats (n = 6/group). The PAF antagonist BN 52021 4 mg/kg pretreatment significantly ($p < 0.05$) decreased leukocyte adhesion (From [34] with permission)

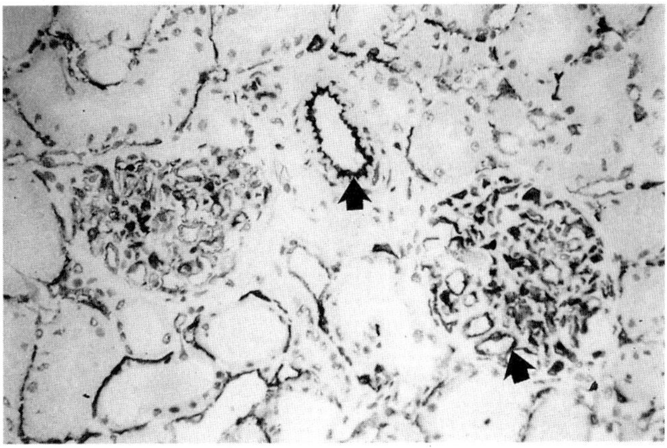

Fig. 8. Immunohistochemical evidence of ELAM-1 expression in kidney samples both a capillary and arterial endothelial cells during sepsis in baboons.

Endothelial leukocyte adhesion molecules (ELAM-1) serve to bind PMN via a sialyl-Lewis-X structure (Fig. 5) [36]. ELAM-1 is not present on unstimulated endothelial cells *in vitro* and may transiently be induced (peak at 4 - 6 h) by LPS, IL-1 or TNF. We have seldom seen ELAM-1 expression in trauma where cytokine release was minimal in the polytraumatic situation in (baboon) models [14]. In sepsis, we have previously shown massive cytokine release [8]. This might explain the differences in endothelial activation. Furthermore, concentrations of endotoxin circulating in the plasma are several long-steps higher in sepsis than in trauma (S. Bahrami, unpublished results). Nevertheless, small amounts of endotoxin seen after polytrauma due to bacterial translocation might account for the few positive endothelial stainings encountered in the trauma animals [8].

ELAM-1 expression may serve as a marker of endothelial activation (as suggested by Pober and Cotran) [35], and is one of the possible preconditions that lead to leukocyte-related endothelial damage. Our data certainly do not permit the clear conclusion that ELAM-1 antigen expression causes EC leakiness. However, a recent study on immunecomplex-induced alveolitis suggests that *in vivo* blocking of ELAM-1 with MoAb has favorable therapeutic effects [37].

Leukostatis of Organs

Probably the most evident sign of EC-leukocyte activation and interactions is leukostasis. We have previously demonstrated this event both in the expe-

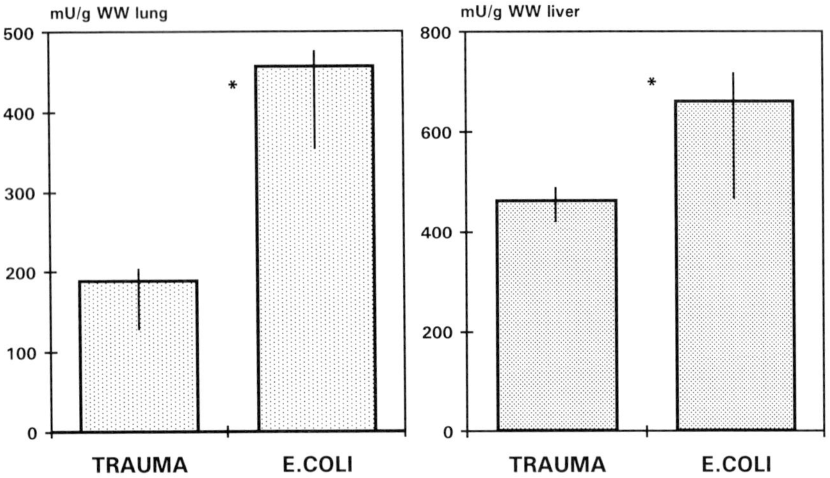

Fig. 9. Myeloperoxidase accumulation as a sign of massive leukostasis was found (a) in the lung and (b) in the liver both after polytrauma and bacteremia, but leukostasis was significantly higher in the sepsis situation. (From [41] with permission)

rimental [38] as well as in the clinical [39] posttraumatic situations. Similar to the canine model, in our baboon model (originally based on Pretorius et al. [40]) leukostasis was found by measurement of myeloperoxidase content in lung and liver tissue. This technique was also used to study baboons after live *E. coli* bacteremia in a hyperdynamic setting [41]. When these two model situations were compared, significantly more leukostasis has been found in the sepsis situation (Fig. 9). Leukostasis is the net effect of three different events. Beside activation of leukocytes and endothelial cells, the balance between PMN-endothelial adhesive forces and hemodynamic dispersal forces is of major importance [42]. The shear forces are decreased in the postcapillary venules during shock. Margination of leukocytes and their adhesion to the endothelium occur almost exclusively in postcapillary venules [43]. House et al. [43] have provided experimental proof that adherence mainly depends on an increase in adhesive forces rather than on diminished shear stresses. Such diminished shear stress is found when blood flow is reduced, e.g. due to hypovolemia as in our polytrauma model, and when a reduction of cardiac output down to one third of normal values occurs. It has to be noted that despite an increase in cardiac output with reinfusion and (over) normalization of blood flow, leukostasis could not be significantly reduced [44], probably due to adhesion phenomena.

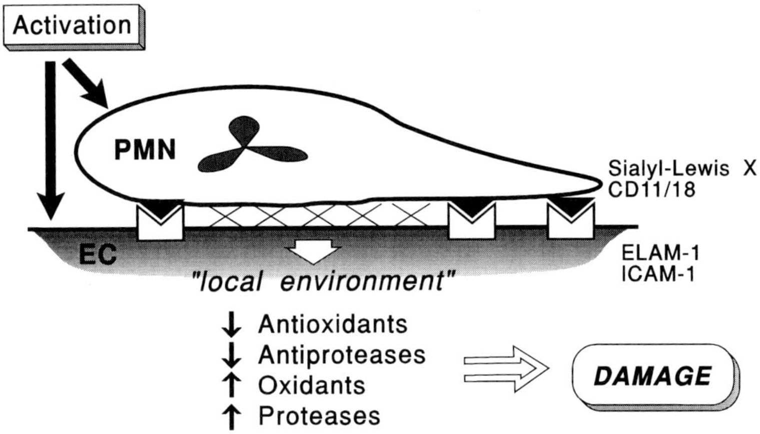

Fig. 10. Formation of a microenvironment due to the adherence of PMN to the endothelium all (EC) and the associated potential membrane damage

Conclusion

Endothelial-leukocyte interactions seem to constitute the prerequisite both for PMN extravasation and EC damage. Since EC alteration or damage causes permeability changes and ultimately edema formation, the EC-leukocyte interactions are of central importance in shock-induced organ damage. According to the current working hypothesis, adhering and activated PMN might be crucial in EC damage, since a microenvironment is formed (Fig. 10), mediators are released locally, and damage occurs without a sufficiently neutralizing capacity (antiproteases, antioxidants). This type of damage is attributed to the effect of oxygen radicals, proteases or both [45].

References

1. Goris RJA, te Boekhorst TPA, Nuytinck JKS, Gimbrere JSF (1985) Multiple organ failure: Generalized auto-destructive inflammation? Arch Surg 120:1109–1115
2. Heideman M, Kaijser B, Gelin LE (1978) Complement activation and hematologic hemodynamic and respiratory reactions early after soft tissue injury. J Trauma 18:696–700
3. Bengtsson A, Lannsjo W, Heideman M (1987) Complement and anaphylatoxin responses to cross clamping of the aorta studies during general anesthesia with or without extradural blockade. Brit J Anaesth 59:1093–1097
4. Zilow G, Naser W, Rutz R, Burger R (1989) Quantitation of the anaphylatoxin C3a in the presence of C3 by a novel sandwich ELISA using monoclonal antibody to a C3a neoepitope. J Immunol Meth 121:261–268

5. Neumann S, Hunzer G, Heinrich N, Lang H (1984). PMN elastase assay: Enzyme immunoassay for human polymorphonuclear elastase complexes with alpha-1 proteinase inhibitor. J Clin Chem Clin Biochem 22:693–697
6. Nuytinck JKS, Goris RJA, Redl H, Schlag G, van Munster PJJ (1986) Posttraumatic complications and inflammatory mediators. Arch Surg 121:886–890
7. Lang H, Jochum M, Fritz H, Redl H (1989) Validity of the elastase assay in intensive care medicine. Prog Clin Biol Res 308:701–706
8. Redl H, Dinges HP, Buurman WA, et al. (1991) Expression of endothelial-leukocyte adhesion molecule-1 in septic but not traumatic/hypovolemic shock in the baboon. Am J Pathol 139:461–466
9. Ayala A, Perrin MM, Meldrum DR, Ertel W, Chaudry IH (1990) Hemorrhage induces an increase in serum TNF which is not associated with elevated levels of endotoxin. Cytokine 2:170–174
10. Colletti LM, Burtch GD, Remick DG, Kunkel SL, Strieter RM, Campbell DA (1990) Role of tumor necrosis factor alpha in the pathophysiologic alterations after hepatic ischemia reperfusion injury in the rat. Transplantation 49:268–272
11. Schlag G, Redl H, Dinges HP, Davies J, Radmore K (1991) Bacterial translocation in baboon model of hypovolemic traumatic shock. In: Schlag G, Redl H (eds) Shock, Sepsis, and Organ Failure. Second Wiggers Bernard Conference, Springer Verlag, Berlin-Heidelberg, pp 53–83
12. Tracey KJ, Fong Y, Hesse DG, et al. (1987) Anti-cachectin TNF monoclonal antibodies prevent septic shock during lethal bacteremia. Nature 330:662–664
13. Schlag G, Redl H, Davies J (1991) TNF antibodies (CB0006) in a subchronic septic model in baboons to prevent multi organ failure. Circ Shock 34:164–165
14. Redl H, Schlag G, Bahrami S, Schade U, Ceska M, Stütz P (1991) Plasma neutrophil-activating peptide-1/interleukin-8 and neutrophil elastase in a primate bacteremia model. J Infect Dis 164:383–388
15. Van Zee KJ, DeForge LE, Fischer E, et al. (1991) IL-8 in septic shock, endotoxemia, and after IL-1 administration. J Immunol 146:3478–3482
16. Fong Y, Tracey KJ, Moldawer LL, et al. (1989) Antibodies to cachectin/tumor necrosis factor reduce interleukin-1 beta and interleukin-6 appearance during lethal bacteremia. J Exp Med 170:1627–1633
17. Redl H, Schlag G, Dinges HP, Buurman WA, Ceska M, Davies J (1991) TNF dependent ELAM-1 expression and IL-8 release in baboon septicemia. Circ Shock 34:92 (Abs.)
18. Heflin AC Jr, Brigham KL (1981) Prevention by granulocyte depletion of increased vascular permeability of sheep lung following endotoxemia. J Clin Invest 68:1253–1260
19. Flick MR, Peral G, Staub NC (1981) Leukocytes are required for increased lung microvascular permeability after microemboli in sheep. Circ Res 48:344–351
20. Shasby DM, Fox RB, Haranda RN, Repine JE (1982) Reduction of the edema of acute hyperoxic lung injury by granulocyte depletion. J Appl Physiol 52:1237–1239
21. Johnson A, Malik AB (1980) Effect of granulocytopenia on extravascular lung water content after micro-embolization. Am Rev Resp Dis 122:561–566
22. Heath Ca, Lai L, Bizios R, Malik AB (1986) Pulmonary hemodynamic effects of antisheep serum-induced leukopenia. J Leuk Biol 3:385–392
23. Winn R, Maunder R, Chi E, Harlan J (1987) Neutrophil depletion does not prevent lung edema after endotoxin infusion in goats. J Appl Physiol 62:116–121
24. Worthen S, Haslett C, Rees AJ, Gumbay RS, Henson JE, Henson PM (1987) Neutrophil-mediated pulmonary vascular injury. Synergistic effect of trace amounts of lipopolysaccharide and neutrophil stimuli on vascular permeability and neutrophil sequestration in the lung. Am Rev Resp Dis 136:19–28
25. Tonnesen MG, Anderson DC, Springer TA, Knedler A, Avdi N, Henson PM (1989) Adherence of neutrophil to cultured human microvascular endothelial cells. Stimulation by chemotactic peptides and lipid mediators and dependence upon the Mac-1, LFA-1, p150,95 glycoprotein family. J Clin Invest 83:637–646

26. Harlan JM, Killen PD, Snecal F, et al. (1985) The role of neutrophil membrane glycoprotein GP-150 in neutrophil adherence to endothelium in vitro. Blood 66:167–178
27. Wallis WJ, Hickstein DD, Schwartz BR, et al. (1986) Monoclonal antibody defined functional epitopes on the adhesion promoting glycoprotein complex (CDw18) of human neutrophils. Blood 67:1007–1013
28. Bierer BE, Burakoff SJ (1988) T-cell adhesion molecules. FASEB J 2:2584–2590
29. Arnaout MA, Lanier LL, Faller DV (1988) Relative contribution of the leukocyte molecules Mol, LFA-1, and p150,95 (LeuM5) in adhesion of granulocytes and monocytes to vascular endothelium is tissue- and stimulus-specific. J Cell Physiol 137:305–309
30. Schlag G, Redl H (1990) Endothelium as the interface between blood and organ in the evolution of organ failure. In: Schlag G, Redl H, Siegel JH (eds) Shock, Sepsis, and Organ Failure. First Wiggers Bernard Conference, Springer Verlag, Berlin, Heidelberg, pp 210–271
31. Lewis MS, Whatley RE, Cain P, McIntyre TM, Prescott SM, Zimmermann GA (1988) Hydrogen peroxide stimulates the synthesis of platelet activating factor by endothelium and induces endothelial cell dependent neutrophil adhesion. J Clin Invest 82:2045–2055
32. Geng JG, Bevilacqua MP, Moore KL, et al. (1990) Rapid neutrophil adhesion to activated endothelium mediated by GMP-140. Nature 343:757–760
33. Marzi I, Bühren V, Schüttler A, Trentz O (1991) Recombinant human superoxide dismutase (rh-SOD) to reduce multiple organ failure after trauma – results of a prospective clinical trial. Circ Shock 34:145 (Abs.)
34. Bühren V, Maier B, Hower R, Holzmann A, Redl H, Marzi I (1991) PAF antagonist BN52021 reduces hepatic leukocyte adhesion following intestinal ischemia. Circ Shock 34:134–135
35. Pober JS, Cotran RS (1990) The role of endothelial cells in inflammation. Transplantation 50:537–544
36. Phillips ML, Nudelman E, Gaeta FCA, et al. (1990) ELAM 1 mediates cell adhesion by recognition of a carbohydrate ligand Sialyl Le-x. Science 250:1130–1135
37. Mulligan MS,Varani J, Dame MK, et al. (1991) Role of endothelial-leukocyte adhesion molecule 1 (ELAM-1) in neutrophil-mediated lung injury in rats. J Clin Invest 88:1396–1406
38. Schlag G, Redl H (1980) Die Leukostase in der Lunge beim hypovolämisch-traumatischen Schock. Anaesthesist 29:606–612
39. Redl H, Dinges HP, Schlag G (1987) Quantitative estimation of leukostasis in the posttraumatic lung - canine and human autopsy data. In: Schlag G, Redl H (eds) Progress in Clinical and Biological Research, Pathophysiological Role of Mediators and Mediator Inhibitors in Shock. Vol. 236A: First Vienna Shock Forum, Alan R Liss Inc, New York, pp 43–53
40. Pretorius JP, Schlag G, Redl H, et al. (1987) The lung in shock as a result of hypovolemic-traumatic shock in baboons. J Trauma 27:1344–1352
41. Redl H, Schlag G, Dinges HP, et al. (1991) Trauma and sepsis induced activation of granulocytes, monocytes/macrophages and endothelial cells in primates. In: Schlag G, Redl H, Siegel JH, Traber DL (eds) Shock, Sepsis, and Organ Failure – Second Wiggers Bernard Conference, Springer-Verlag, Berlin, Heidelberg, pp 297–313
42. Mayrovitz H, Wiedeman M, Tuma R (1977) Factors influencing leukocyte adherence in microvessels. Throm Haemostas 38:823–830
43. House SD, Lipowsky HH (1987) Leukocyte-endothelium adhesion: Microhemodynamics in mesentery of the cat. Microvasc Res 34:363–379
44. Redl H, Schlag G, Hammerschmidt DE (1984) Quantitative assessment of leukostasis in experimental hypovolemic-traumatic shock. Acta Chir Scand 150:113–117
45. Varani J, Ginsburg I, Schuger L, et al. (1989) Endothelial cell killing by neutrophils. Synergistic interaction of oxygen products and proteases. Am J Pathol 135:435–438
46. Springer TA (1990) Adhesion receptors of the immune system. Nature 346:425–434

Oxyradical Pathogenesis in Sepsis

J. J. Zimmerman

Introduction

Evidence implicating the participation of toxic oxygen radical species in the pathogenesis of sepsis is rapidly accumulating. Currently most of this information relates to cell culture and animal models, although some human clinical interventional studies employing oxygen radical scavengers are beginning to appear. This chapter will summarize a variety of evidence which indicates oxygen radical pathogenesis in sepsis and alludes to how this data may be utilized in the near future to design novel sepsis therapeutic agents.

Sources of Oxyradicals in Sepsis

Although microbes and their associated toxins initiate sepsis, a ferocious host inflammatory response largely defines the character and magnitude of sepsis [1,2]. The inflammatory response is multifactorial; toxic oxygen radicals appear to play an important role in this multifaceted inflammatory auto-injury. In sepsis the source of oxyradical species are numerous, four have received the greatest attention (Fig. 1). Various aspects of eicosanoid metabolism are known to generate reactive oxygen species. Moreover, toxic oxygen radicals can in themselves stimulate eicosanoid metabolic pathways. One such oxygen radical generating reaction involves the catalysis of prostaglandin G_2 to prostaglandin H_2 by prostaglandin hydroperoxidase. Obviously both the oxygen radical byproducts as well as eicosanoid metabolic imbalance may contribute to sepsis pathophysiology [3].

Continuous electron bleed from electron transport chains results in incomplete reduction of molecular oxygen. Oxyradical generation from the mitochondrial electron transport chain has been investigated most thoroughly in this regard. NADH dehydrogenase as well as the ubiquinone-cytochrome b complex are two areas where superoxide anion is known to be generated. It has been estimated that perhaps one in every 1.000–10.000 molecules of oxygen participating in the mitochondrial electron transport chain is incompletely reduced and results in generation of superoxide anion. Numerous abnormalities relative to the mitochondrial electron transport chain have been described in the setting of sepsis [4-6]. It is not unreasonable to expect that

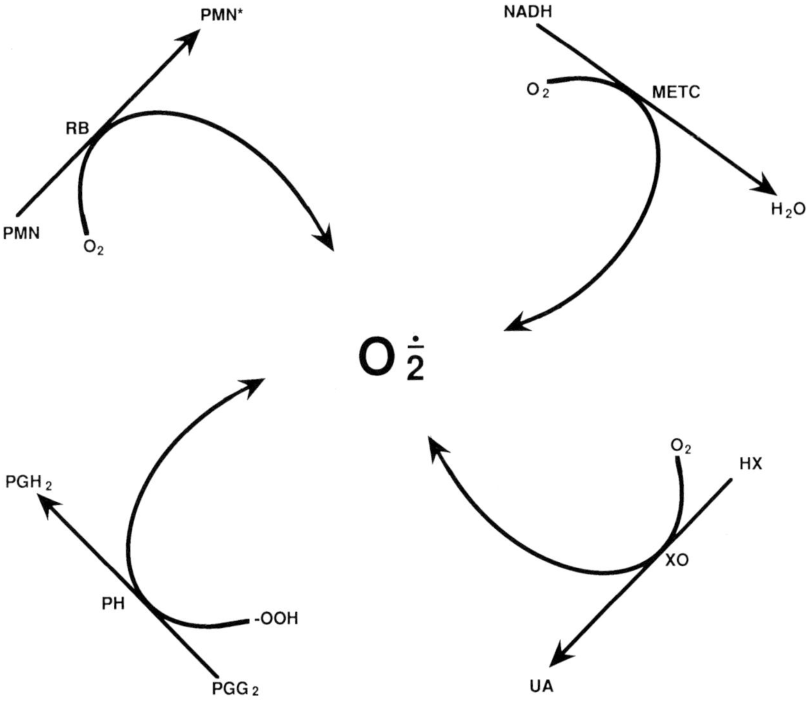

Fig. 1. Sources of oxyradical ($O_2^{\bullet-}$, superoxide anion) generation during sepsis. *PMN:* polymorphonuclear leukocyte; *PMN*:* activated polymorphonuclear leukocyte; *RB:* respiratory burst; *METC:* mitochondrial electron transport chain; *HX:* hypoxanthine; *XO:* xanthine oxidase; *UA:* uric acid; *-OOH:* peroxyl functional group; *PGG2*: prostaglandin G_2; *PH:* prostaglandin hydroperoxidase; *PGH2*: prostaglandin H_2

altered oxygen utilization in sepsis relative to energy substrate catabolism might in fact contribute to the sepsis oxyradical burden.

Because the gross hemodynamic instability as well as changes in microcirculatory perfusion, ischemia/reperfusion states would be predicted to accompany sepsis. With ischemia, there is a progressive accumulation of xanthine and hypoxanthine as a result of critical extraction of high energy phosphate compounds by the cell. Xanthine dehydrogenase is concomitantly converted to xanthine oxidase by the action of intracellular proteases (activated following ischemia-mediated cellular calcium influx) or perhaps by neutrophil elastase. With reintroduction of perfusion and hence oxygen, the stage is set for a burst of superoxide anion production concomitant with the conversion of the xanthine substrates to uric acid [7]. This may represent an important source of oxyradicals in endothelial cells which experience ischemia/reperfusion insults directly.

An important source of oxyradicals, particularly in sepsis, is the respiratory burst of phagocytic leukocytes, especially polymorphonuclear leukocytes

[8,9]. Clinically, neutrophils are known to be in an activated state in septic patients as evidenced by "toxic granulations" revealed by light microscopy. Neutrophil priming as well as activation can occur following exposure to endotoxin or a variety of cytokines (TNF-α, IL-1, IFN-γ) [10,11]. As part of the activation process, NADPH oxidoreductase complex situated on the plasma membrane of neutrophils becomes activated. This enzyme complex is responsible for synthesis of the parent toxic oxygen species, namely superoxide anion. This species may be further metabolized to an array of other reactive species including hydrogen peroxide, hydroxyl radical, hypohalous acids, and N-chloroamines (Fig. 2). Some investigators [12-14] have provided evidence for enhanced superoxide production by neutrophils during sepsis. Interestingly, other investigators have noted that when neutrophils are isolated from septic patients and directly analyzed *in vitro* for superoxide production, their activity appears to be suppressed [15,16]. Utilizing flow cytometry techniques, neutrophils isolated from septic patients have been demonstrated to exhibit various levels of activation as quantitated by hydrogen-peroxide dependent dichlorofluorescein fluorescence [17]. On the one hand, this data may represent a situation in which "exhausted", previously *in vivo* activated neutrophils are resistant to additional *in vitro* stimulation. Alternately, it has also been demonstrated that there appears to be a factor(s) in septic plasma that may directly inhibit the production of superoxide anion by normal neutrophils [18].

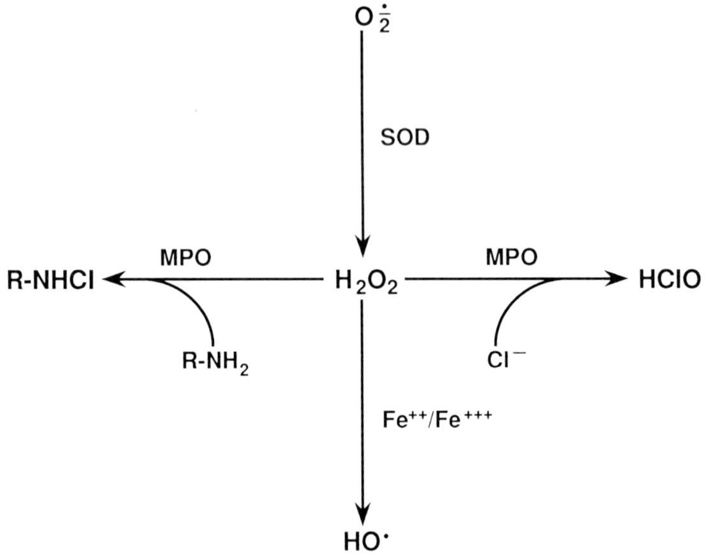

Fig. 2. Interconversion of oxyradicals and related species. SOD: superoxide dismutase; MPO: myeloperoxidase; R-NHCl: N-chloroamine; Fe++/Fe+++: iron redox couple in Fenton reaction

Neutrophils are known to leukosequestrate in various organs in sepsis, particularly the lungs. Their aggregation implies activation of chemotaxis as well as membrane glycoprotein expression which facilitates binding to endothelial cells [19,20]. With this close approximation of leukocyte and endothelial cell and activation of the neutrophil, the stage is set for possible inflammation mediated host autoinjury [21]. In an attempt to clear foreign antigen, the neutrophil may actually impart significant damage to the host milieu as well. It should be appreciated that in addition to release of oxyradicals, a variety of other toxic constituents may be degranulated by activated neutrophils and participate in a synergistic manner with oxyradicals in host autoinjury. At least in the case of animal models of sepsis-induced pulmonary injury, neutrophil depletion frequently results in amelioration of injury.

Molecular Targets of Oxyradicals

Lipids represent a large pool of oxyradical-susceptible macromolecules because they reflect the bulk of lipid bilayer mass in plasma membranes and intracellular organelles (Fig. 3). Polyunsaturated fatty acids are especially susceptible to oxidant injury because of readily extractable allyl methylene hydrogens and because of the ability to form conjugated systems to stabilize the odd electron [22]. Peroxidized phospholipid fatty acids are more readily hydrolyzed by phospholipase A_2 [23]. Resulting lysophospholipids display

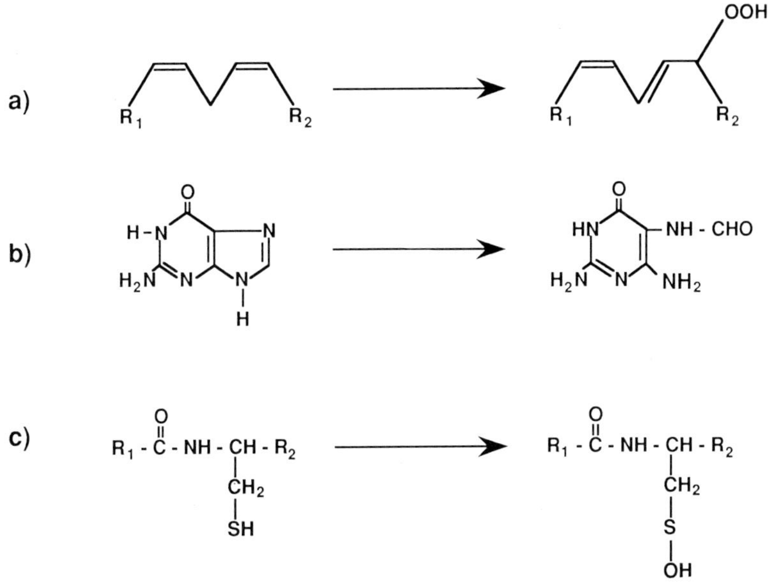

Fig. 3. Examples of common oxidant injury in **a)** polyunsaturated fatty acids (lipid peroxidation), **b)** nucleic acids (2,6-diamino-4-hydroxy-5-formamidopyrimidine from guanine); and **c)** amino-acids (sulfenic acid functional group from cysteine reduced sulfhydryl)

marked detergent activity which can potentiate the oxyradical injury. It should be noted that with respect to lipid peroxidation, once commenced, the process may become autocatalytic. Accordingly, an initiating oxyradical insult may be amplified by free radical chain reactions. Introduction of a polar peroxyl functional group (or the reduced hydroxyl derivative) into the hydrophobic fatty acid aliphatic tail would be expected to induce structural chaos. Moreover, lipid peroxides are known to undergo cyclic intramolecular rearrangement to yield secondary cleavage products including malondialdehyde and the hydroxyalkenyls (e.g. 4-hydroxynonenal). These aldehyde derivatives are highly reactive and cytotoxic and mutagenic [24].

All proteins may be subject to oxidant injury which may result in fragmentation or denaturation of tertiary structure which in turns enhances susceptibility to proteolytic degradation. All amino-acids are sensitive to oxidant injury, although those containing sulfur are particularly susceptible [25]. Oxidant injury leads to alterations in both structure and function of proteins. Protein injury may occur directly by oxyradical mediated damage or indirectly through the action of lipid hydroperoxides, especially if the protein is embedded within a lipid bilayer [26]. The best studied example of protein alteration by oxyradicals involves the inactivation of alpha-1 protease inhibitor. Exposure of this essential plasma antiprotease to oxidant stress, (e.g. neutrophil myeloperoxidase production of HCIO) results in oxidation of a critical, active site methionine residue [27]. Modification of primary structure results in a molecule which will not bind elastase, this resulting in free elastase activity. Oxyradicals from activated neutrophils can also inhibit phosphatidylcholine synthesis in alveolar type II cells [28] and membrane-bound Na^+-K^+-ATPase (Julin CM, Zimmerman JJ, et al. submitted). Oxyradicals are similarly known to inhibit glyceraldehyde-3-phosphate dehydrogenase [29], and glycerol-3-phosphate acyltransferase [30].

Probably, the most ominous oxyradical injury involves alteration of the cellular genome. Base alterations as well as DNA nicks have been demonstrated following nucleic acid oxidant stress [31]. Activation of various DNA repair enzymes is seen concomitant with nucleic acid oxidant damage [32]. In addition to the potential for impaired growth and differentiation as a result of this type of injury, it has also been demonstrated that oxidant-mediated nucleic acid alteration can result in both mutagenesis and carcinogenesis [33].

Cellular Toxicity of Oxyradicals

Based on the information summarized above, it is not surprising that oxidant stress can lead to pertubation of the organization of membranes. Electron paramagnetic resonance studies of porcine endothelial cells have demonstrated increased fluidity following oxidant stress [34]. Numerous investigations employing cell culture techniques have consistently reported oxidant-mediated cell membrane damage as assessed by leakage of ^{51}Cr or lactic dehydro-

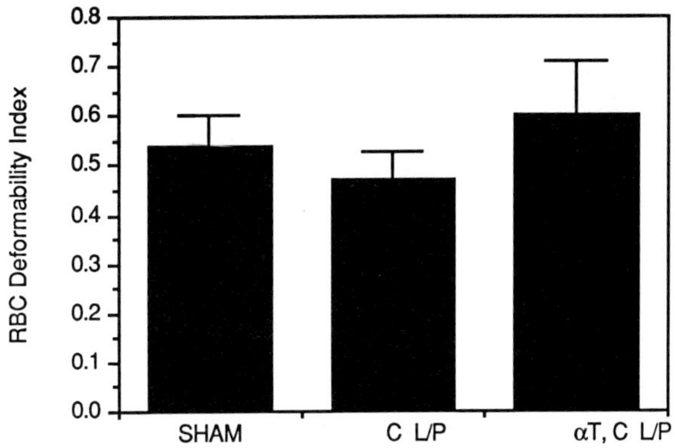

Fig. 4. Aberrations in erythrocyte deformability produced during murine sepsis and protection by alpha-tocopherol (Adapted from [38] with permission). C L/P: cecal ligation and perforation; αT: alpha-tocopherol pretreatment. Bars represent mean ± SD. C L/P values demonstrated $p < 0.05$ compared to sham or αT, C L/P groups

genase from the cytosol [35,36]. In addition to alterations of the plasmalemma, the cardiac sarcoplasmic reticulum has also been proposed as an oxyradical target during endotoxin shock, and may in part account for the myocardial impairment characteristic of sepsis [37]. Erythrocyte membranes have similarly been shown to be susceptible to oxidant stress; the resulting alterations in erythrocyte deformability may account for some of the microperfusion deficits seen in sepsis (Fig. 4) [38]. As a result of plasma membrane and organelle membrane alterations, it has been shown that oxyradicals can mediate calcium overload in endothelial cells. This process, which is postulated to involve both lipid peroxidation as well as protein cross-links results in the production of cation ionophores [39]. As has been previously noted, oxygen radicals may stimulate both intracellular proteolysis as well as lipid peroxidation [40].

Oxyradical-Mediated Microvascular Injury

Oxidant stress may result in alterations in vascular reactivity [41]. By activating the arachidonate pathway, oxyradicals may initiate the production of various vasonconstrictor molecules. On the other hand, direct interaction with guanylate cyclase can lead to vasodilation. Clinically, the hallmark of sepsis is diffuse capillary leak which almost certainly is mediatd in part by oxyradicals. Utilizing a Syrian hamster cheek pouch model and analysis of microvascular suffusate, it has been demonstrated that endotoxin infusion results in a significant increase in leaky sites as well as microvascular clearance of fluorescent-labeled dextran (molecular weight 150.000) [42]. Pretreating the animals with dimethylsulfoxide or high dose allopurinol (oxygen radical scavenging activity) resulted in significant diminution of the

Table 1. Effect of oxyradical scavengers on endotoxin-mediated capillary leak in the hamster cheek pouch model (Adapted from [19], with permission)

	leaky Sites (sites/cm^2)	FITC-D Clearance (ml/min x 10^{-6})
NaCl Control	7 ± 6	7 ± 5
LPS Suffusion	45 ± 18	20 ± 6
LPS & DMSO	9 ± 5	8 ± 2
LPS & Allopurinol	11 ± 7	9 ± 4
LPS & Allopurinol & DMSO	11 ± 6	7 ± 1

FITC-D: fluorescent labeled dextran; *LPS:* lipopolysaccharide;
DMSO: dimethylsulfoxide

endotoxin mediated pathology (Table 1). Endotoxin can initiate endothelial oxidant stress in the presence or absence of neutrophils [43].

Adult respiratory distress sydrome (ARDS) represents the most studied capillary leak phenomena associated with sepsis. Infusion of lipopolysaccharide (LPS) or an agent which causes systemic activation of neutrophils (phorbol myristic acetate) results in pulmonary leukosequestration, extravascular lung water accumulation, and enhanced protein permeability across the pulmonary endothelium, and is associated with a concomitant increase of lung parenchyma lipid peroxidation products [44]. Similarly, it has also been shown that free radicals are associated with the development of gastrointestinal damage in *E. coli* sepsis [45].Gastric mucosal damage noted after *E. coli* infusion into cats was associated with hypotension, impaired cardiac output, and increased pulmonary artery pressure. In this setting, copper-zinc superoxide dismutase had no effects on the hemodynamics of the model but was shown to decrease significantly the gastric mucosal damage.

Demonstration of Oxyradicals in Sepsis

Classically, the association between sepsis and oxygen radicals has been most frequently evaluated by quantitating the appearance of thiobarbituric acid reactive species (TBARS) and conjugated dienes. TBARS reflect the condensation between malondialdehyde (OHC-CH_2-CHO), a β-scission byproduct of lipid peroxidation, and 2 molecules of thiobarbituric acid. The resulting adduct displays a high extinction coefficient at 530 nm [46]. Conjugated dienes refers to the conjugated double bond configuration that results during polyunsaturated fatty acid peroxidation, which may be quantitated by absorbance at 234 nm [47]. Both of these markers reflect lipid peroxidation and both tests may involve a number of confounding variables. A great deal of information relative to oxyradicals and sepsis utilizing these two markers has been gleaned from the chronic lung lymph fistula sheep model [48,49]. Utilizing this now well characterized system, it has been demonstrated that the early pulmonary hypertensive phase following endotoxin infusion is almost certainly mediated by thromboxane A_2, and that the subsequent pulmonary vascular leak phase probably involves neutrophil-mediated oxidant stress. Employing this model (there have been a multitude of related experiments), increases in lung TBARS and plasma conjugated dienes can frequently be associated with physiological markers of increased pulmonary capillary permeability. Following endotoxin administration, systemic neutropenia is characteristically associated with pulmonary leukosequestration, again implicating the neutrophil as a prime player in the endotoxin-mediated pulmonary injury. Pathological changes in the lungs have been associated with a rise in tissue TBARS.

A similar model of sepsis in guinea pigs has revealed evidence of pulmonary oxidant stress in bronchoalveolar lavage fluid (BALF) [50]. For example, extent of pulmonary edema as a result of *E. coli* peritonitis/sepsis correlates with TBARS in BALF. In addition to the increased TBARS in BALF (as well as lung parenchyma), increased leakage of albumin and accumulation of neutrophils were also noted in these specimens. The increase in TBARS correlated with an increase in lung water, and permeability indices as well as histologic data which ascertained a neutrophil alveolitis. This type of experiment is important because similar investigative approaches (i.e. BALF) might be utilized in humans with sepsis-associated ARDS.

In an overwhelming lethal model of *E. coli* canine septic shock, fluorescent products of lipid peroxidation have been shown to accumulate in serum during the septic insult [51]. The 200% rise in fluorescent lipid peroxidation products during sepsis was prevented by pretreatment with antioxidants. Granulocyte depletion did not alter the appearance of the lipid peroxidation marker implicating that other sources of oxyradicals are more important in this particular model (e.g. tissue ischemia reperfusion).

Appearance of lipid peroxidation products has been evaluated in septic human patients utilizing an extremely sensitive assay involving the activation of cyclooxygenase by hydroperoxides [52]. Interestingly, the highest level of hydroperoxides were found in arterial blood in patients whose primary septic focus was pneumonia as compared to pulmonary arterial blood for patients whose primary septic focus was an abdominal infection. Thus, the absolute value of the arterial minus pulmonary artery concentration of oxidant stress marker may be the appropriate way of examining plasma for evidence of oxyradical stress.

Because of intramolecular rearrangement and β-scission reactions, lipid peroxides generate other small molecular weight compounds such as ethane and penthane, in addition to malondialdehyde [53]. In fact, it has been shown in a mouse model of sepsis that exhaled ethane correlated with hepatic homogenate TBARS [54]. This non-invasive assessment of oxidant stress will almost certainly evolve in future clinical investigations examining the role of oxidant

Table 2. Plasma TBARS and alpha-tocopherol levels in controls and septic patients (Adapted from [31] with permission)

	TBARS (nmol MDA/ml)	αT (mg/ml)
Control (n=40)	7.36 ± 1.99	1.05 ± 0.28
Septic (n=7)	10.60 ± 2.29	0.64 ± 0.25

TBARS: thiobarbituric acid reactive species; MDA: malondialdehyde; αT: alpha-tocopherol

stress in human sepsis, as the technique has already demonstrated applicability in both adult [55] and pediatric [56] critically ill patients.

Glutathione and glutathione peroxidase represent essential elements of the antioxidant armentarium. Apparent consumption of glutathione has been demonstrated in a sheep model where consecutive samples were obtained by liver biopsy during progression of sepsis [57].

Similarly consumption of alpha-tocopherol, the key hydrophobic membrane antioxidant, has also been noted in a rat model of sepsis involving cecal ligation and puncture. A decrease in alpha-tocopherol was associated with an increase in lipid peroxidation products (TBARS) in plasma and most organs [58]. In septic humans, apparent alpha-tocopherol consumption has been noted to correlate inversely with plasma peroxidation products (TBARS) (Table 2) [59]. As septic patients improve clinically as quantitated by increases in APACHE scores, plasma alpha-tocopherol levels normalize even in the absence of exogenous supplementation [60].

All of the above techniques examine the result of oxidant stress rather than the actual perpetrator molecules. However, electron paramagnetic resonance with spin trapping has been utilized to demonstrate that carbon-centered radical spin adducts characteristic of lipid peroxides may be quantitated *in vivo*, in real time, in both the heart and liver during endotoxemia [61].

Therapeutic Potential of Oxyradical Scavengers

Because animal models most closely approximate the human situation, therapeutic trials involving oxyradical scavengers in animals are numerous. It should be appreciated, however, that a great deal of information relative to subtleties of the pathogenesis of oxyradical injury, as well as initial trials with oxyradical scavengers, have employed cell culture techniques [62]. As has been previously noted, isolated details of cellular function and structure can be monitored utilizing cell culture technique. An important aspect of these studies has been the appreciation of the relative endothelial penetration of various oxyradical scavengers under scrutiny. By conjugating otherwise highly hydrophilic species (e.g. superoxide dismutase) to hydrophobic carrier molecules (e.g. polyethylene glycol) [63], or by incorporating such species into liposomes [64], the delivery to and uptake of various high molecular weight oxyradical scavengers by endothelial cells can be enhanced significantly. Basically those agents which demonstrate the greatest capacity to penetrate the endothelial cell membrane appear to function best as oxyradical scavengers during endotoxemia [65].

Mention has been made of the susceptibility of sulfur containing aminoacids to oxidant stress, and the role of glutathione and glutathione peroxidase. A variety of low molecular weight sulfhydryl agents are available as therapeutic intervention for endotoxin-mediated oxidant stress. N-acetylcysteine has been demonstrated to inhibit lipid peroxidation as well as extravasation of labeled albumin in a porcine model of *E. coli* sepsis [66]. However, no alterations in survival could be ascertained. Other investigators have also noted that low molecular weight sulfhydryl agents can decrease markers of oxidant stress but have no effect on altering sepsis-associated hemodynamics or ultimate survival.

Dimethylsulfoxide (DMSO) has also been investigated as a possible therapeutic agent in sepsis. DMSO is thought to scavenge hydroxyl radical which is generated from superoxide anion and hydrogen peroxide through the transition metal-catalyzed Fenton reaction. In a rat model of sepsis employing IV administration of *E. Coli* LPS, pre-administration of intraperitoneal DMSO was shown to abolish early hypotension, reverse lactate accumulation, eliminate hypoglycemia, and prevent characteristic hemorrhagic lesions of the small intestine [67]. In a related study, this agent was also shown to prevent pathologic, hepatic, and cardiac ultrastructural changes related to the septic insult. It should be appreciated that DMSO itself induces a number of hemodynamic alterations independent of the septic insult.

Nitrone compounds originally employed as spin trapping agents for electron paramagnetic resonance spectroscopy, have also been analyzed as therapeutic agents in endotoxin-associated oxidant stress. Published results utilizing these agents have been truly impressive with significant improvement in survival noted even when agents were given following the endotoxin insult [68,69].

Therapeutic use of vitamin E (alpha-tocopherol) [70] has similarly been investigated in animal models of endotoxin shock. In a mouse model, pretreatment with vitamin E was shown to reduce the level of hepatic lipid peroxide markers (TBARS) as well as lactic accumulation during sepsis [71]. In a related study examining *E. coli* or staphylococcal peritonitis in septic guinea pigs, vitamin E, but not ascorbate, was shown to have a significant effect on reducing mortality [72]. However, this protective effect was lost at very high pharmacological doses of vitamin E, an observation which may be explained by the neutrophil inhibitory effect of vitamin E at high concentrations.

Like alpha-tocopherol, coenzyme Q10 represents another naturally occurring compound that may have protective effects relative to oxidant stress associated with sepsis [73]. In canine sepsis, pretreatment with coenzyme Q10 has been shown to preserve lung compliance and decrease lactate accumula-

Table 3. Effect of human recombinant superoxide dismutase on endotoxin-mediated pulmonary capillary leak in rats (Adapted from [44], with permission)

	Wet Lung Weight (Mg/100g bw ± SEM	Lung Permeability Index
Controls	532 ± 15	2.11 ± 0.34
Endotoxin	664 ± 46	4.82 ± 0.65
LPS & rHSOD (0.10 mg/kg(min)	617 ± 40	3.28 ± 0.96
LPS & rHSOD (0.22 mg/kg/min)	577 ± 31	2.83 ± 0.55
LPS & rHSOD (0.46 mg/kg/min)	559 ± 39	2.16 ± 0.65

rHSOD: human recombinant superoxide dismutase
LPS: lipopolysaccharide

tion without altering cardiac index or oxygen consumption [74]. In a rat model of sepsis, coenzyme Q10 in combination with alpha-tocopherol was shown to improve survival, preserve ATP levels, and suppress accumulation of lipid peroxidation products in the liver [75]. Whether this compound is acting strictly as a free radical scavenger, or enhancing its natural activity in the mitochondrial electron transport chain is currently not known.

Of the protein oxygen radical scavengers, superoxide dismutase (SOD) has been studied most extensively with regard to a variety of oxidant-mediated injury. SOD, but not N-acetyl cysteine, was shown to increase survival in endotoxic mice [76]. More recently, human recombinant SOD was demonstrated to have a number of dose-related beneficial effects in a rat model of *E. coli* endotoxin shock (Table 3) [77]. Pulmonary vascular permeability index as well as wet lung weight were significantly improved in animals receiving exogenous SOD. Presumed pulmonary oxidant injury in this model was associated with pulmonary neutrophil infiltration. The investigators pointed out that their positive results, utilizing SOD in this model in the face of several other studies which have not demonstrated a protective effect of SOD, were probably due to the five-to-ten fold higher plasma SOD levels obtained in their study as compared to previous ones.

It should be recognized that SOD catalyzes formation of hydrogen peroxide which in itself is a strong oxidant. Accordingly, other investigators have examined the effect of exogenous catalase (CAT) on ameliorating endotoxin-mediated oxidant stress. Most cell culture models investigating oxidant injury report more protection from exogenous CAT then from exogenous SOD. In the sheep lung lymph fistula model, pretreatment with intraperitoneal CAT prior to endotoxin infusion has been shown to attenuate pulmonary artery pressure, lung lymph flow, lung/plasma protein ratio, peripheral neutropenia, and hypoxemia [78]. Related studies in sheep have shown that exogenous CAT attenuates the rise in plasma markers of both thromboxane A_2 and prostacycline as well as plasma conjugated dienes [79]. In this investigation, lung parenchymal lipid peroxidation markers (TBARS) and extravascular lung water were held at baseline in animals pretreated with CAT.

The logical simultaneous use of SOD and CAT has also been investigated. This combination would lead to the rapid metabolism of superoxide through the hydrogen peroxide intermediate to water and oxygen. Both substrates for the Fenton reaction would also be more rapidly cleared. The characterized superoxide anion inhibition of CAT provides still another possible mechanism of synergy between the two enzymes [80]. In a model of endotoxemia in rats, the combination of SOD and CAT significantly improved survival and inhibited the rise in hepatic TBARS [81]. Although exogenous vitamin E and glutathione were also demonstrated to decrease hepatic TBARS in this model, they had no affect on survival.

Endogenous levels of the protein oxyradical scavengers may be enhanced via exposure to endotoxin. In reality this induction probably occurs via induction of cytokine expression. TNF-α, IL-1, and IFN-γ have all been shown to enhance expression of protein oxygen radical scavengers [82]. Toxic oxygen species themselves (e.g. hydrogen peroxide) may activate antioxidant responsive elements. For example, it has recently been shown that the five prime flanking region of glutathione S-transferase which regulates the transcription of the transferase and is responsible for controlling the basal level

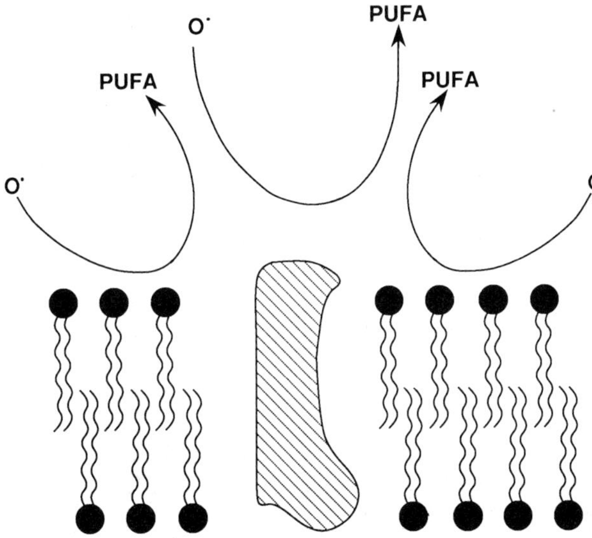

Fig. 5. Polyunsaturated fatty acids (PUFA) acting as free radical (O·) sinks. This schematic depiction of the "alternate hypothesis" [84] proposes that excess PUFA may trap free radicals, thus diverting oxyradical stress away from crucial membrane lipids or proteins (and nucleic acids)

of enzyme, is responsive to hydrogen peroxide [83]. This is one example of an antioxidant responsive element, which are cis-acting regulatory elements which encode proteins important in defense against oxidative stress.

It is possible that polyunsaturated fatty acids (PUFA) may represent a defense as well as target relative to oxidant stress. In this regard, a so-called "alternate hypothesis" has been advanced which speculates that animals fed diets rich in polyunsaturated fatty acids may be protected from oxyradical insult by virtue of the excess PUFA acting as oxyradical traps or sinks (Fig. 5) [84]. This possibility has been actively investigated with respect to hyperoxic lung injury but not in the case of endotoxin-mediated oxidant stress. However, this observation along with previous investigations relative to alpha-tocopherol underscore the importance of nutritional considerations in septic patients.

Conclusions

Abundant evidence in cell culture and animal models strongly implicates the key role of toxic oxygen metabolites in the pathogenesis of sepsis. Therapeutic trails utilizing oxyradical scavengers will undoubtedly eventually provide the critical care physician with additional drugs which have great potential to reduce morbidity and mortality in sepsis.

References

1. Freeman Ba, Crapo JD (1982) Free radicals and tissue injury. Lab Invest 47:412–426
2. Cross AR, Jones OTG (1991) Enzymatic mechanisms of superoxide production. Biochim Biophys Acta 1057:281–298
3. Pittet JF, Morel DR (1991) Imbalance between plasma levels of thromoxane β_2 and 6-keto-prostaglandin F1α during subacute endotoxin-induced hyperdynamic sepsis or multiple organ failure syndrome in sheep. Circ Shock 35:65–77
4. Shimahara Y, Ozawa K, Takeshi I, Ukikusa M, Tobe T (1982) Role of mitochondrial enhancement in maintaining hepatic energy charge level in endotoxin shock. J Surg Res 33:314–323
5. Mela-Riker L, Tavakoli H (1983) Mitochondrial function in shock. Am J Emerg Med 2:2–7
6. Schaefer CF, Lerner MR, Biber B (1991) Dose-related reduction of intenstinal cytochrome c,a_3 induced by endotoxin in rats Circ Shock 33:17–25
7. McCord JM (1985) Oxygen-derived free radicals in postischemic tissue injury. N Engl J Med 312:159–163
8. Babior BM (1984) Oxidants from phagocytes: Agents of defense and destruction. Blood 64:959–966
9. Morel F, Doussiere J, Vignais PV (1991) The superoxide-generating oxidase of phagocytic cells. Physiological, molecular, and pathological aspects. Eur J Biochem 201:523–546
10. Wewers MD, Rinehart JJ, She Z-W, et al. (1990) Tumor necrosis factor infusions in human prime neutrophils for hypochlorous acid production. Am J Physiol 259:267–282
11. Aida Y, Pabst MJ (1990) Priming of neutrophils by lipopolysaccharide for enhanced release of superoxide. J Immunol 145:3017–3025
12. Zimmermann GA, Renzetti AD, Hill HR (1983) Functional and metabolic activity of granulocytes from patients with adult respiratory distress syndrome. Am Rev Respir Dis 127:290–300

13. Hallgren R, Borg T, Venge P, Modig J (1984) Signs of neutrophil and eosinophil activation in adult respiratory distress syndrome. Crit Care Med 12:14–18
14. Simons RK, Maier RN, Lennard S (1987) Neutrophil function in a rat model of endotoxin-induced lung injury. Arch Surg 122:197–203
15. Solomkin JS, Brodt JK, Antrum RM (1985) Suppressed neutrophil oxidative activity in sepsis: A receptor-mediated regulatory response. J Surg Res 39:300–304
16. Zimmerman JJ, Shelhamer JH, Parrillo JE (1985) Quantitative analysis of polymorphonuclear leukocyte superoxide anion generation in critically ill children. Cirt Care Med 14:143–150
17. Bass DA, Olbrantz P, Szejda P, et al. (1986) Subpopulations of neutrophils with increased oxidative product formation in blood of patients with infection. J Immunol 136:860–866
18. Zimmerman JJ, Millard JR, Farrin-Rusk C (1989) Septic plasma suppresses superoxide anion synthesis by normal homologous polymorphonuclear leukocytes. Crit Care Med 17:1241–1246
19. Smith CW (1990) Molecular determinants of neutrophil adhesion. Am J Respir Cell Mol Biol 2:487–489
20. Albelda SM (1991) Endothelial and epithelial cell adhesion molecules. Am J Resp Cell Mol Biol 4:195–203
21. Harlan JM (1985) Leukocyte-endothelial interactions. Blood 65:513–523
22. Gardner HW (1989) Oxygen radical chemistry of polyunsaturated fatty acids. Free Rad Biol Med 7:65–86
23. Sevanian A, Kim E (1985) Phospholipase A_2 dependent release of fatty acids from peroxidized membranes. Free Rad Biol Med 1:263–271
24. Esterbauer H, Cheeseman KH (1990) Determination of aldehydic lipid peroxidation products: Malonaldehyde and 4-hydroxynonenal. Meth Enzymol 186:407–421
25. Davies KJA (1987) Protein damage and degradation by oxygen radicals. J Biol Chem 262:9895–9901
26. Hunt JV, Dean RT (1989) Free radical-mediated degradation of proteins: The protective and deleterious effects of membranes. Biochem Biophys Res Commun 162:1076–1084
27. Clark RA, Stone PJ, Hag AE, Calore JD, Franzblau C (1981) Myeloperoxidase-catalyzed inactivation of α_1 protease inhibitor by human neutrophils. J Biol Chem 256:3348–3353
28. Zimmerman JJ, Lewandoski JR (1991) Acitvated polymorphonuclear leukocytes inhibit phosphatidylcholine synthesis in cultured type II alveolar cells. Pediatr Pulmonol 10:164–171
29. Hyslop PA, Hinshaw DB, Halsey WA, et al. (1988) Mechanisms of oxidant mediated cell injury. The glycolytic and mitochondrial pathways of ADP phosphorylation are major intracellular targets inactivated by hydrogen peroxide. J Biol Chem 263:1665–1676
30. Holm BA, Matalon S, Finkelstein JN, Natter RH (1988) Type II pneumocyte changes during hyperoxic lung injury and recovery. J Appl Physiol 65:2672–2678
31. Spragg RG (1991) DNA strand break formation following exposure of bovine pulmonary artery and aortic endothelial cells to reactive oxygen products. Am J Respir Cell Mol Biol 4:4–10
32. Berger NA (1991) Oxidant-induced cytotoxicity: A Challenge for metabolic modulation. Am J Respir Cell Mol Biol 4:1–3
33. Imlay JA, Linn S (1988) DNA damage and oxygen radical toxicity. Science 240:1302–1309
34. Freeman BA, Rosen GM, Barber MJ (1986) Superoxide pertubation of the organization of vascular endothelial cell membranes. J Biol Chem 261:6590–6593
35. Weiss SJ, Young J, LoBuglio AF, Slivka A (1981) Role of hydrogen peroxide in neutrophil-mediated destruction of cultured endothelial cells. J Clin Invest 68:714–721
36. Kirkland JB (1991) Lipid peroxidation, protein thiol oxidation and DNA damage in hydrogen peroxide-induced injury to endothelial cells: Role of activation of poly (ADP-ribose) polymerase. Biochim Biophys Acta 1092:319–325
37. Manson NH, Hess ML (1983) Interaction of oxygen free radicals and cardiac sarcoplasmic reticulum: Proposed role in the pathogenesis of endotoxin shock. Circ Shock 10:205–213
38. Powell RJ, Machiedo GW, Rush BF, Dikdon G (1991) Oxygen free radicals: Effect on red cell deformity in sepsis. Crit Care Med 19:732–735
39. Franceschi D, Graham D, Sarasua M, et al. (1990) Mechanisms of oxygen free radical-induced calcium overload in endothelial cells. Surgery 108:292–297

40. Davies KJA, Goldberg AL (1987) Oxygen radicals stimulate intracellular proteolysis and lipid peroxidation by independent mechanisms in erythrocytes. J Biol Chem 262:8220–8226
41. Gurtner GH, Burke-Wolin T (1991) Interactions of oxidant stress and vascular reactivity. Am J Physiol 260:207–211
42. Matsuda T, Eccleston CA, Rubinstein I, Rennard SI, Joyner WL (1991) Antioxidants attenuate endotoxin-induced microvascular leakage of macromolecules in vivo. J Appl Physiol 70:1483–1489
43. Chang S, Lauterberg B, Voclkel N (1988) Endotoxin causes neutrophil independent oxidant stress in rats. J Appl Physiol 65:358–367
44. Wong C, Flynn J, Demling RH (1984) Role of oxygen radicals in endotoxin-induced lung injury. Arch Surg 119:77–82
45. Arvidsson S, Falt K, Marklund S, Haglund U (1985) Role of free oxygen radicals in the development of gastrointestinal mucosal damage in Escherichia coli sepsis. Circ Shock 16:383–393
46. Janero DR (1990) Malondialdehyde and thiobarbituric acid-reactivity as diagnostic indices of lipid peroxidation and peroxidative tissue injury. Free Rad Biol Med 9:515–540
47. Recknagel RO, Glende EA (1984) Spectrophotometric detection of lipid conjugated dienes. Meth Enzymol 105:331–340
48. Demling R, Lalonde C (1989) Relationship between lung injury and lung lipid peroxidation caused by recurrent endotoxemia. Am Rev Respir Dis 139:1118–1124
49. Demling R, Lalonde C, Daryani R, Zhu P, Knox J, Youn YK (1991) Relationship between the lung and systemic response to endotoxin: Comparison of physiologic change and the degree of lipid peroxidation. Circ Shock 34:364–370
50. Ishizaka A, Stephens K, Tazelaar H, Hall EW, O'Hanley P, Raffin TA (1988) Pulmonary edema after Escherichia coli peritonitis correlates with thiobarbituric acid reactive materials in bronchoalveolar lavage fluid. Am Rev Respir Dis 137:783–789
51. Morgan RA, Manning PB, Coran AG, et al. (1988) Oxygen free radical activity during live E. coli septic shock in the dog. Circ Shock 25:319–323
52. Keen RR, Stella L, Flanigan DP, Lands WEM (1991) Differential detection of plasma hydroperoxides in sepsis. Crit Care Med 19:1114–1119
53. Wade CR, van Rij AM (1985) In vivo lipid peroxidation in man as measured by respiratory excretion of ethane, pentane and other low-molecular-weight hydrocarbons. Anal Biochem 150:1–7
54. Peavy DL, Fairchild EJ (1986) Evidence for lipid peroxidation in endotoxin poisoned mice. Infect Immun 52:613–616
55. Baldwin SR, Simon RH, Grum CM, Ketai LH, Boder LA, Devall LJ (1986) Oxidant activity in expired breath of patients with adult respiratory distress syndrome. Lancet 1:11–14
56. Pikanen OM, Hallman M, Andersson SM (1990) Correlation of free oxygen radical-induced lipid peroxidation with outcome in very low birth weight infants. J Pediatr 116:760–764
57. Keller GA, Barke R, Harty JT, Humprey E, Simmons RL (1985) Decreased hepatic glutathione levels in septic shock. Arch Surg 120:941–945
58. Takeda K, Shimada Y, Okada T, Amano M, Sakai T, Yoshiya I (1986) Lipid peroxidation in experimental septic rats. Crit Care Med 14:719–723
59. Takeda K, Shimada Y, Amano M, Sakai T, Okada T, Yoshiya (1984) Plasma lipid peroxides and alpha-tocopherol in critically ill patients. Crit Care Med 12:957–959
60. Toonen TR, Lewandoski JR, Zimmerman JJ (1991) Longitudinal analysis of plasma tocopherol levels in patients with septic shock. Clin Res 39:688
61. Brackett DL, Lai EK, Lerner MR, et al. (1989) Spin trapping of free radicals produced in vivo in heart and liver during endotoxemia. Free Rad Res Commun 7:315–324
62. Brigham K, Meyrick B, Berry L, Repine J (1987) Antioxidants protect cultured bovine lung endothelial cells from injury by endotoxin. J Appl Physiol 63:840–850
63. Walther FJ, Wade AB, Warburton D, Forman HJ (1991) Augmentation of superoxide dismutase and catalase activity in alveolar type II cells. Am J Respir Cell Mol Biol 4:364–368
64. Buckley BJ, Tanswell AK, Freeman BA (1987) Liposome-mediated augmentation of catalase in alveolar type II cells protects against H_2O_2 injury. J Appl Physiol 63:359–367

65. McKechnie K, Fuhrman BL, Parratt (1986) Modification by oxygen free radical scavengers of the metabolic and cardiovascular effects of endotoxin infusion in conscious rats. Circ Shock 19:429–439
66. Groeneveld ABJ, den Hollander W, Straub J, Nauta JJP, Thijs LG (1990) Effects of N-acetylcysteine and terbutaline treatment on hemodynamics and regional albumin extravasation in porcine septic shock. Circ Shock 30:185–205
67. Bracket DJ, Lerner MR, Wilson MF (1991) Dimethyl sulfoxide antagonizes hypotensive, metabolic, and pathogenic responses induced by endotoxin. Circ Shock 33:156–163
68. Novelli GP, Angiolini P, Livi P, et al. (1989) Oxygen-derived free radicals in the pathogenesis of experimental shock. Resuscitation 18:195–205
69. Hamburger SA, McCay PB (1989) Endotoxin–induced mortality in rats is reduced by nitrones. Circ Shock 29:329–334
70. Chow CK (1991) Vitamin E and oxidative stress. Free Rad Biol Med 11:215–232
71. Sugino K, Dohi Y, Yamada K, et al. (1987) The role of lipid peroxidation in endotoxin-induced hepatic damage and the protective effect of antioxidants. Surgery 101:746–752
72. Peck MD, Alexander JW (1991) Survival in septic guinea pigs is influenced by vitamin E, but not by vitamin C in enteral diets. J Parent Ent Nutr 15:433–436
73. Beyer RE (1990) The participation of coenzyme Q in free radical production and antioxidation. Free Rad Biol Med 8:545–565
74. Yasumoto K, Inada Y (1986) Effect of coenzyme Q10 on endotoxin shock in dogs. Crit Care Med 14:570–574
75. Sugino K, Dohi K, Yamada K, Kawasaki T (1987) The role of lipid peroxidation in endotoxin-induced hepatic damage and the protective effects of antioxidants. Surgery 101:746–752
76. Broner CW, Shenep JL, Stidham GL, Stokes DC, Hildner WK (1988) Effect of scavengers of oxygen-derived free radicals on mortality in endotoxin-challenged mice. Crit Care Med 16:848–852
77. Schneider J, Friderichs E, Heintz K, Flohe L (1990) Effects of recombinant human superoxide dismutase on increased lung vascular permeability and respiratory disorder in endotoxemic rats. Circ Shock 30:97–106
78. Milligan SA, Hoeffel JM, Goldstein IM, Flick MR (1988) Effect of catalase on endotoxin-induced acute lung injury in unanesthetized sheep. Am Rev Respir Dis 137:420–428
79. Seekamp A, Lalonde C, Zhu D, Demling R (1988) Catalase prevents prostanoid release and lung lipid peroxidation after endotoxemia in sheep. J Appl Physiol 65:1210–1216
80. Kono Y, Fridovich I (1982) Superoxide radical inhibits catalase. J Biol Chem 257:5751–5754
81. Kunimoto F, Morita T, Ogawa R, Fujita T (1987) Inhibiton of lipid peroxidation improves survival rate of endotoxic rats. Circ Shock 21:15–22
82. Harris CA, Derbin KS, Hunte-McDonough B (1991) Manganese superoxide dismutase is induced by IFN-γ in multiple cell types. Synergistic induction by IFN-γ and tumor necrosis factor or IL-1. J Immunol 147:149–154
83. Rushmore TH, Morton MR, Pickett CB (1991) The antioxidant responsive element. Activation by oxidant stress and identification of the DNA consensus sequence required for functional activity. J Biol Chem 266:11632–11639
84. Sosenko IRS, Innis S, Frank L (1988) Polyunsaturated fatty acids and protection of newborn rats from oxygen toxicity. J Pediatr 112:630–637

PAF, Cytokines and Cell to Cell Interactions in Shock and Sepsis

D. Hosford, M. Koltai, and P. Braquet

Introduction

Despite considerable advances in the treatment of shock and sepsis in the past decade, high rates of morbidity and mortality still remain associated with these conditions. The relative lack of effective pharmacological interventions highlights the extremely complex biochemical and pathophysiological events which occur in these disorders. Among the various mediators implicated in endotoxemia, there is much evidence to suggest that, together with various cytokines, leukotrienes, thromboxane and proteases, the inflammatory and chemotactic autacoid, platelet activating factor (PAF), plays an important role.

PAF and PAF Antagonists

PAF is a potent autacoid mediator implicated in a diverse range of human pathologies, particularly inflammatory conditions [1,2]. Originally isolated from antigen-stimulated rabbit basophils and characterized structurally as 1-0-alkyl-2(R)-acetyl-glycero-3-phosphocholine, the alkyl phospholipid is now known to be produced by, and act on, a variety of cell types including neutrophils (PMN), eosinophils, monocytes, macrophages, platelets and endothelial cells.

Studies on the pathophysiological role of PAF have been facilitated by a variety of compounds which can specifically inhibit the binding of PAF to its receptors in various cells and tissues [1,2]. PAF antagonists can be broadly divided into two groups. Synthetic inhibitors include SRI 63-441, SRI 63-119, CV-3988 and BN 52111, which are related to the PAF framework and compounds such as BN 52730, BN 52739, YM 461, RP 52770 and the triazolo-thienodiazepines, WEB 2086 and WEB 2347 which are unrelated to the PAF structure [3]. Many natural compounds and their synthetic derivatives are also potent PAF antagonists. This group includes the terpenes, BN 52021 and swietemahonin, lignans such as kadsurenone and its synthetic derivative L-652-731 and gliotoxin-related compounds produced by various fungi and bacteria.

PAF and Physiological Changes in Shock and Sepsis

The role of PAF in shock has recently been reviewed [4]. It is now well documented that an infusion of PAF is able to mimic the shock state. For example, in guinea pigs PAF administration produces hypotension, bronchoconstriction, thrombocytopenia and death [5]. In dogs the mediator induces hypotension, myocardial contractility impairment, decreased coronary artery flow, systemic and pulmonary vascular changes, renal dysfunction, hemoconcentration and metabolic acidosis [6]. Leukopenia and thrombocytopenia following PAF infusion have also been observed in this species. A broad range of PAF antagonists protect against shock induced by infusion of the mediator in a variety of animal models [1,2], for example BN 52021 [7], CV-6209, WEB 2086 [8] and L-652,731 inhibit PAF-induced hypotension in rats.

The microvascular damage, decrease in blood volume, and increase in plasma extravasation observed in shock are of particular importance to the present discussion [9]. These vascular permeability impairments have also been reported in sepsis in dogs [10]. PAF induces hemoconcentration, plasma extravasation and edema formation in rats [11], guinea pigs [12] and sheep [13]. Locally injected, PAF induces plasma extravasation in guinea pigs and rabbit skin, and intense plasma leakage and sludge in the rabbit retina [14].

More detailed *in vitro* studies have examined the activity of PAF as an inducer of increased microvascular permeability [15,16]. A direct agonistic activity of the mediator on endothelial cells has been suggested by experiments showing that PAF stimulates Ca^{2+} influx-efflux in cultured human endothelial cells [17]. Indeed, recent studies have shown that PAF, but not its deacetylated and biologically inactive metabolite lyso-PAF, dose dependently (0.1 to 10 nM), induces cultured human endothelial cells to retract and lose reciprocal contact and promotes (^{125}I)-albumin diffusion in endothelial cells grown on fibronectin-coated polycarbonate filters [18]. We have also observed impairment of endothelial cells by PAF *in vivo*. Following 5-10 min superfusion with the autacoid [10^{-7} M] in the mesenteric bed of anesthetized guinea pigs, retraction of endothelial cells occurs in the area corresponding to the site of application of PAF, resulting in exposure of the sub-intimal tissue to the blood stream and substantial thrombus formation involving platelets, monocytes and eosinophils, cell infiltration and diapedesis. Formation of blebs and interstitial edema also accompany these PAF-induced changes [19].

In guinea pigs superfused with tumor necrosis factor (TNF), a subsequent injection of a low dose of PAF in the mesenteric bed dramatically enhances thrombosis. This enhanced activity of PAF by pretreatment with TNF occurred at doses at which PAF and TNF given alone, or PAF prior to TNF, did not significantly affect thrombogenesis. BN 52021 or anti-TNF antibodies inhibited this synergism [15]. This result suggests that TNF primes the effect of PAF on the endothelial cell wall, an affect also observed *in vitro*. In guinea pigs superfused in the mesenteric bed with a non-thrombogenic dose of *Salmonella enteritidis* lipopolysaccharide (LPS), subsequent injection of a low dose of PAF (which does not induce a thrombogenic effect *per se*) produced an extensive thrombus [19], suggesting that LPS primes the effect of PAF.

Vascular endothelial cells synthesize and release PAF in response to various stimuli [20]. While in response to stimuli such as thrombin, histamine. ATP and leukotrienes the release of PAF is rapid and transient, a new pathway has recently been elucidated that requires protein synthesis and is primed by IL-1 and TNF [21]. In this pathway, PAF is synthesized *de novo* in endothelial cells with maximal output occurring a few hours after the addition of the two monokines. Thus, while there is very good evidence showing that at higher concentrations PAF itself can induce the endothelial alterations apparent in shock, interactions between low concentrations of PAF and TNF (which may be ineffective *per se)* may be crucial in initiating vascular damage in the very early phases of shock.

In this chapter, we will consider the possible interactions between, PAF, cytokines, LPS, and PMN, and monocytes and macrophages which contribute to the deleterious cascade of events comprising the pathology of these disorders.

Effects of PAF on PMN In Vitro

Tissue damage mediated by free radical production is of considerable importance in shock and sepsis. Neutrophils appear to be a crucial cell type with regard to free radical generation. In the inflammatory microenvironment, these cells become activated by various agonists, adhere to the endothelial surface and release lysosomal proteases. Activated neutrophils also undergo a "respiratory burst", which results in the reduction of molecular oxygen to superoxide [22]. This latter product is rapidly converted to hydrogen peroxide and toxic free radicals which damage the endothelium. PAF is known to be a potent chemotactic agent for neutrophils, inducing superoxide release, aggregation and degranulation in this cell type [15,16]

PAF Production by Neutrophils

While numerous authors have detailed PAF release from neutrophils, several recent studies have attempted to elucidate the mechanisms involved in this process. In human PMN, A23187 stimulats PLA_2 and fatty acyl-CoA acetyltransferase resulting in a stimulated deacylation/reacylation cycle leading to PAF synthesis [23]. The role of PKC and Ca^{2+} in the formation and action of PAF was also studied [24]. PAF itself was able to enhance the release of newly synthesized PAF as measured by $[^3H]$ acetate incorporation in human neutrophils. The non-metabolisable bioactive PAF analogue C-PAF, but not lyso-PAF, enhanced the release of newly synthesized PAF. These responses were inhibited by ginkgolide B. Formyl-methionyl-leucyl-phenylalanine (fMLP), a synthetic chemotactic peptide, also stimulated *de novo* PAF generation. PAF release was potentiated by granulocyte-monocyte colony stimulating factor (GM-CSF) which has recently been implicated as transmembrane signaling factor [25], Na^+/H^+ activator in PMN and macrophages, and enhances PMN exudation at the inflammatory site [26]. The intracellular Ca^{2+} ($[Ca^{2+}]i$) chelator BAPTA inhibited the rise of $[CA^{2+}]_i$ and the release of PAF but not the Na^+/H^+ antiport activity. Pertussis toxin inhibited PAF release but not the rise of free $[Ca^{2+}]_i$ concentration in neutrophils [27.]

These results suggest that functional pertussis toxin-sensitive guanine nucleotide regulatory protein and/or one or more of the changes produced by PLC activation are necessary for PAF release. It appears that PAF release requires a coordinated action of receptor-coupled G-proteins, Ca^{2+} and other parameters. Addition of opsonised particles to human neutrophils leads to a biphasic elevation of cytosolic free Ca^{2+} concentration. This rise during the second phase is pronounced in comparison to the first phase. The second rise was not observed in the presence of WEB 2086, indicating that PAF can act as an intracellular messenger affecting Ca^{2+} homeostasis in human PMN.

In PAF-stimulated human PMN, the sensitive photoprotein aequorin as a Ca^{2+} indicator was used to clarify further the relative importance of $[Ca^{2+}]_i$ and extracellular Ca^{2+} $[Ca^{2+}]_e$ in PMN function [28]. PAF elicited a concentration-dependent Ca^{2+} mobilisation abolished by ethylene glycol-bis(b-aminoethyl ether) N,N,N'N'-tetraacetic acid (EGTA), suggesting that almost all Ca^{2+} mobilised by PAF derives from the external medium. Platelets loaded with aequorin were stimulated by PAF in the presence of autologous PMN. Separate platelet and PMN suspensions were poorly aggregated, while mixed cellular suspensions showed an amplified aggregatory response. PAF induced a concentration-dependent increase of Ca^{2+} mobilisation in aequorin-loaded platelets, and the presence of PAF further increased Ca^{2+} release. Platelet thromboxane (TX) B_2 production was also increased in the presence of PMN. Ginkgolide B dose-dependently inhibited PAF-induced Ca^{2+} mobilisation, aggregation and TXB_2 production.

In a recent study [28], Ro 19-3704 directly inhibited IgE-dependent mediator release from rat basophil leukemia cells by a mechanism independent of its PAF antagonist properties, pointing to the significance of eventual non-specific effects of PAF receptor antagonists.

Effect of PAF and Cytokine Interactions on Neutrophil Activation

Similarly to PAF, TNF also enhances neutrophil superoxide production and adherence [29]. TNF may also indirectly regulate eosinophil cytotoxicity via its effect on the release of other cytokines and growth factors. In addition to directly modulating neutrophil activity, at very low concentrations both PAF and TNF can "prime" neutrophils to respond in an enhanced manner to subsequent agonistic stimuli that would otherwise be ineffectual. Amplified responses including aggregation, adhesiveness, superoxide production and elastase release have been reported using N-formyl-methionyl-leucyl phenylalanine as the inducing agonist following priming with PAF [30].

Work from our laboratory [31] has shown that PAF markedly amplifies superoxide production by TNF-stimulated human PMN. PAF antagonists not only inhibited the PAF amplification, but also partially decreased superoxide production elicited solely by TNF, indicating the involvement of endogenous PAF in this process. Pretreatment of the PMN with pertussis toxin or cholera toxin reduced the PAF amplification of superoxide production in TNF-stimulated PMN, implicating G-proteins sensitive to both toxins in the amplification process.

PAF and Protease Production by PMN in Shock and Sepsis

The release of lysomal enzymes, particularly proteases, by neutrophils in shock and sepsis is of considerable interest. In endotoxemia a marked increase in plasma proteolytic activity is observed, for example during septic shock in man [32] and in endotoxin-induced shock in animal models. In addition, PAF injection in the rat induces a rapid and significant increase in plasma protease activity, for example in the rat [33]. Endotoxin may stimulate phospholipase A_2 resulting in PAF production, which would in turn lead to cell activation and release of lysomal enzymes. As phospholipase A_2 can also be activated by various proteases, a positive feedback cycle is created, increasing the deleterious effects of the toxin. PAF antagonists may act by inactivating this feedback loop. Indeed, as demonstrated by Etienne et al. [34], BN 52021 inhibits both the PAF- and endotoxin-induced plasma protease activity in the rat.

Effects of PAF on Monocytes/Macrophages In Vitro

PAF Production by Monocytes

Monocytes and macrophages provide a major source of TNF and other cytokines following stimulation by endotoxin or LPS, thus numerous *in vitro* studies have utilized this cell type. Stewart and Phillips [34] demonstrated that adherent guinea pig macrophages contained cell-associated PAF whose level was increased following stimulation by fMLP, endotoxin and ionophore A 23187. However, only endotoxin and A 23187 caused release of detectable amounts of PAF into the extracellular medium. In contrast, Worthen et al. [30] found that while exposure of neutrophils to low concentrations of LPS produced a small but significant increase in intracellular PAF levels, release of the mediator was not detected.

Rylander and Beijer [36] examined the production of PAF in alveolar macrophages (AM) and neutrophils recovered by bronchial lavage from guinea pigs exposed to aerosolized bacterial LPS. The amount of cell-associated PAF was estimated by measuring serotonin release from rabbit platelets. An increased and dose-related production was found in AM for as long as 2 h after a 40-min exposure. No production was detectable after 4 h and increasing the exposure time did not prolong the response. When a second exposure was given, no PAF could be detected until the time interval between the 2 exposures was 72 h.

Studies on [^{3}H]-arachidonic acid turnover in LPS stimulated human monocyte-derived macrophages by Leslie and Detty [37] support the evidence that the bacterial toxin can increase PAF production. The latter authors found that relative to unstimulated cells, there was a preferential, dose-dependent loss of [^{3}H]-arachidonic acid from phosphatidylcholine [PC] and phosphatidylinositol [PI] in cells exposed to LPS, which was maximal between 1 and 3 h after adding the toxin. In addition, LPS induced a 35% decrease in the molar quantity of PI in the macrophages but had no effect on the quantity of PC, phosphatidylethanolamine or phosphatidylserine.

PAF concentration-dependently modified cAMP levels in human peritoneal macrophages [1]. In human peripheral blood mononuclear leucocytes labelled with [^{3}H]inositol PAF rapidly but transiently stimulated phosphoinositol hydrolysis and inositol-1,4,5-triphosphate (IP_3) formation. The response paralleled the time course of PAF-induced Ca^{2+} mobilisation, and was inhibited by L-659,989, but remained unaltered by pertussis toxin or cholera toxin. These data suggest that PAF receptors in human peripheral blood mononuclear cells may be coupled through a pertussis toxin-insensitive guanine nucleotide binding protein to a phosphoinositide-specific PLC.

Adherent guinea pig alveolar macrophages stimulated by fMLP *in vitro* released PAF and various eicosanoids [38]. Indomethacin suppressed TXB_2 generation, and BW A137C (a selective lipoxygenase inhibitor) abolished LTB_4 secretion, but none of these drugs influenced PAF release indicating that fMLP-induced PAF release is independent of eicosanoid generation. Alternatively, eicosanoid generation appeared to be dependent on intracellular PAF concentration in guinea pig resident peritoneal macrophages. Adherent macrophages contained cell-associated PAF whose level was increased by fMLP, endotoxin and A23187, however only endotoxin and A23187 caused the release of detectable amounts of PAF into the extracellular medium. Exogenous PAF and each of the above stimuli increased PGI_2 generation in resident macrophages. WEB 2086 and CV-6209 reduced both basal and stimulated PGI_2 production, and in addition WEB 2086 inhibited fMLP- and PAF-induced superoxide anion generation. Responses to A23187 were not inhibited by either antagonist. Ginkgolide B and WEB 2086 prevented PAF-stimulated LT synthesis in human monocytes [39]. More recently, an analysis of PAF metabolism by monocytes indicated that methoxy-PAF is substantially more resistant than PAF to degradation by acethylhydrolyses, thus its activating effect may be stronger for *in vivo* immunotherapy.

The formation of eicosanoids may be a primary route through which PAF exerts effects during endotoxemia. Morris and Moore [40] showed that in cultured horse peritoneal macrophages, PAF and endotoxin significantly increased TXB_2 concentrations. TXA_2 release by endotoxin was not prevented by SRI 63-441, and even it enhanced macrophage TXA_2 and PGI_2 synthesis, suggesting that PAF may induce TXA_2 release through a pathway which may not be related to the presence of specific PAF binding sites. These results should be confirmed by other PAF antagonists.

PAF Priming of Monocytes and Effects of PAF Antagonists

While it is important to consider the direct influence of LPS on PAF production, it is essential to have some understanding of the interactions between PAF and mediators associated with shock. PAF is synthesized and frequently secreted by a variety of cells types in response to mediators and cytokines, particularly TNF. This body information has been reviewed in depth [15,16] and does not require further elaboration here; rather it is more pertinent to consider more subtle interactions such as priming and amplification.

With regard to cytokines, it has been demonstrated that PAF is able to enhance interleukin 1 (IL-1) production in human monocytes treated with endotoxin. PAF was shown to increase the release of IL-1 with a multiphasic dose-response curve. When the cells were treated with PAF and endotoxin in combination, these two stimuli interacted synergistically. Immunostaining of proteins isolated from PAF-stimulated cells revealed that PAF and endotoxin increased intracellular IL-1 precursors and thus increased the levels of this cytokine by facilitating its synthesis. The production of TNF by human platelet-free monocytes, isolated by counterflow elutriation, was analyzed following stimulation with endotoxin in the absence or presence of graded concentration ranges of PAF [41]. Two concentration ranges showed significant increase in TNF production. A major enhancement was observed at 10^{-8} to 10^{-6}M which was blocked by BN 52021, while a second enhancement was seen at 10^{-15} to 10^{-14}M PAF, which was insensitive to BN 52021. These results suggest that PAF can directly modulate cytokine production by human monocytes possibly by interacting with two types of receptor.

The effects of PAF in the induction and priming of TNF secretion in peripheral blood monocytes have recently been studied [42]. Unlike gamma-interferon and endotoxin, the addition of PAF to freshly isolated monocytes triggered a rapid, concentration-dependent TNF secretion in the absence of induction of macrophage-mediated cytotoxicity. While biologically active and cytotoxic TNF was detected early after PAF addition, the cytotoxic activity declined thereafter, though the antigenic activity remained constant. Monocytes primed with PAF responded by secreting TNF to both pokeweed mitogen and concanavalin A, representing unspecific stimuli, but responded poorly to specific stimulation by PAF, endotoxin and gamma-interferon. These findings suggest that PAF may mediate part of its biological activity via the macrophage and further, monocyte secretion of PAF can in turn regulate monocyte function, thereby contributing to the inflammatory response.

Other studies have shown that preincubation of rat spleen macrophages with 10 fM PAF (which had no effect *per se*) prior to stimulation with 20 μg/ml LPS markedly increased production of IL-1 by the cells, relative to that induced by LPS alone [44]. Association of 1 μg/ml pertussis toxin with PAF suppressed the enhancing effect of PAF on IL-1 release, again implicating pertussis toxin sensitive G-proteins in the priming process. Furthermore, while concentrations of PAF lower than 0.1 μM were unable to elicit release of leukotriene B_4 (LTB_4) from human PMN, however preincubation with GM-CSF both increased LTB_4 synthesis by 10 fold in PMN incubated with 0.1 - 1 μM PAF and stimulated LTB_4 release in cells exposed to 1 μM PAF.

An alternative approach to investigate interactions between various cytokines and PAF is to study how treatment with this autacoid can influence cytokine production. In Sprague-Dawley rats, long-term treatment with PAF loaded intravenously with alzet minipumps into the jugular vein was used to address this question [44]. After treatment with 0.5, 1, 4.5, 9, or 28 mg PAF or

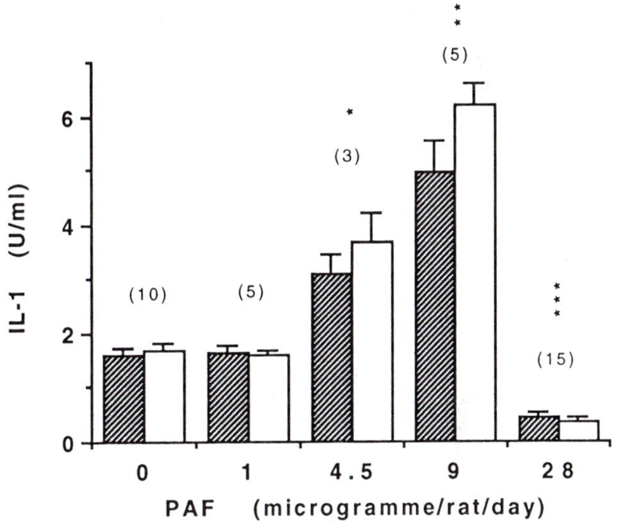

Fig. 1. Representative interaction between PAF and release of the cytokine IL-1 in rat spleen cells. Effect of chronic infusion of various doses of PAF on the *ex vivo* release of IL-1 induced upon LPS. Alzet minipumps containing different doses of PAF or solvent alone were placed under the back skin of rats and connected to the jugular vein. After 7 days, the rats were killed and spleen macrophages from each rat were collected and stimulated with 20 μg LPS. Released (hatched columns) and cell-associated IL-1 activities (open columns) were determined using the thymocyte proliferation assay. Each supernatant from separate rats was measured in triplicate. Results are expressed as IL-1 U/ml and as mean ± SEM of the number of animals indicated in parentheses. $^*p<0.05$, $^{**}p<0.01$, and $^{***}p<0.001$. Note a typical dose-effect relationship in the range of 1-9 mg/rat/day PAF; after 28 mg/rat day of PAF the response became down-regulated.

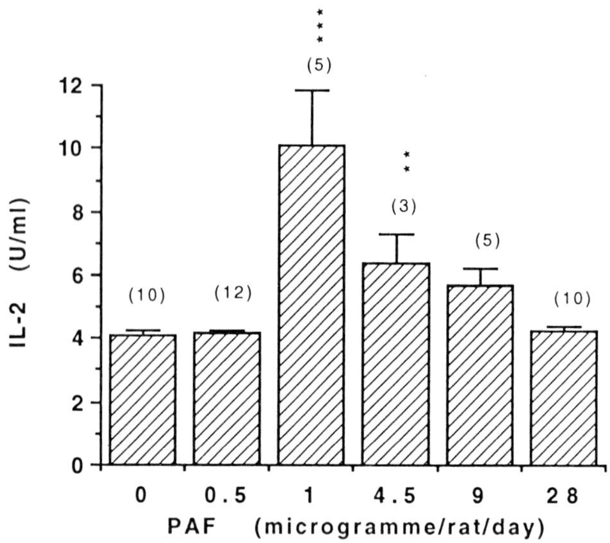

Fig. 2. Representative interaction between PAF and release of the cytokine IL-2 in rat spleen cells. Effect of chronic infusion of various doses of PAF on the *ex vivo* release of IL-2 induced upon nitogen stimulation. Alzet minipumps containing different doses of PAF or solvent alone were placed under the back skin of rats and connected to the jugular vein. After 7 days, the rats were killed and spleen macrophages from each rat were collected. Whole spleen mononuclear cells from each rat obtained after Ficoll gradients were stimulated with 15 mg Con A for 24 h, and the cell-free supernatants were collected and assayed separatley for IL-2 activity. Each supernatant from separate rats was measured in triplicate. Results are expressed as IL-2U/ml and as mean æ SEM of the number of animals indicadet in parentheses.**p<0.01, and ***p<0.001. Note the significant increase in IL-2 release after treatment with 1 μg/rat/day of PAF, whereas higher doses induced grasually decreasing cytokine release.

solvent, spleen mononuclear cells were isolated from Ficoll gradients and the adherent and non-adherent cell fractions were separated before determination of basal and stimulated IL-1 and IL-2 production, respectively. Adherent splenocytes from rats having received 28 mg PAF exhibited a decreased capability to produce IL-1 as compared to those from vehicle-treated animals. In contrast, adherent splenocytes from rats having received 9 or 4.5 mg PAF yielded higher amounts of released and cell-associated IL-1 activity upon LPS stimulation (Fig. 1). Statistically significant increases in IL-2 production were observed when whole spleen mononuclear cells from rats administered with 1 or 4.5 mg PAF were stimulated with Con A (Fig. 2). BN 52021 given orally twice a day in 5 mg/kg doses throughout the experimental period inhibited the effect of 28 mg and 1 mg PAF on IL-1 and IL-2 release, respectively.

Importance of PAF and Monocytes/PMN in Shock and Sepsis In Vitro

PAF Production in Shock and Sepsis

Numerous reports have demonstrated that the mediator is produced in various shock states. Gram-negative sepsis is a major cause of severe circulatory shock, which can be mimicked in animal models by the infusion of either living bacteria or bacterial endotoxin. Inarrea et al. [44] showed that shock triggered by i.p. injections in the rat of 2 x 10^8 colony forming units (CFU) of *E. coli* produced septicemia with 50% mortality. There was also a dose-dependent increase in vascular permeability accompanied by the appearance of PAF in the peritoneal and spleen cells of the intoxicated animals. Similarly, a marked rise in circulating blood levels of PAF 10 min after IV injection of endotoxin in rats was also reported.

We have also recently demonstrated that PAF appears in rat blood samples after IV injection of *Salmonella enteritidis,* while it is not present in control animals. Similar findings have been reported by Buxton et al. [45] using *in situ* perfused rat livers challenged with soluble IgG aggregates. In this experimental system, PAF activity was detected in the effluent following IgG challenge.

Rylander and Beijer [36] showed that inhalation of endotoxin in guinea pigs produced a dose-dependent production of PAF by alveolar macrophages, while Fitzgerald et al. [38] noted that sensitized, isolated and perfused guinea pig lungs released 3 times more PAF when challenged with antigen relative to control preparations. In addition, markedly elevated levels of PAF have been reported in experimental animal model where endotoxin was used to induce intestinal lesions.

In a recent study using isolated, buffer-perfused rabbit lungs, free of plasma and circulating blood cells, Salzer and McCall [47] demonstrated that LPS synergized with PAF to injure the lung. In lungs perfused for 2 h with LPS-free buffer (less than 100 pg/ml), stimulation with 1, 10 or 100 nM PAF produced transient pulmonary hypertension and minimal edema. Lungs perfused for 2 h with buffer containing 100 ng/ml of *Escherichia coli* LPS had slight elevation of pulmonary artery pressure (PAP) but did not develop edema. In contrast, lungs exposed to 100 ng/ml of LPS for 2 h had marked increases in PAP and developed significant edema when stimulated with PAF. LPS treatment increased capillary filtration coefficient, suggesting that capillary leak contributed to pulmonary edema. LPS-primed, PAF-stimulated lungs had enhanced production of thromboxane B_2 (TXB_2) and 6-keto-prostaglandin F1-alpha. These studies indicate that LPS primes the lung for enhanced injury in response to PAF by amplifying the synthesis and release of thromboxane in lung tissue.

Finally, several recent reports have demonstrated increased levels of PAF in human shock. Studies by Bussolino et al. [48] have shown an elevated intravascular release of the mediator in children with sepsis, while Lopez-Diez et al. [49] have examined the possible involvement of PAF in human endotoxemia by determining *ex vivo* PAF binding to platelets of the patients, complemented with extraction and chemical characterization of PAF obtained from these cells. Platelets from 12 healthy human volunteers had 281 ± 63 freely accessible PAF high affinity binding sites per platelet, whereas this number was 49 ± 37 PAF-receptors per platelet, in a group of 13 patients with septicemia. Patients with sepsis also possessed significant amounts of PAF associated to their platelets, whereas this mediator could not be isolated from platelets of control individuals. PAF was also assayed in whole blood samples and found at high concentrations in sepsis patients.

In a recent study, Arditi et al. [50] detected TNF in the cerebrospinal fluid (CSF) of 33 of 38 children with bacterial meningitis, but not in any of 15 children with viral meningitis. In children with bacterial meningitis, TNF in the CSF correlated with CSF bacterial density, CSF protein, endotoxin (LPS) in gram-negative disease, and consecutive febrile hospital days. TNF levels in the CSF greater than 1000 pg/ml were associated with seizures. Furthermore, a higher proportion of children who died had detectable plasma TNF activity as compared with survivors. PAF in the CSF was also higher in 19 children with *Haemophilus influenzae* meningitis than in 17 controls, and correlated with bacterial density and CSF levels of LPS and TNF. Thus it appears that elevated CSF levels of TNF and PAF are often present in children with bacterial meningitis and are associated with seizures and severity of disease.

The above studies demonstrate increased levels of PAF release in human sepsis and that occupancy of PAF receptors and high amounts of platelet-associated PAF are also characteristic of patients with sepsis. The evidence reviewed in this section strongly indicates that increased levels of PAF are a feature of shock and sepsis, and that these elevated levels correlate with the outcome of the condition.

Effects of PAF Antagonists in Shock and Sepsis

The finding of increased levels of PAF in endotoxemia suggested that PAF antagonists may be effective in counteracting this pathology. Indeed, this hypothesis has been suggested by numerous experimental studies. In shock induced by *Salmonella enteritidis* endotoxin [7,34], a significant dose-dependent inhibition of the lethality was observed with BN 52021 treatment (5-20 mg/kg), total protection being provided by the highest dose of the drug. This effect was associated with a reduced increase in body temperature suggesting that BN 52021 has an effect on the release of IL-1. In guinea pigs injected with *Salmonella typhimurium* endotoxin, a similar protection was also afforded by BN 52021 and other PAF antagonists including CV 3988 [51], kadsurenone, L-652,731, SRI 63-072 and SRI 63-441, WEB 2086 [52] and the new hetrapazine-derived antagonists BN 52730 and BN 52739 [53].

In endotoxemic conscious rats and dogs, Fletcher et al. [54] have demonstrated that BN 52021 beneficially attenuates the late systemic hypotension and circulatory dysfuntion, respectively in these species. Similarly in the rat, Rabinovici et al. [55] found that pretreatment of the animals with BN 50739 prevented endotoxin-induced hemoconcentration, reduced 24 h mortality from 100 to 60 % and partially protected against the hypotensive response to endotoxin. LPS-induced elevation of thromboxane and TNF was also attenuated, although leukopenia and thrombocytopenia remained unchanged. In addition, the antagonist reduced TNF-induced mortality by 65 %, but did not alter hematological responses to the cytokine. BN 50739 was also effective in preventing the early phase of LPS-induced thrombocytopenia and thromboxane elevation in the rabbit [53]. The antagonist reduced the 24 hour mortality from 75 to 22 %, and post-treatment with the drug increased the 10 hour survival rate from 33 to 87 %. However, LPS-induced leukopenia and increase in plasmatic TNF levels were not affected in this species by the antagonist.

In dog endotoxemia, BN 52021 had no beneficial effects on the early hypotension (1-2 min) following administration of endotoxin, but beneficially attenuated the continued decrease in blood pressure and cardiac output [56]. Interestingly, the systemic vascular resistance was slightly decreased by BN 52021 at 1-2 min, while the early endotoxin-induced increase in pulmonary vascular resistance was inhibited. The finding that the PAF antagonist prevented the early rise in pulmonary vascular resistance relative to that observed in untreated endotoxemic animals suggests that PAF may be directly or indirectly involved as a pulmonary vasoconstrictor in dog endotoxemia. Although the effects of the PAF antagonist on the hemodynamic and metabolic events in dog endotoxemia were variable, pretreatment with BN 52021 dramatically improved the permanent survival rate from 0 % to 100 % in this model [56]. Other studies by this group on endotoxemic conscious rats have shown that in addition to improving survival, BN 52021 also prevents the release of thromboxane B_2 and prostaglandin E_2 observed in untreated endotoxemic rats [49]. These latter data suggest that the actions of PAF in endotoxemia may be partly mediated by generation of these eicosanoids.

The protection afforded by PAF antagonists against endotoxin-induced changes in carbohydrate metabolism has been investigated by Lang et al. [57]. In chronically catheterized conscious rats, endotoxin (100 µg/100 g body weight) induced a transient 30-35 % reduction in mean arterial blood pressure (MABP), while in animals treated with SRI 63-441, a synthetic PAF antagonist containing a tetrahydofuran ring and a quaternary moiety, MABP was only reduced by 14-18 %. Endotoxin increased plasma glucose and lactate levels as well as the rate of glucose appearance (Ra). The PAF antogonist reduced the hyperglycemia by 60-75 %, partially inhibited the hyperlactacidemia and significantly reduced the elevation in glucose Ra. Although a similar degree of hyperglucagonemia and plasma insulin was observed in endotoxemic rats whether treated or not with the PAF antagonist, plasma catecholamine levels were significantly lower (30-70%) in endotoxemic rats receiving SRI 63-441. These results indicate that enhanced PAF production following endotoxin administration may be partly responsible for the initial changes in blood pressure, but that the role of PAF as a mediator of endotoxin-induced glucose dyshomeostasis are secondary to its hemodynamic effects [57].

Since the demonstration that administration of PAF either as a bolus or continuous infusion [58] induces increases in pulmonary vascular permeability in sheep, several workers have used this model to assess the effects of PAF antagonists both against endotoxin- and PAF-induced shock. Toyofuko et al. [59] reported that the PAF antagonist, ONO-6240, had little effect on pulmonary hypertension and lung lymph balance in ovine endotoxemia, but other researchers using structurally different PAF antagonists have reported significant protective effects of the compounds. Endotoxin infusion (1.3 µg/kg over 30 min) caused a rapid, transient rise in pulmonary arterial pressure (Ppa) and pulmonary vascular resistance (PVR), while arterial pO_2 decreased. A 5 h infusion of SRI 63-441 (20 mg/kg/h) blocked the early rise in Ppa and PVR and fall in arterial pO_2, but had no effect on the late phase pulmonary hypertension or hypoxemia.The drug also abolished the early and attenuated the late increase in lung lymph flow observed in ovine endotoxemia. Similar results have been obtained with WEB 2086 [8], which attenuated the late increase in permeability mediated lymph flow, bud did not prevent the early pulmonary hypertension after bolus LPS administration. BN 52021 is also able to attenuate the early rise in Ppa, the duration of the pulmonary hypertension and the increased thromboxane levels following LPS administration in the sheep. Increases in lymph flow were also beneficially modulated, although high doses of the drug only achieved a 38 % survival rate, dexamethasone treatment resulting in 100 % survival.

In accordance with the protection afforded by PAF antogonists at the general physiological level, these compounds are able to inhibit the effects of endotoxin on specific organs and tissues. Baum et al. [60] have tested the hypothesis that LPS-induced myocardial dysfunction is mediated by PAF or cyclooxygenase-derived metabolites of arachidonic acid. These investigators used ether-anesthetized rats injected IV with normal saline, ibuprofen (cyclooxygenase inhibitor; 15 mg/kg), or the PAF receptor antagonist (SDZ 64-688; 5 mg/kg). Thirty min later, the rats were injected IV with saline or *Escherichia coli* LPS (20 mg/kg). After 2 h, atria was harvested, connected to an isometric force transducer-amplifier-recorder apparatus, and maintained *in vitro* in oxygenated Krebs-Henseleit buffer. Force of contraction indexed to body weight was significantly lower in the LPS group than in the group which received saline. Pretreatment with ibuprofen did not affect this adverse effect of LPS however, pretreatment with SDZ 64-688 improved the deleterious effect of LPS on contractility. These results support the notion that LPS-induced myocardial dysfunction in the rat is mediated, at least partly, by PAF.

In the guinea pig, endotoxin administered by aerosol, induces platelet accumulation and increased vascular permeability in the lung, effects also induced by treatment with PAF. Both these effects of PAF and endotoxin were prevented by WEB 2086, BN 52021 and the ginkgolide mixture BN 56203 [61]. Furthermore, SRI 63-441 inhibited endotoxin induced pulmonary edema and lung microvascular damage in the rat [62].

Recently, we have shown [63] that lung parenchymal strips from guinea pigs treated with endotoxin exhibit specific desensitization to PAF, an effect not observed in animals also administered with BN 52021, which indicates PAF production in endotoxemia. In a similar model using *E. Coli* endotoxin, BN 52021 inhibits the endotoxin-induced tracheal hyperreactivity to histamine in the guinea pig suggesting that PAF may be important in inducing this process. PAF antagonists are also effective in other models of endotoxin-induced pulmonary dysfunction. In the pig, intravenous infusion of LPS for 5 h induces a marked increase in pulmonary arterial blood pressure. Animals concomitantly treated with WEB 2086 had significantly reduced pulmonary hypertension relative to those not receiving the drug, although the PAF antagonist did not affect the systemic hypotension. A sharp decline in peripheral white blood cell counts also occurred following LPS infusion, a process which was retarded by the treatment with WEB 2086. The endotoxin-induced deterioration in both gas exchange and inspiratory pressure were also partially prevented by the drug.

PAF antagonists also inhibit the oliguric acute renal failure associated with decreased renal blood flow (RBF) and glomerular filtration rate (GFR) induced by endotoxin in the rat [64]. For example, both BN 52021 and SRI 63-675 are able to inhibit the endotoxin-induced vascular escape and alterations in RBF, thus producing significant improvement in renal function.

Gastrointestinal hemorrhage is another feature associated with septic shock, a condition which can also be produced in several species by injection of PAF or bacterial endotoxin [65]. Hsueh et al. [46] also noted increased production of the mediator in the bowel of endotoxemic animals. Accordingly, PAF antagonists including CV-3988, RO-193704 and BN 52021, are able to significantly reduce the endotoxin-induced gastro-intestinal damage in the rat [66]. It has also been demonstrated that rats treated with PAF or endotoxin develop ischemic bowel necrosis associated with shock. In this model, the morphological changes of TNF-induced bowel lesions were indistinguishable from those caused by PAF. TNF induced PAF production in bowel tissue, and the effects of TNF and endotoxin on PAF production in the intestine were additive. Furthermore, TNF and endotoxin were synergistic in inducing bowel necrosis, and TNF-induced bowel necrosis was partly due to PAF release, since SRI 63-119 had a protective effect.

In a more recent study, Sun et al. [67] examined the effect of *in vivo* priming on TNF and PAF levels in LPS-induced shock. Rats were primed with intraperitoneal injection of zymosan 24 h before, or Bacillus Calmette-Guerin [BCG] 12 to 15 days before intravenous injection of a low dose of LPS (0.5 mg/kg). Results showed that non-primed animals developed mild hypotension and moderate leukopenia in response to LPS. In contrast, zymosan-primed rats developed shock and marked leukopenia, and more severe bowel injury than non-primed rats. In addition, following LPS injection, zymosan-primed animals had higher TNF and PAF levels than non-primed rats. Pretreatment of the animal with the PAF antagonist SRI 63-441 markedly ameliorated the hypotension and tissue injury. Interestingly, BCG-primed rats did not show aggravation of LPS-induced hypotension and only levels of TNF (but not PAF) in these animals were increased. Thus, it appears that TNF release alone, without a sufficient increase in PAF, is unable to cause severe hypotension in this model.

The mediatory role of PAF in intestinal inflammation and ulceration has also been investigated. Using the rat model of colitis, the effects of treatment with BN 52021 in comparison with WEB 2086 and WEB 2170, were studied in endotoxin-induced ulceration by measuring PAF biosynthesis and changes in vascular permeability. In agreement with previous findings [68], PAF antagonists were found to accelerate healing of chronic colitis, thereby suggesting a role for PAF in the mechanism of intestinal ulceration induced by endotoxin.

Finally, the effects of endotoxin on the brain include both alterations in cerebral blood flow (CBF) and a fall in respiratory control ratio (state 3/state 4 of the respiratory chain; RCR). In dogs administered IV with endotoxin, Ekstrom-Jodal et al. [10] observed decreased CBF and increased cerebral metabolism. In further studies, this group demonstrated increased permeability of the blood-brain barrier following endotoxin treatment [62].

The considerable body of evidence reviewed in this section indicates the very high probalility that PAF antagonists are capable of protecting against endotoxemia, both with regard to general physiological and hemodynamic alterations, and shock-induced changes experienced by specific organs.

Mechanisms of PAF-induced Effects in Shock and Sepsis

Mechanisms of PAF and Monocyte/PMN Interactions

There is evidence indicating possible interactions between PAF, cytokines and various cell types during shock and sepsis, and the effect of PAF antagonists in these conditions. Based on the accumulated data, a complex interaction between LPS, PAF proteases, TNF and other cytokines is of fundamental importance in initiating the pathological changes not only in shock and sepsis, but also in a variety of other inflammatory conditions [15,16].

Shock and ischemia are characterized by endothelial injury, bleb formation, plasma leakage, hemodynamic alterations and eventually vascular collapse and end-organ failure. The primary event in these train of events is cellular activation leading to the adherence of blood cells such as platelets, PMN, eosinophils and monocytes to the endothelial surface followed by their aggregation, infiltration and degranulation. In addition to directly eliciting cell chemotaxis and free radical production, PAF can also induce the release of various inflammatory cytokines such as TNF. We havc shown that PAF stimulates TNF production from peripheral blood derived monocytes and at picomolar concentrations amplifies lipopolysaccharide-induced TNF production, effects inhibited by various PAF antagonists. PAF also acts synergistically with γ-interferon (γ-IFN) to increase the monocyte cytotoxicity. PAF can modulate the production of both IL-1 and interleukin 2 (IL-2) [43] from rat monocytes and lymphocytes respectively, cytokines which in turn elicit the release of other mediators and growth factors.

Apart from inducing vascular damage via infiltration and degranulation of various blood cells, PAF [15,16], IL-1 and TNF [70] also exert direct effects on the vascular system, causing hypotension when they are administered *in vivo*. Furthermore, while it has been known for some time that endothelial cells produce PAF when stimulated with various agonists such as thrombin, it has recently been established that TNF, IL-1 and lymphotoxin, but not IL-2, IL-3, IL-6, γ-IFN and colony stimulating factors, induce cultured endothelial cells to synthesize PAF, the majority of which remains associated with the cells [21]. GM-CSF, another cytokine produced by activated T cells, endothelial cells and fibroblasts stimulated by TNF, is also able to prime the PAF-induced production of both superoxide [31] and leukotrienes [25,70] from human polymorphonuclear leukocytes. This suggests that GM-CSF may also be involved in the PAF/cytokine interactions during shock and ischemia.

Thus it seems that in these conditions, complex interactions may arise between mediators and cells which eventually give rise to microvascular damage. The fact that PAF and various cytokines cannot only induce the release of each other, but also their own generation *in vivo* indicates that self-generating positive feedback cycles may become established. We propose that PAF and TNF play pivotal roles in the formation of initial loops, which subsequently recruit other cytokines and growth factors into the feedback network [15,16]. For example, a situation can be envisaged where in the inflammatory micro-environment PAF primes the release of IL-1 and TNF from activated monocytes and leukotriene, and free radical production from stimulated polymorphonuclear cells. PAF also activates platelets to form thrombin and ATP which in turn, as IL-1 and TNF, act on the endothelium to produce more PAF resulting in increased neutrophil chemotaxis. These cells may then be primed by TNF for PAF-induced superoxide generation. In addition, PAF generated by the endothelium may amplify the TNF- and IL-1-activated production of IL-6 and GM-CSF from endothelial cells.

This latter growth factor which is also produced by stimulated monocytes, potently enhances release of superoxide and leukotriene C_4 by eosinophils [71]. Furthermore, in combination with IL-3, it elicits monocyte cytotoxity by inducing TNF secretion from this cell type.

The priming ability of these mediators indicates the extreme sensitivity of the inflammatory process and the rigid controls which must usually operate to stop excessive inflammatory responses. It may be that an equilibrium exists between the mediators involved in the priming and feedback processes

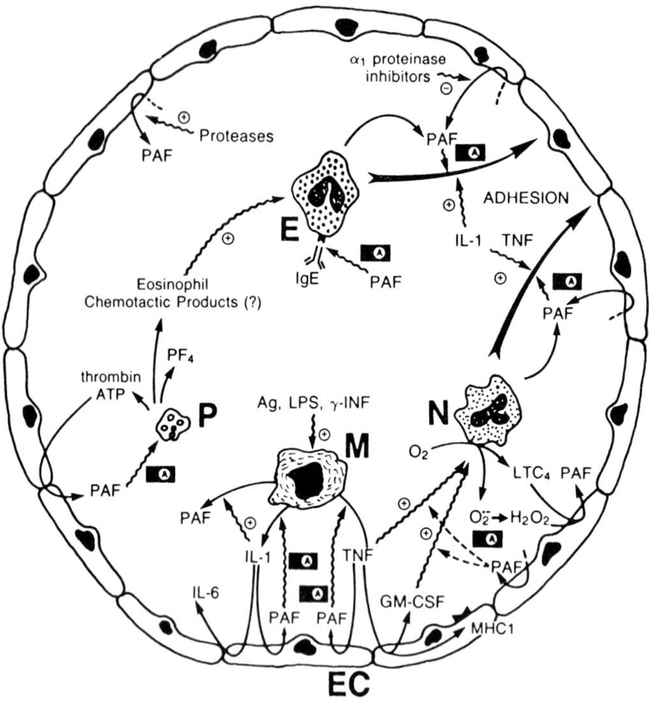

Fig. 3 Some examples of intravascular PAF/cytokine feedback processes. Clockwise: PAF amplifies thrombin and ATP generation by platelet (P) and IL-1 and TNF production from macrophages (M), vectors which stimulate endothelial cells (EC) to produce more PAF. IL-1 may further stimulate IL production by EC, while TNF induces release of GM-CSF. These two latter mediators may subsequently elicit superoxide anion and leukotriene production by neutrophils (N), a process amplified by PAF. Adhesion of N and eosinophils (E) to the endothelium by IL-1 and TNF is amplified by PAF release by EC. PAF may also prime IgE-dependent E cytotoxicity and indirectly influence E chemotaxis by modulating the release of chemotactic products from P. Proteases may play an important role in PAF generation by the endothelium.

and internal mechanisms which down regulate these loops and confine cytotoxic reactions to a specific site. Indeed, several endogenous inhibitors of PAF, TNF, IL-1 and IL-2 have been reported [15,16]. Under normal physiological conditions, a balance may be maintained between cytotoxic and inhibitory mechanisms, which would strictly control the inflammatory process and prevent endothelial injury. In contrast, in pathologies such as shock and ischemia where there may be an overloading of the system by excessive mediator production or a critical reduction in inhibitory factors, the feedback cycles may become unregulated and the toxicity converted into a systemic process, resulting in free radical production, endothelial damage, cell infiltration, vascular leakage and microcirculatory collapse. This fine balance between the protection and destruction of the processes maintaining life is reminiscent of the catastrophe theory (Fig. 3).

Therapeutic Strategies in Shock and Organ Failure

PAF antagonists are currently being evaluated clinically and may constitute valuable drugs in diseases where control of the inflammatory response has to be reinstated therapeutically. In common with the numerous other drugs already employed for the treatment or inflammation, the end result of PAF antagonist action is protection of vascular integrity. While PAF inhibitors probably achieve this result by inhibiting the priming, amplification and feedback processes described in this review, other agents effective in shock and ischemia may produce a similar vascular protection via their own individual mechanisms of action.

With regard to the development of potential therapeutic regimes for shock and ischemia, it should be emphasized that PAF antagonists alone are only capable of blocking the pathological processes directly or indirectly dependent on PAF, no matter how diverse these may be. The vast majority of other anti-inflammatory drugs also only act through inhibition of a single mediator, synthetic pathway or process. As proposed in this chapter, the complex multi-component nature of the deleterious processes operating in shock and ischemia suggests that more successful therapeutic regimes may consist of a combination of drugs possibly including protease inhibitors, calcium antagonists, prostacyclin analogues, inhibitors of interleukins and growth factors, anti-TNF antibodies and PAF antagonists.

It is also extremely important to note that any drug therapy should endeavor to offer vascular protection as rapidly as possible. This is not only of critical importance for the immediate outcome of the condition but also for the future prognosis. Indeed, endothelium that has sustained previous damage may be particulary prone to future injury. Recently, it has been shown that the recovery of balloon denudated pig endothelim is not complete as the cells lose the ability to produce endothelium-derived relaxing factor and possibly other relexant agents. EDRF also reduces platelet aggregation and the inability of previously damaged endothelial cells to produce such factors suppressive to the activity of the feedback mediators, makes regenerated endothelium markedly more susceptible to further inflammatory damage.

In addition to combinations of drugs, the other possible pharmacological approach to the treatment of shock and ischemia is the design of compounds which possess a dual or multi-inhibitory activity. Our laboratory is currently developing such drugs, and studies on animal models with compounds acting as PAF antagonists/anti-proteases or PAF antagonists/5-lipoxygenase inhibitors have produced very encouraging results. Despite the technical difficulties of combining various inhibitory properties in one molecule, we believe that this approach offers great potential for the therapy of shock, ischemia and other inflammatory diseases.

Conclusion

Although the precise mechanism by which PAF antagonists protect against shock and sepsis remains unclear, it is becoming apparent that a complex interaction occurs between PAF, proteases and cytokines, which, if uncontrolled, leads to circulatory collapse. It appears that PAF antagonists, which are effective in counteracting shock and ischemia because of their indirect anti-protease activity and their ability to inhibit deleterious PAF/cytokine auto-generated feedback processes, may offer considerable potential for the treatment of these conditions in man.

References

1. Braquet P, Touqui L, Shen TS, Vargaftig BB (1987) Perspectives in platelet-activating factor research. Pharmacol Reviews 39:97–145
2. Koltai M, Hosford D, Guinot P, Esanu A, Braquet P (1991) PAF : A review of its effects, antagonists and possible future clinical implications. Drugs 42:I-9–29, II-174–204
3. Hosford D, Braquet P (1990) Antagonists of platelet-activating factor : Chemistry, pharmacology and clinical applications. Prog Med Chem 27:325–380
4. Hosford D, Braquet P (1990) The potential role of platelet-activating factor in shock and ischemia. J Critical Care 5:1–17
5. Vargaftig BB, Lefort J, Chignard M, Benveniste J (1981) Platelet-activating factor induces a platelet-dependent bronchoconstriction unrelated to the formation of prostaglandin derivatives. Eur J Pharmacol 65:185–192
6. Bessin P, Bonnet J, Appfel D, et al. (1983) Acute circulatory collapse caused by platelet-activating factor (PAF-acether) in dogs. Eur J Pharmacol 86:403–413
7. Adnot S, Lefort J, Lagente V, Braquet P, Vargaftig BB (1986) Interference of BN 52021 a PAF-acether antagonist with endotoxin-induced hypotension in the guinea pig. Pharmacol Res Comm 18:197–200
8. Purvis AW, Christman C, McPherson CD, et al. (1988) WEB 2086 a platelet activating factor receptor antagonist attenuates the response to endotoxin in awake sheep. Am Rev Resp Dis 137:99–100
9. Wedmore CV, Williams TJ (1981) Platelet-activating factor (PAF), a secretory product of polymorphonuclear leukocytes increases vascular permeability in rabbit skin. Br J Pharmacol 19:916–917
10. Ekstrom-Jodal B, Haggendal J, Larsson LE, Westerlind A (1982) Cerebral blood flow and oxygen uptake in endotoxin shock: An experimental study in dogs. Acta Anaesthesiol Scan 26:163–170
11. Hwang SB, Lam MH, Lee CL, Shen TY (1986) Release of platelet activating factor and its involvement in the first phase of carrageenin-induced rat foot edema. Eur J Pharmacol 120:33–41
12. Beijer L, Botting J, Crook P (1988) The involvement of platelet activating factor in endotoxin-induced pulmonary platelet recruitment in the guinea pig. Br J Pharmacol 92:803–808
13. Burhop KE, van der Zee H, Bizios R, Kaplan JE, Malik AB (1986) Pulmonary responses to platelet-activating factor in awake sheep and the role of cyclooxygenase metabolites. Am Rev Resp Dis 134:548–554
14. Braquet P, Vidal RF, Braquet M, Hamard H, Vargaftig BB (1984) Involvement of leukotrienes and PAF-acether in the increase microvascular permeability of the rabbit retina. Agents Actions 15:82–85

15. Braquet P, Paubert-Braquet M, Bourgain R, Bussolino F, Hosford D (1989) PAF/cytokine autogenerated feedback networks in microvascular immune injury consequences in shock ischemia and graft rejection. J Lipid Mediators 1:75–112
16. Braquet P, Paubert-Braquet M, Koltai M, et al. (1989) Is there a case for PAF antagonists in the treatment of ischemic states? Trends Pharmacol Sci 10:23–30
17. Bussolino F, Aglietta M, Sanavio F, Stacchini A, Lauri D, Camussi G (1985) Alkylether phosphoglycerides influence calcium fluxes into human endothelial cells. J Immunol 135:2748–2755
18. Bussolino F, Cammussi G, Aglietta M, et al. (1987) Human endothelial cells are a target for platelet-activating factor. J Immunol 139:2439–2446
19. Bourgain RH, Maes L, Braquet P, Andries R, Touqui L, Braquet M (1985) The effect of 1-0-alkyl-2-acetyl-sn-glycero-3-phosphocholine (PAF-acether) on the arterial wall. Prostaglandins 30:185–197
20. Camussi G, Aglietta M, Malavasi F, et al. (1983) The release of platelet-activating factor from human endothelial cells in culture. J Immunol 131:2397–2403
21. Bussolino F, Camussi G, Baglioni C (1988) Synthesis and release of platelet-activating factor by human vascular endothelial cells treated with tumor necrosis factor or interleukin 1α. J Bio Chem 263:11856–11861
22. Malech HL, Gallin JI (1987) Neutrophils in human diseases. New Eng J Med 11:687–694
23. Gomes-Cambronero J, Durstin M, Molski TF, Naccache PH, Sha-afi RI (1989) Calcium is necessary for the platelet-activating factor release in human neutrophils stimulated by physiological stimuli : Role of G-proteins. J Biol Chem 264:12699–12704
24. Vallance SJ, Downes CP, Cragoe EJ, Whetton AD (1990) Granulocyte-macrophage colony-stimulating factor can stimulate macrophage proliferation via persistent activation of Na+/H+ antiport activation. Biochem J 265:359–364
25. DiPersico JF, Belling P, Williams R (1988) Human granulocyte-macrophage colony-stimulating factor and other cytokines primes human neutrophils for enhanced arachidonic acid release and leukotriene B4 synthesis. J Immunol 140:4315–4322
26. Mock BH, English D (1990) Granulocyte-macrophage colony-stimulating factor enhances exudation of neutrophils to sites on inflammatory challenge in vivo. J Lipid Mediators 2:137–141
27. Marquis O, Robaut C, Cavero I (1989) Evidence for the existence and ionic modulation of platelet-activating factor receptors mediating degranulatory responses in human polymorphonuclear leukocytes. J Pharm Exp Therap 250:293–300
28. Gilfillan AM, Wiggan GA, Hope WC, Patel BJ, Welton AF (1990) Ro 19-3704 directly inhibits immunogolulin E-dependent mediator release by a mechanism independent of its platelet-activating factor antagonist properties. Eur J Pharmacol 176:255–262
29. Berkow RL, Wang D, Larrich JW (1987) Enhancement of neutrophil superoxide production by preincubation with recombinant human tumor necrosis factor. J Immunol 139:3780–3791
30. Worthen GS, Seccombe JF, Clay KL, Guthrie LA, Johnston RB (1988) The priming of neutrophils by lipopolysaccharide for production of intracellular platelet-activating factor. J Immunol 140:3553–3559
31. Paubert-Braquet M, Hosford D, Koltz P, Guilbaud J, Braquet P (1990) Tumor necrosis factor a primes the platelet-activating factor-induced superoxide production by human neutrophils : possible involvement of G proteins. J Lipid Mediators 2:1–14
32. Caridis DT, Reinhold RB, Woodruff PW, Fine J (1972) Endotoxemia in man. Lancet 1:1381–1385
33. Etienne A, Hecquet F, Guilmard C, Soulard C, Braquet P (1987) A potential link between platelet-activating factor and plasma protease activity in endotoxemia. Int J Tiss Reac 9:19–26
34. Etienne A, Hecquet F, Soulard C, Spinnewyn B, Clostre F, Braquet P (1985) In vivo inhibition of plasma protein leakage and Salmonella enteritidis-induced mortality in the rat by a specific PAF acether antagonist BN 52021. Agents Actions 17:368–370
35. Stewart AG, Phillips WA (1989) Intracellular platelet-activating factor regulates eicosanoid genertion in guinea pig resident peritoneal macrophages. Br J Pharmacol 98:141–148

36. Rylander R, Beijer L (1987) Inhalation of endotoxin stimulates alveolar macrophage production of platelet-activating factor. Am Rev Respir Dis 135:83–86
37. Leslie CC, Detty DM (1986) Arachidonic acid turnover in response to lipopolysaccharide and opsonized zymosan in human monocyte-derived macrophages. Biochem J 236:251–259
38. Fitzgerald MF, Moncada S, Parente L (1989) The anaphylactic release of platelet-activating factor from perfused guinea pig lungs. Br J Pharmacol 88:149–153
39. Fauler J, Sielhorst G, Frölich JC (1989) Platelet-activating factor induces the production of leukotrienes by human monocytes. Biochim Biophys Acta 1013:80–85
40. Morris DD, Moore JN (1989) Equine peritoneal macrophage production of thromboxane and prostacyclin in response to platelet-activating factor and its receptor antagonist SRI 63–441. Circ Shock 28:149–158
41. Poubelle PE, Gingras D, Demers C, et al. (1991) Platelet-activating factor (PAF-acether) enhances the recombinant production of tumour necrosis factor-alpha and interleukin-1 by subsets of human monocytes. Immunology 72:181–187
42. Bonavida B, Mencia-Huerta JM, Braquet P (1990) Effects of platelet-activating factor on peripheral blood monocytes : Induction and priming for TNF secretion. J Lipid Mediators 2:65–76
43. Pignol B, Hénane S, Sorlin B, Rola-Pleszczynski M, Mencia-Huerta JM, Braquet P (1990) Effect of long-term treatment with platelet-activating factor on IL-1 and IL-2 production by rat spleen cells. J Immunol 145:980–984
44. Inarrea P, Gomes-Cambronero J, Pascual J, Ponte MC, Hernando L, Sanchez-Crespo M (1985) Synthesis of PAF-acether and blood volume changes in gram-negative sepsis. Immunopharmacol 9:45–52
45. Buxton DB, Fisher RA, Hanahan DJ, Olsen MS (1986) Platelet-activating factor-mediated vasconstriction and glyco-genolysis in the perfused rat liver. J Biol chem 261:644–649
46. Hsueh W, Gonzalez-Crussi F, Arroyave J (1987) Platelet-activating factor an endogenous mediator for bowel necrosis in endotoxemia. FASEB J 1:403–405
47. Salzer WL, McCall CE (1990) Primed stimulation of isolated perfused rabbit lung by endotoxin and platelet activating factor induces enhanced production of thromboxane and lung injury. J Clin Invest 85:1135–1143
48. Bussolino F, Porcellinin MG, Varese L, Bosia A (1987) Intravascular release of platelet-activating factor in children with sepsis. Thrombos Res 48:619–620
49. Lopez-Diez F, Nieto ML, Fernandez-Gallardo S, Gijon MA, Sanchez-Crespo M (1989) Occupancy of platelet receptors for platelet-activating factor in patients with septicemia. J Clin Invest 83:1733–1740
50. Arditi M, Manogue KR, Caplan M, Yogev R (1990) Cerebrospinal fluid cachectin/tumor necrosis factor-alpha and platelet-activating factor concentrations and severity of bacterial meningitis in children. J Infect Dis 162:139–147
51. Terashita Z, Imura Y, Nishikawa Kand Sumida S (1985) Is platelet activating factor (PAF) a mediator of endotoxin shock? Eur J Pharmacol 109:257–261
52. Casals-Stenzel J, Muacevic G, Heuer H (1987) Pharmacological actions of WEB 2086 a new specific antagonist of platelet-activating factor. J Pharmacol. Exp Ther 241:974–981
53. Yue TI, Farhat M, Rabinovici R, Perera PU, Vogel SN, Feuerstein G (1990) Protective effect of BN 50739 a new PAF antagonist in endotoxin-treated rabbits. J Pharmacol Exp Ther 254:976–981
54. Fletcher JR, Di Simone BS, Earnest MA (1990) Platelet-activating factor receptor antagonist improves survival and attentuates eicosanoid release in severe endotoxemia. Ann Surg 211:312–316
55. Rabinovici R, Yue TL, Farhat M, et al. (1990) Platelet-activating factor (PAF) and tumor necrosis factor (PAF) and tumor necrosis factor (TNF) interactions in endotoxemic shock. Studies with BN 50739, a novel PAF antagonist. J Pharmacol Exp Ther 255:256–263
56. Earnest MA, DiSimone AG, Fletcher JR (1990) The effects of BN 52021 a PAF receptor antagonist in canine endotoxemia in Ginkgolides In: Braquet P (Ed) Chemistry Biology Pharmacology and Clinical Perspectives Vol 2, Barcelona pp 463–470
57. Lang CH, Dobrescu C, Hargrove DM, Bagby C, Spitzer JJ (1988) Attenuation of endotoxin-induced increase in glucose metabolism by platelet-activating factor antagonist. Circ Shock 23:179–188

58. Burhop KE, Garcia JGN, Selig WM, et al. (1986) Platelet-activating factor increases lung vascular permeability to protein. J Appl Physiol 61:2210–2217
59. Toyofuku T, Kubo K, Kobayashi T, Kusama S (1986) Effects of ONO-6240 a platelet-activating factor antagonist on endotoxin shock in unanesthetized sheep. Prostaglandins 31:271–281
60. Baum TD, Hard SO, Feldman HS, Latka CA, Fink MP (1990) Endotoxin-induced myocardial depression in rats: effect of ibuprofen and SDZ 64-688 a platelet activating factor receptor antagonist. J Surg Res 48:629–634
61. Beijer L, Bottig J, Crook P (1988) The involvement of platelet activating factor in endotoxin-induced pulmonary platelet recruitment in the guinea-pig. Br J Pharmacol 92:803–808
62. Chang SW, Feddersen CO, Henson PM, Voelkel NF (1987) Platelet-activating factor mediates hemodynamic changes and lung injury in endotoxin-treated rats. J Clin Invest 79:1498–1509
63. Touvay C, Vilain B, Carre C, Mencia-Huerta JM, Braquet P (1989) Role of platelet-activating factor (PAF) in the bronchopulmonary alterations induced by endotoxin effects on beta-adrenoceptors. In: Braquet P (ed) Ginkolides: Chemistry Biology Pharmacology and Clinical Perspectives Vol 1, JR Prous, Barcelona, pp 477–486
64. Tolins JP, Vercellotti GM, Wilkowske M, Ha B, Jacob HS, Raij L (1989) The role of platelet-activating factor in endotoxemic acute renal failure in the male rat, J Lab Clin Med 113:316–324
65. Gonzales-Crussi F, Hsueh W (1983) Experimental model of ischemic bowel necrosis: The role of platelet-activating factor and endotoxin. Am J Path 112:127–135
66 Wallace JL, Steel G, Whittle BJR (1987) Evidence for platelet-activating factor as as mediator of endotoxin-induced gastrointestinal damage in the rat. Effects of three platelet-activating factor antagonists. Gastroenterology 93:765–773
67. SunX, Hsueh W (1988) Bowel necrosis induced by tumor necrosis factor in rats is mediated by platelet-activating factor. J Clin Invest 81:1328–1331
68. Wallace JL, Braquet P, Ibbotson GC, Mc Naughton WK, Cirino G (1989) Assessment of the role of platelet-activating factor in an animal model of inflammatory bowel disease. J Lipid Mediators 1:13–23
69. Weinberg JR, Wright DJM, Guz A (1988) Interleukin-1β and tumor necrosis factor cause hypotension in the conscious rabbit. Clinical Sci 75:251–254
70. Dahinden CA, Zirgg I, Malif FE (1988) Leukotriene production in human neutrophils primed by recombinant human granulocyte/macrophage colony-stimulating factor and stimulated with the complement component C5A and FMLP as second signals. J Exp Med 167:1281–1295
71. Silberstein DJ, Owen WF, Gasson JC (1986) Enhancement of human eosinophil cytotoxicity and leukotriene synthesis by biosynthetic (recombinant) granulocyte-macrophage colony stimulating factor. J Immunol 137:3290–3294

Nitric Oxide as a Mediator of the Vascular Derangements of Sepsis and Endotoxemia

J.R. Parratt and J.C. Stoclet

Introduction

It is a concept, fundamental to physiology and pharmacology, that if a cellular recognition site exists for a chemical quite foreign to the body, then a similar recognition site, or receptor, might also be the means by which an endogenous ligand, similar to that foreign chemical, also results in cellular activation. Thus, the demonstration of specific recognition sites for morphine led to the search for, and discovery of, endogenous opioid-like peptides.. More recently, there has been increasing evidence for the presence within the body of an "endogenous digitalis". It is now well over a century since T. Lauder Brunton described the beneficial effects of amyl nitrite in patients with angina pectoris, and less than 30 years ago since the precise vascular and cellular mechanisms of action of organic nitrates and nitrites were elucidated. The finding that this depends on activation of soluble guanylyl cyclase within vascular smooth muscle cells, with a subsequent formation of an intracellular second messenger, cyclic 3-5-guanosine monophosphate (cGMP), was one of the factors that led eventually to the discovery of an "endogenous nitrodilator" nitric oxide (NO), the formation of which is responsible for the action of clinically useful nitrodilators such as glyceryl trinitrate, nitroprusside and sydnonimines such as molsidomine (and its active metabolite SIN-1) which act on the blood vessel walls by "donating" NO. Endogneous NO is now known to be produced from the amino-acid L-arginine in a variety of cells [1] including vascular endothelium [2, 3], macrophages [4], neutrophils [5, 6] and platelets [7, 8]. In endothelial cells, it is this endogenous nitrodilator, NO (or a closely related compound releasing this free radical) that is responsible of the effects of the endothelium-derived relaxing factor (EDRF) originally described by Furchgott and Zawadzki in 1980 [9], who discovered that the ability of acetycholine to relax vascular smooth muscle depended on the integrity of the endothelium and the release from it of a diffusible substance.

Over the past three years there has been increasing evidence that it is the excessive generation of NO that is primarily responsible for the loss of vascular tone and the "unrelenting hypotension" observed both in patients with the sepsis syndrome and in experimental animals in which sepsis has been induced by a combination of caecal ligation and perforation or in which one of the primary mediators of sepsis (endotoxin) has been administered. The purpose of this chapter is to summarize briefly the experimental evidence (there is only scant clinical evidence at present) for the view that NO is an important mediator of the vascular derangement characteristic of clinical sepsis and endotoxemia, and which contribute to mortality in such patients [10, 11].

Loss of Vascular Tone is an Early Consequence of Endotoxin Release or Administration

The present author [12] observed nearly twenty years ago that following the administration of a bolus dose of *E.coli* endotoxin to anesthetized cats, the positive inotropic and pressor responses to injected catecholamines such as epinephrine and norepinephrine, were markedly depressed within 1 to 2 h of the onset of endotoxemia. Although subsequent experiments were more concerned with determining the mechanism of the reduced cardiac responses to catecholamines (and to other positive inotropic agents), it became clear that this reduced vascular responsiveness was a general phenomenon in that it occurred in response to calcium [13]. Further, certain vasodilator responses, such as those to the phosphodiesterase inhibitor quazodine [14] were more marked following administration of endotoxin. That altered vascular responses following the administration of endotoxin are retained if blood vessels are removed from such animals and examined in an isolated organ bath was first demonstrated by the United States Navy group in Bethesda [15]. They showed for example, that if they removed blood vessels from rats administered endotoxin, the ability to respond to norepinephrine was impaired in comparison with the same vessels removed from control rats. This finding was important for two reasons. First, it showed that the large number of circulating vasodilator mediators released in shock [16] are unlikely to be involved in this phenomenon because whatever mechanism is responsible is still present when the vessel is isolated and removed from this chemical environment. Presumably then, the loss of vascular responsiveness is due either to the *local* release of a powerful vasodilator substance in response to endotoxin, or to some fundamental defect in the ability of vascular smooth muscle cells to contract. For reasons that will be clear later, the first of these explanations is the most likely. The second reason for the importance of the finding of the Bethesda group is that, if this loss of vascular responsiveness can be observed *in vitro*, then it is much easier to determine the mechanisms involved. It was studied involving such isolated vessels that has led to the hypothesis that it is the local formation of the potent vasodilator substance NO that is responsible for the loss of vascular responsiveness under conditions of endotoxemia and sepsis.

Most of these studies have been carried out using large arteries, such as the thoracic aorta, removed from rats administered quite large doses of endotoxin several hours previously. It became clar that this loss of responsiveness is a general phenomenon. Bigaud et al. [17] examined the effects of a

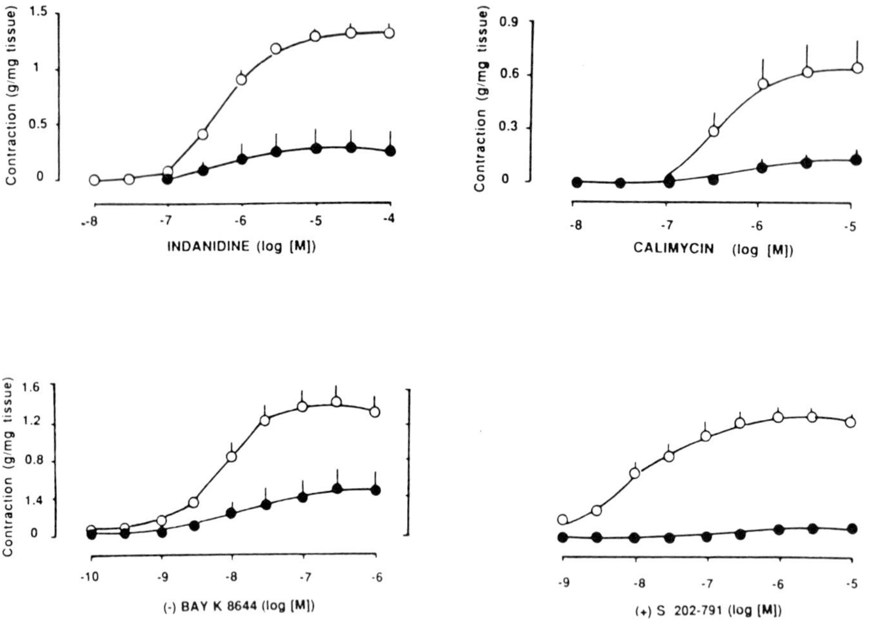

Fig. 1. Cumulative concentration-effect curves for (top left) the α_1-adrenoceptor agonist indanidine, the calcium ionophore calimycin and the calcium agonists BAY K 8644 and (+) S 202-791 in endothelium-denuded aortic rings taken from control (○) and LPS-pretreated (●) rats. The vertical bars represent s.e. mean of 6-7 observations (From [17] with permission)

wide variety of vasoconstrictor agents in such isolated aorta preparations and observed that the vessels were much less responsive to agents acting through specific receptors (e.g. specific α_1-adrenoceptor agonists such as indamidine and phenylephrine, both of which induce calcium entry into cells through calcium channels and stimulate intracellular calcium release from the sarcoplasmic reticulum through an inositol-1,4,-triphosphate, IP_3 sensitive mechanism), calcium ionophores such as calimycin (A23817) which "carry" calcium ions across the membrane, calcium agonists acting on specific channels (such as BAY K 8644 and (+) S 202-791), as well as calcium itself in the presence of a potassium chloride depolarizing solution (Fig. 1). However, it is of considerable interest that the contractile responses to endothelin [18] and to caffeine are either unaffected or only slightly modified. The importance of this observation is that it reveals that the ability of smooth muscle to contract is not dimished by lipopolysaccharide (LPS) and that there is therefore no fundamental defect of the vascular contractile apparatus.

This reduction in responsiveness, for example to norepinephrine, in thoracic aorta removed from animals given endotoxin several hours previously, is seen whether or not the endothelium is present and is also evident after the cyclooxygenase pathway of arachidonic acid metabolism has been inhibited. The first demonstration that this loss of responsiveness was due to activa-

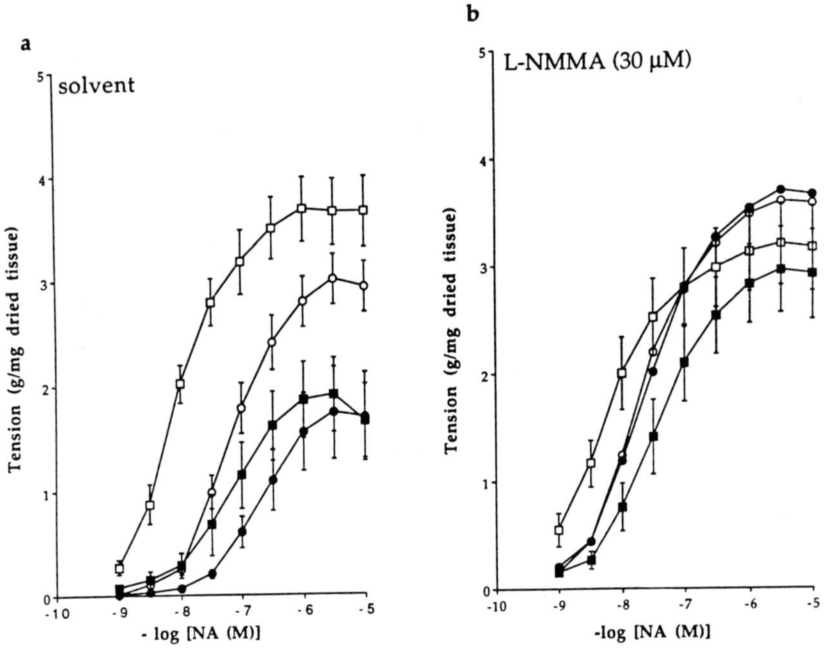

Fig. 2. Concentration-response curves for norepinephrine (NA) in aortic rings, with (○,●) and without (❑, ■) endothelium, from control (open symbols) and LPS-treated rats (filled symbols) in the presence of (**a**) solvent and (**b**) N^G-monomethyl-L-arginine (L-NMMA, 30 μM). Results are presented as the mean ± s.e. mean, n = 8. The inhibitor of the L-arginine NO pathway restores responsiveness to norepinephrine in rats administered endotoxin.

tion, by endotoxin, of the L-arginine NO pathway were the studies of Fleming et al. (Fig. 2) [19]. These results revealed that inhibitors of the L-arginine NO pathway such as N^G-monomethyl-L-arginine (L-NMMA) or N^G-nitro-L-arginine methyl ester (L-NAME) restored responsiveness to norepinephrine. These experiments, and others designed to further explore the mechanism of activation of the L-arginine NO pathway by endotoxemia, are described in more detail below.

Evidence that the Loss of Vascular Responsiveness in Sepsis and Endotoxemia Involves Activation of L-arginine NO Pathway

Changes in Vasoconstrictor Responses Induced by LPS in vivo; Evidence of this is Due to NO Production

In experimental animals, the administration of LPS (endotoxin) or the induction of sepsis by a combination of caecal ligation together with perforation,

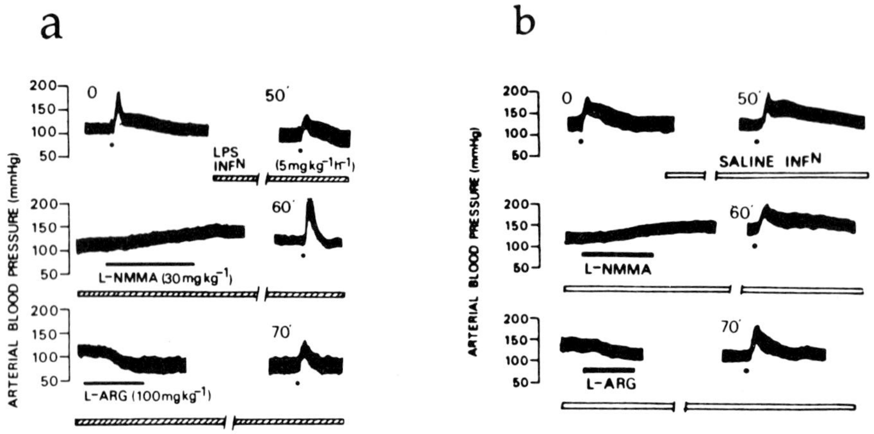

Fig. 3. Pressor responses to norepinephrine (●) in anesthetized rats before and during an infusion of bacterial LPS derived from *E. coli* (5 mg/kg/h) (**a**) or solvent (saline, **b**). Responses to norepinephrine (1 μg kg at the closed circles) were depressed 50 min after commencing the infusion of LPS but were restored to normal (middle panel) following the administration of the L-arginine analogue L-NMMA (30 mg/kg). Administration of the substrate (L-arginine, 100 mg/kg) resulted in a return of depressed responses to norepinephrine. (From [29] with permission)

reduces vasoconstrictor responses to a variety of pressor agents [12, 13, 20-27]. The pressor responses to sympathetic nerve stimulation are also markedly reduced by endotoxin e.g. in the pithed rat studies of Gray et al. [28]. Although there is some evidence that prostaglandin production contributes to this loss of responsiveness [28], it now seems clear that NO generation is primarily responsible. For example, in the anesthetized rat preparation, pressor responses to norepinephrine are reduced within 1 h of the commencement of an infusion of *E. coli* endotoxin, in a dose (5 mg/kg/h) too small to modify significantly arterial blood pressure (Fig. 3) [29, 30]. The pressor responses to norepinephrine are restored following the infusion of inhibitors of the L-arginine NO pathway such as L-NMMA or L-NAME. These themselves increase systemic arterial blood pressure either by inhibiting the basal release of NO from endothelial cells or via an effect on the central nervous system to remove the "break" on central sympathetic neurones. If L-arginine, the precursor of NO, is then infused, blood pressure decreases and there is again a reduced responsiveness to norepinephrine (Fig. 3).

This interaction between endotoxin, inhibitors of the L-arginine NO pathway and the NO precursors, L-arginine, is quite specific. Thus, pressor responses to norephinephrine are only restored by L-NMMA but not by D-NMMA (Fig. 4), and these restored pressor responses are reversed by L-arginine but not by D-arginine. Inhibition of the L-arginine NO pathway has no effect on pressor responses to norepinephrine in the absence of endotoxin (Fig. 4). Further, vascular hyporesponsiveness to norepinephrine is unaffected by inhibition of the cyclooxygenase pathway; L-NAME increases blood pressure and restores norepinephrine responsiveness following administra-

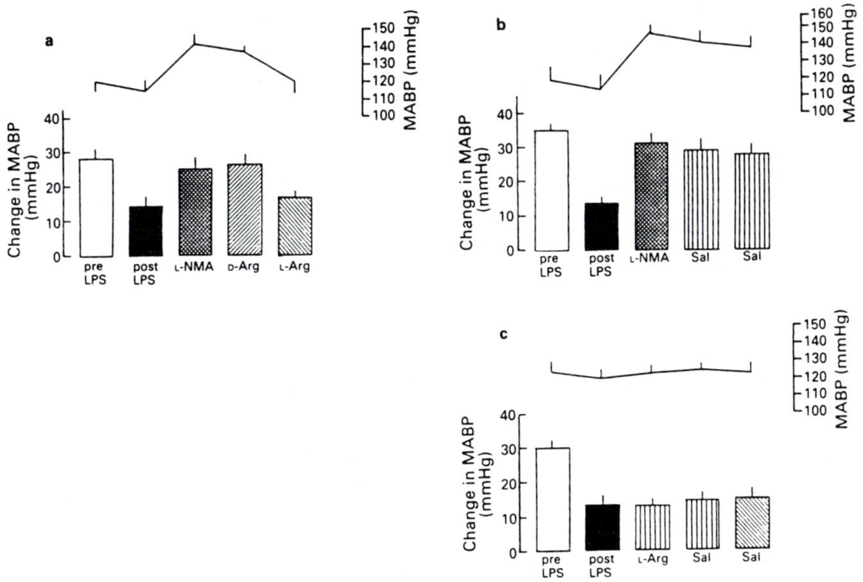

Fig. 4. Stability of the effects of L-NMMA (30 mg/kg) on MABP (line graphs) and pressor responses to norepinephrine (NA, 300 ng/kg, histograms) and their reversal by L- but not D-arginine (100 mg /kg) during continuous infusion of *E. coli* LPS, (10 mg/kg/h) in anesthetized rats. The increase in MABP and restoration of responsiveness By L-NMMA (L-NMA) in (**a**) are both reversed by subsequent administration of L (L-Arg) but no D-arginine (D-Arg). (**b**) Shows them both maintained during saline (Sal) administration. In (**c**), both the MABP and LPS-induced depression of responsiveness are maintained during the time period of the experiment and MABP is not reduced, nor the hyporesponsiveness to NA enhanced, by provision of additional L-arginine (100 mg/kg). Values are the mean of 6-7 experiments; vertical lines show standard errors of the mean. *$P < 0.05$ compared to pre-infusion value. (From [27] with permission)

tion of a dose of indomethacin sufficient to prevent the production of prostaglandins from arachidonic acid [27].

As one might expect from these results, inhibitors of the L-arginine NO pathway such as L-NAME also restore to normal pressor responses to sympathetic nerve stimulation. These studies were performed in a pithed rat preparation which allows electrical stimulation of the spinal sympathetic flow [31]. This results in pressor responses which are frequency dependent. Such pressor responses are inhibited by endotoxin and restored by either L-NAME or vasopressin [32]. These results are however complicated by the finding that, unlike in anesthetized rats, responsiveness to norepinephrine and to sympathetic nerve stimulation is enhanced in the absence of endotoxin by both L-NAME and vasopressin. This is presumably due to an increased availability of calcium to the contractile elements.

We know little at present concerning whether vasoconstrictor responses to sympathetic nerve stimulation are altered in all vascular beds innervated by vasoconstrictor fibres or whether some vascular beds are affected more than others. This is being determined by measuring blood flow in various vascular beds following sympathetic nerve stimulation under conditions of endotoxemia (unpublished data). The renal and mesenteric vascular beds are certainly among those involved. In isolated hearts, Smith et al. [33] have shown that the coronary vasoconstriction induced by the thromboxane-mimetic U46619 are reduced by endotoxin, and that this loss of responsiveness is reversed by dexamethasone.

The above studies have been primarily concerned with determining the mechanism of the loss of vascular reactivity which occurs following endotoxin administration. There is also evidence that NO generation is involved in the early marked reduction in blood pressure which occurs following the administration of large bolus doses of endotoxin [34]. Thiemermann and Vane [34] showed that the administration of an inhibitor of NO production from L-arginine, N^G-monomethyl-L-arginine (NeArg) both increased blood pressure and attenuated the profound hypotension which resulted from the administration of *E. coli* endotoxin. The difficulty with such studies is that, following the administration of the inhibitor of the L-arginine NO pathway, systemic arterial blood pressure is considerably higher than in the controls. Indeed, from their published results, one could argue that there is little difference between the hypotensive response to endotoxin following administration of the inhibitor as compared to that in those rats given endotoxin alone. The same inhibitor also attenuates the hypotension induced by the cytotoxic protein tumor necrosis factor (TNF) [35] which is released from macrophages by endotoxin. The marked hypotension induced by large bolus doses of endotoxin or TNF could be quite unrelated to the subsequent loss of vascular responsiveness to norepinephrine and sympathetic nerve stimulation. That there is a dissociation between these two phenomenon is clear from studies with platelet activating factor (PAF). The hypotension associated with administration of this substance is blocked by various antagonists although the loss in vascular responsiveness induced by endotoxin is unaffected by such antagonists [36]. Further, the available evidence (see below) is that the loss of vascular responsiveness to norepinephrine is due to the time and concentration dependent induction of a NO synthase which differs from the constitutive enzyme. It is difficult to imagine how such an enzyme could be so rapidly induced by a bolus injection of endotoxin; indeed, there is considerable evidence against such an early induction.

Evidence that the L-arginine NO Pathway is Stimulated in Blood Vessels Removed from Endotoxin-treated Animals

As outlined above, a loss of vascular responsiveness to norepinephrine and to other vasoconstrictor agents can be demonstrated in vessels removed from animals in which sepsis has been induced or from animals (usually rats) given endotoxin [15, 17, 37-40]. This *ex vivo* effect is illustrated in Figure 2.

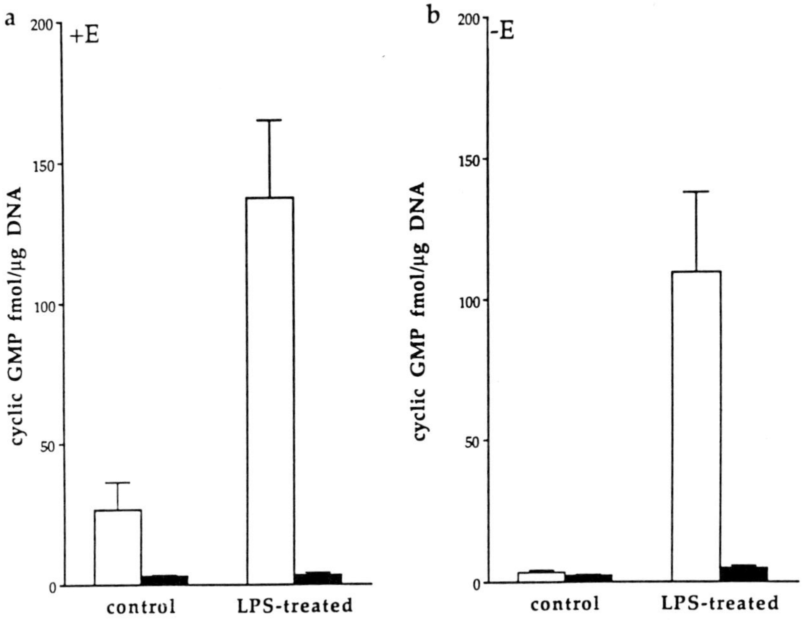

Fig. 5. Histogram depicting the cyclic GMP content in aortic rings, (**a**) with and (**b**) without endothelium, from control and LPS-treated rats contracted with norepinephrine (10 μM) in the presence (filled columns) and absence (open columns) of L-NAME (300 μM). Results are presented as the mean ± s.e. mean, n = 5 (From unpublished studies by I Fleming)

As with the *in vivo* experiments, responsiveness to norepinephrine is restored by inhibitors of the L-arginine NO pathway such as L-NMMA or L-NAME. Again, this restoration is stereospecific (D-NMMA is ineffective) and the effect of the inhibitor can be overcome by addition to the organ bath of L-arginine but not D-arginine. This implies either substrate exhaustion or some defect in the transport of L-arginine into vascular smooth muscle cells.

Other evidence that the L-arginine NO pathway is activated comes from parallel measurements of the cGMP content of vessels removed from rats administered endotoxin [41] and from the effects of inhibitors of soluble guanylyl cyclase, which is the enzyme responsible for its production from GTP. Two such inhibitors have been used, methylene blue [42] and 6-anilo-5,8-quinolinedione (LY83583) which both inhibit the enzyme and destroy NO [43]. In vessels taken from LPS-treated rats, and whether endothelium was present or not, cGMP content was significantly higher than that in aortic rings taken from control rats (Fig. 5). This increase in cGMP was not seen if inhibitors of the L-arginine NO pathway were present, but levels were again elevated on addition of L-arginine. As with inhibitors of the L-arginine NO pathway, responsiveness to norepinephrine in such isolated vessels was restored by either methylene blue or LY83583, an effect again independent of the presence of a functional endothelium.

Evidence that the L-arginine NO Pathway is Activated in Normal Blood Vessels Incubated In Vitro with Endotoxin

When aortic rings are taken from normal rats with intact endothelium and incubated in medium containing endotoxin-stimulated peritoneal macrophages, responses to norepinephrine are markedly depressed [44]. We now know that this reduced responsiveness to norepinephrine is also due to activation of the L-arginine NO pathway [45] because the contraction-response curves, which are shifted downward and to the right following incubation, are restored by L- but not D-NMMA and by methylene blue. Further, the loss of responsiveness is associated with the appearance of NO synthase activity in media-adventitia homogenates of rat aorta incubated with endotoxin [46].

Possible Sources of NO Generated in Blood Vessels by Endotoxin

What is the source of NO generated in vessels in the presence of endotoxin? The most obvious cellular source of NO in blood vessels is the endothelium. Indeed, NO accounts for much of the biological activity of endothelium-derived relaxing factor originally described in 1980 by Furchgott and Zawadzki [9]. Their experiments showed that certain vasodilator agents, such as acetylcholine, relaxed blood vessels with an intact endothelium but that this relaxation was abolished, or even converted to a constrictor response, if the endothelium was mechanically removed by gentle rubbing. A number of substances are now known to depend, for their vasodilator action *in vivo*, on an ability to NO from endothelial cells. This NO then diffuses to the underlying smooth muscle cells to stimulate soluble guanylyl cyclase and elevate cGMP. Endothelium-derived NO, together with prostacyclin, accounts for most of the protectice effects of the endothelium, which include not only vasodilatation but also inhibition of platelet adhesion and aggregation. There is marked synergism in this respect between these two endothelium-derived substances. It was somewhat surprising in our own early experiments to discover that norepinephrine responses could be restored to normal in blood vessels removed from endotoxin treated rats even when the endothelium was removed. This implied that the NO generated as a result of endotoxin administration was derived from cellular sources other than the endothelium [19]. Tissue macrophages are a likely source but there is also recent evidence that vascular smooth muscle cells can themselves generate NO in the presence of endotoxin. Such studies do not of course imply that under *in vivo* conditions, the endothelium is unimportant in determining this loss of responsiveness to vasoconstrictor agents. However, it does imply that endotoxin is able to induce an enzyme capable of generating NO in a variety of cells. This would have widespread implications for patients with the sepsis syndrome. We favor the view that the production of NO, initially vasoprotective, eventually becomes grossly exaggerated and out of hand. This may be because there is considerable evidence that endotoxin, after initial stimulation of the endothelium, then results in the functional and mechanical deterioration of this protective cellular barrier. As Kang and Williams [47] have shown, endotoxin is ultimately cytotoxic to endothelial cells, inducing both functional impairment of endothelium-dependent responses, physical lesions and detachment with resultant alterations in permeability. It is possible that this cytotoxicity is mediated by the excessive local generation of NO.

Impaired Vasodilator Responses Following Sepsis and Endotoxemia

There is evidence for a role of the L-arginine NO pathway in the modification that occurs to vasodilator responses under conditions of endotoxemia. There is early work, in mesenteric arterioles, showing that vasodilator responses to bradykinin, histamine, substance P and acetylcholine are inhibited by endotoxin; this was attributed to endothelial damage [48]. Vasodilator responses to isoprenaline are also impaired [49]. In a more detailed study, Guc et al. [32, 50] found in pithed rats that vasodilator responses to acetylcholine, 5-HT, endothelin and bradykinin were attenuated in rats administered endotoxin, even when the blood pressure was restored by vasopressin. This reduced responsiveness could be due to endothelial dysfunction. We [51] and others [52] have also reported diminished responsiveness to acetylcholine in vessels incubated with LPS under *in vitro* conditions whereas responses to NO and endothelium-independent vasodilators, were unaffected by such incubation. In coronary artery ring preparations, isolated from dogs several hours after administration of endotoxin, responses to acetylcholine were markedly impaired, whereas those to nitroprusside were unaltered [53]. The conclusion from all these studies was that there is an altered endothelium dependent vasodilation in blood vessels during endotoxemia. This, of course, is difficult to reconcile with the evidence, outlined above, that it is the overproduction of NO that is responsible for the reduced vasoconstrictor responses. Working at the Université Louis Pasteur, Fleming has recently obtained results that go a long way to explaining this apparent discrepancy. She incubated normal blood vessels, with or without endothelium, with various doses of endotoxin *in vitro*. There was an initial period of hyper-responsiveness to acetylcholine, at a time when responses to norepinephrine were unaffected. Later, responsiveness to acetylcholine declined. Under these conditions, there thus appears to be a *general* loss of vascular reactivity following the administration of endotoxin; this applies to *both* vasoconstrictor and vasodilator responses.

What are the Mechanisms through which Endotoxin Activates the L-arginine-NO Pathway?

It seems likely that the initial trigger for the stimulation of NO production is through the release of cytokines such as interleukin-1 (IL-1) and TNF, although it is possible that endotoxin might activate the pathway through stimulation of specific receptors on the cell surface.

The evidence that cytokines are involved comes from recent studies by Beasley et al. [52, 54, 55] and by McKenna [56]. They found that incubation of blood vessels, such as the rat aorta, with LPS or with IL-1 leads to an increase in cGMP irrespective of whether the endothelium is present or not. An increase in cGMP was not seen in the presence of guanylyl cyclase inhibitors such as methylene blue and LY83583, or in the presence of hemoglobin which binds NO. In other words, the mechanism of the loss of responsiveness which results from either endotoxin [45] or IL-1 administration is the same; it is due to the induction of an enzyme (NO synthase) which generates NO from L-arginine. The view that LPS induced stimulation of the L-arginine NO pathway is mediated through cytokines is supported by studies showing that the enzyme responsible is the induced form rather that the constitutive form. If isolated blood vessels are incubated with endotoxin (or IL-1) in the presence of the protein synthesis inhibitor cycloheximide, there is no increase in cGMP [57] and no loss of vascular responsiveness. An accumulation of cGMP following incubation with endotoxin is also prevented by the presence of a combination of methotrexate and 2,4-diamino-6-hydroxy-pyridimine which inhibit the synthesis of tetrahydrobiopterin [58], a co-factor for NO synthase. In contrast, the accumulation of cGMP is unaffected by calcium removal or by the calmodulin antagonist calmidazolium, indicating that the NO synthase involved is the induced form rather than the constitutive form.

In studies designed to examine the role of endothelium in determining the loss of vascular responsiveness induced by endotoxin, Fleming has recently demonstrated that loss of responsiveness occurs sooner if the endothelium is present (unpublished data). The presence of endothelium in some way accelerates the process. One explanation for this would be the liberation from the endothelium of TNF [56] which, like IL-1, both decrease vascular responsiveness to norepinephrine [59] and induce an L-NMMA sensitive increase in intracellular cGMP.

We can now summarize the most likely mechanisms of NO generation by endotoxin as follows. Endotoxin induces the release of cytokines (TNF and IL-1) which then, acting on specific receptors, stimulate the formation of a new NO synthase. This process involves protein synthesis. The resultant generation of NO by a variety of cells elevates cGMP by activation of soluble guanylyl cyclase. This results in relaxation of blood vessels and prevents vasoconstrictor responses. Later, the endothelium becomes non-functional, presumably because the large amounts of NO generated locally become cytotoxic to these cells, resulting in both a general loss of vascular responsiveness (to vasodilator as well as vasoconstrictor agents) and to an increase in capillar permeability. NO generation could thus account for most of the vascular derangement observed during sepsis. The abnormal distribution of blood flow under such conditions (such as has been demonstrated, for example, in the myocardium [60]) could be due to a loss of responsiveness to key mediators involved in the regulation of vascular tone, whereas responsiveness to the most powerful of all naturally occurring vasoconstrictors, namely endothelin, is unaffected [18]. Such a situation would have far reaching implications for cardiovascular integrity.

Clinical Sepsis: Is there a Case for Inhibiting the L-arginine NO Pathway?

It is not possible, in the absence of relevant experimental data in animals, to determine what effect inhibiting the L-arginine NO pathway would have on the outcome of clinical sepsis. The essential animal experiments have not as yet been performed. We know nothing about blood flow distribution during endotoxemia when the pathway has been inhibited, nor do we know whether such an approach modifies survival. Such experiments would need to be done in, for example, the chronically instrumented conscious rat model described by McKechnie et al. [61]. On theoretical grounds, there would be a danger of a drastic decrease in gastrointestinal blood flow, already critically reduced during sepsis, if inhibitors of the L-arginine NO pathway were administered. There is already experimental evidence for a detrimental effect of these inhibitors on gastrointestinal vascular integrity under conditions of endotoxemia; NO is crucial for maintaining vascular integrity under these conditions [62]. Because under physiological conditions, NO generation by endothelial cells is also partly responsible for inhibiting platelet adhesion, it is possible that giving inhibitors of the pathway might induce both platelet adhesion to the vessel wall and aggregation. A recent report [63] in an anesthetized rabbit model of endotoxemia comes to the conclusion, based partly on mortality studies, that inhibition of both constitutive and inducible NO synthases during endotoxemia is deleterious but this can be overcome by replacing NO intravenously with a donor of NO such as S-nitroso-N-acetyl-penicillamine. They also suggest that selective inhibition of inducible synthase, for example with dexamethasone, might be beneficial in shock induced by endotoxin.

From what we know about the pathophysiology of septic shock, it would be unlikely that such inhibitors would be beneficial if given in the late stages. However, provided we had a short lasting inhibitor of the pathway which did not cross the blood brain barrier, it might well be worth exploring whether the administration of such a compound during the early, hyperdynamic phase of sepsis when it is difficult to elevate pressure by the infusion of pressor agents. This might interrupt the viscious circle of elevated cardiac output and markedly reduced systemic vascular resistance which, if prolonged, would lead either to early mortality or would contribute importantly to multiple organ failure. It might also be possible to elevate perfusion pressure in the early hyperdynamic phase of sepsis by giving methylene blue, which would inhibit guanylyl cyclase. Almost certainly, by the time this publication appears both these approaches would have been attempted.

Conclusion

There is now little doubt that a major contributor to vascular derangements of endotoxemia and sepsis is the generation in the vascular wall of the powerful dilator nitric oxide, from its precursor L-arginine. Interruption of this pathway, either by the administration of analogues of the precursor such as L-NMMA or L-NAME, or of its target in vascular smooth muscle guanylyl cyclase, using methylene blue, leads to an increase in blood pressure and, more importantly, a restoration of responsiveness to norepinephrine. The precise mechanisms of activation of the pathway are uncertain but almost certainly involve, at least in part, the release of cytokines such a IL-1 and TNF. Whether inhibition of NO production or of its actions is a reasonable approach to the therapy of patients with sepsis is debatable. Even the proper animal experiments have yet to be carried out. However, the early administration of either methylene blue or an analogue of L-arginine might offer an approach to the restoration of perfusion pressure in the very early stages of sepsis.

Acknowledgements. Much of the work described in this review comes from a collaboration between the Department of Physiology and Pharmacology, University of Strathclyde, Glasgow and the Institut de Pharmacologie Moléculaire et Cellulaire, Université Louis Pasteur, Strasbourg supported by the European Economic Commission.

References

1. Moncada S, Palmer RMJ, Higgs EA (1991) Nitric oxide: Physiology, pathophysiology and pharmacology. Pharmacol Rev 43:109–142
2. Palmer RM, Ferrige AG, Moncada S (1987) Nitric oxide release accounts for the biological activity of endothelium-derived relaxing factor. Nature (London) 327:524–526
3. Salvemini D, Korbut R, Anggard E, Vane JR (1990) Immediate release of a nitric oxide-like factor from bovine aortic endothelial cells by Escherichia coli lipopolysaccharide. Proc Natl Acad Sci USA 87:2593–2597
4. Hibbs JR Jr, Taintor RR, Vavrin Z, Rachlin EM (1988) Nitric oxide: A cytotoxic activated macrophage effector molecule. Biochem Biophys Res Commun 157:87–94
5. Rimele TJ, Sturm RJ, Adams LM, et al. (1988) Interaction of neutrophils with vascular smooth muscle: Identification of a neutrophil-derived relaxing factor. J Pharmacol Exp Ther 245:102–111
6. Salvemini D, De Nucci C, Gryglewski RJ, Vane JR (1989) Human neutrophils and mononuclear cells inhibit platelet aggregation by releasing a nitric oxide-like factor. Proc Natl Acad Sci USA 86:6328–6332
7. Radomski MW, Palmer RMJ, Moncada S (1990) An L-arginine/nitric oxide pathway present in human platelets regulates aggregation. Proc Natl Acad Sci USA 87:5193–5197
8. Radomski MW, Palmer RMJ, Moncada S (1990) Characterization of the L-arginine nitric oxide pathway in human platelets. Br J Pharmacol 101:325–328
9. Furchgott RF, Zawadzki JV (1980) The obligatory role of endothelial cells in the relaxation of arterial smooth muscle by acethylcholine. Nature (London) 288:373–376
10. Groeneveld ABJ, Bronsveld W, Thijs LG (1986) Hemodynamic determinants of mortality in human septic shock. Surgery 99:140–152

11. Parratt JR (1989) Alterations in vascular reactivity in sepsis and endotoxemia. In: Vincent JL (ed) Update in intensive care and emergency medicine. Vol 8, Springer, Berlin, pp 299–308
12. Parratt JR (1973) Myocardial and circulatory effects of E. coli endotoxin; modification of responses to catecholamines. Br J Pharmacol 47:12–25
13. McCaig DJ, Parratt JR (1980) Reduced myocardial response to calcium during endotoxin shock in the cat. Circ Shock 7:23–30
14. Parratt JR, Winslow E (1974) The haemodynamic effects of quazodine, a cardiac stimulant, in experimental E. coli endotoxin shock in the cat. Clinical and Experimental Pharm Physiol 1:31–42
15. Pomerantz K, Casey L, Fletcher JR, Ramwell PW (1982) Vascular reactivity in endotoxin shock: Effect of lidocaine or indomethacin pretreatment. Adv Shock Res 7:191–198
16. Parratt JR (1983) Neurohumoral agents and their release in shock. In: Altura AM, Lefer AM, Schumer W (eds) Handbook of Shock and Trauma, Vol 1 (Basic Science), Raven Press, New York, pp 311–336
17. Bigaud M, Julou-Schaeffer G, Parratt JR, Stoclet JC (1990) Endotoxin-induced impairment of vascular smooth muscle contractions elicited by different mechanisms. Eur J Pharmacol 190:185–192
18. Julou-Schaeffer G, Schott C, Parratt JR, Stoclet JC. (1989) Influence of in vivo endotoxin treatment on endothelin-induced contractions of the rat isolated aorta. J Physiol (London) 417:66
19. Fleming I, Gray GA, Julou-Schaeffer G, Parratt JR, Schott C, Stoclet JC (1990) Impaired vascular reactivity in the rat following endotoxin treatment can be endothelium-independent, yet involves the L-arginine pathway. J Physiol London 423:18
20. Archer LT, Black MR, Hinshaw LB (1975) Myocardial failure with altered response to adrenaline in endotoxin shock. Br J Pharmacol 54:145–155
21. Auclair MC, Carli A, Lechat P (1982) Decrease of the hypertensive responses to phenylephrine in the rat submitted to a sublethal dose of E. coli endotoxin. Restoration by indomethacin. J Pharmac (Paris) 13:341
22. Auclair MC, Svinareff P, Schmitt H (1986) Vascular α-adrenoceptor blockade of E. coli endotoxin in the rat. Eur J Pharmacol 127:121–124
23. Auclai MC, Schmitt H (1987) Antagonism by E. coli endotoxin of some cardiovascular effects induced in the rat by two α_2-adrenoceptor agonists. Eur J Pharmacol 141:183–290
24. Fink MP, Homer LD, Fletcher JR (1985) Diminished pressor response to exogenous norepinephrine and angiotensin II in septic, unanesthetized rats: Evidence for a prostaglandin-mediated effect. J Surg Res 38:335–342
25. Schaller MD, Waeber B, Nussberger J, Brunner HR (1985) Angiotensin II, vasopressin and sympathetic activity in conscious rats with endotoxemia. Am J Physiol 249: 1086–1092
26. Evequoz D, Waeber B, Corder R, Nussberger J, Gaillard R, Brunner HR (1987) Markedly reduced blood pressure responsiveness in endotoxemic rats; reversal by neuropeptide Y. Life Sci 41:2573–2580
27. Gray GA, Schott C, Julou-Schaeffer G, Fleming I, Parratt JR, Stoclet JC (1991) An investigation of the effect of inhibitors of the L-arginine pathway on endotoxin-induced vascular hyporeactivity in vivo. Br J Pharmacol 103:1218–1224
28. Gray GA, Furman BL, Parratt JR (1990) Endotoxin-induced impairment of vascular reactivity in pithed rat: Role of arachidonic acid metabolites. Circ Shock 31:395–406
29. Julou-Schaeffer G, Gray GA, Fleming I, Schott C, Parratt JR, Stoclet JC (1990) Loss of vascular responsiveness induced by endotoxin involves the L-arginine pathway. Am J Physiol 295: 1038–1043
30. Julou-Schaeffer G, Gray GA, Fleming I, Parratt JR, Stoclet JC (1991) Activation of the L-arginine pathway is involved in vascular hyporeactivity induced by endotoxin. J Cardiovasc Pharmacol 17: 207–212
31. Gillespie JS, McLaren A, Pollock D (1970) A method of stimulating different segments of the autonomic outflow from the spinal column to various organs in the pithed rat and cat. Br J Pharmacol 40:257–267
32. Guc MO, Gray GA, Furman BL, Parratt JR (1991). Endotoxin-induced impairment of vasodepressor responses in the pithed rat. Eur J Pharmacol 204:63–70

33. Smith REA, Palmer RMJ, Moncada S (1991) Coronary vasodilation induced by endotoxin in the rabbit isolated perfused heart is nitric oxide-dependent and inhibited by dexamethasone. Br J Pharmacol 104:5–6
34. Thiemermann C, Vane JR (1990) Inhibition of nitric oxide synthesis reduces the hypotension induced by bacterial lipopolysaccharides in the rat in vivo. Eur J Pharmacol 182:591–595
35. Kilbourn RG, Gross SS, Jubran A, et al. (1990) N^G-Methyl-L-arginine inhibits tumor necrosis factor-induced hypotension: Implications for the involvement of nitric oxide. Proc Natl Acad Sci USA 87:3629–3632
36. Parratt JR, Furman BL, Bouvier C (1991) Endotoxin induced loss of vascular responsiveness; Role of platelet activating factor. Circ Shock 34:375
37. McKenna TM, Martin FM, Chernow B, Briglia FA (1986) Vascular endothelium contributes to decreased aortic contractility in experimental sepsis. Circ Shock 19:267–273
38. Wakabayashi I, Hatake K, Kakishita E, Nagai K (1987) Diminution of contractile response of the aorta from endotoxin-injected rats. Eur J Pharmacol 141:117–122
39. Wakabayashi I, Hatake K, Kakishita E, Nagai K (1987) Effect of phorbol ester on contractile response of aorta from endotoxin rats. Biochem Biophys Res Commun 150:1115–1121
40. Wakabayashi I, Hatake K, Sakamoto K (1991) Mechanisms ex vivo aortic hyporeactivity in endotoxemic rat. Eur J Pharmacol 199:115–118
41. Fleming I, Julou-Schaeffer G, Gray GA, Parratt JR, Stoclet JC (1991) Evidence that an L-arginine/nitric oxide dependent elevation of tissue cyclic GMP content is involved in depression of vascular reactivity by endotoxin. Br J Pharmacol 103:1047–1052
42. Martin W, Furchgott RF, Villani GM, Jothianandan D (1989) Depression of contractile responses in rat aorta by spontaneously released endothelium-derived relaxing factor (EDRF). J Pharmacol Exp Ther 237:529–538
43. Mulsch A, Busse R, Liebau S, Forstermann U (1988) LY 83583 interferes with the release of endothelium-derived relaxing factor and inhibits soluble guanylate cyclase. J Pharmacol Exp Ther 247:283–288
44. McKenna TM, Reusch DW, Simpkins CO (1988) Macrophage-conditioned medium and interleukin 1 suppress vascular contractility. Circ Shock 25:187–196
45. Fleming I, Gray GA, Julou-Schaeffer G, Parratt JR, Stoclet JC (1990) Incubation with endotoxin activates the L-arginine pathway in vascular tissue. Biochem Biophys Res Commun 171:562–568
46. Rees DD, Cellk S, Palmer RMJ, Moncada S (1990) Dexamethasone prevents the induction by endotoxin of a nitric oxide synthase and the associated effects of vascular tone: An insight into endotoxin shock. Biochem Biophys Res Commun 173:541–547
47. Kang Y-H, Williams R (1991) Endotoxin-induced endothelial injury and subendothelial accumulation of fibronectin in rat aorta. Anat Rec 229:86–102
48. Altura BM, Gebrewold A, Burton RW (1985) Failure of microscopic metarterioles to illicit vasodilator responses to acetylcholine, bradykinin, histamine and substance P after ischemic shock, endotoxemia and trauma: Possible role of endothelial cells. Microcirc Endoth Lymph 2:121–134
49. Auclair MC, Vernimen C, Carli A, Lechat A (1983) Depressed isoprenaline vascular response in endotoxic rats. Eur J Pharmacol 90:143–150
50. Guc MO, Furman BL, Parratt JR (1990) Endotoxin-induced impairment of vasopressor and vasodepressor responses in the pithed rat. Br J Pharmacol 101:913–919
51. Gray GA, Julou-Schaeffer G, Fleming I, Parratt JR, Stoclet JC (1990) Endothelial function is impaired in aortae from lipopolysaccharide (LPS)-treated rats. J Molec Cell Cardiol 22:8
52. Beasley D, Cohen RA, Levinsky NG (1990) Endotoxin inhibits contraction of vascular smooth muscle in vitro. Am J Physiol 258: 1187–1192
53. Parker JL, Keller SR, DeFily DV, Laughlin MH, Novotny MJ, Adams HR (1991) Coronary vascular smooth muscle function in E. coli endotoxemia in dogs. Am J Physiol 260:832–841
54. Beasley D (1990) Interleukin-1 and endotoxin activate soluble guanylate cyclase in vascular smooth muscle. Am J Physiol 259:38–44
55. Beasley D, Schwartz JH, Brenner BM (1991) Interleukin-1 induces prolonged L-arginine-dependent cyclic guanosine monophosphate and nitrite production in rat vascular smooth muscle cells. J Clin Invest 87:602–608

56. McKenna TM (1990) Prolonged exposure of rat aorta to low levels of endotoxin in vitro results in impaired contractility; association with vascular cytokine release. J Clin Invest 86:160–168
57. Fleming I, Gray GA, Parratt JR, Stoclet JC (1991) LPS-induced activation of the L-arginine/NO pathway in endothelium denuded arterial tissue is time dependent and requires de novo protein synthesis. Br J Pharmacol 102:123
58. Werner-Felmayer G, Werner ER, Fuchs D, Hausen A, Reibnegger G, Wachter H (1990) Tetrahydrobiopterin-dependent formation of nitrite and nitrate in murine fibroblasts. J Exp Med 172:1599–1607
59. Busse R, Mulsch A (1990) Induction of nitric oxide synthase by cytokines in vascular smooth muscle cells. FEBS Lett 275:87–90
60. Groeneveld ABJ, van Lambalgen AA, van den Bos GC, Bronsveld W, Nauta JJP, Thijs LG (1991) Maldistribution of heterogeneous coronary blood flow during canine endotoxin shock. Cardiovasc Res 25:80–88
61. McKechnie K, Dean HG, Furman BL, Parratt JR (1985) Plasma catecholamines during endotoxin infusion in conscious unrestrained rats: Effects of adrenal demedullation and/or guanethidine treatment. Circ Shock 17:85–94
62. Hutcheson IR, Whittle BRJ, Boughton-Smith NK (1990) Role of nitric oxide in maintaining vascular integrity in endotoxin-induced acute intestinal damage in the rat. Br J Pharmacol 101:815–820
63. Wright CE, Rees DD, Moncada S (1992) Protective and pathological roles of nitric oxide in endotoxin shock. Cardiovasc Res 26:48–57

Endogenous Opioids and Opioid Antagonists in Endotoxic and Septic Shock: A Current Perspective

J.W. Holaday and N.J. Gurll

Introduction

For several years after their discovery in 1975, the endogenous opioids (or "endorphins") were at the forefront of investigations characterizing the role of peptides in biology and medicine. In 1978, it was first proposed that endogenous opioid systems were involved in endotoxic shock [1] and other forms of critical illnesses. In retrospect, the postulation was simple: that the "morphine-like" substances within the body could be released in excessive amounts by the severe physiological stress of shock and trauma; this "overdose" of endogenous opioids would contribute to the decreased cardiovascular function and organ perfusion that characterize shock [2]. The availability of naloxone (Narcan), a competitive antagonist that selectively blocks or reverses the actions of morphine or endogenous opioids, provided an opportunity to test this hypothesis. The first several preclinical and clinical publications clearly demonstrated that naloxone, administered following the onset of shock, improved arterial pressure and other hemodynamic endpoints and, in some studies, survival. By inference, evidence indicated that the body's own opiate "painkillers" were indeed involved in the pathogenesis of endotoxic or septic shock.

Over the past decade, hundreds of articles and reviews have addressed the potential function of endogenous opioids and their receptors in circulatory shock due to endotoxemia, sepsis, hemorrhage, anaphylaxis and neurogenic causes [2, 3]. However, times change, and the enthusiasm for defining the biological relevance of endorphins and peptides has been replaced by a plethora of research characterizing the role of inflammatory cytokines and other mediators in the etiology of shock and trauma. Nonetheless, the changing tides of scientific enthusiasm do not dictate biological relevance, and it is perhaps opportune at this time to reevaluate the role of endogenous opioids and their receptors in the pathogenesis of circulatory shock.

This chapter will focus on endotoxic and septic shock, and provide a summation of a recent meta-analysis performed by Gurll [4] wherein the available preclinical and clinical literature was critically reviewed according to the Koch-Dale criteria and other objective methods of causal analysis.

Endogenous Opioid Peptides and their Receptors

There are three categories of endogenous opioid peptides – enkephalins, β-endorphin and dynorphins – each of which derives from a distinctly different precursor molecule, and each of which is characterized by distinctive patterns of distribution throughout the central nervous system, the autonomic network and the endocrine system. The first four amino-acids at the "amine" end of these peptide molecules, common to all three families of endogenous opioids, are "Tyr-Gly-Gly-Phe", a sequence that is essential to their opiate-like actions. The fifth amino-acid is either "Met" or "Leu", and serves to distinguish between the pentapeptides "Met-" and "Leu-" enkephalin. The remaining amino-acid sequences of β-endorphin (Tyr-Gly-Gly-Phe-Met, followed by an additional 26 amino-acids) and dynorphins (Tyr-Gly-Gly-Phe-Leu, followed by 8 amino-acids for dynorphin B or 12 amino-acids for dynorphin A) dictate the unique pattern pharmacological and physiological profiles that distinguishes among these endogenous opioid peptides. Thus, the "enkephalin" end of the molecule provides the "opioid" action, and the remaining amino-acids alter their specificities for the three opioid receptor types upon which they primarily act.

Endogenous opioid "systems" constitute not only the three different categories of opioid peptides described above, but also the cellular receptors to which they bind and through which they implement their biological actions. At least five categories of opioid receptors have been described, among which three receptor types are critical to endogenous opioids. Met-enkephalin acts primarily upon μ receptors, Leu-enkephalin acts upon δ receptors, β-endorphin acts upon both μ and δ receptors, and dynorphin A or B act upon κ receptors. Because of the lack of absolute receptor selectivity, these opioid peptide ligands, given adequate concentrations, will "crosstalk" with other opioid receptor types. Evidence is also accumulating to indicate that even these three "opioid receptor" types are not biologically or biochemically distinct, but may instead be different binding surfaces that share a common macromolecular opioid receptor complex [5].

The third components of "endogenous opioid systems" are the second messengers that transduce the receptors' message to the cell's interior. Depending upon the receptor type, opioid receptor occupancy may result in ion (Na+ or Ca++) flux, inhibition of cyclic nucleotides (e.g. cyclic adenosine monophosphate cAMP) or activation of "G" proteins; within the cells, phosphorylation of proteins or other less well defined biochemical processes ultimately translate the opioid message into cellular, and ultimately, organ-level responses.

Endotoxic and Septic Shock

As reviewed in the introduction, extensive information about the role of endogenous opioid peptides in endotoxic or septic shock has been obtained by the use of naloxone, a "universal" competitive opioid receptor antagonist that blocks or reverses opioid responses at all receptor types when adequate concentrations are used. The successful reversal of the signs of circulatory shock by naloxone has served as important inferential evidence to indicate a role of endogenous opioid systems in the pathogenesis of shock [1–4].

Early experiments involved the administration of endotoxin lipopolysaccharide (LPS) as a model of septic shock; subsequent experimentation relied upon more sophisticated models of sepsis, including the intravenous administration of live *E. coli* or the intraperitoneal implantation of fecal pellets. In a typical experiment, once a hypodynamic response was obtained, naloxone was administered. In the initial studies using a rat model of endotoxic hypotension [1], it was shown that naloxone injection resulted in a prompt restoration of the arterial pressure to control levels. Subsequent studies using endotoxin administration to well-instrumented dogs [6] and cynomulgus monkeys [7] clearly demonstrated that naloxone at a dose of 2 mg/kg significantly improved hemodynamic variables as well as survival [8].

Sites and Mechanisms of Endogenous Opioid Actions

Many studies have addressed the potential mechanisms by which endogenous opioids mediate their pathophysiological actions in endotoxic and septic shock [2, 3]. Working backwards from the biochemical to the organ level, it was first necessary to determine whether naloxone and other general opioid antagonists were producing their salutary effects via opioid receptors, by non-opioid receptors or by non-specific (i.e. membrane) effects. Opioid receptors are stereospecific, requiring the (–)isomer to achieve opioid responses; (+)isomers are not biologically active as opioid agonists or antagonists. Through the use of (–) and (+)stereoisomers of naloxone, it was shown that only the (–) isomer successfully antagonized endotoxic shock hypotension in rats [9], providing evidence for an opioid-specific involvement in this model of circulatory shock.

The doses of naloxone required to reverse shock hypotension exceeded by one or two orders of magnitude the doses required to reverse the pharmacological actions of administered opioid alkaloids such as morphine that act upon μ receptors. For that reason, it was suspected that endogenous opioids were acting upon non-μ receptors since far higher concentrations of naloxone are required to reverse opioid actions at δ and κ receptors. The availability of more specific antagonists for the δ and κ receptors provided an opportunity to test this hypothesis. Indeed, the selective μ antagonists, naloxazone (now known as naloxonazine) and β-funaltrexamine (β-FNA) were without effect on endotoxic hypotension, whereas the δ antagonists ICI-154.129 and ICI-174.864 improved arterial pressure whether administered intracerebroventricularly into the brain in microgram doses or intravenously at mg/kg doses [10].

From these studies, it was concluded that δ, not μ, receptors are involved in endogenous opioid actions in endotoxic shock, and that these actions are at least in part mediated within the brain since very low antagonist doses, ineffective when administered systemically, reversed endotoxic shock hypotension when injected into the ventricles of the brain in both rats and dogs [3, 11]. Other studies have shown that endogenous opioids and morphine may act directly on the myocardium to depress contractility [2], and that the intracoronary arterial administration of naloxone can improve myocardial contractility in dogs subjected to hemorrhagic shock [12].

Studies attempting to define the type of endogenous opioid and their site of release in endotoxic and septic shock have been difficult to interpret. Although circulating endorphins and enkephalins both increase dramatically during circulatory shock, and both can act upon δ receptors, the predominant source of these endogenous opioids and their mechanisms of action have yet to be firmly established. Without belaboring the extensive experimental data addressing a potential pituitary, adrenal or autonomic origin of endogenous opioids involved in endotoxemia or sepsis, it appears *unlikely* that pituitary-derived endorphins or adrenal-derived enkephalins are primary factors [3]. Experimental data in a number of shock models are consistent with actions of endogenous opioids to inhibit sympatho-adrenal function; further evidence directly links opioids receptors with catecholamine systems [12, 13]. Lechner et al. [12] have speculated that this interaction is at a second messenger level within the cells of the myocardium where opioids inhibit cAMP, and catecholamines stimulate cAMP. This is consistent with data indicating that naloxone potentiates epinephrine's hypertensive effects in endotoxemic rats [14].

In a series of exceptionally creative studies, it has recently been shown that endorphins can derive directly from circulating lymphocytes, and that endotoxin serves to release these lymphocyte-derived endogenous opioids in concentrations that cause hypotension by actions upon δ opioid receptors [15]. From these studies, it appears likely that a primary source of endogenous opioids in sepsis may be lymphocytes, and that their release of opioid peptides may be part of their orchestrated physiological or pathophysiological actions in circulatory shock, trauma or inflammation. The emerging data linking the disciplines of endocrinology and immunology is now replete with examples that many of the classic "endocrine" hormones localized within circulating lymphocytes, such as endorphins, prolactin and growth hormone, may function as autocrine or paracrine cytokines or growth factors [16].

Meta-Analysis of Existing Literature

An exhaustive review of the preclinical and clinical literature addressing the role of endogenous opioid systems in the pathophysiology of endotoxic and septic shock has been recently completed [4]. Of the many published reports on the role of endorphins in endotoxic and septic shock, 63 primary references were anlayzed (omitting reviews, letters to the editor, case reports, or other published sources with inadequate populations or methods). These studies included rat, dog, cat, sheep, pig, monkey, baboon and man as experimental subjects. Several "nodes" of the decision tree were addressed, including adequacy of the study design, clinical relevance of the model, species relevance, reversal by opioid antagonists, measurement of endogenous opioids, and demonstration that endogenous opioid release was caused by the shock state.

Expressed as a percentage of published reports, 94% used an appropriate study design and 75% used a clinically relevant model, but only 27% used a species that is relevant to human sepsis (rats, dogs and cats were considered inappropriate models). Reversal of a circulatory shock endpoint by opioid antagonists such as naloxone was shown in 77% of the reports (10% failed to demonstrate an effect of naloxone, and 13% had equivocal data). Measurement of endogenous opioids was performed in only 15% of the studies, but each of these studies adequately demonstrated that the endogenous opioid release was caused by the shock state. In approximately 87% of these publications, the authors concluded that endogenous opioids were involved in endotoxic-septic shock. However, based upon the meta-analysis results, only 2% (i.e. only one study) met all criteria and was found to be justified in concluding that endogenous opioids are involved in the pathophysiology of endotoxic-septic shock.

Conclusion

After well over a decade of research addressing a potential role of endogenous opioid systems in the pathophysiology of endotoxic-septic shock, an enormous amount of data using a broad range of species has amassed to indicate that opioid antagonists may be useful in treating human septic shock. Despite many published clinical reports where naloxone was administered to patients with septic shock [4], no clinical trials have yet been reported where adequate doses of naloxone have been used.

Although precise mechanisms require additional clarification, the fundamental observation that naloxone and related opioid antagonists improve the shock state has been reported in over 80% of the published investigations. According to the rigid criteria dictated by a classic meta-analysis, the vast majority of published reports provide only inferential data and do not conclusively demonstrate a cause-effect relationship between endogenous opioids and endotoxic-septic shock. However, there are several criticisms of this technique, including the fact that many journals will not publish negative reports, thus skewing the literature available for meta-analysis.

It is perhaps unfortunate that the process of scientific research emphasizes new discoveries, often prematurely dismissing the old. Today, state-of-the-art research in circulatory shock emphasizes cytokines, monoclonal antibodies, eicosanoids and other sexy mediators. However fickle the scientists, the "true" relevance of mediators is dictated by biology. In the case of endogenous opioids and endotoxic-septic shock, it would be timely for new research addressing interactions between opioid antagonists, for instance, and cytokine release in preclinical models of endotoxemia and septic shock. At the clinical level, it is critical that prospective randomized studies be conducted using opioid antagonists such as naloxone in 1–2 mg/kg doses before firm conclusions can be drawn about the relevance of endogenous opioid systems to septic shock.

References

1. Holaday JW, Faden AI (1978) Naloxone reversal of endotoxin hypotension suggests role of endorphins in shock. Nature 275:450–451
2. Holaday JW, Malcolm DS (1988) Endogenous opioids and other peptides: Evidence for their clinical relevance in shock and CNS injury. In: Chernow B, Holaday JW, Zaloga G, Zaritsky A (eds) Pharmacologic approach to the critically ill patient, 2nd edn. William & Wilkins, Baltimore, pp 718–732
3. Bernton EW, Long JB, Holaday JW (1985) Opioids and neuropeptides: Mechanisms in circulatory shock. Fed Proc 44:290–299
4. Gurll NJ (1992) Endogenous opiates in septic-endotoxic shock. In: Neugebauer E, Holaday JW (eds) Handbook on mediators in septic shock. CRC Press, Florida (in press)
5. Holaday JW, Porreca F, Rothman RB (1991) Functional coupling among opioid receptor types. In: Estefanos F (ed) Opioids in anesthesia II. Butterworth-Heineman, Boston, pp 50–60
6. Reynolds DG, Gurll NJ, Vargish T, Lechner R, Faden AI, Holaday JW (1980) Blockade of opiate receptors with naloxone improves survival and cardiac performance in canine endotoxic shock. Circ Shock 7:39–48
7. Gurll NJ, Reynolds DG, Holaday JW (1988) Evidence for a role of endorphins in the cardiovascular pathophysiology of primate shock. Crit Care Med 16:521–524
8. Gurll NJ (1985) Endorphins in endotoxic shock. In: Proctor RA, Hinshaw LB (eds) Handbook of endotoxin Vol II. Elsevier, Amsterdam, pp 299–310
9. Faden AI, Holaday JW (1980) Naloxone treatment of endotoxin shock: Stereospecificity of physiologic and pharmacologic effects in the rat. J Pharm Exp Ther 212:441–447
10. D'Amato RJ, Holaday JW (1984) Multiple opiate receptors in endotoxic shock: Evidence for d involvement and m – d interactions in vivo. Proc Natl Acad Sci 81:2898–2901
11. Holaday JW (1984) Neuropeptides in shock and traumatic injury: Sites and mechanisms of action. Neuroendo Perspectives 3:161–199
12. Lechner RB, Gurll NJ, Reynolds DG (1985) Naloxone potentiates the cardiovascular effects of catecholamines in canine hemorrhagic shock. Circ Shock 16:347–361
13. Holaday JW (1983) Cardiovascular effects of the endogenous opiate system. Ann Rev Pharm Tox 23:541–594
14. Malcolm DS, Zaloga GP, Willey SC, Holaday JW (1988) Naloxone potentiates epinephrine's hypertensive effects in endotoxemic rats. Circ Shock 25:259–265
15. Harbour DV, Galin FS, Hughes TK, Smith EM, Blalock JE (1991) Role of leukocyte-derived pro-opiomelanocortin peptides in endotoxic shock. Circ Shock 35:181–191
16. Holaday JW, Bryant HU, Kenner JR, Bernton EW (1989) Brain, endocrine and immune interactions: Implications in intensive care. In: Holaday JW, Bihari D (eds) Brain Failure: Update in Intensive Care and Emergency Medicine, vol 9. Springer-Verlag, New York, pp 1–13

Role of Neural Stimuli and Pain

H. Kehlet

Introduction

Despite a tremendous increase in our knowledge on mediators of the response to injury and sepsis, the relative role and interplay of these factors have not been completely outlined. Historically, the release mechanisms have often been divided into those of the nervous system and those involving humoral factors. This chapter is a short update on the role of the nervous system and pain to release the injury response, despite the fact that such a separation from humoral factors is somewhat artificial, as the two systems are linked together in many aspects. The review has not the intention to give a complete bibliography, but rather to bring recent findings in balance with previous data, summarized in recent reviews [1–3]. The review will also be limited to clinical studies of neural release mechanisms and will mostly contain data from elective, operative injury since there is a paucity of data from severely traumatized or septic patients. However, it is felt that knowledge from the elective trauma situation may be of value for the understanding of mediators in severe stress states such as sepsis and multiple organ failure (MOF).

The description of the role of neural stimuli and pain in mediating the response to injury will be discussed based upon studies of neural blockade techniques, as shown in (Fig. 1).

Antagonism of Endogenous Algesic Substances and Activation of Inflammatory Response

Although the exact nature and relative roles of the various signals to initiate, amplify and sustain the neural response has not been evaluated, an interplay exists between the release of the nociceptive signal to trauma and its modification by trauma-induced release of several algesic substances, which may reduce the threshold to initiate an afferent neural response. These factors include histamine, serotonine, kinins, arachidonic cascade metabolites and substance-P, which may facilitate afferent neural stimuli as well as contribute to "post-injury pain hypersensitivity". Furthermore, macrophage-derived factors such as interleukin-1 (IL-1) may facilitate neural traffic due to hyperalgesia [4].

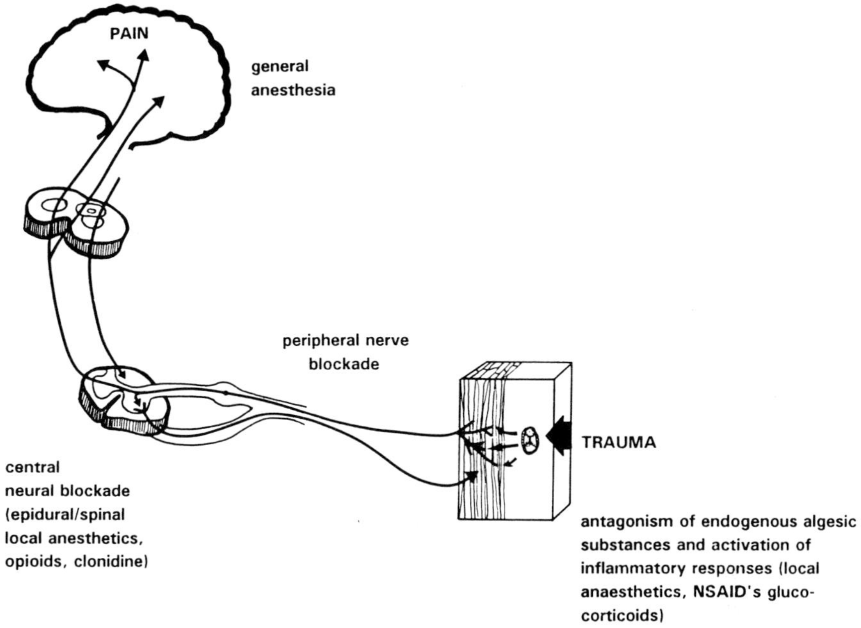

Fig. 1. Measures to provide neural blockade and modification of the injury response

Indirect documentation of the involvement of the peripheral nervous system and the above mentioned factors to initiate the response to clean injury comes from several studies. Thus, application of local anesthetics in the wound may reduce both pain and the pituitary response to surgery [5], probably due to a direct neural effect as well as an anti-inflammatory effect of the local anesthetic, as demonstrated in an experimental peritonitis model [6]. Other studies with instillation of local anesthetics intraperitoneally or intrapleurally have not been successful in reducing the surgical stress response [7–10].

Combination of neural blockade with epidural analgesia and pharmacological blockade with antihistamines, serotonin-2 receptor antagonists, cyclooxygenase inhibition as well as inhibition of fibrinolysis, has not been successful in reducing the acute phase protein response and leukocytic response to herniotomy, despite apparent sufficient neural blockade with abolished cortisol and glucose response [11, 12]. Application of large volumes of incisional bupivacaine with or without local wound hypothermia to about 15°C subcutaneously, did neither influence the leukocytosis response [13].

Thus, activation of the afferent neural stimulus and pain may be modified by several techniques with a peripheral effect. Administration of neural blockade with or without additional pharmacological agents supposed to modify the inflammatory response, have clarified that the pituitary response (cortisol) and the more complex hyperglycemic response may be blocked without concomitant significant reduction of leukocytosis or acute phase protein modification, indicating that these latter responses are released by other factors than neural stimuli.

The role of the nervous system to modify the local inflammatory reaction may have major interests in other disease states, since denervation, surgically or by local anesthetics, and with capsacin or immuno-sympathectomy may reduce swelling, hyperalgesia as well as accumulation of leukocytes following an experimental thermal or chemical injury [14, 15]. Thus, the nervous system may amplify the inflammatory response through the axon reflex leading to neurogenic inflammation [16], which may be important in various pulmonary, gastrointestinal and joint diseases [17, 18].

Peripheral Nerve Blockade

Although several decades have passed since Hume and Egdahl [19] in experimental studies demonstrated the importance of the peripheral nerves to mediate the adrenocortical response to clean trauma, the effect of peripheral nerve blocks have only been addressed in few clinical studies. Paravertebral [20], intercostal [21, 22], or splanchnic blockade [23–25] have only a moderate, if any, inhibitory effect on the classical endocrine metabolic response to abdominal surgery. This finding is not unexpected, since the afferent neural blockade is incomplete, as well as these techniques may not block both somatic and visceral afferent stimuli. Peripheral nerve blockade have not been studied in major injury, but according to experimental studies with major tissue injury, no major effect may be expected [19].

The role of neural stimuli in mediating the response to clean injury has mostly been studied using epidural or spinal anesthesia with local anesthetics. In addition, as information has increased on the biochemistry of nociceptive transmission in the spinal cord [26], information has also been gathered from techniques with more specific nociceptive blockade, such as epidural/intrathecal opioid administration, and α-2 agonist administration. Results from these studies have been of major importance in our understanding of the role of the peripheral and central nervous system in mediating the stress response to surgical injury. A detailed review of these data has been presented previously [1, 3, 27] and will only be summarized here together with recent data.

In studies on surgical procedures in the lower part of the body, pituitary hormones such as growth hormone, arginine vasopressin, adrenocorticotropic hormone, pituitary beta-lipotropin and beta-endorphin, prolactin and thyroid stimulating hormone are blocked or blunted by central neural blockade, while changes in follicle stimulating and luteinising hormone are largely unaffected. Adrenal hormones such as cortisol, aldosterone, renin, as well as catecholamines are also reduced while changes in thyroid hormones are unaffected. No important effect of the neural blockade is seen on insulin, although the postoperative increase in insulin resistance may be improved by epidural bupivacaine [28, 29]. Neural blockade has no effect on postoperative plasma calcitonin gene-related peptide [30]. Data on plasma glucagon are inconclusive, and no data are available on postoperative changes in sex hormones, gastrointestinal hormones or neural transmitters.

Due to the reduction in the classical endocrine response, several metabolic responses are modified. Thus, the hyperglycemic response is blocked, due to combined reduction of hepatic glycogenolysis and gluconeogenesis as well as insulin resistance is improved. Also, isotope studies have demonstrated reduced glucose production and oxidation in surgical patients [31]. Neural blockade reduces plasma changes in lipid metabolic parameters, but no information is available on lipid turn-over and oxidation rate. Neural blockade improves nitrogen economy, since postoperative nitrogen balance is improved [1, 3, 31–33], as well as stable isotope methodology has demonstrated reduced protein brake-down without compromising whole body protein synthesis [34]. Neural blockade also inhibits trauma-induced changes in free amino-acid concentrations in skeletal muscle [35].

Since neural blockade may inhibit various hormones with effects on water- and electrolyte balance (cortisol, aldosterone, arginin-vasopressin, renin, catecholamines), an important effect may be expected on post-traumatic renal function, as well as an effect mediated by the blockade of nervous traffic directly to the kidneys. Unfortunately, this question has only been addressed in very few studies suggesting no major effect except for a less negative potassium balance [1]. A study in patients undergoing aorto-coronary bypass surgery has demonstrated neural blockade to reduce interstitial fluid accumulation and pressure [36].

The effect of neural blockade on hepatic function, as measured by changes in serum enzymes and in acute phase proteins, is small or absent [1, 11, 12, 37]. Postinjury changes in coagulation and fibrinolysis are mostly uninfluenced by neural blockade [1] although a few studies have demonstrated a reduction in thrombocyte aggregation and coagulation, or an increase in fibrinolysis [1, 38–40].

The effect of neural blockade on postoperative immuno-function is small, although a few studies have shown less postoperative lymphopenia and improved function of T-cells, NK-cells and monocytes [1, 41, 42].

It shall be emphasized that most of the studies cited concern surgical procedures in the lower part of the body, and a similar degree of inhibition of injury response has not been demonstrated in a large number of studies during major abdominal and thoracic procedures [1, 3]. The explanation hereto is most likely an insufficient afferent somatic and sympathetic blockade [1, 3, 27]. Thus, a pronounced inhibition of fast conducting neural pathways have been demonstrated during lumbar epidural anesthesia using evoked potentials to peripheral electrical stimulation [43, 44], in contrast to ineffective afferent blockade during thoracic epidural anesthesia [45]. Therefore, studies using neural blockade techniques in upper abdominal or thoracic procedures cannot effectively separate the relative role of the nervous system or humoral factors in mediating the various responses. In an effort to overcome these problems, a recent study used thoracic epidural analgesia with bupivacaine and morphine to block pain stimuli and the catecholamine response, etomidate to block the cortisol and aldosterone response, and somatostatin to block the glucagon response [46]. Subsequently, the hepatic stress response as measured by the functional hepatic nitrogen clearance and urea production was abolished in such patients undergoing cholecystectomy [46]. These findings suggest the nervous system and subsequent changes in the classical catabolic hormones (catecholamines, cortisol and glucagon) to be the most important mediators of the protein catabolic response to clean trauma. Unfortunately, no similar studies are available from patients with severe trauma or sepsis, where effects of various humoral factors and cytokines may become more important.

Of the various neural blocking techniques, continuous spinal anesthesia may be more effective on the cortisol response than epidural anesthesia [47, 48], in accordance with the more effective blockade based upon neurophysiological assessment [49].

In summary, the plenty studies with central neural blockade suggest the nervous system to be the most important release mechanism of the classical endocrine and protein catabolic response, while inflammatory reactions such as leukocytosis, changes in acute phase proteins, and most immunological parameters are unaffected, and therefore released by other (humoral) factors. No studies have investigated the effect of neural blockade on cytokine responses.

The effect of modification of nociceptive transmission by epidural/spinal opioids or α-2 agonists is less pronounced than that obtained during the use of local anesthetics [27, 50, 51], in accordance with the more selective nociceptive blockade by these techniques.

The modulatory effect of central neural blockade with general anesthesia inhibits the perception of an operation, but a vast literature have demonstrated that the various volatile and IV agents in low or moderate doses have no important effect on the stress response [1, 3, 52]. However, high-dose opiate anesthesia has been demonstrated to reduce intraoperative responses [52]. Furthermore, high dose opioid anesthesia administered intraoperatively *and* for 24 h postoperatively in infants had a pronounced inhibitory effect on the classical stress responses [53].

Effect of Pain Relief *per se* on the Injury Response

Of the great number of afferent stimuli released by surgical injury, pain conducting stimuli represent only a part of the total afferent barrage. Accordingly, several studies during abdominal surgery with effective blockade of pain conducting G-fibers but insufficient blockade of fast conducting fibers [27], have shown no clear relationship between pain relief *per se* and the modification of the stress response. Thus, even total pain relief by a combination of neural blockade and systemic non-steroidal anti-inflammatory agents [54] or combined local anesthetics and morphine [27], or systemic on-demand opioid administration [55] may not significantly inhibit the classical endocrine metabolic response. However, the effect of non-steroidal anti-inflammatory drugs on various responses to surgical injury should be further explored, since these drugs may have a major role in the treatment of postoperative pain [56]. Thus, non-steroidal anti-inflammatory drugs have been shown to reduce postoperative nitrogen balance and hemodynamic responses to mesenterial traction [56].

Improved pain relief by addition of a single high-dose preoperative methylprednisolone to an effective epidural regimen may be of advantage, since the hyperthermic, IL-6, prostanoid and acute phase protein responses could be attenuated, as well as pulmonary function and fatigue improved [57, 58].

In summary, pain relief *per se* does not necessarily inhibit the surgical stress response since the nociceptive block is incomplete with most techniques; neural blockade with local anesthetics being the most effective.

Neural Blockade and the Injury Response: Clinical Implications

Although our picture of the role of neural stimuli to mediate the response to clean injury is still incomplete, a vast amount of data suggest that neural stimuli constitute one of the major release mechanisms of this response. Unfortunately, almost all available data come from elective surgery and no important information is available from clinical studies in patients with major (accidental) trauma, MOF or sepsis. However, several experimental studies suggest that neural blockade with epidural local anesthetics may improve survival in hemorrhagic shock [59, 60], although other studies in smaller animals suggest removal of homeostatic controls by neural blockade to be unwise [61].

A summary of data from controlled studies comparing postoperative morbidity in patients receiving different techniques of neural blockade versus general anesthesia suggests such a programme to be attractive, which results in at least some inhibition of the stress response and trauma-induced demands on the organs. Thus, various postoperative morbidity parameters such as blood loss, cardio-pulmonary complications, thromboembolic complications, mortality and gastrointestinal paralysis are reduced [1, 3, 40, 62, 63]. Also, a reduction of postoperative morbidity and septic complications in infants undergoing cardiac surgery during intra- and postoperative high-dose opioid anesthesia with concomitant reduction of the stress response [53] suggests such a strategy to be promising. However, it remains to be determined whether there is a causal relationship between reduction of stress by neural blockade and pain alleviation, and the reduction in morbidity, or whether this is just a coincidental event.

Conclusion

A vast amount of experimental and clinical data have demonstrated neural stimuli from the traumatized area to be the most important release mechanism of the classical endocrine and catabolic response to clean surgical trauma. In contrast, neural blockade has no important effect on inflammatory responses such as leukocytosis, acute phase protein changes and most changes in immunofunction. Unfortunately, no studies are available on the effect of similar neural blockade techniques on the responses in patients with major (accidental) trauma, multiple organ failure or sepsis, conditions where humoral mediators may be more important in the release of the injury response. Since neural blockade has been demonstrated to reduce postoperative morbidity, the role of the nervous system to mediate responses to major injury should be explored.

References

1. Kehlet H (1987) Modification of responses to surgery in anesthesia by neural blockade: Clinical implications. In: Cousins MJ, Bridenbaugh PO (eds) Neural Blockade in Clinical Anesthesia and Management of Pain, 2nd. ed. Lippincott Philadelphia pp 145–188
2. Gann DS, Lilly MP (1983) The neuroendocrine response to multiple trauma. World J Surg 7:101–118
3. Kehlet H (1992) Differential effects of regional vs general anesthesia: Responses to surgery and postoperative outcome. In: Rogers M, Tinker J, Covino B (eds) Principles and Practice of Anesthesiology, C.V. Mosby, St. Louis (in press)
4. Ferreira SH, Lorenzetti BB, Bristow AF, Poole S (1988) Interleukin-1β as a potent hyperalgesic agent antagonized by a tripeptide analogue. Nature 334:698–700
5. Sinclair R, Cassuto J, Högström S, et al. (1988) Topical anesthesia with lidocaine aerosol in the control of postoperative pain. Anesthesiology 68:895–901
6. Rimbäck G, Cassuto J, Wallin G, Westlander G (1988) Inhibition of peritonitis by amide local anesthetics. Anesthesiology 69:881–886
7. Rademaker BMP, Sih IL, Kalkman CJ, et al. (1991) Effects of interpleurally administered bupivacaine 0.5% on opioid analgesis requirements and endocrine response during and after cholecystectomy: A randomized double-blind controlled study. Acta Anaesthesio Scand 35:108–112
8. Scott NB, Mogensen T, Greulich A, Hjortsø N-C, Kehlet H (1988) No effect of continuous i.p. infusion bupivacaine on postoperative analgesia, pulmonary function and the stress response to surgery. Br J Anaesth 61:165–168
9. Scott NB, Mogensen T, Bigler D, Kehlet H (1989) Comparison of continuous intrapleural vs epidural 0.5% bupivacaine on pain, metabolic response and pulmonary function following cholecystectomy. Acta Anaesthesiol Scand 33:535–539
10. Wallin G, Cassuto J, Högström S, Hedner T (1988) Influence of intraperitoneal anaesthesia on pain and the sympathoadrenal response to abdominal surgery. Acta Anaesthesiol Scand 32:553–558
11. Schulze S, Schierbeck J, Sparsø HB, Bisgaard M, Kehlet H (1987) Influence of neural blokkade and indomethacin on leucocyte, temperature and acute-phase protein response to surgery. Acta Chir Scand 153:255–259
12. Schulze S, Drenck NE, Hjortsø E, Kehlet H (1988) Influence of combined neural blockade, H_1- and H_2-receptor and serotonin$_2$-receptor blockade, indomethacin and transexamic acid on leucocyte, temperature and acute phase protein response to surgery. Acta Chir Scand 154:329–333

13. Schulze S, Rye B, Møller IW, Kehlet H (1992) Influence of local anesthesia and local hypothermia on leucocyte, temperature and acute phase protein response to surgery. Dan Med Bull 39:86–89
14. Helme RD, Andrews PV (1985) The effect of nerve lesions on the inflammatory response to injury. J Neurosci Res 13:453–459
15. Levine JD, Dardick SJ, Basbaum AI, Scipio E (1985) Reflex neurogenic inflammation. Contribution of the peripheral nervous system to spatially remote inflammatory responses that follow injury. J Neurosci 5:1380–1386.
16. Chapman LF, Godell H (1964) The participation of the nervous system in the inflammatory reaction. Ann N York Acad Sci 116:990–1017
17. Barnes PJ, Belvisi MG, Rogers DF (1990) Modulation of neurogenic inflammation: Novel approaches to inflammatory disease. TiPS 11:185–189
18. Levine JD, Coderre TJ, Basbaum AI (1988) The peripheral nervous system and the inflammatory process. In: R Dubner, CF Gebhart, MR Bond (eds) Proceedings of the Vth World Congress on Pain. Elsevier Science Publishers, Amsterdam, pp 33–43
19. Hume DM, Egdahl RH (1959) The importance of the brain in the endocrine response to injury. Ann Surg 150:697–704
20. Giesecke K, Hamberger B, Järnberg P-O, Klingstedt C (1988) Paravertebral block during cholecystectomy: Effects on circulatory and hormonal responses. Br J Anaesth 61:652–656
21. Pither CE, Bridenbaugh LD, Reynolds F (1988) Preoperative intercostal nerve block: Effect on the endocrine metabolic response to surgery. Br J Anaesth 60:730–732
22. Scheinin B, Scheinin M, Asantila R, Lindberg R, Viinakäki O (1987) Sympatho-adrenal and pituitary hormone responses during and immediately after thoracic surgery – modulation by four different pain treatments. Acta Anaesthesiol Scand 31:762–767
23. Shirasaka, C, Tsuji H, Asoh T, Yakeuchi Y (1986) Role of the splanchnic nerves in endocrine and metabolic response to abdominal surgery. Br J Surg 73:142–145
24. Tsuji H, Shirasaka C, Asoh Y, Takeuchi T (1983) Influence of splanchnic nerve blockade on endocrine-metabolic responses to upper abdominal surgery. Br J Surg 70:437–439
25. Hamid SK, Scott NB, Sutcliffe NP, et al. (1992) The effect of continuous coeliac plexus blockade plus intermittent wound infiltration with local anaesthesia on pain relief, pulmonary function and the stress response following upper abdominal surgery: A double blind randomized study. Acta Anaesthesiol Scand (in press)
26. Yaksh TL, Hammond PL (1982) Peripheral and central substrates involved in the rostrad transmission of nociceptive information. Pain 13:1–85
27. Kehlet H (1989) Surgical stress: The role of pain and analgesia. Br J Anaesth 63:189–195
28. Magnusson J, Nybell-Lindahl G, Tranberg K-G (1986) Clearance and action of insulin during general or epidural anaesthesia. Clin Nutr 5:159–165
29. Uchida I, Asoh T, Shirasaka C, Tsuji H (1988) Effect of epidural analgesia on postoperative insulin resistance as evaluated by insulin clamp technique. Br J Surg 75:557–562
30. Bythell VE, Lacoumenta S, Breimer LH, Brooks S, Burrin JM, Hall GM (1989) Effects of epidural analgesia on plasma calcitonin gene-related peptide. Acta Anaesthesiol Scand 33:666–669
31. Shaw JHF, Galler L, Holdaway IM, Holdaway CM (1987) The effect of extradural blockade upon glucose and urea kinetics in surgical patients. Surg Gynecol Obstet 165:260–266.
32. Tsuji H, Shirasaka C, Asoh T, Uchida I (1987) Effects of epidural administration of local anaesthetics or morphine on postoperative nitrogen loss and catabolic hormones. Br J Surg 74:421–425
33. Vedrinne C, Vedrinne JM, Guiraud M, Patricet MC, Bouletreau P (1989) Nitrogen sparing effect of epidural administration of local anesthetics in colon surgery. Anesth Analg 69:354–359
34. Carli F, Webster J, Pearson M, et al. (1991) Protein metabolism after abdominal surgery: Effect of 24-h extradural block with local anaesthetic. Br J Anaesth 67:729–734
35. Christensen T, Waaben J, Lindeburg T, et al. (1986) Effect of epidural analgesia on muscle amino-acid pattern after surgery. Acta Chir Scand 152:407–411
36. Rein K-A, Stenseth R, Myhre HO, Levang OW, Krogstad A (1989) The influence of thoracic epidural analgesia on transcapillary fluid balance in subcutaneous tissue. Acta Anaesthesiol Scand 33:79–83

37. Hesselvik F, Brodin B, Håkanson E, Rutberg H, Von Schenck H (1987) Influence of epidural blockade on postoperative plasma fibronectin concentrations. Scand J Clin Lab Invest 47:435–440
38. Odoom JA, Dokter WC, Sturk A, Cate WT, Sih IL, Bovill JG (1988) The influence of epidural analgesia on platelet function and correlation with plasma bupivacaine concentrations. Eur J Anaesthesiol 5:379–382
39. Nielsen TH, Nielsen HK, Husted EC, Hansen LC, Olsen KH, Fjeldborg N (1989) Stress response and platelet function in minor surgery during epidural bupivacaine and general anaesthesia: Effect of epidural morphine addition. Eur J Anaesthesiol 6:409–417
40. Tuman KJ, McCarthy RJ, March RJ, DeLaria GA, Patel RV, Ivankovich AD (1991) Effects of epidural anesthesia and analgesia on coagulation and outcome after major vascular surgery. Anesth Analg 73:696–704
41. Tønnesen E, Wahlgreen C (1988) Influence of extradural and general anaesthesia on natural killer cell activity and lymphocyte subpopulations in patients undergoing hysterectomy. Br J Anaesth 60:500–507
42. Stevenson GW, Hall SC, Rudnick S, Seleny FL, Stevenson HC (1990) The effect of anesthetic agents on the human immune response. Anesthesiology 72:542–552
43. Lund C, Selmar P, Hansen OB, Kehlet H (1987) Effect of intrathecal bupivacaine on somatosensory evoked potentials following dermatomal stimulation. Anesth Analg 66:809–813
44. Lund C, Mogensen T, Hansen OB, Qvitzau S, Kehlet H (1991) Effects of etidocaine administered epidurally on changes in somatosensory evoked potentials after dermatomal stimulation. Reg Anesth 16:38–42
45. Lund C, Hansen OB, Mogensen T, Kehlet H (1987) Effect of thoracic epidural bupivacaine on somatosensory evoked potentials after dermatomal stimulation. Anesth Analg 66:731–734
46. Heindorff H, Schulze S, Mogensen T, Almdal T, Kehlet H, Vilstrup H (1992) Hormonal and neural blockade prevents the postoperative increase in amino-acid clearance and urea synthesis. Surgery 111 (in press)
47. Webster J, Barnard M, Carli F (1991) Metabolic response to colonic surgery: Extradural vs continuous spinal. Br J Anaesth 67:467–469
48. Dahl JB, Rosenberg J, Dirkes WE, Mogensen T, Kehlet H (1990) Prevention on postoperative pain by balanced analgesia. Br J Anaesth 64:518–520
49. Dirkes WE, Rosenberg J, Lund C, Kehlet H (1991) The effect of subarachnoid lidocaine and combined subarachnoid lidocaine and epidural bupivacaine on electrical sensory thresholds. Reg Anesth 16:262–264
50. Lund C, Qvitzau S, Greulich A, Hjortsø N-C, Kehlet H (1989) Effect of epidural clonidine vs morphine on postoperative pain, stress response, cardio-pulmonary function, motor and sensory blockade. Br J Anaesth 63:516–519
51. Camu F, Debucquoy F (1991) Affentanil infusion for postoperative pain: A comparison of epidural and intravenous routes. Anesthesiology 75:171–178
52. Desborough JP, Hall GM (1989) Modification of the hormone and metabolic response to surgery by narcotics and general anaesthesia. Clin Anaesthesiol 3:317–335
53. Anand KJS, Hickey PR (1992) Halothane-morphine compared with high-dose sufentanil for anesthesia and postoperative analgesia in neonatal cardiac surgery. N Engl J Med 326:1–9
54. Schulze S, Roikjaer O, Hasselstrøm L, Jensen NH, Kehlet H (1988) Epidural bupivacaine and morphine plus systemic indomethacin eliminates pain but not systemic response and convalescence after cholecystectomy. Surgery 103:321–327
55. Møller IW, Dinesen K, Søndergård S, Knigge U, Kehlet H (1988) Effect of patient-controlled analgesia on plasma catecholamine, cortisol and glucose concentrations after cholecystectomy. Br J Anaesth 61:160–164
56. Dahl JB, Kehlet H (1991) Non-steroidal anti-inflammatory drugs: Rationale for use in severe postoperative pain. Br J Anaesth 66:703–712
57. Schulze S, Møller IW, Bang U, Rye B, Kehlet H (1990) Effect of combined prednisolone, epidural analgesia and indomethacin on pain, systemic response and convalescence after cholecystectomy. Acta Chir Scand 156:203–209

58. Schulze S, Sommer P, Bigler D, et al. (1992) Effect of combined prednisolone, epidural analgesia and indomethacin on the systemic response after colonic surgery. Arch Surg 127:325–331
59. Shibata K, Yamamoto Y, Murakami S (1989) Effects of epidural anesthesia on cardiovascular response and survival in experimental hemorrhagic shock in dogs. Anesthesiology 71:953–959
60. Shibata K, Yamamoto Y, Kobayashi T, Murakami S (1991) Beneficial effect of upper thoracic epidural anesthesia in experimental hemorrhagic shock in dogs: Influence of circulating catecholamines. Anesthesiology 74:303–308
61. Stoner HB (1986) A role for the central nervous system in the responses to trauma. In: RA Little, KN Frayn (eds) The Scientific Basis for the Care of the Critically Ill. Manchester Universtiy Press, pp 215–229
62. Scott NB, Kehlet H (1988) Regional anaesthesia and surgical morbidity. Br J Surg 75:299–304
63. Kehlet H (1990) Epidural analgesia in surgical practice. Curr Pract Surg 2:223–226

Sepsis and Strenuous Exercise: Common Inflammatory Factors

G. Camus, J. Pincemail, and M. Lamy

Introduction

During the last decade, numerous studies of the effects of exercise on the immune system have been performed. Owing to the development and improvement of techniques for studying immune function *in vitro* as well as *in vivo*, there is at present a large body of data suggesting that strenuous exercise triggers an inflammatory response similar to that occurring in the presence of bacterial infection or tissue injury [1].

Indices of an inflammatory response after exercise include, among others, leukocytosis [2], increases in host defense mediators with pleiotropic biological properties such as cytokines [1, 3-6], and the release of enzymes from various types of leukocytes [5, 7-9].

That such an inflammatory response could occur in healthy subjects submitted to strenuous exercise in the absence of pathological events such as open wounds (and associated infection), macroscopic tissue injury or myopathy, seems at first surprising and rather difficult to understand. The lack of obvious and specific tissue injury and, to some extent, the conflicting results of a few studies with administration of anti-inflammatory drugs led several authors to challenge the hypothesis of an exercise-induced inflammatory response [10]. Nevertheless, the pattern of cellular and humoral changes that emerges from the recent literature dealing with exercise resembles the pattern described for the early stage of sepsis [6]. This possible analogy is substantiated by the significant increase in the plasma levels of the lipopolysaccharide (LPS) endotoxin reported in athletes who took part in a triathlon competition [11]. Although the precise mechanisms responsible for such endotoxemia are unknown and its effects on indicators of a possible associated inflammatory reaction have not been concomitantly studied, its occurrence in healthy subjects makes the concept of an inflammatory response to prolonged exercise more plausible. Although this inflammatory response to exercise is similar to the sepsis response as far as the nature of the involved mediators is concerned, it differs considerably in its magnitude and duration, and its evolution is markedly dissimilar to the septic inflammatory response.

Information concerning the effects of exercise of short duration on the plasma level of LPS are still lacking but such endotoxemia appears unlikely, at least in young healthy subjects who are not exercising in extreme conditions. Therefore, in an attempt to explain the appearance of several indices of immunological and inflammatory reactions reported in subjects submitted to short periods of either maximal or submaximal exercise, we hypothesized that complement activation by microscopic muscle and/or adjacent connective tissue injury could be the common triggering pathway for some of these defense mechanisms [6]. Consistent with this view are our recent results showing a significant relationship between plasma myeloperoxidase concentration (MPO) – a specific marker of polymorphonuclear neutrophils (PMN) activation – and the complement split product C5a [12].

Although these data lend strong support to the hypothesis that strenuous exercise could trigger an inflammatory response via a transient endotoxemia and/or discrete tissue damage, the interrelationship between the inflammatory mediator systems and the possible consequences of their activation has not, until now, been explored. In an attempt to guide further experiments in this field, we examined whether other common factors could exist in the physiological responses to exercise and the early stage of sepsis.

The Host Defense Response to Sepsis

Sepsis is a pathological state characterized by the presence of pathogenic organisms and/or their toxins in the blood or tissues. Components of the bacterial wall – especially the LPS molecule from the outer membrane of

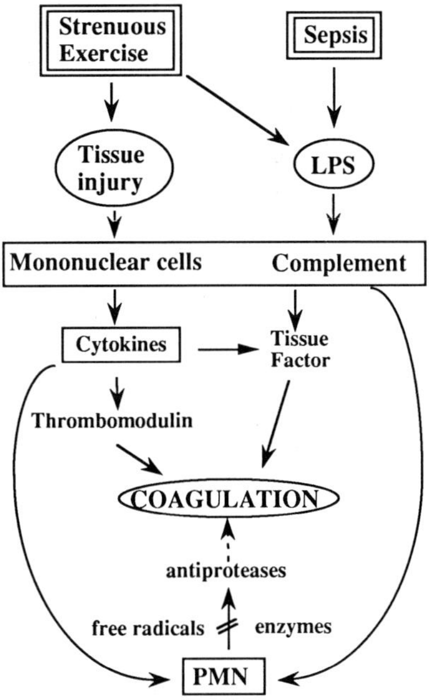

Fig. 1. Schematic diagram showing some possible mechanisms relating the activation of polymorphonuclear (PMN) and mononuclear cells to coagulation and free radical production in both strenuous exercise and sepsis. LPS: lipopolysaccharide; destructive (⇞) or inhibitory (↑) action

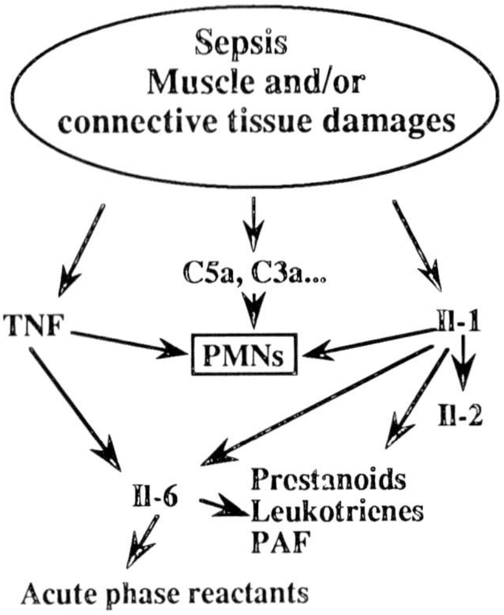

Fig. 2. Possible mechanisms underlying the release of common inflammatory mediators in sepsis and strenuous exercise. PMN: polymorphonuclear neutrophils; TNF: tumor necrosis factor; IL-1, 6: interleukin-1, 6; PAF: platelet activating factor; C3a, C5a: anaphylatoxins from complement cascade.

gram-negative bacteria – are potent activators of cellular and humoral host defense systems [13]. It is well accepted that the extensive activation of these defense systems is responsible for the septic syndrome and septic shock, mainly through the release of various inflammatory and procoagulant mediators. However, sepsis involves many mediators and complex interrelationships between the defense mechanisms. Thus, their precise role remains poorly understood. To better understand data from clinical and laboratory experiments, theoretical models of mediator cascades have been developed. One of the most recent attempts in this field emphasized the roles played by cytokines, by activated PMN and monocytes, and by the proteolytic enzymes derived from complement, coagulation and fibrinolytic cascades (Fig. 1 & 2) [14].

Cytokines

Upon activation by bacterial toxins, blood monocytes and tissue macrophages secrete various cytokines such as interleukins (IL-1, IL-6, IL-8) and tumor necrosis factor (TNF) [14]. Cytokines are highly pro-inflammatory molecules which appear sequentially, and synergistically induce a broad spectrum of biological effects [15]. In response to cytokines, platelet activating factor (PAF) is secreted by endothelial cells. PAF mediates platelet aggregation and secretion, increased vascular permeability and hypotension [16]. IL-1, PAF and TNF are potent stimulators of neutrophil degranulation [14, 17–19].

Complement

Bacterial or fungal polysaccharides also directly activate the complement system primarily via the alternate pathway [13]. Following activation and enzymatic cleavage of C3 and C5 components, the C3a and C5a anaphylatoxins are produced. These anaphylatoxins possess multiple pharmacological properties such as vasodilation, and trigger biological responses from several leukocyte lines [17]. Upon binding to PMN, the activated complement fractions induce chemotaxis, secretion, adherence to endothelium and phagocytosis. C3a and C5a induce histamine release from mast cells and basophils [17]. C5a also stimulates PAF release from PMN and basophils [20].

Complement cleavage products and cytokines are thus among the main factors which could be responsible for PMN activation. This activation has been demonstrated by the increase in the plasma levels of elastase (EL) [8, 9] and myeloperoxidase (MPO] [7, 12] which are enzymes contained in the primary granules of PMN.

Coagulation and Fibrinolytic Cascades

Bacterial products such as LPS can directly activate the contact system of coagulation, which comprises the proteins factors XII and XI, prekallikrein and high molecular weight kininogen [14]. Injury to endothelial cells resulting from the combined actions of cytokines can also activate the contact system by exposing the negatively charged collagen surfaces contained in their basal membrane [21]. This results in the activation of the intrinsic clotting, fibrinolytic, kallikrein-kinin and complement systems [14]. As a consequence, a broad array of compounds, capable of triggering aggregation and degranulation of PMN, increasing vascular permeability and inducing vasodilation is produced. The generation of kallikrein with bradykinin release, the activation of the first component of complement and of the fibrinolytic system are thus further consequences of contact system activation. It has been suggested that the activation of the contact system plays a major role in inducing hypotension and shock [14].

Interactions of endothelial cells with LPS, but also with IL-1 and TNF promote coagulation. These two cytokines probably exert their procoagulant action through inducing tissue factor expression and down regulation of thrombomodulin at the level of endothelial cells. This results in the formation of fibrin and thrombin which lead to disseminated intravascular coagulation [14].

Activation of PMN and Macrophages

One of the most important events in the pathophysiology of sepsis appears to be the massive and uncontrolled activation of PMN and macrophages. These cells are capable of responding to a large variety of compounds, the production of which is increased by sepsis. This enhances their bactericidal properties but also their ability to damage host tissues. Activated PMN and macrophages release lysosomial enzymes and produce various toxic metabolites of molecular oxygen (free radicals), all of which are bactericidal and cytotoxic. They also secrete MPO capable of generating oxidant chlorinated compounds, and several metabolites of arachidonic acids (the prostaglandins and leukotrienes), which exert profound effects on smooth muscle tone and on the function of inflammatory cells [17]. Products of activated PMN and macrophages are not only potent destructors of endothelial cells and other cellular tissue elements but are also inactivators of protease inhibitors. Indeed, the main plasma inhibitor of elastase, α1-proteinase inhibitor, can be inactivated through oxidation by PMN-derived products [14], and it appears that α2-macroglobulin, the main plasma inhibitor for many proteases, is also destroyed by MPO activity (G. Deby-Dupont, personal communication). This could result in increased levels of active elastase with possible cleavage of elastin but also of the serine protease inhibitors (antithrombin III, α2-antiplasmin, C1 esterase inhibitor) which control the coagulation, contact, complement and fibrinolysis systems [14]. Such enzymatic cleavage could amplify the activation of these cascades and facilitate the development of multiple organ failure syndrome.

Other Sources of Free Radicals

Activated PMN are not the only source of free radicals during sepsis. The impairement of microcirculation due to intravascular coagulation and the release of vasoactive substances cause severe tissue ischemia, particularly in the splanchnic bed [22]. The lack of oxygen initiates a chain of adverse events damaging the mitochondrial respiratory chain, impairing the production of adenosine triphosphate, and allowing intracellular influx of Ca^{2+} with activation of protease leading to massive conversion of the enzyme xanthine dehydrogenase into xanthine oxidase. During reoxygenation of ischemic tissue following reperfusion or oxygen therapy, the hypoxanthine accumulated within the cells is metabolized into uric acid by xanthine oxidase with subsequent production of superoxide anion, hydrogen peroxide and hydroxyl radical. Damaged mitochondria contribute to this process [22]. The metabolism of arachidonic acid is another source of free radicals during sepsis [22]. It has indeed been shown that sepsis leads to an increased release of prostanoids into the circulation, and that cyclooxygenase activity is accompanied by the production of oxygen free radicals and their side products.

As pointed out above, these free radical species are capable of causing severe tissue damage via reactions with cellular structures, or by inducing the release of active mediators which amplify the host reactions to endotoxemia.

Main Features of the Inflammatory Response to Strenuous Exercise

An increasing number of studies have shown that the humoral and cellular changes induced by sepsis also occur transiently in healthy subjects submitted to strenuous physical exercise. Furthermore, recent experimental data suggest that exercise-induced PMN activation can be interpreted within the framework of an inflammatory response triggered by muscle damage [6]. This hypothesis, i.e. that muscular exercise could trigger an inflammatory reaction, was first substantiated by animal experiments where histological examination of muscle biopsies revealed the presence of inflammatory cells such as PMN and macrophages in the interstitium, by damages caused to the connective tissue [10].

In man, evidence for the occurrence of an inflammatory response during strenuous muscular exercise relies upon experimental data showing that prolonged exercise is accompanied by metabolic and immunologic changes mimicking those observed in inflammatory or infectious diseases. These similarities include, among others, leukocytosis, PMN activation, biochemical markers, cellular infiltrates, delayed painful sensations (delayed onset muscular soreness, DOMS), muscle swelling, loss of function, ultrastructural damage, hemostatic changes, and free radical production.

Leukocytosis

In most studies, it has been found that exercise generally increases the peripheral white blood cell count (WBC) [2]. However, there are several reports that eccentric exercises such as downhill running, which lead to marked DOMS and significant increases in plasma creatine kinase and lactate dehydrogenase activities [23, 24], were not accompanied by any significant changes in WBC [24, 25]. These results led some authors to conclude that inflammation was not the underlying mechanism of DOMS associated with muscle damage [10]. The origin of these conflicting results remains unclear, but we have recently confirmed that short-term concentric (and eccentric) exercises of 20 min duration were accompanied by a significant increase in the number of PMN (nPMN) [26]. In agreement with other studies, a marked neutrophilia was found in each subject. The largest increase in mean nPMN values (from 2700 ± 900 to 4700 ± 1500 cells/μl) was found at the end of a 20 min exercise test performed by 11 healthy male subjects at 80 % maximal oxygen uptake ($\dot{V}O_2max$) on a cycle ergometer [26]. In these experiments, nPMN remained significantly higher than resting values after 20 min recovery.

Complement and PMN Activation

In agreement with Schaefer et al. [9], we also found that PMN were activated by exercise [7, 12]. This exercise-induced PMN activation was demonstrated by significant increases in the plasma concentrations of MPO [7, 12] and EL (unpublished results). In an attempt to elucidate the mechanisms responsible for this activation, we hypothesized that activation of the complement system could play a role in priming PMN. Therefore, we concomitantly measured MPO and the plasma concentration of a complement split product, C5a anaphylatoxin (C5a) in male subjects submitted to a 20 min exercise at 80 % $\dot{V}O_2$ max on a cycle ergometer. Interestingly, parallel and significant increases of MPO and C5a were found [12]. From the significant relationship between these two variables ($r = 0.65$; $P < 0.001$), we showed that 42% of the variance in MPO were explained by changes in C5a [12]. Although these findings confirm the results of Dufaux and Order [27] and strongly argue for the involvement of complement activation in the process of PMN degranulation, it should be kept in mind that other factors could also play a role in PMN activation, among which are the cytokines.

Cytokines

The release of IL-1 following strenuous exercise was first demonstrated by Cannon and Kluger [28], and confirmed later by the same group [1]. Cannon et al. [3] showed that a downhill run of 45 min at an intensity corresponding to 75% $\dot{V}O_2$ max induced a prolonged increase of IL-1β in muscle tissue. The results reported by Cannon et al. [3] suggest that this cytokine is associated with the inflammatory response to exercise-induced muscle damage.

Whether IL-1 is involved in the early PMN response observed in our subjects is unknown. Other cytokines, such as TNF and IL-6, have been found to be released during exercise. Dufaux and Order [5] have recently observed that a 2.5-h running test was followed by elevation of the plasma concentration of elastase-α1-proteinase inhibitor complexes, neopterin, TNF, and soluble IL-2 receptor. They concluded that PMN, macrophages and T-lymphocytes were activated by exercise. Although the physiological meaning of these changes and the precise underlying mechanisms remain poorly understood, these results give further support to the notion of an exercise-induced inflammatory response, and are consistent with the increase of acute-phase plasma proteins observed after exercise [29, 30]. The experiments dealing with the effects of exercise on the production of cytokines are consistent with those reporting increased blood and muscle concentrations of IL-1 [1, 3], plasma interferon activity [31], blood levels of acute phase reactants [29, 30], MPO [7, 12], elastase-α1-proteinase inhibitor complexes [8, 9], and complement cleavage products [12, 27]. Given these observations, it is tempting to postulate that exercise-induced activation of PMN, as recently demonstrated by the significant increase of MPO [7, 12], could be a further manifestation of an inflammatory response.

Delayed Onset Muscular Soreness

Pain is an important symptom common to acute inflammation and unaccustomed exercise [10], especially eccentric exercise in which muscles are lengthened while developing tension. It has long been suggested that the muscle pain that becomes apparent some hours after the exercise and which may persist for several days is likely due to muscle and/or connective tissue damage [10]. As pointed out by Smith [10], a broad array of substances have been proposed as activators of pain afferents following exercise.

However, most of these potential mediators of exercise-induced painful sensations have not been measured. Therefore, their precise role remains largely hypothetical. Despite the conflicting results of a few studies where anti-inflammatory drugs have been used [10], it has been suggested that muscle pain following strenuous exercise, especially eccentric exercise, could be a further manifestation of the exercise-induced inflammatory response. Consistent with this hypothesis is the similiar time course for increases in PGE_2 and DOMS reported after exercise [10]. According to Smith [10], the sensation of pain could be related to the synthesis of PGE_2 by activated macrophages in injured areas.

Muscle Swelling and Loss of Function

Local tissue edema resulting from increased permeability of small blood vessels is another sign of acute inflammation after exercise [10]. The increase in vascular permeability in damaged rat muscles after negatively biased contractions and the increase in limb volume and intramuscular pressure observed in man several hours after eccentric contractions further emphasize the similarities between exercise and acute inflammation [10].

Decreases in muscle performances after strenuous exercise – especially after eccentric exercise – are well documented and similiar in their time course with the loss of function reported in acute inflammation [10]. In recent experiments performed by Newham et al. [32], it was found that the maximal voluntary force exerted by painful muscle group following eccentric contractions was not increased by superimposed electrical stimulation. From these results, they concluded that the observed loss of force was not due to a reduced ability to fully activate the motor units but rather to injury at the level of the muscle itself.

Hemostatic Changes

The effects of exercise on the hemostatic system are well documented. These effects include an increased coagulability of the blood and an enhanced fibrinolytic activity [33, 34]. Activation of platelets and increase in thrombin activity have been reported after long-term exercise [35]. In addition to a drop in plasma factor VII and an increase in factor VIII activity, Hansen et al. [34] found that the thromboplastin activity of blood monocytes was significantly raised in subjects previously submitted to exercise of various durations. In agreement with other studies, these authors reported an enhancement of fibrinolytic activity, shown by an increased plasma level of tissue plasminogen activator (tPA) and shortened whole blood clot lysis time. Most of the hemostatic changes observed by Hansen et al. [34] and others [33] were found to be persistent, up to several hours after cessation of exercise. The underlying mechanisms of these exercise-induced hemostatic alterations are poorly understood. Interestingly, it has been suggested that muscle tissue damage and endothelial cell disruption could increase the coagulability of the blood through the release of tissue thromboplastins [35] and the direct binding of factor VII to thromboplastin at the site of endothelial cell disruption [34].

According to Hansen et al. [34], proteolytic attack on factor VII by granulocyte elastase or other coagulation factors could also play a role. These authors suggested that the unknown cell mediated component increasing fibrinolytic activity in concert with tPA release could be elastase and cathepsin G released from activated PMN [34].

Free Radicals

Evidence for the generation of free radicals during exercise is limited and to some extent contradictory. Using electron paramagnetic resonance, Davies et al. [36] directly demonstrated that strenuous exercise resulted in free radical signals in rat muscle and liver. Using the same techniqe, Jackson et al. [37] observed greater free radical signals in rat muscle previously stimulated to contract by electrical impulses.

Human observations in this field are based on indirect methods, i.e. the measurement of various reaction products derived from lipid peroxidation [7, 38] and endogenous antioxidants [39, 40].

Among the potential sources of free radicals during exercise are the increased turnover of semiquinone in mitochondria [38], hemoglobin autooxidation [41], xanthine oxidase catalyzed reactions [38] and PMN activation [7]. To date, the relative importance of these potential sources of free radicals and their involvement in exercise-induced lipid peroxidation as a function of exercise intensity and duration are unknown.

In an attempt to verify whether exercise-induced PMN activation could be a significant source of free radicals leading to lipid peroxidation, we compared the PMN response to concentric and eccentric exercise of equal oxygen cost [42]. We assumed that eccentric exercise would exert a greater tension on muscle fibers and/or connective tissue and therefore would trigger a more important activation of PMN than concentric exercise. We compared the changes in MPO and EL induced in 10 subjects by two different exercise tests consisting of uphill walking (concentric exercise) and downhill running (eccentric exercise) at about 60% $\dot{V}O_2max$. It was found that while MPO and EL did not change significantly after uphill walking, these indicators of PMN activation were markedly increased after downhill running [42]. We concluded that the above exercise protocol, leading to a significant PMN activation after downhill running only, could be used in association with the measurement of free radical markers in order to study the possible consequences of PMN activation on lipid peroxidation phenomena during exercise [42].

Comparison between Strenuous Exercise and Sepsis

From this review, it would appear that the inflammatory responses observed during strenuous muscular exercise and the early stage of sepsis display a similar pattern. Exercise and sepsis could have the release of LPS in blood as common triggering factor [11]. In addition, physical exercise can also trigger an inflammatory response, probably mediated by muscle and/or adjacent connective tissue damage similar to that demonstrated by Hikida et al. [43] in marathon runners [44]. Both LPS and muscle damage activate phagocytic

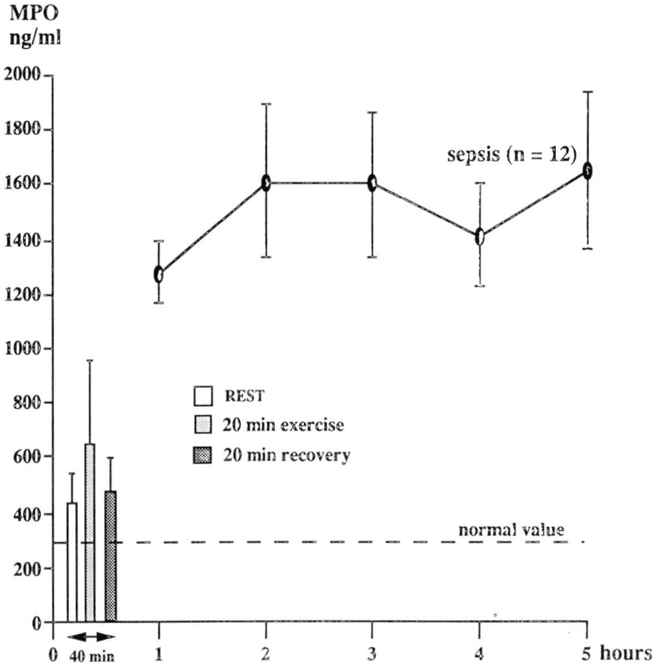

Fig. 3. Mean plasma levels of myeloperoxidase in 12 septic patients treated in the Intensive Care Unit, and in 11 healthy volunteers after strenuous exercise performed on a cycle ergometer (20 min at 80% maximal oxygen uptake). MPO was measured at rest, immediately after exercise, and after 20 min recovery.

cells and the complement cascade, releasing several mediators (Fig. 1), particularly the cytokines, with their multiple effects (hemostatic changes and PMN activation) (Fig. 2). Strenuous exercise and sepsis induce the production of free radicals leading to lipid peroxidation [7, 38]. The extent to which free radicals generated by activated PMN could play a role in lipid peroxidation phenomena during exercise remains to be evaluated. Sjödin et al. [38] have suggested that severe free radical attack could lead to cell necrosis and inflammation.

It is worth emphasizing, however, that the magnitude and duration of PMN activation in sepsis are considerably greater than during strenuous exercise. These differences are illustrated in Fig. 3, where the mean plasma levels of MPO measured in 11 healthy subjects submitted to a dynamic exercise of 20 min duration at 80% $\dot{V}O_2max$ [12] is compared to the MPO values reported in 12 septic patients. A similar conclusion is reached when the mean plasma concentration of IL-6 measured in 8 subjects after a 10 km run (unpublished results) is compared to the values obtained in patients after surgery of graded intensity, and other patients with sepsis and at time of septic shock (Fig. 4) [45, 46].

From these comparisons, it is tempting to consider that in most cases, the inflammatory response to exercise, including exercise-induced lipid peroxidation phenomena and an increase in the coagulability of the blood, have no pathological consequences. It should be pointed out, however, that some data suggest that intracoronary platelet aggregation, coronary spasm and thrombotic events could be responsible for sudden death and myocardial infarction following strenuous exercise [35]. According to Fitzgerald [47], overtraining could increase susceptibility to infection by impairing the immune system. Cannon et al. [4] have shown that PMN are involved in the delayed increase in muscle membrane permeability after damaging exercise. However, strenuous exercise seldomly results in sudden death or severe and persistent inflammation in healthy subjects. As pointed out above, the ma-

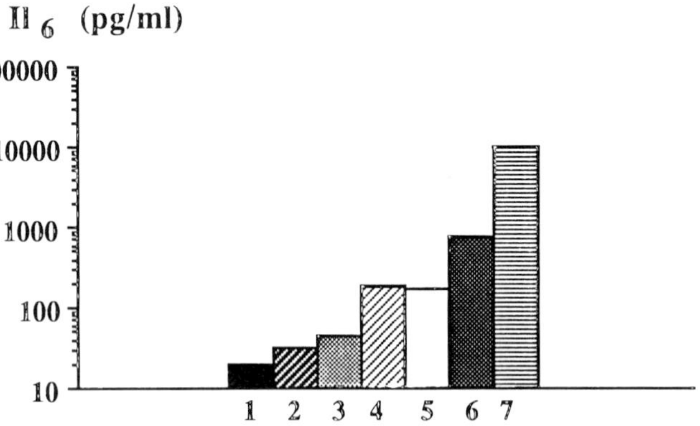

Fig. 4. Mean plasma levels of interleukin-6 ranges from 20 pg/ml after a 10 km run (8 subjects) to 10,049 pg/ml in septic shock patients. Column 1: 10 km run; columns 2 to 5: surgery of graded severity [44]; column 6: sepsis; column 7: septic shock [45].

gnitude and duration of these exercise-induced humoral and cellular changes are quite different from those observed in sepsis. Therefore, further studies are needed in order to define the physiological meaning of the changes occurring during exercise and the extent to which they could be considered as potential hazards, especially for untrained individuals who exerce too vigorously in poorly controlled conditions, or experienced individuals who overtrain.

Conclusions

In agreement with the conclusion of a previous review on a similar topic [6], there are thus a number of elements that suggest more than one analogy between strenuous exercise and the early stage of sepsis. These analogies are based on:

1) an inflammatory response leading to the release of common mediators;
2) hemostatic changes; and
3) free radical production resulting in lipid peroxidation.

Nevertheless, it should be kept in mind that these analogies are qualitative; magnitude and duration of the observed inflammatory reactions are less important during strenuous exercise than during sepsis.

References

1. Cannon JG, Evans WJ, Hughes VA, Meredith CN, Dinarello CA (1986) Physiological mechanisms contributing to increased interleukin-1 secretion. J Appl Physiol 61:1869–1874
2. McCarthy DA, Dale MM (1988) The leucocytosis of exercise. A review and model. Sports Med 6:333–363
3. Cannon JG, Fielding RA, Fiatarone MA, Orencole SF, Dinarello CA, Evans WJ (1989) Increased interleukin 1β in human skeletal muscle after exercise. Am J Physiol 257:451–455
4. Cannon JG, Orencole SF, Fielding RA, et al. (1990) Acute phase response in exercise: Interaction of age and vitamin E on neutrophils and muscle enzyme release. Am J Physiol 259:1214–1219
5. Dufaux B, Order U (1989) Plasma elastase-α1-antitrypsin, neopterin, tumor necrosis factor, and soluble interleukin-2 receptor after prolonged exercise. Int J Sports Med 10:434–438
6. Camus G, Pincemail J, Lamy M (1991) Is there an analogy between sepsis and strenuous physical exercise in the process of neutrophil activation in man: A working hypothesis. In: Vincent JL (ed) Update in intensive Care and Emergency Medicine Vol 14, Springer Verlag, Berlin Heidelberg, pp 206–212
7. Pincemail J, Camus G, Roesgen A, et al. (1990) Exercise induces pentane production and neutrophil activation in humans. Effects of propranolol. Eur J Appl Physiol 61:319–322
8. Hansen JB, Wilsgård L, Østerud B (1991) Biphasic changes in leukocytes induced by strenuous exercise. Eur J Appl Physiol 62:157–161
9. Schaefer RM, Kokot K, Heidland A, Plass R (1987) Jogger's leukocytes. N Engl J Med 316:223–224
10. Smith LL (1991) Acute inflammation: The underlying mechanism in delayed onset muscle soreness? Med Sci Sports Exerc 23:542–551
11. Bosenberg AT, Brock-Utne JG, Gaffin SL, Wells MTB, Blake GTW (1988) Strenuous exercise causes systemic endotoxemia. J Appl Physiol 65:106–108

12. Camus G, Pincemail J, Duchateau J, et al. (1992) Complement and polymorphonuclear neutrophil activation during submaximal dynamic exercise in man. Arch Int Physiol Biochim (Abs) (in press)
13. Morrison DC, Ryan JL (1987) Endotoxins and disease mechanisms. Ann Rev Med 320:365–376
14. Hack CE, Thijs LG (1991) The orchestra of mediators in the pathogenesis of septic shock: A review. In: Vincent JL (ed) Update in intensive care and emergency medicine Vol 14, Springer Verlag, Berlin Heidelberg, pp 232–246
15. Arai K, Lee F, Miyajima A, Miyatake S, Arai N, Yokota T (1990) Cytokines: Coordinators of immune and inflammatory responses. Ann Rev Biochem 59:783–836
16. Parratt JR, Pacitti N (1987) The possible roles of lipoxygenase products of arachidonic acid metabolism and of platelet activating factor in shock. In: Vincent JL, Thijs LG (eds) Update in intensive care and emergency medicine Vol 4, Springer Verlag, Berlin Heidelberg, pp 74–88
17. Larsen GL, Henson PM (1983) Mediators of inflammation. Ann Rev Immunol 1:335–359
18. Gay JC (1990) Priming of neutrophil oxidative responses by platelet-activating factors. J Lipid Mediat 2:161–175
19. Shalaby MB, Aggarwal BB, Rinderkwecht E, Svedersky LP, Finkle BS, Palladino MA (1985) Activation of human polymorphonuclear neutrophil functions by interferon-gamma and tumor necrosis factors. J Immunol 135:2069–2073
20. Yancey KB (1988) Biological properties of human C5a: Selected in vitro and in vivo studies. Clin Exp Immunol 71:207–210
21. Aasen AO (1987) The role of proteolytic enzyme systems with particular emphasis on the plasma kallikrein-kinin system during septicemia and septic shock. In: Vincent JL, Thijs LG (eds) Update in intensive care and emmergency medicine Vol 4, Springer Verlag, Berlin Heidelberg pp 116–128
22. Schoenberg MH (1987) The participation of oxygen free radicals in septic shock. In: Vincent JL, Thijs LG (eds) Update in intensive care and emergency medicine Vol 4, Springer Verlag, Berlin Heidelberg pp 108–115
23. Maughan RJ, Donnelly AE, Gleeson M, et al. (1989) Delayed-onset muscle damage and lipid peroxidation in man following a downhill run. Muscle & Nerve 12:332–336
24. Schwane JA, Johnson SR, Vandenakker CB, Armstrong RB (1983) Delayed-onset muscular soreness and plasma CPK and LDH activities after downhill running. Med Sci Sports Exerc 15:51–56
25. Bobbert MF, Hollander AP, Huijing PA (1986) Factors in delayed onset soreness of man. Med Sci Sports Exerc 18:75–81
26. Camus G, Sondag D, Maggipinto J, et al. (1991) Mobilisation des leucocytes lors de l'exercice dynamique sous-maximum. Arch Int Physiol Biochim 99:419–423
27. Dufaux B, Order U (1989) Complement activation after prolonged exercise. Clin Chim Acta 179:45–50
28. Cannon JG, Kluger MJ (1983) Endogenous pyrogen activity in human plasma after exercise. Science Wash DC 220:617–619
29. Liesen H, Dufaux B, Hollmann W (1977) Modifications of serum glycoproteins the days following prolonged physical exercise and the influence of physical training. Eur J Appl Physiol 37:243–254
30. Taylor C, Rogers G, Goodman C, et al. (1987) Hematologic, iron-related, and acute-phase protein responses to sustained strenuous exercise. J Appl Physiol 62:464–469
31. Viti A, Muscettola M, Paulescu L, Bocci V, Almi A (1985) Effect of exercise on plasma interferon levels. J Appl Physiol 59:426–428
32. Newham DJ, Jones DA, Clarkson PM (1987) Repeated high force eccentric exercise: Effects on muscle pain and damage. J Appl Physiol 63:1381–1386
33. Wheeler ME, Davis GL, Gillespie WJ, Bern MM (1986) Physiological changes in hemostasis associated with acute exercise. J Appl Physiol 60:986–990

34. Hansen JB, Wilsgård L, Olsen JO, Østerud B (1990) Formation and persistence of procoagulant and fibrinolytic activities in circulation after strenuous physical exercise. Thromb Haemost 64:385–389
35. Röcker L, Drygas WK, Heyduck B (1986) Blood platelet activation and increase in thrombin activity following a marathon race. Eur J Appl Physiol 55:374–380
36. Davies KJA, Quintanilha AT, Brooks GA, Packer L (1982) Free radicals and tissue damage produced by exercise. Biochem Biophys Res Commun 107:1198–1205
37. Jackson MJ, Edwards RHT, Symons MCR (1985) Electron spin resonance studies of intact mammalian skeletal muscle. Biochim Biophys Acta 847:185–190
38. Sjödin B, Westing YH, Apple FS (1990) Biochemical mechanisms for oxygen free formation during exercise. Sports Med 10:236–254
39. Pincemail J, Deby C, Camus G, et al. (1988) Tocopherol mobilization during intensive exercise. Eur J Appl Physiol 57:189–191
40. Duthie GG, Robertson JD, Maughan RJ, Morrice PC (1990) Blood antioxidant status and erythrocyte lipid peroxidation following distance running. Arch Biochem Biophys 282:78–83
41. Hochstein P, Jain SK (1981) Association of lipid peroxidation and polymerization of membrane proteins with erythrocyte aging. Fed proc 40:183–188
42. Camus G, Pincemail J, Ledent M, et al. (1992) Plasma levels of polymorphonuclear elastase and myeloperoxidase after uphill walking and downhill running at similar energy cost. Int J Sports Med (in press)
43. Hikida RS, Staron RS, Hagerman FC, Sherman WN, Costill DL (1983) Muscle fiber necrosis associated with human marathon runners. J Neurol Sci 59:185–203
44. Armstrong RB (1986) Muscle damage and endurance events. Sports Med 3:370–381
45. Damas P, leclercq P, Vrindts Y, et al. (1992) The metabolic response after abdominal surgery. Acta Anaesth Scand (in press)
46. Damas P, Ledoux D, Nys M, et al. (1992) Cytokines serum levels during severe sepsis in human. IL-6 as a marker of severity. Ann Surg 215:356–362
47. Fitzgerald L (1991) Overtraining increases the susceptibility to infection. Int J Sports Med 12:5–8

The Gut-Liver Axis in Multiple Organ Failure

J.C. Marshall

Introduction

Advances in the management of acute life-threatening illness have resulted in progressively improving rates of survival for a broad spectrum of disorders. These same advances, directed against the immediate threat to survival posed, for example, by bleeding, infection, or acute organ system failure, have profoundly altered patterns of morbidity and mortality in critical illness. In the wake of increasing success in the management of acute physiological instability has arisen a new series of clinical challenges: those that result not from the original injury but from the host response to injury, and from the therapeutic measures taken to achieve short term survival.

Rapid resuscitation, timely transport, and aggressive surgical intervention following multiple trauma, for example, effected a reduction in immediate mortality related to hemorrhagic shock, but simultaneously set the stage for the emergence of a new post-resuscitation syndrome: the adult respiratory distress syndrome (ARDS); support of the lung by mechanical ventilation, in turn, created a new series of problems including barotrauma and ventilator-associated pneumonia. The development of total parenteral nutrition has permitted prolonged survival in the absence of oral intake, but at the cost of TPN-induced cholestasis and liver dysfunction. The early control of life-threatening infections by physiological support and potent antimicrobial agents was a necessary prelude to the emergence of superinfection with organisms such as coagulase-negative *Staphylococci* and *Candida*. These new clinical challenges, arising in the wake of the treatment of a primary life-threatening disorder, comprise the post-resuscitation syndrome known variously as multiple organ failure (MOF) or multiple organ dysfunction syndrome (MODS), now the leading cause of ICU mortality [1].

MOF is best conceptualized as a syndrome of altered homeostasis which develops in the wake of a life-threatening insult, and which arises as a result of the *response* to the original insult or its treatment. The syndrome is intimately related to infection and the host septic response, mediated in turn by products of host immune cells- cytokines, prostanoids, and intermediates of oxygen and nitrogen. These mediators can produce both organ injury and an acquired state of immune dysfunction which, in concert with the influences of invasive monitoring devices and broad spectrum antibiotics, predisposes to the development of superinfection, and perpetuation of the syndrome.

This paradigm, injury resulting from the response to prior injury, defines the syndrome of MOF and establishes a conceptual framework for the present review of the gut-liver axis as a potential second insult in the pathogenesis of MOF, and in particular, in the pathogenesis of the state of altered immune homeostasis which characterizes the syndrome.

The Gut in Critical Illness: An Historical Perspective

The concept that the gastrointestinal (GI) tract is central to the systemic derangements associated with acute illness can be traced back four millennia. The Egyptians believed that a toxic factor of intestinal origin, designated as WHDW (and pronounced 'ukhedu'), could pass into the body producing illness or death [2]. Similar ideas were propounded by the Greeks, and the word 'sepsis' as used by Hippocrates and Aristotle denoted a process of putrefaction occurring within the colon and differentiated from the companion process of 'pepsis' or digestion [3].

Metchnikoff, at the turn of this century, proposed that a spectrum of problems ranging from puerperal fever to premature senility arose as a consequence of the absorption of toxins produced by the intestinal flora [4]. His concepts led to the popular belief that dietary supplementation with yogurt could promote longevity by modifying gut flora and stimlated a brief period of enthusiasm for even more drastic measures. The British surgeon, Sir Arbuthnot Lane, advocated colectomy as the treatment for chronic intestinal stasis [5], a practise lampooned in Shaw's play *A Doctor's Dilemma*.

Studies by Fine and others, beginning around 1950, demonstrated that bacteria could pass from the intestine into the peritoneal cavity in the setting of a sterile chemical peritonitis [6], and implicated a factor of intestinal origin in the lethality associated with hemorrhagic shock [7, 8]. This factor proved to be gram-negative bacterial endotoxin [9]. It was shown, moreover, that not only was the gut a source of endotoxin, it also contributed to the lethality of endotoxemia, since a 90% enterectomy significantly improved rates of survival following endotoxin infusion in a canine model [10]. The concept that the gut can amplify injury in critical illness thus dates back a quarter of a century.

Contemporary interest in the gut in critical illness stems from a series of observations regarding infection in the critically ill. ICU-acquired infections often develop in the absence of a well-defined reservoir of the causative organisms, and involve a microbial spectrum which is fundamentally different from the flora of community-acquired infections [11–13]. Control of infection does not necessarily result in diminution of the associated septic response or in a reduction in mortality [14, 15]. The MOF syndrome classically arises in patients with uncontrolled intraabdominal infection in whom the infectious focus lies immediately adjacent to the GI tract [16], yet control of that infection frequently fails to reverse organ failure [17].

We and others have hypothesized that interactions between the GI tract and the liver contribute to the evolution and expression of the MOF syndrome [18–21]. Briefly sketched, the gut hypothesis proposes in alternate mechanism for the initiation and perpetuation of the host septic response. Critical illness and its management alters normal patterns of proximal GI colonization with the result that the gut becomes overgrown with common ICU pathogens. These organisms can enter the host and produce foci of invasive ICU-acquired infection either by aspiration of contaminated gastric secretions or by translocation across an altered mucosal barrier. Additionally, however, interactions between microorganisms or their products and immune cells in the gut mucosa and liver may trigger the local release of the biochemical mediators of the septic response. The resultant mediator cascade, initiated within the gut mucosa or liver becomes manifest as a systemic syndrome of clinical sepsis and its ultimate consequence, organ dysfunction, in the absence of demonstrable invasive infection.

Altered Proximal GI Flora in Critical Illness

In health, the proximal GI tract is sterile or lightly colonized with gram-positive organisms and *Lactobacilli* [22]. Hypochlorhydria, as a consequence of medical [23] or surgical [24] vagotomy or in conjunction with pernicious anemia [25], is associated with significant overgrowth by gram-negative organisms. Small bowel overgrowth with gram-negatives is also evident in the patient with liver disease [26, 27].

Colonization of the upper GI tract develops rapidly following admission to an ICU [28, 29]. Its causes are multifactorial. Human studies have shown that the use of acid-reducing measures for the prophylaxis of stress ulceration predisposes to gram-negative bacterial overgrowth [30, 31], however since gram-positive organisms and fungi are also found in increased numbers, other causes are likely. In animal models, peritonitis [32], interruption of bile flow [33], and disruption of the normal microbial ecology with broad spectrum antibiotics [34, 35] all produce gut microbial overgrowth.

In a study of 34 critically ill patients admitted to a surgical ICU, we found *Candida, Pseudomonas, S. epidermidis,* and the enterococcus to be the most common species colonizing the upper GI tract, with mean concentrations ranging from 10^4 to 10^7 CFU/ml of GI fluid [36]. Gut colonization was significantly associated with the development of invasive infection with *Candida, Pseudomonas,* and *S. epidermidis*; these infections included not only pneumonia, but also recurrent peritonitis, urinary tract infections, and bacteremias.

Interactions between Gut Flora and the Host

The relationship between the indigenous GI flora and the normal host is a symbiotic one: the host provides nutrients and optimal conditions for microbial growth, the organism, in turn, exerts multiple beneficial influences on systemic homeostasis. Studies in germfree animals, for example, have shown that an intact microbial flora is a prerequisite for normal morphologic development of the small bowel and an important factor in the regulation of the rate of intestinal transit [37].

The indigenous intestinal flora plays a critical role in normal immunologic development. The spleen of the germfree animal contains fewer T helper cells [38], and unlike their conventional counterparts, these animals fail to develop normal delayed type hypersensitivity responses following immunization with sheep red blood cells [39]. Neutrophils [40] and macrophages [41] from the germfree animal display impaired chemotaxis in response to an inflammatory stimulus. Germfree animals are highly susceptible to infection with *S. aureus* or *Klebsiella*, yet resistant to doses of endotoxin which are lethal to conventional animals [42]. Gram-negative colonization of the GI tract has also been shown to regulate macrophage-mediated suppression of the secondary antibody response [43].

The indigenous gastrointestinal flora has been implicated in a diverse group of diseases which share, as a common feature, abnormalities in immune regulation. Experimental liver injury resulting from either dietary deficiency of choline [44] or administration of carbon tetrachloride [45] can be minimized by antimicrobial therapy directed against intestinal gram-negative aerobes, and in particular, by neutralization of gut endotoxin. Similarly, the liver injury resulting following infection with Frog Virus 3 is largely prevented by prior colectomy [46]. Autoimmune thyroiditis in susceptible animals is attenuated by oral antibiotics; restoration of the normal gram-negative flora results in exacerbation of the thyroiditis [47]. Intestinal bacterial products also appear to play a role in the pathogenesis of experimental arthritis [48, 49].

Profound dysregulation of normal immunologic responsiveness is a prominent feature of MOF [50]; changes in the gut flora potentially contribute to this state by one of four mechanisms:

1. aspiration of contaminated upper GI fluids resulting in pneumonia and its sequelae;
2. translocation of viable microorganisms across the gut mucosa producing invasive infection with its sequelae;
3. absorption of endotoxin into the portal vein resulting in the release of mediator molecules from Kupffer cells and hepatocytes, and
4. local activation of immunologically competent cells in the gut mucosa with the release of regulatory mediators into the mesenteric lymphatics or portal vein.

Aspiration Pneumonitis and its Sequelae

Subclinical aspiration of colonized gastric secretions is an important cause of pneumonia in the intubated ICU patient [30, 31, 51, 52]. Aspirated microorganisms can proliferate in the lung, producing local tissue injury, or spread hematogenously or via lymphatics to other sites in the body. They also interact with local host phagocytic cells, predominantly alveolar macrophages and neutrophils, and the biochemical products of these interactions in turn can induce local and distant tissue injury.

Alveolar macrophages release tumor necrosis factor (TNF) and interleukin-1 (IL-1) in response to bacterial endotoxin stimulation both *in vivo* [53] and *in vitro* [54]; in fact, LPS-triggered alveolar macrophages release substantially more TNF than Kupffer cells do [55]. Endotoxin also stimulates alveolar macrophages to release a potent neutrophil chemo-attractant (likely the cytokine IL-8), resulting in augmented accumulation of neutrophils in the alveoli [56, 57]. Both TNF [58] and neutrophil products [59] induce the characteristic lung injury of ARDS in the experimental animal.

Alveolar macrophages also exert an important immunoregulatory influence *in vivo*, downregulating the response of lymphocytes to activation by antigen or mitogen [60, 61].

Bacterial Translocation

Extensive studies both in animals [62–65] and humans [66–68] have shown that bacterial translocation, the passage of intact, viable bacteria through the GI tract into sterile host tissues, is a common phenomenon when normal physiological homeostasis is disrupted. The factors promoting translocation in the experimental animal (shock, trauma, hemorrhage, malnutrition, absence of enteral feeding, endotoxemia, and obstructive jaundice), are factors which are commonly present in the critically ill patient [69]. Moreover, translocating bacterial species include all of the common isolates from ICU-acquired infections: *Pseudomonas* [70], *Candida* [66], coagulase-negative *Staphylococci* and the enterococcus [64].

It is well-established that bacterial translocation occurs; it is less clear whether it is a mechanism of disease or an epiphenomenon. Transient bacteremia can be detected in patients undergoing sigmoidoscopy [71] or colonoscopy [72] in the absence of obvious systemic sequelae; on the other hand, translocation of *Candida* by oral ingestion of a large fungal inoculum by a healthy human volunteer resulted in significant systemic upset [66]. Disruption of the normal GI flora, particularly the anaerobic flora, can cause bacterial translocation. Translocation induced by gut overgrowth with *E. coli* is associated with suppression of lymphocyte proliferation *in vitro* [73] and of delayed hypersensitivity responsiveness *in vivo* [74] as well as with augmentation of Kupffer cell procoagulant activity

[75]. On the other hand, suppression of gut flora by oral non-absorbed antibiotics does not improve outcome in experimental models of burn wound infection [76] or zymosan peritonitis [77], despite a reduction in rates of bacterialtranslocation.

Absorption of Endotoxin

Bacteria identified by culture of host tissues represent only a very small proportion of the body burden of bacteria or bacterial products present in models of bacterial translocation, since nonviable organisms outnumber viable organisms by a factor of as much as one hundred to one [78]. The physiological effects seen in association with bacterial translocation may, therefore, be a consequence of the absorption of endotoxin, rather than the translocation of live organisms.

Despite the presence of large amounts of endotoxin within the gut lumen, the normal gut mucosa forms an effective barrier, and systemic absorption of endotoxin is minimal [79]. Increased passage of endotoxin across the gut mucosa occurs under circumstances similar to those which facilitate bacterial translocation. Absorption of endotoxin has been documented in experimental models following surgery [80] and hemorrhagic shock [81], and in the presence of small bowel obstruction [82]. Systemic endotoxemia, presumably of gut origin, can be demonstrated in human burn victims [83] and in patients with inflammatory bowel disease [84]. The portal vein appears to be the most important route of uptake of endotoxin absorbed from the GI tract [85]. Concentrations of endotoxin in the portal blood are elevated following cecal perforation [85] and small bowel obstruction [82] in experimental animals. Few data are available regarding portal endotoxemia in humans. Low level portal endotoxemia has been detected in otherwise healthy humans undergoing laparotomy [86] and in patients with liver disease [87]. On the other hand, endotoxin was not found in portal blood in the first five days following abdominal trauma [88], nor in patients who do not have concomitant GI disease [89]. It is probable that if portal endotoxemia occurs normally, it does so intermittently or at only very low concentrations.

Local Activation of Gut Associated Lymphoid Tissues

The GI tract is a complex immunoregulatory organ which has evolved to serve a dual role: the exclusion of potentially harmful microorganisms from the environment and the downregulation of injurious immune reactions to ingested foodstuffs. Gut associated lymphoid tissues (GALT) are found throughout the length of the GI tract and include lymphocytes, mast cells, macrophages, and specialized sampling and effector cells such as the Paneth cell and the M cell.

Table 1. Soluble Immunoregulatory Products of the GALT

Cell Source	Mediator
Mucosal T cells	IL-2, 4, 5, Interferon gamma, IL-6, TNF
Mucosal mast cells	TNF, histamine
Macrophages	IL-1, Granulocyte-macrophage CSF
Paneth cells	TNF, Lysozyme, Defensins
Neural tissues	Neuropeptides- VIP, Somatostatin, Substance P
Dietary casein	Beta casomorphin

Intestinal lymphocytes comprise three separate compartments: the intraepithelial lymphocytes which are almost exclusively T cells, the majority of which are CD8 positive [90]; the lamina propria lymphocytes which include both T and B cells [91]; and the specialized aggregations of lymphocytes known as Peyer's patches. Lymphocytes of the GALT differ from those found in the peripheral circulation in a number of important respects. In rodents, T cells bearing the gamma/delta receptor predominate among the intraepithelial lymphocytes [92], although the same is not true in humas [93]. Intestinal T cells, unlike their circulating counterparts, are preferentially activated via the CD2 rather than the CD3 receptor [94]. They produce large amounts of IL-5 which regulates B cell differentiation to secrete IgA [95]. Production of this cytokine is usually associated with the Th2 subset of helper T cells, however CD8+ gamma/delta intraepithelial T cells also produce IL-5 both constitutively and in response to engagement of the CD3 or CD8 receptor [96]. A unique subset of T cells found in Peyer's patches, the contrasuppressor T cell, plays an important role in facilitating local immune responses in the face of immune interactions which induce systemic tolerance [97].

Intercellular signalling by the release of soluble mediators is critical to the coordination and expression of mucosal immunity [98]. Cells of the gut associated lymphoid tissues are a rich source of immunologically active mediator molecules (Table 1). In addition to IL-5, normal intestinal T cells release interferon gamma, TNF [99], IL-2 and -4 [94], and IL-6 [95]. These same cytokines may contribute to local disease. Increased numbers of cells secreting TNF are seen in patients with Crohn's disease [100] and local mucosal injury in graft versus host disease can be prevented by antibodies directed against interferon gamma [101]. Macrophages are found throughout the GI tract and are likely the source of increased amounts of IL-1 and GM-CSF produced by intestinal mononuclear cells from patients with inflammatory bowel disease [102].

Other cell populations in the gut mucosa play a role in local immunity. An important antibacterial role for Paneth cells is suggested by the fact that they express mRNA for TNF, and have been shown to contain both lysozyme and antibacterial defensins [103]. Mucosal mast cells also synthesize and release large quantities of TNF [104]. Moreover, neuropeptides such as substance P [90] and even exogenous compounds such as the milk-derived peptide beta-casomorphin [105] are able to exert a significant regulatory influence on immune responses within the intestinal mucosa.

The influence of the luminal flora on the production and release of cytokines by the GALT has not been studied, although emerging data regarding the rich immunoregulatory repertoire of these tissues suggest that interactions between the GALT and its environment are highly probable.

The Liver and the Mediator Response of MOF

The fetal liver is an important organ of extramedullary hematopoeisis. This function ceases by the time of birth, however the liver retains a critical role as an effector of antibacterial immunity, and a regulator of systemic immune homeostasis. It also figures prominently in the metabolic and immunologic alterations accompanying the septic response.

A variety of stimuli including infection, tissue injury, sterile inflammation, and pregnancy evoke a characteristic pattern of altered hepatocyte protein synthesis known as the acute phase response. Synthesis of acute phase reactants such as C reactive protein, alpha-1 antitrypsin, fibrinogen, ceruloplasmin, ferritin, and haptoglobin is increased, while the synthesis of albumin, LDL, and HDL is decreased. The acute phase response is highly

Table 2. Secretory Products of Kupffer Cells

Cytokines	IL-1 IL-6 IL-8 TNF Interferon Alpha/Beta Transforming Growth Factor Beta
Bioactive Lipids	Prostaglandin D2 Prostaglandin E2 Thromboxane A2 PAF
Cytokine Inhibitors	IL-1 inhibitor
Complement Components	
Reactive Oxygen Intermediates	
Reactive Nitrogen Intermediates	

conserved, being found in invertebrates as well as vertebrates [106], although its biological role is poorly understood. Certain of the acute phase reactants, notably C reactive protein [107] and alpha-1 antitrypsin [108] demonstrate immunmodulatory activity *in vitro*, while the negative acute phase reactant high density lipoprotein binds endotoxin and slows its removal by the reticuloendothelial system [109]. Whether these represent adaptive responses to invasive infection, maladaptive responses which impair host defense, or mere *in vitro* curiosities is unknown.

The acute phase response is initiated by IL-6, a major secretory product of endotoxin-activated Kupffer cells [110]. Activated Kupffer cells release a remarkable array of biologically active mediators including the proinflammatory cytokines IL-1, IL-6, and TNF, prostaglandins, thromboxane A2, platelet activating factor (PAF), and intermediates of oxygen and nitrogen (Table 2) [111, 112]. Kupffer cell products may act in an autocrine fashion to regulate subsequent Kupffer cell mediator release [113], in a paracrine fashion to alter hepatocyte protein synthesis [114] or release of factors such as nitric oxide [115], or in an endocrine fashion, affecting remote organs following their release into the systemic circulation [116].

The Kupffer cell mass comprises more than 70% of the total population of macrophages and monocytes in the human, and may, therefore, be the major site of synthesis of macrophage-derived mediators of MOF [112]. Indeed, studies in human volunteers show that systemic endotoxemia results in the release of TNF and IL-6 from the splanchnic circulation, splanchnic production accounting for as much as one half of total TNF release under these circumstances [117]. Hepatocyte products with immunoregulatory potential have also been described [118, 119], and liver injury is associated with a spectrum of immunologic abnormalities very similar to those occurring in MOF [120].

The liver plays an important role in antigen-specific tolerance. Portal administration of antigen results in suppression of both cell-mediated [121] and humoral [122] responses following subsequent immunization, and portal drainage of an allograft permits prolonged graft survival [123]. The mechanism is unknown, but may involve the release of an antigen-specific serum factor [124].

The Gut, The Liver, and Immune Dysfunction in MOF

MOF is associated with a complex spectrum of immunologic abnormalities and an enhanced susceptibility to invasive infection [112]. Impairment of cell-mediated immunity, manifested by a reduction in delayed type hypersensitivity (DTH) responsiveness *in vivo* [125] and of mitogen-stimulated lymphocyte proliferation *in vitro* [126], is a particularly prominent feature. We have investigated the potential contribution of gut-liver interactions to this systemic state of altered immune responsiveness.

Table 3. Differential Effects of Portal and Systemic Bacteremia on the Experimental Delayed Hypersensitivity Response. (Adapted from [128, 129] with permission)

Infusion	(DTH as % of Non-operated Controls) IVC	Route of Infusion: Portal	p.
Saline	59 ± 7	63 ± 6	NS
Live *E. coli*	59 ± 4	41 ± 9*	< 0.05
Killed *Ps.aeruginosa*	61 ± 4	48 ± 3*	< 0.05
Live *S. fecalis*	49 ± 5*	60 ± 4	< 0.05
Carrageenan	61 ± 4	79 ± 8*	< 0.05

Mean ± SEM

In rats which have been presensitized to the experimental antigen, keyhole limpet hemocyanin (KLH), the induction of peritonitis by cecal ligation without puncture produces significant suppression of DTH reactivity to KLH, and massive jejunal overgrowth with *E. coli*. By suppressing the animal's endogenous *E. coli* with oral antibiotics and then repopulating the gut with antibiotic-resistant *E. coli*, we were able to show that the small bowel overgrowth induced by cecal ligation contributed to the observed DTH suppression [32]. Similarly, prolonged feeding of killed *Pseudomonas* or *Candida*, but not *S. epidermidis* or sheep red blood cells, resulted in significant suppression of DTH responsiveness [127], independent of bacterial viability.

Suppression of *in vivo* and *in vitro* cell-mediated immunity could also be induced by infusion of gram-negative bacteria into the portal vein, but not into the systemic circulation. Rats received an infusion of organisms into either the systemic circulation via the infrahepatic vena cava, or the portal circulation via the portal vein (Table 3). When the challenge organism was live *E. coli* or killed *Pseudomonas aeruginosa*, delayed hypersensitivity responses were significantly depressed in portally-infused animals, whereas responses in systemically-infused animals did not differ from control values; suppression was not seen when the organism was a gram-positive bacterium, *S. fecalis*. *In vivo* ablation of Kupffer cell responsiveness by administration of carrageenan significantly reduced the magnitude of DTH suppression resulting from surgery [128, 129].

Suppression of mitogen-stimulated lymphocyte proliferation was also evident 24 h following portal but not systemic infusion of killed *Pseudomonas* (Fig. 1). Splenocytes isolated from portally-infused animals failed to proliferate when stimulated *in vitro* with the T cell mitogen, concanavalin A, and responses to the B cell mitogen LPS were reduced; splenocytes from systemically-infused animals responded normally to mitogenic stimulation. The suppressive influence present in the cultures of spleen cells from portally-infused animals could be removed by depletion of splenic adherent cells. Mo-

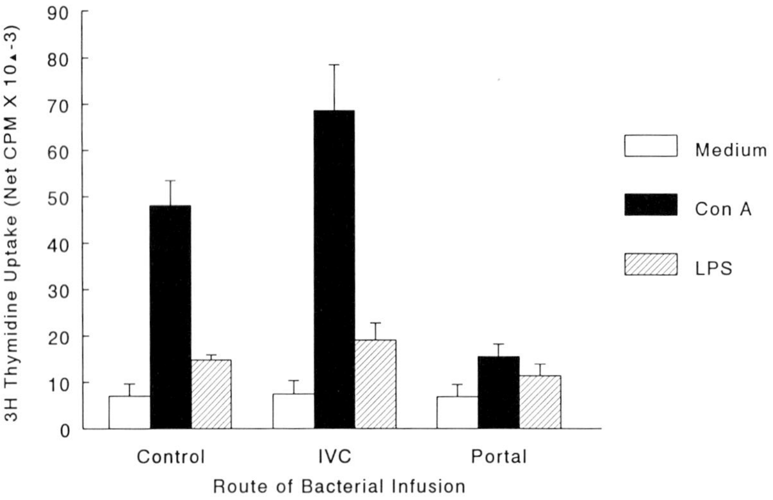

Fig. 1. Suppression of the proliferative response to the mitogens Con A and LPS of splenocytes isolated from rats 24 h following infusion of 3 x 10^8 killed *Pseudomonas aeruginosa* into either the infrahepatic vena cava or the portal vein. Responses in systemically (IVC) infused animals do not differ from those of their non-operated controls; portal infusion, however, induced marked suppression of *in vitro* proliferation.

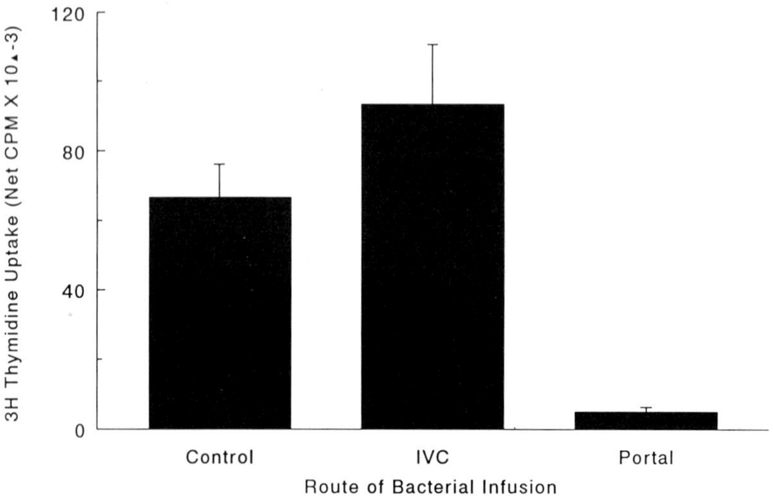

Fig. 2. Alveolar macrophages isolated from rats 24 h following infusion of *Pseudomonas aeruginosa* into the infrahepatic vena cava or portal vein. Macrophages from portally-infused animals release a potent soluble suppressor factor which can inhibit the mitogen-induced proliferative response of isolated splenocytes.

reover, alveolar macrophages harvested from portally-infused animals were shown to secrete significant amounts of a soluble factor which could almost completely inhibit proliferation of normal control splenocytes (Fig. 2) [130].

These studies demonstrate a potential role for the liver as a component of a biological cascade initiated by portal endotoxemia and resulting in the release of an immunosuppressive factor from remote macrophage populations. Endotoxin itself is not responsible for this suppressive influence, since LPS actually stimulates splenocyte proliferation in a dose-dependent fashion. Rather the process appears to involve the release of an hepatic factor which in turn promotes the release of a second factor or factors from remote macrophages. The identity of this second factor is under investigation: suppression can be overcome by a blocking antibody to transforming growth factor beta, but although TGFβ is necessary for suppression, it alone is not sufficient to induce suppression of the degree seen in the model.

Conclusion

The gut-liver paradigm provides a different perspective on the pathogenesis of the state of altered immune homeostasis which characterizes MOF. If classical invasive infection produces morbidity as a result of the interaction of invading organisms with host immune cells, an alternate pathway for this process may occur in the critically ill as a consequence of interactions between an altered gut flora and immune cells in the liver. The clinical importance of this gut-liver axis is, at present, impossible to quantitate in the absence of effective gut-directed interventions which might selectively inhibit it. Moreover, animal models of critical illness fail in many important respects to model the complex organ system interactions which characterize MOF as it evolves in the critically ill patient receiving intensive monitoring and therapy and maximal organ system support.

Clinical studies have largely focused on the role of the gut as a source of invasive infection in critical illness. A number of reports suggest that the risk of ICU-acquired infection can be minimized by measures taken to prevent gut bacterial overgrowth, although even this is controversial. Whether such measures can also attenuate the host response which produces organ dysfunction is unknown. Support of the gut mucosa by early enteral feeding has been shown to reduce rates of infectious complications, to reduce post-trauma bacteremia, febrile episodes, and pulmonary failure, and to attenuate the acute phase response following trauma. Yet it remains to be proven that enteral feeding can prevent MOF.

For the present, the most promising therapeutic advances seem to lie in the area of selective manipulation of the putative mediators of organ injury, independent of their anatomic site of production or of the pathological processes which triggered their release. Ultimately the importance of the gut-liver axis may lie not in the specific avenues it opens for novel means of therapy, but in the emphasis it focuses on the dynamic and constantly changing nature of the problems which lie at the frontiers of critical care.

Acknowledgments. This work was supported in part by the grants from the Physician's Services Incorporated Foundation, Ontario Canada and the Canadian Association of General Surgeons.

References

1. Marshall JC (1991) Multiorgan Failure. In: Wilmore DW, Brennan MF, Harken AH, Holcroft JW, Meakins JL (eds) Care of the Surgical Patient. Volume I Critical Care. Scientific American, New York. pp 1–20
2. Chen TSN, Chen PSY (1989) Intestinal autointoxication: a medical leitmotif. J Clin Gastroenterol 11:434–441
3. Majno G (1991) The ancient riddle of sepsis. J Infect Dis 163:937–945
4. Metchnikoff E (1905) The Nature of Man. Studies in Optimistic Philosophy. GP. Putnam's Sons, New York and London
5. Lane WA (1912) A clinical lecture on chronic intestinal stasis. BMJ 1:989–993
6. Schweinburg FB, Seligman AM, Fine J (1950) Transmural migration of intestinal bacteria. A study based on the use of radioactive Escherichia coli. N Engl J Med 242:747–751
7. Lillehei RC (1957) The intestinal factor in irreversible hemorrhagic shock. Surgery 42:1043–1054
8. Fine J, Frank ED, Ravin HA, Rutenberg SH, Schweinburg FB (1959) The bacterial factor in traumatic shock. N Engl J Med 260:214–220
9. Schweinburg FB, Fine J (1960) Evidence for lethal endotoxemia as the fundamental feature of irreversibility in three types of traumatic shock. J Exp Med 112:793–800
10. Evans WE, Darin JC (1966) Effect of enterectomy in endotoxin shock. Surgery 60:1026–1029
11. Garrison RN, Fry DE, Berberich S, Polk HC (1982) Enterococcal bacteremia. Clinical implications and determinants of death. Ann Surg 196:43–47
12. Dyess DL, Garrison RN, Fry DE (1985) Candida sepsis. Implications of polymicrobial bloodborne infection. Arch Surg 120:345–348
13. Marshall JC, Christou NV, Horn H, Meakins JL (1988) The microbiology of multiple organ failure. The proximal GI tract as an occult reservoir of pathogens. Arch Surg 123:309–315
14. Craven DE, Kunches LM, Kilinsky V, Lichtenberg DA, Make BJ, McCabe WR (1986) Risk factors for pneumonia and fatality in patients receiving continuous mechanical ventilation. Am Rev Respir Dis 133:792–796
15. Marshall J, Sweeney D (1990) Microbial infection and the septic response in critical surgical illness. Sepsis, not infection, determines outcome. Arch Surg 125:17–23
16. Polk HC, Shields CL (1977) Remote organ failure: A valid sign of occult intra-abdominal infection. Surgery 81:310–313
17. Norton LW (1985) Does drainage of intra-abdominal pus reverse multiple organ failure? Am J Surg 149:347–350
18. Carrico CJ, Meakins JL, Marshall JC, Fry D, Maier RV (1986) Multiple-organ-failure-syndrome. The GI tract: The "motor" of MOF. Arch Surg 121:196–208
19. Border JR, Hassett J, LaDuca J, et al. (1987) The gut origin septic states in blunt multiple trauma (ISS=40) in the ICU. Ann Surg 206:427–448
20. Wilmore DW, Smith RJ, O'Dwyer ST, Jacobs DO, Ziegler TR, Wang XD (1988) The gut: A central organ after surgical stress. Surgery 104:917–923
21. Deitch EA (1988) Does the gut protect us or injure us when ill in the ICU? In: Cerra F (ed) Perspectives in Critical Care, Quality Medical, St. Louis pp 1–32
22. Drasar BS, Shiner M, McLeod GM (1969) Studies on the intestinal flora. I. The bacterial flora of the gastronintestinal tract in healthy and achlorhydric persons. Gastroenterology 56:71–79
23. Stockbrugger RW, Cotton PB, Eugenides N, Bartholomew BA, Hill MJ, Walters CL (1982) Intragastric nitrates, nitrosamines, and bacterial overgrowth during cimetidine treatment. Gut 23:1048–1054
24. Greenlee HB, Vivit R, Paez J, Dietz A (1971) Bacterial flora of the jejunum following peptic ulcer surgery. Arch Surg 102:260–265

25. Gianella RA, Broitman SA, Zamcheck N (1972) Gastric acid barrier to ingested microorganisms in man: Studies in vivo and in vitro. Gut 13:251–256
26. Martini GA, Phear EA, Ruebner B, Sherlock S (1957) The bacterial content of the small intestine in normal and cirrhotic subjects: Relation to methionine toxicity. Clin Sci 16:35–51
27. Bode JC, Bode C, Heidelbach R, Durr HK, Martini GA (1984) Jejunal microflora in patients with chronic alcohol abuse. Hepato-gastroenterol 31:30–34
28. Garvey BM, McCambley JA, Tuxen DV (1989) Effects of gastric alkalization on bacterial colonization in critically ill patients. Crit Care Med 17:211–216
29. Marshall JC (1991) The ecology and immunology of the gastrointestinal tract in health and critical illness. J Hosp Infect 19 (Suppl C):7–17
30. du Moulin GC, Hedley-White J, Paterson DG, Lisbon A (1982) Aspiration of gastric bacteria in antacid-treated patients: A frequent cause of postoperative colonisation of the airway. Lancet 1:242–244
31. Driks MR, Craven DE, Celli BR, et al (1987) Nosocomial pneumonia in intubated patients given sucralfate as compared with antacids or histamine type 2 blockers. N Engl J Med 317:1376–1382
32. Marshall JC, Christou NV, Meakins JL (1988) Small bowel bacterial overgrowth and systemic immunosuppression in experimental peritonitis. Surgery 104:404–411
33. Deitch EA, Sittig K, Li M, Berg RD, Specian D (1990) Obstructive jaundice promotes bacterial translocation from the gut. Am J Surg 159:79–84
34. Kennedy MJ, Volz PA (1985) Ecology of Candida albicans gut colonization: Inhibition of Candida adhesion, colonization, and dissemination from the gastrointestinal tract by bacterial antagonism. Infect Immun 49:654–663
35. Hentges DJ, Stein AJ, Casey SW, Que JU (1985) Protective role of intestinal flora against infection with Pseudomonas aeruginosa in mice: Influence of antibiotics on colonization resistance. Infect Immun 47:118–122
36. Marshall JC, Christou NV, de Santis M, Meakins JL (1987) Proximal gastrointestinal flora and systemic infection in the critically ill surgical patient. Surg Forum 38:89–91
37. Abrams GD (1988) Impact of the intestinal microflora on intestinal structure and function. In: Hentges DJ (ed) Human Intestinal Microflora in Health and Disease, Academic Press Inc, New York. pp 292–310
38. Ohwaki M, Yasutake N, Yasui H, Ogura R (1977) A comparative study on the humoral immune responses in germfree and conventional mice. Immunology 32:43–48
39. MacDonald TT, Carter PB (1979) Requirements for a bacterial flora before mice generate cells capable of mediating the delayed hypersensitivity reaction to sheep red blood cells. J Immunol 122:2624–2629
40. Abrams GD, Bishop JE (1965) Normal flora and leukocyte mobilization. Arch Pathol 79:213–217
41. Morland B, Smievoll AI, Midtvedt T (1979) Comparison of peritoneal macrophages from germfree and conventional mice. Infect Immun 26:1129–1136
42. Dubos RJ, Schaedler RW (1960) The effect of the intestinal flora on the growth rate of mice and on their susceptibility to experimental infections. J Exp Med 111:407–417
43. Mattingly JA, Eardley DD, Kemp JD, Gershon K (1979) Induction of suppressor cells in rat spleen: Influence of microbial stimulation. J Immunol 122:787–790
44. Rutenburg AM, Sonnenblick E, Koven I, Aprahamian HA, Reiner L, Fine J (1957) The role of intestinal bacteria in the development of dietary cirrhosis in rats. J Exp Med 106:1–14
45. Nolan JP, Leibowitz AI (1978) Endotoxin and the liver. III. Modification of acute carbon tetrachloride injury by polymyxin B- an antiendotoxin. Gastroenterology 75:445–449
46. Gut JP, Schmitt S, Bingen A, Anton M, Kirn A (1982) Protective effect of colectomy in frog virus 3 hepatitis of rats: Possible role of endotoxin. J Infect Dis 146:594–605
47. Penhale WJ, Young PR (1988) The influence of the normal microbial flora on the susceptibility of rats to experimental autoimmune thyroiditis. Clin Exp Immunol 72:288–292
48. Midtvedt T (1987) Intestinal bacteria and rheumatic disease. Scand J Rheumatol 64 (Suppl):49–54

49. Severijnen AJ, van Kleef R, Hazenberg MP, van de Merwe JP (1990) Chronic arthritis induced in rats by cell wall fragments of Eubacterium species from the human intestinal flora. Infect Immun 58:523–528
50. Abraham E (1989) host defense abnormalities after hemorrhage, trauma, and burns. Crit Care med 17:934–939
51. Craven DE, Driks MR (1987) Nosocomial pneumonia in the intubated patient. Semin Resp Infect 2:20–33
52. Kingston GW, Phang PT, Leathley MJ (1991) Increased incidence of nosocomial pneumonia in mechanically ventilated patients with subclinical aspiration. Am J Surg 161:589–592
53. Tabor DR, Burchett SK, Jacobs RF (1988) Enhanced production of monokines by canine alveolar macrophages in response to endotoxin-induced shock. Proc Soc Exp Biol Med 187:408–415
54. Becker S, Devlin RB, Haskill JS (1989) Differential production of tumor necrosis factor, macrophage colony stimulating factor, and interleukin-1 by human alveolar macrophages. J Leuk Biol 45:353–361
55. Callery MP, Kamei T, Mangino MJ, Flye MW (1991) Organ interactions in sepsis. Host defense and the hepatic pulmonary macrophage axis. Arch Surg 126:28–32
56. Harmsen AG (1988) Role of alveolar macrophages in lipopolysaccharide-induced neutrophil accumulation. Infect Immun 56:1858–1863
57. Christman JW, Petras SF, Vacek PM, Davis GS (1989) Rat alveolar macrophage production of chemoattractants for neutrophils: response to Escherichia coli endotoxin. Infect Immun 57:810–816
58. Ferrari-Baliviera E, Mealy K, Smith RJ, Wilmore DW (1989) Tumor necrosis factor induces adult respiratory distress syndrome in rats. Arch Surg 124:1400–1405
59. Mallick AA, Ishizaka A, Stephens KE, Hatherill JR, Tazelaar HD, Raffin TA (1989) Multiple organ damage caused by tumor necrosis factor and prevented by prior neutrophil depletion. Chest 95:1114–1120
60. Twomey JJ, Laughter A, Brown MF (1983) A comparison of the regulatory effects of human monocytes, pulmonary alveolar macrophages (PAMs) and spleen macrophages upon lymphocyte responses. Clin Exp Immunol 52:449–454
61. Holt PG (1986) Downregulation of immune responses in the lower respiratory tract: The role of alveolar macrophages. Clin Exp Immunol 63:261–270
62. Berg RD (1981) Promotion of the translocation of enteric bacteria from the gastrointestinal tracts of mice by oral treatment with penicillin, clindamycin, or metronidazole. Infect Immun 33:854–861
63. Deitch EA, Winterton J, Li M, Berg R (1987) The gut as a portal of entry for bacteremia. Role of protein malnutrition. Ann Surg 205:681–692
64. Wells CL, Rotstein OD, Pruett TL, Simmons RL (1986) Intestinal bacteria translocate into experimental intra-abdominal abscesses. Arch Surg 121:102–107
65. Alexander JW, Gianotti L, Pyles T, Carey MA, Babcock GF (1991) Distribution and survival of Escherichia coli translocating from the intestine after thermal injury. Ann Surg 213:558–567
66. Krause W, Matheis H, Wulf K (1969) Fungaemia and funguria after oral administration of Candida albicans. Lancet 1:598–599
67. Gaussorgues PH, Gueugniaud PY, Vedrinne JM, Salord F, Mercatello A, Robert D (1986) Septicémies dans les suites immédiates des arrêts cardio-circulatoires. Réan Soins Intens Med Urg 2:67–69
68. Deitch EA (1989) Simple intestinal obstruction causes bacterial translocation in man. Arch Surg 124:699–701
69. Wells CL, Maddaus MA, Simmons RL (1988) Proposed mechanisms for the translocation of intestinal bacteria. Rev Infect Dis 10:958–979
70. Howerton EE, Kolmen N (1972) The intestinal tract as a portal of entry of Pseudomonas in burned rats. J Trauma 12:335–340
71. LeFrock JL, Ellis CA, Turchik JB, Weinstein L (1973) Transient bacteremia associated with sigmoidoscopy. N Engl J Med 289:467–469
72. Dickman MD, Farrell R, Higgs RH, Wright LE, Humphries TJ, Wojcik JD (1976) Colonoscopy associated bacteremia. Surg Gynecol Obstet 142:173–176

73. Deitch EA, Xu D, Qi L, Berg RD (1991) Bacterial translocation from the gut impairs systemic immunity. Surgery 109:269–276
74. Marshall JC, Christou NV, Meakins JL (1988) Small-bowel bacterial overgrowth and systemic immunosuppression in experimental peritonitis. Surgery 104:404–411
75. Sullivan BJ, Swallow CJ, Girotti MJ, Rotstein OD (1991) Bacterial translocation induces procoagulant activity in tissue macrophages. A potential mechanism for end-organ dysfunction. Arch Surg 126:586–590
76. Jones WG, Barber AE, Minei JP, Fahey TJ, Shires GT III, Shires GT (1990) Antibiotic prophylaxis diminishes bacterial translocation but not mortality in experimental burn wound sepsis. J Trauma 30:737–740
77. Goris RJA, van Bebber IPT, Mollen RMH, Koopman JP (1991) Does selective decontamination of the gastrointestinal tract prevent multiple organ failure? Arch Surg 126:561–565
78. Alexander JW, Gianotti L, Pyles T, Carey MA, Babcock GF (1991) Distribution and survival of Escherichia coli translocating from the intestine after thermal injury. Ann Surg 213:558–567
79. Berczi I, Bertok L, Baindtner K, Vere B (1968) Failure of oral Escherichia coli endotoxin to induce either specific tolerance or toxic symptoms in rats. J Pathol Bact 96:481–486
80. Gans H, Matsumoto M (1974) The escape of endotoxin from the intestine. Surg Gynecol Obstet 139:395–402
81. Rush BF, Sori AJ, Murphy TF, Smith S, Flanagan JJ Jr, Machiedo GW (1988) Endotoxemia and bacteremia during hemorrhagic shock. Ann Surg 207:549–554
82. Roscher R, Oettinger W, Beger HG (1988) Bacterial microflora, endogenous endotoxin, and prostaglandins in small bowel obstruction. Am J Surg 155:348–355
83. Winchurch RA, Thupari JN, Munster AM (1987) Endotoxemia in burn patients: Levels of circulating endotoxins are related to burn size. Surgery 102:808–812
84. Wellman W, Fink PC, Benner F, Schmidt FW (1986) Endotoxaemia in active Crohn's disease. Treatment with whole gut irrigation and 5-aminosalicyclic acid. Gut 27:814–820
85. Cuevas P, Fine J (1972) Route of absorption of endotoxin from the intestine in nonseptic shock. J Reticuloendothelial Soc 11:536–538
86. Jacob AI, Goldberg PK, Bloom N, Degenshein GA, Kozinn PJ (1977) Endotoxin and bacteria in portal blood. Gastroenterology 72:1268–1270
87. Prytz H, Holst-Christensen J, Korner B, Liehr H (1976) Portal venous and systemic endotoxemia in patients without liver disease and systemic endotoxemia in patients with cirrhosis. Scand J Gastroenterol 11:857–863
88. Moore FA, Moore EE, Poggetti R, et al. (1991) Gut bacterial translocation via the portal vein: A clinical perspective with major torso trauma. J Trauma 31:629–638
89. Brearly S, Harris RI, Stone PCW, Keighly MRB (1985) Endotoxin level in portal and systemic blood. Dig Surg 2:70–72
90. Bienenstock J, Ernst PB, Underdown BJ (1987) The gastrointestinal tract as an immunologic organ: State of the art. Ann Allergy 59:17–20
91. Elson CO, Kagnoff MF, Fiocchi C, Befus AD, Targan S (1986) Intestinal immunity and inflammation: Recent progress. Gastroenterology 91:746–768
92. Bonneville M, Janeway CA, Ito K, et al. (1988) Intestinal intraepithelial lymphocytes are a distinct set of gamma/delta T cells. Nature 336:479–481
93. Groh V, Porcelli S, Fabbi M, et al. (1989). Human lymphocytes bearing T cell receptor gamma/delta are phenotypically diverse and evenly distributed throughout the lymphoid system. J Exp Med 169:1277–1294
94. Pirzer UC, Schurmann G, Post S, Betzler M, Meuer SC (1990) Differential responsiveness to CD3-Ti vs. CD2-dependent activation of human intestinal T lymphocytes. Eur J Immunol 20:2339–2342
95. James SP, Kwan WC, Sneller MC (1990) T cells in inductive and effector compartments of the intestinal mucosal immune system of nonhuman primates differ in lymphokine mRNA expression, lymphokine utilization, and regulatory function. J Immunol 144:1251–1256
96. Taguchi T, Aicher WK, Fujihashi K, et al. (1991) Novel function for intestinal intraepithelial lymphocytes. Murine CD3+, gamma/delta TCR+ T cells produce IFN-gamma and IL-5. J Immunol 147:3736–3744

97. Kawanishi H, Kiely J (1988) In vitro induction of a contrasuppressor immunoregulatory network by polyclonally activated T cells derived from murine Peyer's patches. Immunology 63:415–421
98. MacDonald TT, Dillon SB (1988) Chemical mediators of cellular communication. In: Heyworth MF, Jones AL (Eds) Immunology of the Gastrointestinal Tract and Liver, Raven Press Ltd., New York
99. Deem RL, Shanahan F, Targan SR (1991) Triggered human mucosal T cells release tumor necrosis factor-alpha and interferon-gamma which kill human colonic epithelial cells. Clin Exp Immunol 83:79–84
100. MacDonald TT, Hutchings P, Choy M-Y, Murch S, Cooke A (1990) Tumour necrosis factor-alpha and interferon-gamma production measured at the single cell level in normal and inflamed human intestine. Clin Exp Immunol 81:301–305
101. Mowat AMcI (1989) Antibodies to IFN- prevent immunologically mediated intestinal damage in murine graft-versus-host reaction. Immunology 68:18–23
102. Pullman WE, Elsbury S, Kobayashi M, Hapel AJ, Doe WF (1992) Enhanced mucosal cytokine production in inflammatory bowel disease. Gastroenterology 102:529–537
103. Keshav S, Lawson L, Chung LP, Stein M, Perry VH, Gordon S (1990) Tumor necrosis factor mRNA localized to Paneth cells of normal murine intestinal epithelium by in situ hybridization. J Exp Med 171:327–332
104. Bissonette EY, Befus AD (1990) Inhibition of mast cell-mediated cytotoxicity by IFN-alpha/beta and gamma. J Immunol 145:3385–3390
105. Elitsur Y, Luk DG (1991) Beta-casomorphin (BCM) and human colonic lamina propria lymphocyte proliferation. Clin Exp Immunoll 85:493–497
106. Pepys MB, Baltz ML (1983) Acute phase proteins with special reference to C reactive protein and related proteins (pentaxins) and serum amyloid A protein. Adv Immunol 34:141–212
107. Vetter ML, Gewurz H, Hansen B, James K, Baum LL (1983) Effects of C-reactive protein on human lymphocyte responsiveness. J Immunol 130:2121–2126
108. Arora PK, Miller HC (1978) Alpha 1 antitrypsin is an effector of immunological stasis. Nature 274:589–590
109. Munford RS, Andersen JM, Dietschy JM (1981) Site of tissue binding and uptake in vivo of bacterial lipopolysaccharide-high density lipoprotein complexes. Studies in the rat and squirrel monkey. J Clin Invest 68:1503–1513.
110. Gauldie J, Richards C, Harnish D, Lansdorp P, Baumann H (1987) Interferon B-2/B cell stimulating factor type 2 shares identity with monocyte-derived hepatocyte stimulating factor and regulates the major acute phase protein response in liver cells. Proc Natl Acad Sci 84:7251–7255
111. Decker K (1990) Biologically active products of stimulated liver macrophages (Kupffer cells). Eur J Biochem 192:245–261
112. Marshall JC, Bryden K, Murdoch J (1992) The Gut-liver axis in multiple organ failure: Kupffer cell modulation of systemic immune responses. In: Matuschak GM (ed) Multiple Systems Organ Failure: Hepatic Regulation of Systemic Host Defense. Marcel Dekker Inc, New York. (in press)
113. Callery MP, Mangino MJ, Kamei T, Flye MW (1990) Interleukin-6 production by endotoxin-stimulated Kupffer cells is regulated by prostaglandin E2. J Surg Res 48:523–527
114. Keller GA, West MA, Cerra FB (1985) Macrophage-mediated modulation of hepatic function in multiple-system failure. J Surg Res 39:555–563
115. Curran RD, Billiar TR, Stuehr DJ, Hofmann K, Simmons RL (1989) Hepatocytes produce nitrogen oxides from L-arginine in response to inflammatory products of Kupffer cells. J Exp Med 170:1769–1774
116. Colletti LM, Remick DG, Burtch DG, Kunkel SL, Strieter RM, Campbell DA (1990) Role of tumor necrosis factor alpha in the pathophysiologic alterations after hepatic ischemia/reperfusion injury in the rat. J Clin Invest 85:1936–1943
117. Fong Y, Marano MA, Moldawer LL, et al. (1990) The acute splanchnic and peripheral tissue metabolic response to endotoxin in humans. J Clin Invest 85:1896–1904

118. Chisari FV, Nakamura M, Milich DR, Han K, Molden D, Leroux-Roels GG (1985) Production of two distinct and independent hepatic immunoregulatory molecules by the perfused rat liver. Hepatology 5:735–743
119. Baumgardner GL, Billiar T, So SK, et al. (1989) In vitro immunosuppressive effects of murine hepatocyte cytosol. Transplantation Proc 21:1154–1155
120. Thomas HC (1977) The immune response in hepatic cirrhosis: Animal and human studies. Proc Roy Soc Med 70:521–525
121. Cantor HM, Dumont AE (1967) Hepatic suppression of sensitization to antigen absorbed into the portal system. Nature 215:744–745
122. Callery MP, Kamei T, Flye MW (1989) The effect of portacaval shunt on delayed-hypersensitivity responses following antigen feeding. J Surg Res 46:391–394
123. Boeckx W, Sobis H, Lacquet A, Gruwez J, Vandeputte M (1975) Prolongation of allogeneic heart graft survival in the rat after implantation on portal vein. Transplantation 19:145–149
124. Fujiwara H, Qian J-H, Satoh S, Kokudo S, Ikegami R, Hamaoka T (1986) Studies on the induction of tolerance to alloantigens. II. The generation of serum factor(s) able to transfer alloantigen-specific tolerance for delayed-type hypersensitivity by portal venous inoculation with allogeneic cells. J Immunol 136:2763–2768
125. Christou NV (1985) Host defence mechanisms in surgical patients: A correlative study of the delayed hypersensitivity skin-test response, granulocyte function and sepsis. Can J Surg 28:39–49
126. Keane RM, Birmingham W, Shatney CM, Winchurch RA, Munster AM (1983) Prediction of sepsis in the multitraumatic patient by assays of lymphocyte responsiveness. Surg Gynecol Obstet 156:163–167
127. Marshall JC, Christou NV, Meakins JL (1988) Immunomodulation by altered gastrointestinal tract flora. The effects of orally administered, killed Staphylococcus epidermidis, Candida, and Pseudomonas on systemic immune responses. Arch Surg 123:1465–1469
128. Marshall JC, Lee C, Meakins JL, Michel RP, Christou NV (1987) Kupffer cell modulation of the systemic immune response. Arch Surg 122:191–196
129. Marshall JC, Rode H, Christou NV, Meakins JL (1988) In vivo activation of Kupffer cells by endotoxin causes suppression of nonspecific, but not specific, systemic immunity. Surg Forum 39.111–113
130. Marshall JC, Ribeiro MA, Chu PTY, Sheiner PA, Rotstein OD (1992) Portal endotoxemia triggers the release of an immunosuppressive factor from splenic and alveolar macrophages. J Sung Res (in press)

Secondary Hepatic Dysfunction: Clinical Epidemiology, Pathogenesis and Current Therapeutic Approaches

S. Migliori and F. B. Cerra

Introduction

Hepatic dysfunction after trauma, surgery or infection is a common clinical event. This dysfunction is often evident within hours to a few days of injury, referred to as primary heptic dysfunction. The etiologies are usually related to the injury or to the shock and resuscitation response, e. g. hypoxia, direct tissue injury, endotoxemia.

Another variety of hepatic dysfunction has been described after these same injuries, referred to as secondary hepatic dysfunction or failure. This form of dysfunction occurs several days after injury and in the setting of a systemic inflammatory response and multiple organ dysfunction. In many patients, this dysfunction transforms into frank hepatic failure and death ensues. The etiology of this secondary hepatic dysfunction remains somewhat obscure. This chapter will attempt to present the clinical framework within which it occurs and its clinical characteristics, discuss some of the current thinking about its pathogenesis, and provide a basis for the standard and new therapeutic approaches to prevent the occurrence of and to treat the dysfunction once it is present.

Clinical Framework and Characteristics

Fig. 1 summarizes the response patterns to tissue injury. Following an injury event, there is a metabolic ebb phase usually associated with compromise of the microcirculatory perfusion. Within several hours of resuscitation, the flow phase response occurs. After a single, uncomplicated injury, this response tends to peak on day 3-5 and to abate by day 7-10 post-injury. With a severe injury in a compromised host, the response can proceed rapidly to death. With the occurrence of a complication, the response continues and organ dysfunction appears; and the process abates when the complication is corrected, as in the drainage of an abscess. In other settings of significant and persistent tissue injury, the response continues unabated, multiple organs fail and the patient expires. These patterns were originally described following polytrauma [1] but have now been observed after infections and septic shock [2-4], severe hypovolemia with or without shock [5-7], in the presence of inadequate resuscitation [8,9], and in the presence of severe inflammation as in pancreatitis [2].

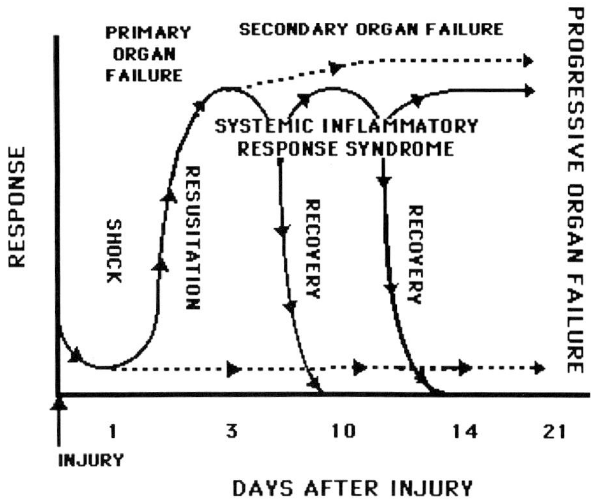

Fig. 1. Trauma, shock, infection, and tissue damage can induce a response best described as a systemic inflammatory response. This response has a number of clinical patterns; this figure summarizes these patterns

Once the response becomes manifest, the clinical characteristics are not distinguishable by etiology [2,4]. The local characteristics of an infection or an injury can clearly aid in diagnosis. However, in the presence of the systemic response, the usual clinical signs, symptoms and laboratory tests are not helpful in distinguishing the presence or absence of infection, traumatic injury, or perfusion-related injury. Hence, the concept of the systemic inflammatory response syndrome (SIRS) (hypermetabolism, hyperdynamic state, and sepsis syndrome) has evolved, with the term sepsis reserved for SIRS where there is evidence for a response to microorganisms or microorganisms in tissue where there should not be any [8].

Two general clinical pathways are followed (Fig. 2) [9,10]. In the first, frequently seen after a primary pulmonary initiating event such as aspiration, the progressive multiple organ dysfunction is a terminal event, becoming manifest only within a few days of death. In the second, commonly seen in septic shock with ARDS, the multiple organ dysfunction is present nearly from the time of injury, is stable for a 7-10 day period, and then becomes progressive. The transition to progressive multiple organ failure (MOF) is a significant prognostic event. It heralds a change in mortality risk from the 40-60% range to the 90-100% range.

Several clinical settings are associated with the transition from SIRS to the development of secondary organ dysfunction, including a persistent perfusion deficit, an unrecognized perfusion deficit, persistent flow-dependent oxygen consumption, a persistent focus of infection, the combination of a perfusion deficit and a persistent or new septic focus, a persistent inflammatory focus in the absence of infection such as acute fulminant pancreatitis (Fig. 3) [11-16] summarizes the common chemical indicators of this clinical course.

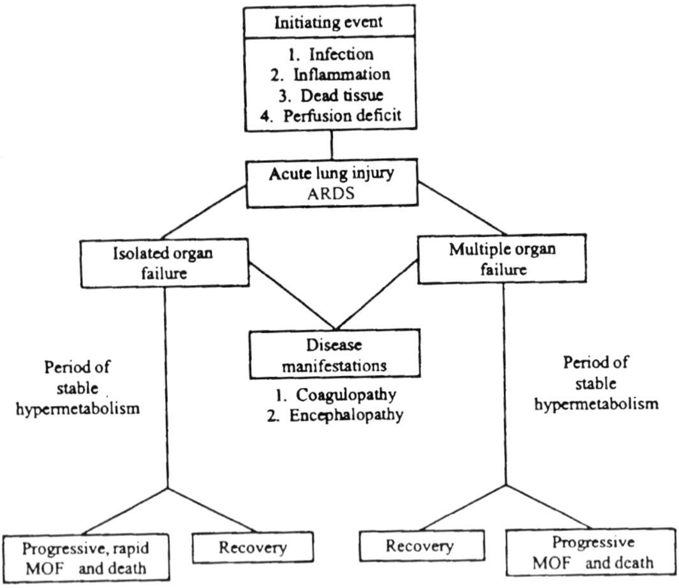

Fig. 2. Two general patterns of clinical response have been observed. In one, the clinical picture is dominated by pulmonary failure; in the other, by multiple organ failure

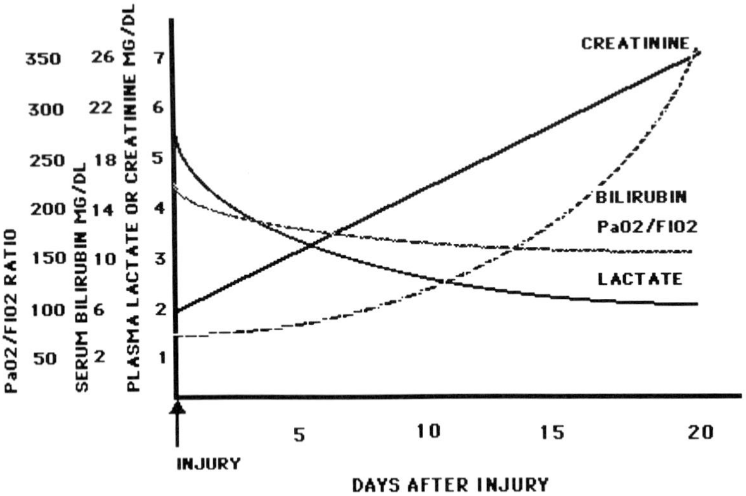

Fig. 3. The most commonly observed pattern of secondary hepatic failure is depicted. It manifests over time and is usually heralded by a progressive rise in serum bilirubin (secondary hepatic failure)

Within this context, hepatic dysfunction and failure occur. The patients manifest such abnormalities as progressive jaundice, biliary stasis, reduced hepatic amino-acid extraction and reduced hepatic and total body protein synthesis in the presence of nutrition support, increased hepatic triglyceride production with reduced peripheral triglyceride clearance, increased ureagenesis even in the absence of protein loading, reduced hepatic redox potential as reflected in the betahydroxybutyrate/acetoacetate ratio, and terminally, a failure of glucose release and hypoglycemia (Table 1) [2,4,12,17-19]. The physiologic and metabolic responses have been studied and characterized in a number of publications. These responses are summarized in Table 2 and represent the clinical manifestations of the inflammatory process. As such, their manifestation indicates the presence of SIRS and they function as outcomes to be explained by pathogenic mechanisms and for evaluating the response to therapeutic intervention.

Pathogenesis

The pathogenesis of the liver dysfunction is complex and changes over time (Table 6). This section will concentrate on mechanisms of regulation and provide examples of those mechanisms. It will focus on the post-resuscitative SIRS response and the transition to progressive organ failure.

A number of agents have been described that appear to be involved in the regulation of liver metabolism. These include substrate induction, macrohormones, cytokines, autocoids, and chemical mediators such as nitric oxide. They regulate and modulate different aspects of liver cell metabolism such as gluconeogenesis, protein synthesis, biotransformation and detoxification reactions, and ketone body synthesis. They originate from within and without the liver itself and act as hormone, paracrine, and autocrine agents. Ultimately, their mechanism of action affects second messenger generation, gene regulation, and/or energy production, distribution, or allocation.

Ketone Bodies

It has been nearly a universal finding that sepsis and inflammation in the absence of type I diabetes mellitus is associated with an absence of ketonemia and ketouria [2,4-20-23]. This has been interpreted as a reflection of a reduction in hepatic synthesis, putatively due to the associated increased levels of circulating insulin. During the SIRS response, the ratio of betahydroxybutyrate to acetoacetate is usually normal, reflecting a normal mitochondrial redox potential. When progressive organ failure occurs, the respiratory quotient can spontaneously exceed one, the very low density lipoprotein (VLDL) output from the liver increases, and the ketone body ratio progressively rises. This response probably reflects a falling mitochondrial redox potential.

Table 1. Characteristics of the liver dysfunction-failure of SIRS/MOF

Category	Characteristics
A. Clinical setting	persistent systemic inflammation after injury (hyperdynamic and hypermetabolic); persistent net catabolism and loss of lean body mass; wound failure; nosocomial infections
B. Clinical findings	jaundice; biliary dilatation and sledge; acalculous cholecystitis; coagulopathy; decreasing serum albumin and transferrin; increase in acute phase proteins early and a decrease in serum concentrations late in time-course; progressive nonresponsiveness of the visceral proteins to exogenous nutrition
C. Chemical findings	rising serum bilirubin; decreasing serum albumin and transferrin; increased and then decreased amino-acid extraction; decreased ketone body production with a progressive fall in betahydroxybutyrate/acetoacetate ratio;

Table 2. Characteristics of the systemic inflammatory response

Characteristic	Starvation	Systemic inflammation
oxygen consumption	-	++
cardiac output	-	++
systemic vascular resistance	NC	--
gluconeogenesis	-	+++
ketonemia	+++	-
proteolysis	+	+++
ureagenesis	+	++
total nitrogen excretion	+	+++
net catabolism	+	+++
lipolysis	+	++
acute phase protein synthesis	+	++
rate of malnutrition developing	+	+++
neuroendocrine activation	-	++
cytokine production	-	++

- = decreased, + = increased, NC = no change

Table 3. Effect of starvation and cecal ligation peritonitis on liver ketone body production

Characteristic	18 h fasting		66 h fasting	
	Control	Septic	Control	Septic
Liver blood flow, ml/kg/min	23±6	23±4	24±5	93±10*
Plasma ketone level, uM/l	10±2	13±5	30±9	30±19
Liver FFa delivery, uM/kg/min	9.7±7.5	15.9±9.3*	13.9±9	29±17.2
Liver ketone production, uM/kg/min	7±1.6	1.9±2.2*	4.5±5	6.2±5.1

* = $p < 0.05$

One of the problems in these studies is that the gut is both a major producer and user of ketone bodies. In a chronic *in vivo* canine model of peritonitis employing cecal ligation and puncture, the effects of bowel ketone metabolism can be controlled for. In this setting, over a 2-3 day period relative to control, hepatic blood flow increased, free fatty acid (FFA) delivery to the liver increased, hepatic ketone production (release) was initially suppressed but returned to control levels over the 2-3 day observation period. This latter return of liver ketone body release to control levels was felt to reflect the increased FFA supply to the liver in the septic state [20] (Table 3).

Hepatic FFA oxidation, through which ketogenesis occurs, is a mitochondrial function. This beta-oxidation process of long chain fatty acids is rate-limited at the step regulated by the enzyme carnitine palmitoyltransferase (CPT). This enzyme is the key portion of the transport of long chain acyl-Co-A-fatty acids from cytosol into the mitochondria where beta-oxidation occurs. In a rat model of cecal ligation and puncture (CLP) sepsis, plasma beta-hydroxybutyrate was reduced, CPT activity was decreased, and CPT gene transcription (mRNA) was decreased [24]. In the absence of sepsis, beta-agonists such as dobutamine, increased CPT gene expression and activity, and ketone body release. Additional studies in the CLP model have indicated a regulatory role for nuclear proteins of the leucine zipper class: c-FOS transcription and translation was increased; c-FOS appeared to inhibit c-JUN induced CPT gene expression [25].

Protein Synthesis

In the unstimulated state, the hepatocyte performs basal functions that are constitutive in nature, maintain the energy charge, and normalize its environment. For the liver cells to perform their functions, some form of signa-

Table 4. Functions of acute phase proteins during the inflammatory response

Acute phase protein	Response
A. Major Increase in Production	
1. C-reactive protein	opsonization
2. alpha-2-macroglobulin	antiproteinase, cytokine transport
3. cystein proteinase inhibitor	antiproteinase transport,
4. alpha-1-acid glycoprotein	such as drugs
B. Some Increase in Production	
1. haptoglobin	hemoglobin binding, particulary iron
2. ceruloplasmin	oxygen radical scavenger, transport
3. fibrinogen	coagulation
4. hemopexin	hemoglobin binding, particularly iron
5. alpha-1-proteinase inhibitor	antiproteinase
C. Decrease in Production	
1. albumin	transport
2. transferrin	transport

ling or directing needs to occur. This regulatory need has been discussed for ketone body production; this section will focus on some of the regulatory mechanisms involved in the regulation of hepatocellular protein synthesis. A number of such factors have been identified that regulate acute phase and nonacute phase protein synthesis. These include cortisol, cytokine, eicosanoid, and environmental factors such as the Kupffer cell, interstitial matrix components, lipopolysaccharide (LPS), and tissue oxygen tension.

The usual response in post-traumatic inflammatory states in characterized by increased net protein synthesis, a fractional increase in acute phase protein synthesis; a fractional decrease in the synthesis of non-acute phase protein such as albumin and transferrin; an increase in amino-acid clearance, and an increase in urea formation. When the transition to progressive hepatic failure occurs, the net synthesis of hepatocellular protein decreases with a decrease in both acute phase and non-acute phase protein synthesis, a decrease in amino-acid clearance, and a marked increase in the rate of ureagenesis [2,4].

The increased synthesis and release of acute phase proteins is characteristic of the acute inflammatory response [26,27]. Most of these reactants are glycoproteins and appear to have survival benefit and to perform a variety of functions. Some of these functions are summarized in Table 4.

Cortisol has long been recognized as being a necessary component of the regulation of the acute phase protein response. Cortisol interacts with hepatocytes by a transmembrane receptor with the activation of protein kinase. Its presence also appears to be necessary for the regulatory interaction be-

Table 5. Cytokine regulation of inflammatory proteins in hepatocytes (From [27] with permission)

Interaction	Acute phase proteins effected
A. IL-6 and IL-1 stimulation	C-reactive proteine, serum amyloid A, haptoglobin hemopexin, complement factor 3, alpha-1-glycoprotein
B. IL-6 stimulation	fibrinogen, ceruloplasmin, cysteine proteinase inhibitor, haptoglobin (human), alpha-2-macroglobulin
C. IL-1 and IL-6 synergy	complement factor 3, haptoglobin (rat), alpha-1 acid glycoprotein
D. IL-1 and IL-6 inhibition	fibrinogen, alpha-2-macroglobulin, cysteine proteinase inhibitor

tween hepatocytes and interleukin 6 (IL-6) [28]. Most of the acute phase proteins appear to have this requirement; most of the genes for the acute phase proteins appear to have a regulatory element for glucocorticoid in their respective promoter regions [29]. Cortisol has also been observed in cell culture to override the protein synthesis suppression of LPS on hepatocytes [30].

Perhaps the greatest modulator of acute phase protein synthesis in the inflammatory response is cytokine, particularly, IL-6, and tumor necrosis factor (TNF) [31-33]. The prototype pathway is one of specific receptor activation (g-protein system) with second messenger generation (phosphoinositol, diazoglycerol, calcium, protein kinase) and molecular regulation, through transcriptional mechanisms with modulation by the various groups of nuclear proteins. Protein kinase C does not appear to play a major role in the cytokine-induced acute phase protein response [27]. It appears as if different cytokines regulate different acute phase proteins; the cytokine interaction in timing and in amount affects the acute phase protein activated. A summary of these phenomena are presented in Table 5.

Hepatocytes exist in close proximetry to other cells such as Kuppfer cells, endothelial cells, and lipocytes; to matrix elements such as fibronectin, laminin, collagen and heparin and heparan; and are exposed in shock states to reductions in oxygen tension and increased amounts of LPS. All of these factors effect total liver cell protein synthesis and release; and the relative synthesis of acute phase and non-acute phase protein.

LPS acts directly and indirectly on hepatocellular protein synthesis. LPS can directly promote an acute phase response for a 23 Kd protein in rat and mouse hepatocytes [34]. The phenomenon is dose dependent and appears to be mediated through protein kinase C. The indirect interaction between hepatocytes and LPS occurs through macrophages [30]. The activated macrophage (or endothelial cell) releases cytokine. A number of agents can prime the macrophage for this response, including interferon, platelet activating

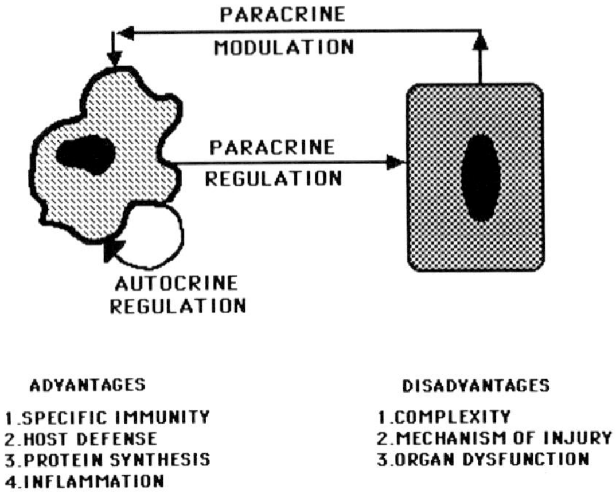

Fig. 4. Cell to cell communication is an important mechanism of regulating hepatocellular protein synthesis. Excessive or persistent inflammation, however, is associated with organ dysfunction and failure

factor (PAF), and hypoxia [35]. The response of the macrophage to LPS is dose dependent and mediated primarily through protein kinase C. The factors released by the activated macrophage in response to LPS include IL-1, IL-6, TNF, PGE_2 and nitric oxide.

When Kuppfer cells are placed in proximetry to hepatocytes, the basal rate of synthesis of hepatocellular secretory protein doubles with an increase in acute phase proteins and a relative decrease in the rate of albumin release [36]. With increasing doses of LPS, there is a progressive decrease in the hepatocellular protein synthesis of acute and non-acute phase proteins. This effect can be overridden by increases doses of dexamethazone or such matrix components as heparan or laminin (Matrigel) [37]. Supernatant transfer experiments indicate that the active mediators are in the Kuppfer cell supernate, and include IL-1, IL-6, TNF, PgE_2, and nitric oxide. Interestingly, the reverse supernate transfer from hepatocytes to Kuppfer cells enhances the Kuppfer cell release of the same mediators. Thus, the Kuppfer cells and the hepatocytes engage in two-way communication in the regulation of acute phase protein synthesis, an example of paracrine regulation (Fig. 4). In the presence of hypoxia, LPS induces the Kuppfer cells to release growth factors in addition to eicosanoids and monokines. Fibroblast growth factor is released under such conditions and stimulates fibroblast mitosis [35].

Gluconeogenesis

Gluconeogenesis is increased during the acute inflammatory response. This increase correlates with the increased glucose release and hyperglycemia characteristic of the process. The rate limiting step in gluconeogenesis is at the step of phosphoenolpyruvate carboxykinase (PEPCK). *In vitro,* IL-6 can inhibit PEPCK [38]. This phenomenon may account for the hypoglycemia observed in severe sepsis or the late stages of MOF.

Transition to Liver Failure

The characteristics of the transition to liver failure have been previously presented. The pathogenesis mechanisms for the transition remain largely hypothesis. In cell culture systems, it has yet to be demonstrated that the activated Kuppfer cell can injure the hepatocyte in some lethal or irreversible way. That hepatocyte injury can be induced by high amounts of such factors as TNF, has been observed. However, considerable question is raised as to whether these doses are relevant in the intact liver.

The area of greatest interest in this transition is that of molecular regulation and gene-mediated cell death. There are two lines of experimentation that are unfolding. In one, it is hypothesized that the accumulated injuries reach a threshold at which genetic self-destruction occurs, a phenomenon referred to as apoptosis [39,40]. The other approach concerns itself with hierarchically regulated cell death. During the homeostatic response, the synthesis of constitutive proteins (e.g. enzymes, structural) and acute phase proteins is expressed. When a threshold of injury occurs, the heat shock genes become expressed. Their expression may then obligate substrate and energy utilization such that constitutive synthetic function becomes compromised and individual cells begin to fail [39,40].

It is not necessary to hypothesize that individual cell death needs to occur in order to explain organism death from progressive MOF. Rather, only enough cell dysfunction needs to be present to interfere with organ function in a way that is incompatible with life in itself; or upsets inter-organ balance in a way that is not consistent with the function of other organs.

Therapeutic Approaches

Prevention remains the major therapeutic approach to organ dysfunction after injury, and for the secondary hepatic dysfunction and progressive organ failure after injury. The basic approach consists of three types of therapy: source control, restoration and maintenance of oxygen transport, and metabolic support (Fig. 5).

Whenever possible, complete control or removal of the cause of the inflammatory response should be performed, as in surgical control of bleeding, early drainage of an abscess, full-thickness burn excision and skin grafting for third degree burns, and early stabilization and fixation of fractures in trauma patients. These efforts are aimed at minimizing the soft tissue injury, and thus the degree of inflammatory response.

Rapid, effective resuscitation needs to be achieved concomitantly with source control. With the recognition of subclinical flow-dependent oxygen consumption in such settings as pancreatitits, ARDS, and septic and volume shock, and its relationship to SIRS-MOF, increased emphasis is placed on invasive techniques of resuscitation during the shock response, using oxygen consumption criteria [41-43]. Clinically relevant, flow-dependent oxygen

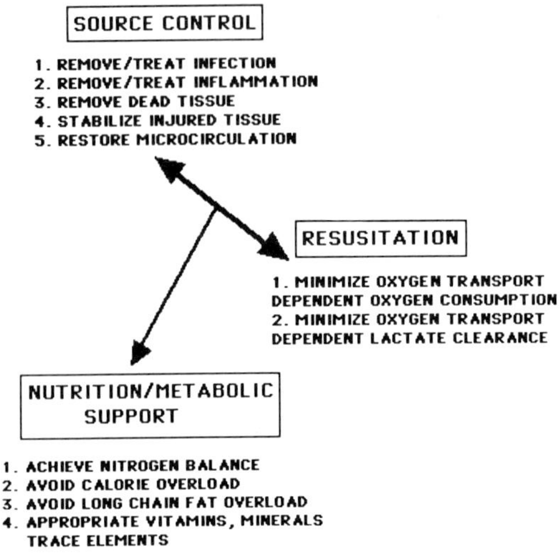

Fig. 5. The general approach to therapy is prevention and consists of control of the source, resuscitation, and the institution of appropriate nutrition/metabolic support.

consumption is treated with a comprehensive approach. Oxygen content is increased by maintaining an arterial oxygen tension that will maintain over 90% saturation of the arterial hemoglobin, and maintaining a hemoglobin in the 11-12 g% range. Oxygen consumption is then measured and flow increased until there is no clinically relevant increase in oxygen consumption, and the lactate/pyruvate ratio or plasma lactate returns to a normal range. In elective, high cardiovascular risk patients, studies also indicate a decrease in mortality, infectious complications and progressive MOF when these same principles are used [41].

Malnutrition is both a co-morbidity/co-mortality and a primary manifestation of SIRS-MOF. Current nutrition support does not alter the course of the disease process itself. Rather, standard nutrition support effectively minimizes the risk of single nutrient and generalized nutrient deficiency, resulting in a reduction in morbidity and mortality. Several principles have evolved [2,20,44-47]: provide 25-30 total calories/kg/day with 3-5 gm/kg/day as glucose; maintain a respiratory quotient under 0.9; provide long-chain, polyunsaturated w-6 fatty acids in doses less than 1.5 gm/kg/day [20]; start amino-acids, preferably the modified stress formulas at 1.5 gm/kg/day and promote nitrogen retention by adjusting the dose of amino-acids every 5-7 days to achieve nitrogen equilibrium; the enteral route is the preferred route of administration [44-47].

This approach to treatment has resulted in significant reductions in morbidity and mortality when it is effectively applied by knowledgeable practitioners. Nonetheless, the morbidity and mortality rates remain substantially elevated even in the younger age groups. Based on the concept that the inflammatory response may also contribute to the morbidity, mortality and resource costs, therapies are becoming directed at modulating the inflammatory response. These therapies are both specific and nonspecific. Specific therapy is targeted against a defined mediator, such as endotoxin,

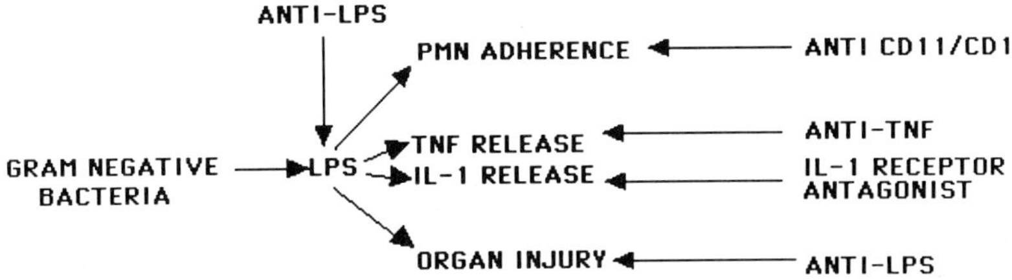

Fig. 6. One approach to therapy is to prevent or limit the response early in the cascade of mediator activation. Anti-endotoxin antibody, although the precise mechanism of action is unknown, is associated with a reduction in mortality and MOF in clinical use.

IL-1 receptors or TNF. Nonspecific therapy is directed at more generalized processes, such as second messenger generation (Fig. 6,7).

One of the best studied specific therapies is that of antibodies directed against endotoxin [48,49]. The rationale is that such therapy will prevent or ameliorate direct cell injury from LPS as well as a reduction in the injury from the inflammatory response that occurs. When administered to new ICU admissions who have infection with sepsis and gram-negative bacteremia, a reduction in mortality was observed. Currently, a number of monoclonal antibodies targeted to interfere with various points in the evolution of the inflammatory response are in clinical testing. They include antibodies designed to interfere with PMN adherence (anti CD18 or CD11), IL-1 receptors, or that bind TNF. Data is not yet available for analysis.

A number of questions and concerns remain related to dosing, the timing of their use, adverse reactions, whether or not there will be reasonable efficacy because they are too well targeted, leaving many alternate mediator pathways available; and whether or not cost-effectiveness will be demonstrable. For those reasons, less-targeted therapies are also being evaluated. These are designed to modulate the mechanisms through which the inflammatory process occurs or manifests itself, such as second messenger

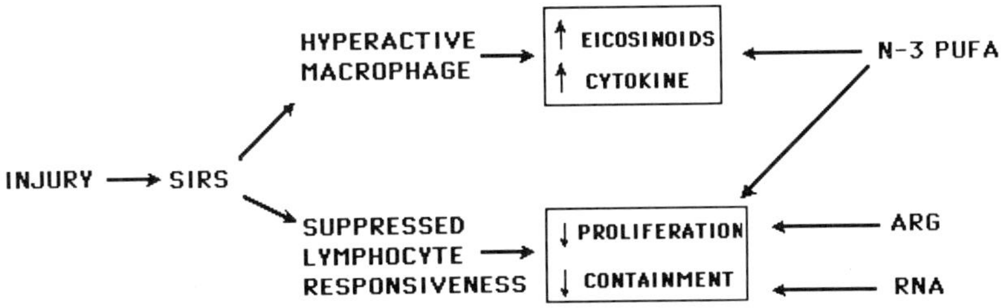

Fig. 7. Another approach to therapy is less specific and designed to modulate mechanisms that mediate SIRS. n-3 polyunsaturated fatty acids represent one such therapy, appears to have its effects by altering membrane fluidity, second messenger generation, and eicosanoid and cytokine release.

generation, antigen processing, or the proliferation response to specific antigen presentation.

The best studied nonspecific therapies are nutrients which use is designed to suppress the overactive macrophage and reduce the output of interleukin, TNF and eicosanoids such as PGE_2 and LTB_4, to stimulate lymphocyte proliferation in response to specific antigen stimulation, and to alter second messenger generation, particularly through the receptor mediated g-protein system. These therapies include n-3 PUFA such as eicosapentanoic acid (EPA) and docasahexanoic acid (DHA), arginine, uracil or ribonucleic acid (RNA). Arginine is considered a conditionally essential amino-acid. It is a potent secretogogue influencing many endocrine glands and has been observed to restore antigen-induced lymphocyte blastogenesis in immunosuppressed and postoperative cancer patients. The precise mechanism of these effects remains to be elucidated [50-55].

Nucleotides are precursors of deoxyribonucleic acid (DNA) and ribonucleic acid (RNA) [56]. The liver is probably the major source of preformed purines and pyrimidines for other tissues, although nucleotides are also reutilized through salvage pathways in such tissues as gut mucosa [57]. The absence of dietary nucleotides results in suppression of cellular immune responses [58]. Uracil, unlike adenine, can restore delayed type hypersensitivity response to various foreign antigens in mice, reduce abscess formation, enhance T-lymphocyte proliferation in tissue allograft models, and reverse the immunosuppression associated with blood transfusion [59,60]. It has also been suggested that dietary nucleotides are effective in macrophage activation of the T helper/inducer population [60].

n-3 polyunsaturated fatty acids (PUFA) alter the lipid composition of cell membranes, and effect membrane fluidity, second messenger generation, and the pattern of eicosanoid and cytokine synthesis and release [61-63]. Generally, the n-3 PUFA products are less potent than those of n-6 PUFA. A relative excess of linoleic acid substrate, a n-6 PUFA, stimulates PGE_2 production, which decreases the ability of cytokines to stimulate IL-2 synthesis by lymphocytes. The release of dienoic eicosanoids and TNF and IL-1 release by Kupffer cells is directly related to the amount of n-6 PUFA, n-3 PUFA and the n-3/n-6 PUFA ratio in the cell membrane [61,63-69]. The incorporation of the PUFA's into cell membranes can occur within hours of ingestion and become stabilized within 2-4 days [64,65]. In animal models, n-3 PUFA incorporation into cell membranes of liver cells and Kupffer cells was associated with a reduction in mortality in the presence of cecal ligation and puncture peritonitis [20].

Clinical trials with these agents as part of an enteral nutrition regimen have demonstrated restoration and enhancement of the *in vitro* tests of immune function, improved nutritional outcomes, and significant reductions in length of stay and nosocomial infection rates [69,70].

Unquestionably, combination therapies will be tested. These therapies will be designed to effect multiple points of the inflammatory response concurrently and sequentially, and specifically and nonspecifically. Whether they will have efficacy and be reasonably cost-effective await the clinical trials.

Conclusion

Secondary hepatic dysfunction is a major clinical event that occurs several days after an episode of shock and resuscitation following a significant tissue injury. In many patients, it proceeds to frank hepatic failure and death. The origin of this secondary hepatic failure remains somewhat controversial and appears to involve a number of mechanisms that regulate hepatic function. In this post-resuscitative phase of the inflammatory response, the dominant mechanisms appear to be related to cytokine modulation of gluconeogenesis, ketosis and protein synthesis in the presence of activated Kupffer cells and activated endothelial cells. The liver cells also actively participate in this regulation with cell to cell communication between themselves and the macrophages. In addition, other hormones such as cortisol and environmental factors such as endotoxin, pH, lactate, the prevailing oxygen tension and the interaction of matrix components all serve to modulate the regulatory functions. The primary mechanisms of regulation appear to be through second messenger generation and gene function (transcription and translation). The transition to frank organ failure remains hypothesis, with altered gene regulation being the focus of active research.

The major treatment of secondary hepatic failure remains prevention. The approach is through source control, rapid circulatory resuscitation, and aggressive nutrition/metabolic support. More recent approaches employ specific and nonspecific therapy. Specific therapy is directed toward specific mediators such as TNF or LPS. Nonspecific therapies are directed at mechanisms of mediator action such as second messenger generation or gene regulation. The nonspecific approach employs such nutrients as n-3 PUFA, arginine, and uracil. The clinical efficacy of both these specific and nonspecific therapies remains to be elucidated.

References

1. Baue AE (1975) Multiple, progressive or sequential systems failure: A syndrome of the 1970's. Arch Surgery 110:779–781
2. Cerra F (1987) Hypermetabolism, organ failure, and metabolic support. Surgery 101(1):1–14
3. Pine RW, Wertz MJ, Lennard ES, et al. (1983) Determinants of organ malfunction or death in patients with intraabdominal sepsis. Arch Surgery 118:242
4. Siegel JH, Cerra FB, Border JR, et al. (1979) Physiological and metabolic correlation in human sepsis.Surgery 806:409
5. Tilney N, Bailey G, Morgan A (1973) Sequential systems failure after rupture of abdominal aortic aneurysms. Ann Surgery 118:117
6. Baker CC, Oppenheimer L, Stephans B, et al. (1980) Epidemiology of trauma deaths. Am J Surg 140:144

7. Goris RJA, Draisma J (1982) Causes of death after blunt trauma. J Trauma 22:141
8. ACCP-SCCM Consensus Conference (1992) Definitions for sepsis and organ failure and guidelines for the use of innovative therapies in sepsis. Chest 101:1644–1655
9. Barton R, Cerra FB (1989) The hypermetabolism multiple system organ failure. Chest 96:1153–1160
10. Cerra FB, Negro F, Eyer S (1990) Multiple organ failure syndrome: pattens and effect of current therapy. In: Vincent IL (ed), Update in Intensive Care and Emergency Medicine Vol 10, Springer-Verlag, Berlin, pp 22–31
11. Goris RJA, Draisma J (1982): Causes of death after blunt trauma. J Trauma 22:141
12. Moyer ED, Border JR, Cerra FB, et al. (1981) Multiple systems organ failure VI: Death predictors in the trauma-septic state - the most critical determinants. J Trauma 21(10):862–869
13. Cerra FB, Siegel JH, Coleman B, Border JR, McMenamy RH (1980) Septic autocannibalism, a failure of exogenous nutritional support. Ann Surg 192:570–580
14. Bihari D, Smithies M, Gimson A, et al. (1987) The effects of vasodilation with prostacyclin on oxygen delivery and uptake in critically ill patients. New Engl J Med 317:397
15. Gutierrez G, Pohil R (1986) Oxygen consumption is linearly related to the oxygen supply in critically ill patients. J Crit Care Med 1:45
16. Danek S, Lynch J, Weg J, et al. (1980) The dependence of oxygen uptake on oxygen delivery in the adult respiratory distress syndrome. Am Rev Respir Dis 122:387
17. Cerra FB, Siegel JH, Border JR, Peters DM, McMenamy RH (1979) Correlations between metabolic and cardiopulmonary measurements in patients after trauma, general surgery and sepsis. J Trauma 19:621–629
18. Moyer ED, McMenamy RH, Cerra FB, et al. (1982) Multiple systems organ failure III: Contrasts in plasma amino acid profiles in septic trauma patients who subsequently survive and do not survive - Effect of intravenous amino acids. J Trauma 21(4):263–274
19. Moyer ED, Border JR, Cerra FB, (1981) Multiple systems organ failure IV: Imbalances in plasma amino acids associated with exogenous albumin in the trauma-septic patient. J Trauma 21:543–547
20. Cerra FB, Alden PA, Negro F, et al. (1988) Sepsis and exogenous lipid modulation. JPEN 12:63S–69S
21. Williamson CH (1981) Regulation of ketone body metabolism and the effect of injury. Acta Chir Scan 507:22–29
22. Neufeld HA, Pace JG, Kaminski MV, et al. (1980) A probable endocrine basis for the depression of ketone bodies during infections or inflammatory states in rats. Endocrinology 107:596–601.
23. Neufeld HA, Pace JA, White FE (1976) The effect of bacterial infections on ketone concentrations in rat liver and blood and on free fatty acid concentrations in rat blood. Metabolism 25:877–884
24. Barke RA, Brady PS, Brady LJ (1991) The effect of peritoneal sepsis on hepatic gene expression and hepatic mitochondrial long chain fatty acid oxidation in rats. Surg Forum 42:62–64
25. Barke RA, Brady PS, Roy S, Charboneau R, Brady L (1992) The possible inhibitory role of the leucine-zipper DNA binding protein c-FOS in the regulation of hepatic gene expression following sepsis. Surgery (in press)
26. Gallin JI (1983) Inflammation. In: Paul WE (ed), Fundamentals of Immunology, Raven Press, pp 721–733
27. Gaudie J, Baumann H (1992) Cytokines and acute phase protein expression. In: Kimball ES (ed), Cytokines and Inflammation. CRC Press pp 275–305
28. Baumann H, Richards C, Gaudie J (1987) Interaction among hepatocyte-stimulating factors interleukin 1, and glucocorticoids for regulation of acute stimulating factors interleukin 1, and glucocorticoids for regulation of acute phase plasma proteins in human hepatoma cells. J Immunol 139:4122–4128
29. Baumann H, Maquat LE (1986) Localization of DNA sequences involved in dexametasone-dependent expression of the rat alpha 1 aci glycoprotein gene. Mol Cell Biol 6:2551–2561
30. West MA, Keller G, Hyland B, et al. (1985) Hepatocyte function in sepsis: Kupffer cells mediate in biphasic protein synthesis response in hepatocytes after endotoxin and killed E coli. Surgery 98:388–395

31. Dinarello (1984) Interleukin-1 and the pathogenesis of the acute-phase response. New Engl J Med 311:341–344
32. Vilcek LEJ (1987) Biology of disease TNF and IL-1: Cytokines with multiple overlapping biological activities. Lab Invest 56:234–248
33. Le J, Weinstein D, Gubler U, and Vilcek J (1987) Induction of membrane-associated interleukin-1 by tumor necrosis factor in human fibroblasts. J Immunol 138:2137–2142
34. Mazuski JE, Platt JL, West MA, et al. (1988) Direct effects of endotoxin on hepatocytes. Arch Surgery 123:340–344
35. Bankey P, Fiegel B, Singh R, Knighton D, Cerra FB (1989) Hypoxia and endotoxin induce macrophage-mediated suppression of fibroblast proliferation. J Trauma 29:972–980
36. Mazuski JE, Bankey PE, Carlson A, Cerra FB (1988) Hepatocytes release factors that can modulate macrophage IL-1 secretion and proliferation. Surgical Forum 39:13–15
37. Bissel DM, Arenson DM, Maher JJ, Roll FJ (1987) Support of cultured hepatocytes by a laminin-rich gel. Evidence for a functionally significant subendothelial matrix in normal rat liver. J Clin Invest 79:801–812
38. Hill MR, Stith RD, McCallum RE (1989) Mechanism of action of interferon beta2/interleukin 6 on induction of hepatic liver enzymes. Ann N Y Acad Sci 557:502–505
39. De Maio A, Buchman T (1991) Molecular Biology of Circulatory Shock IV: translation and secretion of HEP G2 cell proteins are independently attenuated during heat shock. Surgery 34:329–335
40. Buchman TG, Cabin DE, Vickers S, et al. (1990) Molecular Biology of Circulatory Shock II: Expression of four groups of hepatic genes is enhanced following resuscitation from cardiogenic shock.Surgery 108:902–912
41. Berlauk JF, Abrams JH, Gilmour IJ, O'Connor SR, Knighton DR, Cerra FB (1991) Preoperative optimization of cardiovascular hemodynamics improves outcome in peripheral vascular surgery. Ann Surg 214:289–299
42. Shoemaker WC (1985) Hemodynamic and oxygen transport patterns in septic shock: physiologic mechanisms and therapeutic implications. In: Sibbald W, Sprung C (eds): New Horizons: Perspectives in Sepsis and Septic Shock. Society of Critical Care Medicine pp 203–234
43. Shoemaker W, Appel PL, Kram HB (1989) Tissue oxygen debt as a determinant of lethal and nonlethal postoperative organ failure. J Crit Care Med 16:1117–1121
44. Cerra FB, Hirsch J, Mullen K, Blackburn G, Luther W (1987) The effect of stress level, amino acid formula, and nitrogen dose on nitrogen retention in traumatic and septic stress. Ann Surg 205:282–287
45. Bower RHR, Muggin-Sullam M, Fischer J (1986) Branched chain amino acid-enriched solutions in the septic patient. Ann Surg 203:13–21
46. Moore EE, Dunn EL, Jones TN (1981) Immediate jejunostomy feeding after major abdominal trauma. Arch Surg 116:681
47. Cerra FB, McPherson J, Konstantinides FN, Konstantinides NN, Teasley KM (1988) Enteral nutrition does not prevent multiple organ failure syndrome after sepsis. Surgery 104:727–733
48. Dunn DL, Ferguson RM (1982) Immunotherapy of gram-negative sepsis: Enhanced survival in a guinea pig model by use of rabbit antiserum to Escherichia coli J5. Surgery 92:212
49. Ziegler EJ, Fisher CJ Jr, Sprung CL, et al. (1991) Treatment of gram-negative bacteremia and septic shock with HA-1A human monoclonal antibody against endotoxin. N Engl J Med 324:429–436
50. Barbul A, Sisto DA, Wasserkrug HL, et al. (1981) Metabolic and immune effects of arginine in post-injury hyperalimentation. J Trauma 21:970–974
51. Barbul A, Wasserkrug HL, Sisto DA, et al. (1980) Thymic and immune stimulatory actions of arginine. JPEN 4:446–449
52. Saito H, Trocki O, Wang S, et al. (1987) Metabolic and immune effects of dietary arginine supplementation after burn. Arch Surg 122:784–789
53. Barbul A, Sisto DA, Wasserkrug HL, et al. (1981) Arginine stimulates lymphocyte immune response in healthy humans. Surgery 90:244–251.
54. Reynolds JV, Thom AK, Zhang SM, et al. (1988) Arginine, protein calorie malnutrition and cancer. J Surg Res 45:513–522
55. Barbul A (1990) Arginine and immune function. Nutrition 6:53–58

56. Zöllner N, Gröbner W (1977) Dietary feedback regulation of purine and pyrimidine biosynthesis in man. In: Elliott K, Fitzsimons D, (eds). Purine and Pyrimidine Metabolism. Amsterdam, pp 165–178
57. Sonada T, Tatibana M (1978) Metabolic fate of pyrimidines and purines in dietary nucleic acids ingested by mice. Biochem Biophys Acta 521:55–66
58. Kulkarni AD, Fanslow WC, Rudolph FB, et al. (1986) Effect of dietary nucleotides on response to bacterial infections. JPEN 10:169–171
59. Kulkarni SS, Bhateley DC, Zander AR, et al. (1984) Functional impairment of T lymphocytes in mouse radiation chimeras by a nucleotide-free diet. Exp Hematol 12:694–699
60. Rudolph FB, Kulkarni AD, Fanslow WC, et al. (1990) Role of RNA as a dietary source of pyrimidines and purines in immune function. Nutrition 6:45–52
61. Kinsella J, Lakesh B, Boughton S (1990) Dietary PUFA and eicosanoids potential effects on the modulation of inflammation and immune cells. Nutrition 6:24–45
62. Spector AA, Yorek MA (1985) Membrane lipid composition and cellular functions. J Lipid Res 26:1015–1019
63. Kremer JM, Michalek AV, Kininger L, et al. (1985) Effect of manipulation of dietary fatty acids on clinical manifestations of rheumatoid arthritis. Lancet 1:184–187
64. Holman RT (1964): Nutritional and metabolic interrelationships between fatty acids. Fed Proc 23:1062–1067
65. Holman RT (1986) Control of polyunsaturated acids in tissue lipids. J Am Coll Nut 5: 236–265
66. Billiar TJ, Bankey PE, Svingen BA, et al. (1988): Fatty acid intake and Kupffer cell function alters eicosanoid and monopkine production to endotoxin stimulation. Surgery 104:343–349
67. Cook JA, Halushka PV (1989) Arachidonic acid metabolism in septic shock. In: Bihari DJ, Cerra FB (eds), New Horizons: Multiple Organ Failure. Society of Critical Care Medicine, pp 101–124
68. Cerra FB, Lehman S, Konstantinides N, Konstantinides F, Shronts EP, Holman R (1990) Effect of enteral nutrient on in vitro tests of immune function in ICU patients: A premilinary report. Nutrition 6:84–87
69. Lieberman M, Shou J, Torres BS, Daly J (1990) Effects of nutrient substrates on immune function. Nutrition 6:88–92

Cardiac Effects of the Mediators of Sepsis

J.L. Vincent and G. Berlot

Introduction

Like other forms of acute circulatory failure, septic shock is characterized by an imbalance between oxygen demand and oxygen supply. As a result, tissue hypoxia occurs, as reflected by the development of anaerobic metabolism and elevated blood lactate levels. Many clinical studies have indicated that in contrast to physiological conditions, oxygen uptake (VO_2) can remain dependent on oxygen delivery (DO_2) in patients with septic shock, even though cardiac output and DO_2 are generally normal or elevated.

The degree of severity of this imbalance between oxygen demand and supply is thought to be directly related to poor outcome. The VO_2/DO_2 dependency phenomenon could be a relatively transient phenomenon, so that its presence is not clearly related to survival. However, the degree of severity of the oxygen debt is directly reflected by the blood lactate levels, and the magnitude and the duration of the hyperlactatemia have been correlated with survival [1,2]. An increase in oxygen demand, an alteration in oxygen extraction and a reduction in myocardial contractility have been implicated in the development of septic shock [3].

The release of the various mediators of sepsis can be implicated in all three alterations. Several clinical studies have correlated the importance of the release of the various cytokines to the severity of the sepsis and the mortality rates [4-6]. Therefore, it is attractive to explore the interdependence between the immunological response and the tissue hypoxia in an attempt to eventually combine them in a unique pathophysiological defect (Fig. 1).

The therapeutic aspects of these two facets of septic shock are different. The optimization of the oxygen delivery has led to the proposal to increase DO_2 to supranormal levels in all patients at risk [7] or to tailor this therapy according to repeated measurements of blood lactate levels and oxygen-derived variables [8]. Focus on an exaggerated immunological reponse can lead to various forms of immunotherapy which have been tested, which are currently under trial, or which will be tested in the future. The present chapter will attempt to present some link between these hemodynamic and immunological alterations of severe sepsis, with a particular emphasis on the effects of the mediators of sepsis on the myocardial function. It will also discuss the possible hemodynamic effects of some forms of therapy directed against the mediators of sepsis.

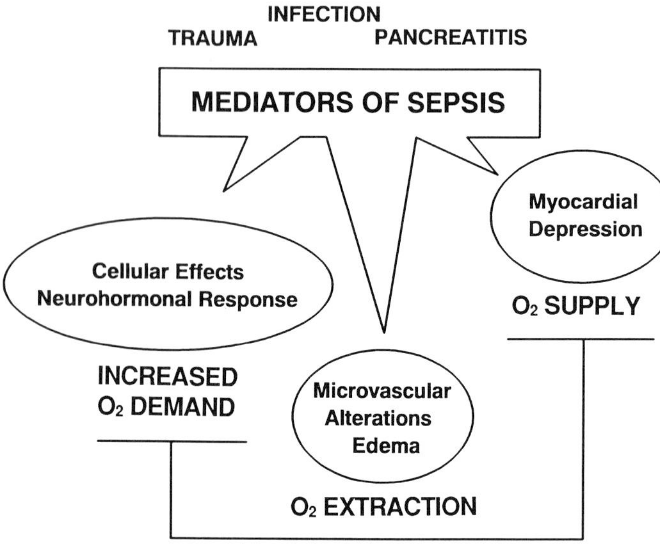

Fig. 1. The mediators of sepsis can influence each of the three major hemodynamic alterations characterizing severe sepsis: the increased oxygen demand, the altered oxygen extraction, and the myocardial depression.

Role of Tissue Hypoxia in Triggering the Mediators Response

The persistence of tissue hypoxia can represent an important trigger of the inflammatory response. Macrophage stimulation is known to be enhanced in hypoxic conditions [9,10]. Lactic acidosis has been suggested to increase the secretion and the transcription of TNF [11]. Acute circulatory failure triggers a strong sympathetic response, and the stimulation of the alpha-adrenergic receptors is known to increase the TNF release [12]. This enhanced inflammatory stimulation could, in turn, alter the oxygen balance of the tissues. Importantly, TNF release has been demonstrated after ischemia/reperfusion, even in the absence of sepsis. After 90 min of lobar hepatic ischemia in rats, Colletti et al. [13] observed that TNF was measurable during the reperfusion period in the plasma, but endotoxin was not. Pulmonary and hepatic injury was documented, and was furthermore prevented by the previous administration of anti-TNF antiserum [13].

The increased microvascular permeability observed during ischemia/reperfusion can be attenuated by agents increasing cyclic AMP, like isoproterenol, forskolin or dibutyryl-cAMP [14]. Adrenergic agents could limit the lesions also by promoting blood flow. Demling et al. [15] recently showed in awake sheep that dobutamine infusion could limit the oxidant-induced lung tissue lipid peroxidation, but did not reverse the increased permeability which was already present.

At a regional level, the release of the mediators could be implicated in the persistent ischemia to the gut, which could alter the integrity of the intestinal mucosa. The resulting translocation of bacteria and their products into the circulation could activate the cascade of the inflammatory mediators.

Role of the Mediators in the Development of Tissue Hypoxia

The Increased Oxygen Demand

The release of various mediators of sepsis is largely implicated in the inflammatory reaction which results in an increase in the cellular oxygen requirements. This hypermetabolic reaction is essential to promote host defense mechanisms and tissue repair. Interleukin 1 (IL-1) and other cytokines stimulate the hyperthermia which increases the cellular oxygen requirements. Their stimulation of the hypothalamic and adrenal glands, results in the release of growth hormone, ACTH, cortisol, glucagon, catecholamines and arachidonic acid metabolites [16,17]. The administration of small doses of TNF in rats produces significant increases in glucose, lactate, and triglycerides, and decreases in branched chain amino-acids [16]. Administration of TNF as part of a cancer therapeutic trial enhanced energy expenditure, with elevated CO_2 production, increased protein metabolism and lipolysis [18].

In early septic states, when cellular ATP stores are well maintained, ATP can be utilized at an increased rate, as indicated by a decrease in phosphocreatine levels in the muscle. The sometimes important cellular catabolism has been called "septic autocannibalism" [19]. TNF is known to promote muscle catabolism [20,21] inducing cachexia in animals like in patients with cancer. Its association with heart failure has been implicated with some catabolic effects as well [22].Although a cleavage product of IL-1 has been also implicated, IL-1 does not seem to increase muscle proteolysis [23]. Some of these catabolic effects could be also mediated by prostanoids [24].

The Altered Oxygen Extraction

The role played by the cascade of mediators on the alterations in extraction capabilities is quite complex. The capillary obstruction associated with the activation of leukocytes, platelets and other cellular elements, the decreased arteriolar responsiveness to adrenergic stimulation and the endothelial cells injury resulting in the development of interstitial edema can all participate in these alterations. TNF and other cytokines are known to induce endothelial cells adhesion properties and to increase adherence, sequestration and activation of neutrophils in the microvasculature.

Therefore, the alterations in extraction capabilities are related to a complex interplay between the activation of various cell types, the release of the mediators, and the secondary alterations in endothelial cells function with subsequent development of interstitial edema.

The cytokines have been implicated in the reduction in vascular tone that characterized sepsis. In rat cremaster muscle, Vicaut et al. [25] observed that TNF has acute vasodilating effects which are greatest for the small arterioles. The TNF administration by itself did not acutely alter the response of arterioles to vasopressive agents [25]. Hollenberg et al. [26] observed that TNF induces the relaxation of rat aortic rings, by direct effects on the endothelium and the smooth muscle. IL-1 also has been shown to directly reduce the reactivity of the vascular smooth muscle *in vitro* [27]. These effects of TNF and IL-1 could be at least in part indirectly mediated by the release of prostacyclin [25], which itself has been implicated in the sepsis-related vasodilation. In *in vitro* studies on rat aortic rings, the administration of ibuprofen was not found to influence the TNF-mediated relaxation [26]. Various studies showed that ibuprofen administration prevents the sepsis-related reduction in systemic vascular resistance. The release of nitric oxide (NO) (which accounts for the activity of the endothelium dependent relaxing factor) has also been implicated, as TNF can activate the NO-synthesis [28].

Some relationship has been established between the degree of vasodilation and the severity of sepsis. In animals, McKenna et al. [27] showed a direct relation between the amount of endotoxin administered and the loss of vascular response to norepinephrine stimulation. In patients, the severity of vasodilation is directly related to the severity of sepsis. Several groups of investigators [29-31] observed a lower systemic vascular resistance in the non-survivors than in the survivors from septic shock. A relationship between oxygen extraction capabilities and outcome is less well established.

The Altered Oxygen Transport

Cytokines could alter oxygen delivery by reducing the arterial oxygen content of the blood. In particular, the release of TNF has been implicated in the development of acute respiratory failure associated with sepsis [32]. However, the resulting hypoxemia is relatively easily recognized and compensated by oxygen therapy or mechanical ventilation. More insidious and less easily recognized is the development of myocardial depression.

Many experimental studies have indicated that the myocardial contractility was altered early after the administration of endotoxin or live bacteria in a variety of animal models [33]. Several mechanisms have been implicated, including the presence of alterations in the myocardial cell membrane or in the contractile apparatus, the development of myocardial edema, or in more severe cases, the development of myocardial hypoxia.

Although endotoxin does not seem to have any direct effect on the myocardium, its administration in volunteers results in an acute impairement of the cardiac function [34]. Several substances with negative inotropic properties have been described (Table 1). Various mediators of sepsis have been recently incriminated (Table 2).

Table 1. Some endogenous substances with myocardial depressant effects

Myocardial depressant factor (MDF)	Lefer at al. 1970	(83)
Early lipid-soluble cardiodepressant factor (ECDF)	Carli et al. 1980	(84)
Myocardial depressant substance (MDS)	Parrillo et al. 1985	(85)
Cardiodepressant factor (CDF)	Hallström et al. 1991	(86)

Table 2. Some mediators of sepsis with myocardial depressant effects

Tumor necrosis factor
Interleukin-1
Interleukin-2
Interferon-gamma
Platelet activating factor
Thromboxane
Leukotrienes
Oxygen free radicals

Several studies indicated that the administration of TNF or IL-1 in animals resulted in a significant reduction in arterial pressure and in cardiac output. However, the relative effects on venous return and on myocardial contractility was not always individualized in these studies. The effects of TNF on myocardial function were studied more specifically in dogs by Natanson et al. [35] who demonstrated that the administration of TNF, like the administration of endotoxin, decreases the ventricular ejection fraction. Other investigators recently reported comparable findings [36,37]. Administration of TNF in volunteers results in similar effects as those of endotoxin [38]. TNF also reduces the contractility of isolated myocytes [39]. *In vivo* administration of TNF in guinea pigs induces left atrial dysfunction demonstrated *ex vivo* [40]. Sometimes profound myocardial depression has been reported in patients receiving TNF as part of a cancer therapy [41]. It is intriguing to speculate that the increased TNF activity noted in some patients with heart failure [22] could contribute to the impairment of their cardiac function.

These effects of TNF could be mediated by a large variety of substances. TNF induces the release of other cytokines, PAF [42] or arachidonic acid metabolites [43].

IL-2 is another cytokine synthesized primarily by helper T-cells, which exerts multiple effects on the immune system. Their primary action is to activate natural killer cells. Administration of IL-2 as part of therapy has been shown to produce a hyperdynamic state associated with a reduction in myocardial contractility, as indicated by a decrease in left ventricular ejection fraction [44].

The administration of interferon also results in myocardial depression [45]. Repeated interferon administration in cancer patients can result in even more complex cardiac effects, including dilated cardiomyopathy, arrhythmias and ischemic heart disease. In most of the patients, this cardiac toxicity is reversible after the cessation of the therapy [46]. However, IL-6 administration has no detectable hemodynamic effect [47].

The mechanisms implicated in the cytokines-induced myocardial depression could be multiple. Cytokines could impair myocardial function by inducing a vasodilation that could reduce coronary blood flow. This phenomenon does not seem to be predominant, however, as the global coronary blood flow is usually well preserved and lactate production by the myocardium is not usually observed in clinical septic shock [48,49].

A direct or indirect effect of cytokines on the microvasculature, the endothelial cells and the myocardial cells is more likely. This hypothesis is supported by the observation that TNF reduces the contractility of isolated myocytes [39].Some of the effects of cytokines on the myocardial cells have been recently well elucidated. Both TNF and IL-1 inhibit the myocardial response to beta-adrenergic stimulation by an impairment of signal transduction [50,51]. Some studies have concluded to homologous desensitization, implicating that the receptor itself is affected [52]. Others reported that TNF can upregulate the Gi in the myocardium [53]. In some others, the adenylate cyclase activity was also reduced and the administration of propranolol had protective effects [54-56].

The effects of these cytokines could be mediated by complex mechanisms involving various cell elements and a number of released substances.This complex interrelation precludes the individualization of a single responsible mediator. Cytokines are known to induce the adherence of the leukocytes to the myocytes by CD18 dependent mechanisms and monoclonal antibodies that inhibit leukocyte adhesion reducing the myocardial reperfusion injury in dogs [57]. Activated leukocytes like T-lymphocytes can damage the myocardium [58].

Arachidonic acid metabolites could be implicated. The administration of OKY-046, a potent thromboxane synthase inhibitor, has been shown to prevent hte reduction in myocardial contractility otherwise observed after endotoxin administration by an alteration in the end-systolic pressure/diameter relationship and the dP/dtmax [59]. Thromboxane synthase inhibitors have been shown to improve myocardial function also following experimental cardiopulmonary bypass [60]. Leukotrienes are also known to present vasoconstrictive properties which could result in analogous effects [61]. Ibuprofen has been reported to have a protective effect on the myocardium during endotoxic shock [62].

Platelet activating factor (PAF) could also play a role. Chang et al. [63] have observed a parallelism between the decrease in cardiac output and the increase in PAF levels. PAF inhibitors have been shown to reduce the degree of myocardial depression [63,64]. PAF itself can increase the synthesis of arachidonic acid metabolites. Moore et al. [65] recently reported that the administration of a PAF receptor antagonist in lethal canine endotoxemia attenuated the release of thromboxane and improved survival.

The release of oxygen free radicals under the influence of the leukocytes activation is also likely to be implicated. Oxygen free radicals can alter the endothelial cells function, induce microvascular permeability changes and interstitial edema. They can also alter the sensitivity of the adrenergic receptors [66]. There is ample evidence that oxygen free radicals released during reperfusion following an ischemic event can alter the function of the heart like other organs. Myocardial function can be also altered following ischemia or hypoxia and reperfusion of the liver [67].

These effects of the cytokines on the myocardium could be enhanced by vasoconstricting effects of the mediators on the splanchnic circulation, resulting in gut ischemia, translocation of bacterial products and further release of cytokines. Oxygen radicals and eicosanoids have been implicated in the development of gut ischemia. Leukotrienes receptors antagonists have been shown to reduce the intestinal mucosal acidosis [68]. PAF could also reduce blood flow to the mesenteric circulation [69], even though a protective effect of PAF antagonists on the endotoxin-induced translocation has been questioned [70].

Right ventricular failure can be of particular importance in septic shock. Pulmonary hypertension is known to follow the administration of endotoxin in animals and to be associated with sepsis in man. The release of thromboxane [71], leukotrienes and PAF [72] have been implicated in the phenomenon. TNF itself has been reported recently to have vasodilating effects on the lung vasculature, when it was administered to perfused lung lobes [73]. Right ventricular dysfunction has been reported to develop early in the course of septic shock related to peritonitis. In addition, the degree of right ventricular impairment was found to be more severe in the non-survivors than in the survivors [74]. A more recent study using thermodilution measurements of right ventricular ejection fraction in patients with septic shock again indicated a stronger myocardial dysfunction in the non-survivors [31]. However, the pulmonary artery pressures were similar in the two groups, so that differences in contractility were incriminated.

Both the intensity of the immunological response and the severity of the myocardial depression are directly related to the severity of sepsis.A variety of experimental and clinical studies have shown that the myocardial depression was more severe in the more septic individuals. In particular, Mc Donough et al. [75] observed that the reduction in myocardial contractility was directly proportional to the amount of endotoxin administered to the animal. Several clinical studies reported that non-survivors from shock had a more severe ventricular impairment, as expressed by the relationship between ventricular stroke work and cardiac filling pressure [74,76] or by a lower right ventricular ejection fraction [31,77]. In the studies by Parker et al. [30], the left ventricular ejection fraction did not show the same pattern, probably because left ventricular ejection fraction is influenced not only by contractility but also by the left ventricular afterload, and the systemic vascular resistance is also lower in non-survivors [29-31].

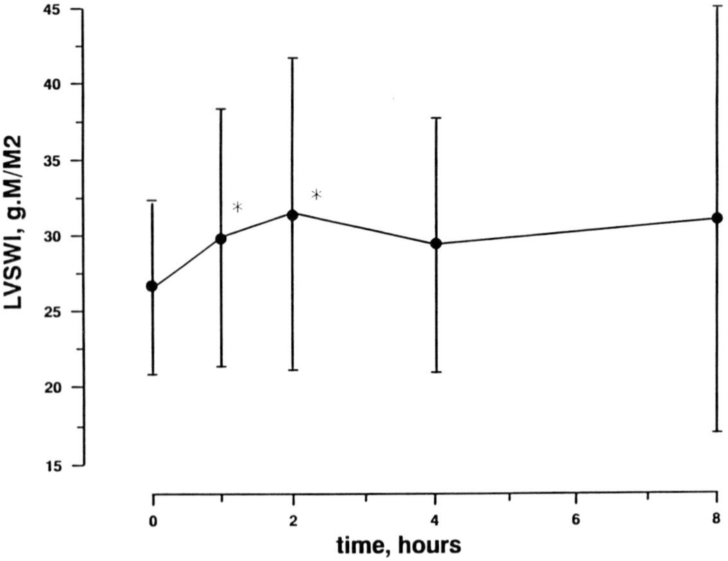

Fig. 2. Increase in left ventricular stroke work index following administration of anti-TNF antibodies in 10 patients with septic shock. (From [80] with permission.)

The effects of the inhibitors of this immunological response are expected to counterbalance this negative influence on myocardial contractility. In animals, the administration of anti-TNF antibodies was followed by a global cardiovascular improvement [78]. A preliminary report from Exley et al. [79] indicated that anti-TNF antibodies might increase blood pressure and reduce the vasopressor requirement in patients with septic shock. There was a simultaneous decrease in core temperature and in heart rate. A pilot study from our group [80] tended to confirm an increase in arterial pressure and a reduction in heart rate in 10 septic shock patients who received anti-TNF antibodies as part of a therapeutic trial. In addition, the data suggested that anti-TNF antibodies improved myocardial function, as indicated by an increase in ventricular stroke work (Fig. 2).

IL-1ra has been reported to improve left ventricular function in animals [81]. Some studies have suggested that the removal of some mediators by hemofiltration or plasmapheresis might improve cardiac function. Although some clinical studies have been also encouraging [82], well controlled prospective studies are still lacking.

Conclusions

The mediators of sepsis are implicated in the increased oxygen demand, the altered oxygen extraction and the reduced myocardial contractility that characterize severe sepsis. As all these factors are incriminated in the imbalance

Table 3. Relation betweenhemodynamic alterations of sepsis, influence of cytokines and their relation to outcome

Hemodynamic alterations	Influence of cytokines	Relation to outcome
Increased oxygen demand	yes	?
Peripheral vasodilation	yes	yes
Altered oxygen extraction	likely	likely
Myocardial depression	yes	yes
Increased capillary pemeability	yes	yes

between oxygen demand and oxygen supply, the magnitude of the immunological response and the degree of tissue hypoxia are likely to be interrelated (Table 3). Ultimate prognosis of septic shock has been related to the magnitude of the immunological response and to the severity of the tissue hypoxia.

References

1. Bakker J, Vincent JL (1991) The oxygen supply dependency phenomenon is associated with increased blood lactate levels. J Crit Care 6:152–159
2. Bakker J, Coffernils M, Leon M, Gris P, Vincent JL (1991) Blood lactate levels are superior to oxygen derived variables in predicting outcome in human septic shock. Chest 99:956–962
3. Vincent JL (1991) Diagnostic and medical management/supportive care of patients with gram-negative bacteremia and septic shock. Infect Dis Clin North Am 5:807–816
4. Damas P, Reuter A, Gysen P, Demonty J, Lamy M, Franchimont P (1989) Tumor necrosis factor and interleukin-1 serum levels during severe sepsis in humans. Crit Care Med 17:975–979
5. Calandra T, Baumgartner JD, Grau DG, et al. (1990) Prognostic values of tumor necrosis factor/cachectin, interleukin-1, interferon-alpha, and interferon-gamma in the serum of patients with septic shock. J Infect Dis 161:982–987
6. Pinsky MR, Vincent JL, Kahn RJ, Schandene L, Dupont E, Content J (1990) Inflammatory mediators of septic shock in man. Am Rev Respir Dis 141(Abs):A512
7. Shoemaker WC, Appel PL, Kram HB, Waxman K, Lee T (1988) Prospective trial of supranormal values of survivors as therapeutic goals in high-risk surgical patients. Chest 94:1176–1186
8. Vincent JL (1991) Advances in the concepts of intensive care. Am Heart J 121:1859–1865
9. Ghezzi P, Dinarello CA, Bianchi M (1991) Hypoxia increases IL-1 and TNF production by human mononuclear cells. Cytokine 3:189–194
10. Stellin G, Waxman K, Yamamoto R, Granger G (1991) Hypoxia stimulates release of tumor necrosis factor from human macrophages.Crit Care Med 4:S57
11. Jensen JG, Buresh C, Norton JA (1990) Lactic acidosis increases tumor necrosis factor secretion and transcription in vitro. J Surg Res 49:350–353
12. Spengler RN, Allen RM, Remick DG, Strieter RM, Kunkel SL (1990) Stimulation of alpha-adrenergic receptor augments the production of macrophage-drived tumor necrosis factor. J Immunol 145:1430–1434
13. Colletti LM, Remick DG, Burtch GD, Kunkel SL, Strieter RM, Campbell Da Jr (1990) Role of tumor necrosis factor-alpha in the pathophysiologic alterations after hepatic ischemia/reperfusion injury in the rat. J Clin Invest 85:1936–1943
14. Walman A, Parker S, Traystman R, Furtner G (1984) Isoproterenol protects against pulmonary edema in endotoxin lung injury. Anesthesiology 61:3–8

15. Demling RH, Knox J, Youn YK, Daryani R, LaLonde C (1992) Effect of dobutamine infusion on endotoxin-induced lipid peroxidation in awake sheep. Surgery 111:79–85
16. Darling G, Goldstein DS, Stull R, Gorschboth CM, Norton JA (1989) Tumor necrosis factor: Immune endocrine interaction. Surgery 106:1155–1160
17. Tracey KJ, Lowry SF, Fahey TS, et al. (1987) Cachectin/tumor necrosis factor induces lethal shock and stress hormone responses in the dog. Surg Gynecol Obstet 164:415–421
18. Starnes HF, Warren RS, Jeevanandam M, et al. (1988) Tumor necrosis factor and the acute metabolic response to tissue injury in man. J Clin Invest 82:1321–1325
19. Cerra FB (1989) Hypermetabolism, organ failure, and metabolic support. Surgery 191:1–6
20. Flores EA, Bistrian BR, Pomposelli JJ, Dinarello CA, Blackburn GL, Istfan NW (1989) Infusion of tumor necrosis factor/cachectin promotes muscle catabolism in the rat. J Clin Invest 83:1614–1622
21. Michie HR, Spriggs DR, Manogue KR, et al. (1988) Tumor necrosis factor and endotoxin induce similar metabolic responses in human beings. Surgery 104:280–286
22. Levine B, Kalman J, Mayer L, Fillit HM, Packer M (1990) Elevated circulating levels of tumor necrosis factor in severe chronic heart failure. N Engl J Med 323:236–241
23. Goodman MN (1991) Tumor necrosis factor induces skeletal muscle protein breakdown in rats. Am J Physiol 260:727–730
24. Baracos V, Rodemann P, Dinarello CA, et al. (1983) Stimulation of muscle protein degradation and prostaglandin E2 release by leukocytic pyrogen (interleukin-1). A mechanism for the increased degradation of muscle proteins during fever. N Engl J Med 308:553–558
25. Vicaut E, Hou X, Payen D, Bousseau A, Tedgui A (1991) Acute effects of tumor necrosis factor on the microcirculation in rat cremaster muscle. J Clin Invest 87:1537–1540
26. Hollenberg SM, Cunnion RE, Parrillo JE (1991) The effect of tumor necrosis factor on vascular smooth muscle. Chest 100:1133–1137
27. McKenna T (1990) Prolonged exposure of rat aorta to low levels of endotoxin in vitro results in impaired contractility. J Clin Invest 86:160–168
28. Kilbourn RG, Gross SS, Jubran A, et al. (1990) NG-methyl-L-arginine inhibits tumor necrosis factor-induced hypotension: Implications for the involvement of nitric oxide. Proc Natl Acad Sci USA 87:3629–3632
29. Groeneveld AB, Bronsveld W, Thijs LG 81986) Hemodynamic determinants of mortality in human septic shock. Surgery 99:140–152
30. Parker MM, Suffredini AF, Natanson C, Ognibene FP, Shelhamer JH, Parrillo JE (1989) Responses of left ventricular function in survivors and nonsurvivors of septic shock. J Crit Care 4:19–25
31. Vincent JL, Gris P, Coffernils M, et al. (1992) Myocardial depression and decreased vascular tone characterize fatal course from septic shock. Surgery (in press).
32. Stephens KE, Ishizaka A, Larrick JW, Raffin TA (1988) Tumor necrosis factor causes increased pulmonary permeability and edema. Am Rev Respir Dis 137:1364–1370
33. Abel FL (1989) Myocardial function in sepsis and endotoxin shock. Am J Physiol 257:R1265-R1281
34. Suffredini AF, Fromm RE, Parker MM, et al. (1989) The cardiovascular response of normal humans to the administration of endotoxin. N Engl J Med 321:280–287
35. Natanson C, Eichenholz PW, Danner RL, et al. (1989) Endotoxin and tumor necrosis factor challenges in dogs stimulate the cardiovascular profile of human septic shock. J Exp Med 169:823–832
36. Pagani FD, Baker LS, Knox MA, et al. (1991) Tumor necrosis factor alpha causes diastolic creep and reversible left ventricular systolic dysfunction in conscious dogs. Surg Forum 41:40–43
37. Horibe M, Tezuka S, Okada K (1991) Changes in Emax after administration of tumor necrosis factor. Circ Shock (Abs) 34:22
38. Schirmer JM, Fry DE (1989) Recombinant human tumor necrosis factor produces hemodynamic changes characteristic of sepsis and endotoxemia. Arch Surg 124:445–448
39. Hollemberg SM, Cunnion RE, Lawrence M, Kelly JL, Parrillo JE (1989) Tumor necrosis factor depress myocardial cell function: Results using an in vitro assay of myocyte performance. Clin Res 37:528–534

40. Heard SO, Perkins MW, Fink MP (1992) Tumor necrosis factor-alpha causes myocardial depression in guinea pigs. Crit Care Med 20:523–527
41. Hegewisch S, Weh JH, Hossfeld DK (1990) TNF-induced cardiomyopathy. Lancet (Letter) 1:294–295
42. Bakker J (1992) Serial blood lactate levels can predict multiple organ failure in septic shock patients. Crit Care Med (Abs) (in press)
43. Roubin R, Elsas PP, Fiers W, Dessein AJ (1987) Recombinant human tumor necrosis factor (rTNF) endhances leukotriene biosynthesis in neutrophils and eosinophils stimulated with the Ca_2^+ ionophore A23187. Clin Exp Immunol 70:484–490
44. Ognibene FP, Parker MM, Natanson C, Shelhamer JH, Parrillo JE (1988) Depressed left ventricular performance. Response to volume infusion in patients with sepsis and septic shock. Chest 93:903–910
45. Deyton LR, Walker RE, Konvacs JA, et al. (1989) Reversible cardiac dysfunction associated with interferon alpha therapy in AIDS patients with Kaposi's sarcoma. N Engl J Med 321:1246–1249
46. Sonnenblick M, Rosin A (1991) Cardiotoxicity of interferon. Chest 99:557–561
47. Preiser JC, Schmartz D, Van der Linden P, et al. (1991) IL-6 administration has no acute hemodynamic effect in the dog. Cytokine 3:1–4
48. Cunnion RE, Schaer GL, Parker MM, Natanson C, Parrillo JE (1986) The coronary circulation in human septic shock. Circulation 73:637–644
49. Dhainaut JF, Huyghebaert MF, Monsallier JF, et al. (1987) Coronary hemodynamics and myocardial metabolism of lactate, free fatty acids, glucose, and ketones in patients with septic shock. Circulation 75:533–541
50. Gulick T, Chung MK, Pieper SJ, Lange LG, Schreiner GF (1989) Interleukin 1 and tumor necrosis factor inhibit cardiac myocyte beta-adrenergic responsiveness. Proc Natl Acad Sci USA 86:6753–6757
51. Chung MK, Gulick TS, Rotondo RE, Schreiner GF, Lange LG (1990) Mechanism of cytokine inhibition of beta-adrenergic agonist stimulation of cyclic AMP in rat cardiac myocytes - Impairment of signal transduction. Circ Res 67:753–763
52. Notterman D. Steinberg C, Metakis L, Singh M (1991) Tumor necrosis factor (TNF) produces homologous desensitization of the beta-adrenergic receptor complex. Crit Care Med 19:S74
53. Reithmann C, Gierschik P, Werdan K, Jakobs KH (1991) Tumor necrosis factor alpha up-regulates Gi alpha and G beta proteins and adenylate cyclase responsiveness in rat cardiomyocytes. Eur J Pharmacol 206:53–60
54. Mak IT, Kramer JH, Freedman AM, Tse SYH, Weglicki WB (1990) Oxygen radical-mediated injury of myocytes – Protection by propranolol. J Mol Cell Cardiol 22:687–695
55. Massey KD, Burton K (1990) Free radical damage in neonatal rat cardiac myocyte cultures: Effects of alpha-tocopherol, trolox, and phytol. Free Radical Biol Med 8:449–458
56. Wagenknecht B, Hug M, Freudenrich C, et al. (1990) Cardiodepressive and cardiotoxic effects of oxygen free radicals in cultured heart muscle cells. J Mol Cell Cardiol 22:S51
57. Simpson PJ, Todd RF, Fantone JC, Mickelson JK, Griffin JD, Lucchesi BR (1988) Reduction of experimental canine myocardial reperfusion injury by a monoclonal antibody (anti-MO1, anti-CD11b) that inhibits leukocyte adhesion. J Clin Invest 81:624–629
58. Woodley SL, McMillan M, Shelby J, et al. (1991) Myocyte injury and contraction abnormalities produced by cytoxic T lymphocytes. Circulation 83:1410–1418
59. Fujioka K, Sugi K, Isago T, et al. (1991) Thromboxane synthase inhibition and cardiopulmonary function during endotoxemia in sheep. J Appl Physiol 71: 1376–1381
60. Kulatilake N, Gonzalez-Lavin L, Grover GJ (1991) Thromboxane A2 receptor blockade improves contractile function following cardiopulmonary bypass in dogs and pigs. J Surg Res 51:336–340
61. Etemadi AR, Tempel GE, Farah BA, Wise WC, Halushka PV, Cook JA (1987) Beneficial effects of a leukotriene antagonist on endotoxin-induced acute hemodynamic alterations. Circ Shock 22:55–63
62. Soulsby ME, Jacobs ER, Perlmutter BH, Bone RG (1984) Protection of myocardial function during endotoxin shock by ibuprofen. Prostaglandins Leukotrienes Med 13:295–305

63. Chang SW, Feddersen CO, Henson PM, Voelkel NF (1987) Platelet-activating factor mediates hemodynamic changes and lung injury in endotoxin-treated rats. J Clin Invest 79:1498:1509
64. Doebber TW, Wu MS, Robbins JC, Choy BM, Chang MN, Shen TY (1985) Platelet-activating factor (PAF) involvement in endotoxin-induced hypotension in rats. Studies with PAF-receptor antagonist kadsurenone. Biochem Biophys Res Commun 127:799–808
65. Moore JM, Earnest MA, DiSimone AG, Abumrad NN, Fletcher JR (1991) A PAF receptor antagonist, BN 52021 attenuates thromboxane release and improves survival in lethal canine endotoxemia. Circ Shock 35:53–59
66. Kaneko M, Chapman DC, Ganguly PK, Beamish RE, Dhalla NS (1991) Modification of cardiac adrenergic receptors by oxygen free radicals. Am J Physiol 260:821–826
67. Pretto EO (1991) Cardiac function after hepatic ischemia-anoxia and reperfusion injury: A new experimental model. Crit Care Med 19:1188–1193
68. Cohn SM, Fink MP, Lee PC, et al. (1990) LY 171883 preserves mesenteric perfusion in porcine endotoxin shock. J Surg Res 49:37
69. Qi M, Jones SB (1990) Contribution of platelet activating factor to hemodynamic and sympathetic responses to bacterial endotoxin in conscious rats. Circ Shock 32:153–163
70. Deitch EA, Ma L, MA JW, et al. (1989) Inhibition of endotoxin-induced bacterial translocation in mice. J Clin Invest 84:36–41
71. Snapper JR, Hutchinson AA, Ogletree ML, Brigham KL (1983) Effects of cyclooxygenase inhibitors on the alterations in lung mechanics caused by endotoxemia in the unanesthetized sheep. J Clin Invest 72:63–76
72. Horvath CJ, Kaplan JE, Asrar BM (1991) Role of platelet-activating factor in mediating tumor necrosis factor alpha-induced pulmonary vasoconstriction and plasma-lymph protein transport. Am Rev Respir Dis 144:1337–1341
73. Mayers I, Johnson D, Hurst T, To T (1991) Interactions of tumor necrosis factor and granulocytes with pulmonary vascular resistance. J Appl Physiol 71:2338–2345
74. Vincent JL, Weil MH, Puri V, Carlson RW (1981) Circulatory shock associated with purulent peritonitis. Am J Surg 142:262–270
75. McDonough KW, Brumfield BA, Lang CH (1986) In vitro myocardial performance after lethal and nonlethal doses of endotoxin. Am J Physiol 250:H240–H246
76. D'Orio V, Mendes P,Saad G, Marcelle R (1990) Accuracy in early prediction of prognosis of patients with septic shock by analysis of simple indices: Prospective study. Crit Care Med 18:1339–1345
77. Vincent JL, Frank RN, Contempre B, Kahn RJ (1989) Right ventricular dysfunction in septic shock: Assesment by measurements of right ventricular ejection fraction using the thermodilution technique. Acta Anaesthesiol Scand 33:34–38
78. Tracey KJ, Wei H, Manogue KR, et al. (1988) Cachectin/tumor necrosis factor induces cachexia, anemia and inflammation. J Exp Med 167:1211–1214
79. Exley AR, Cohen J, Buurman WA, et al. (1900) Monoclonal antibody to TNF in severe septic shock. Lancet (Letter) 2:1275–1277
80. Vincent JL, Bakker J, Marécaux G, Schandene L, Kahn RJ, Dupont E (1992) Anti-TNF antibodies administration increases myocardial contractility in septic shock patients. Chest 101:810–815
81. Fisher CJ (1992). J Clin Invest (in press)
82. Barzilay E, Kessler D, Lesmes C, et al. (1988) Sequential plasmafilter dialysis with slow continuous hemofiltration: Additional treatment for sepsis induced AOSF treatment. J Crit Care 3:163–166
83. Lefer AM (1970) Role of a myocardial depressant factor in the pathogenesis of circulatory shock. Fed Proc 29:1836–1847
84. Carli A, Auclair MC, Vernimmen C, Jourdon P (1979) Reversal of calcium of rat heart cell dysfunction induced by human sera in septic shock. Circ Shock 6:147–151
85. Parrillo JE, Burch C, Shelhamer JH (1985) A circulating myocardial depressant substance in humans with septic shock. J Clin Invest 76:1539–1553
86. Hallström S, Koidl B, Müller U, Werdan K, Schlag G (1991) A cardiodepressant factor isolated from blood blocks Ca2+ current in cardiomyocytes. Heart Circ Physiol 29:869–876

The Peripheral Vasculature

C. Bernard, A. Tedgui, and D. Payen

Introduction

The hemodynamic profile of septic shock in humans has been well described [1] and some authors have suggested that the severity and profile of these physiological changes are predictive of survival in surgical patients [2,3]. However, others failed to find these correlations in non-surgical patients [4], and hemodynamic data from clinical and experimental literature questioned these patterns. Briefly, one can discuss the respective role of direct or indirect effects of sepsis on the observed hemodynamic patterns in human and animal models. The hyperkinetic status is characterized by an elevated cardiac output and low peripheral vascular resistances combined with hypotension. This might result from septic injury, reflex activation, and often resuscitation especially fluid administration.

If the modification of the cardiac function during severe sepsis has been extensively demonstrated [5], the peripheral vasculature impairment remains relatively unclear. The available data demonstrate a broad range of alterations in vascular responsiveness complicating sepsis from vasoplegia to vasoconstriction. This imprecision may result from:

1) the difference in sepsis model, especially the species used and the type of septic injury;
2) the use of anesthetic agents which may interfere with vasoregulation;
3) the importance of fluid resuscitation before measurements;
4) the study perfomed early or late after septic injury;
5) the predominance or not of myocardial failure on peripheral vascular failure;
6) the differences between regional circulations; and
7) the *in vitro* studies.

This chapter will focus on peripheral vessel hemodynamics and mechanisms leading to vascular failure during severe sepsis considering the vessel as an organ.

Hemodynamic Aspects

Hemodynamic Patterns during Septic Shock

In addition to cardiac dysfunction, septic shock is generally associated with vasoplegia, which concerns arterioles and veins. The heterogeneity of vasodilation is the main factor of abnormal distribution of flow between organs [6,7]. For some authors, vasoplegia correlates with outcome of septic shock [3,8], but in different ways. Depending on the parameter used, hypotension with high cardiac output is associated with a higher rate of survivors [9,4], whereas the ability to reduce vasoplegia during a cardiac output decrease indicates a better outcome [3].

Although the capacitive circulation, i.e. the veins, has received little attention in sepsis, few data demonstrate an increase in systemic effective compliance from 2.3 to 4.5 ml/mm Hg.kg [10]. The combination of an arterial and venous vasodilation should be analyzed in the light of venous return concept.

AC Guyton et al. [11] emphasized that the regulation of cardiac output is determined by the interaction between the vasculature and the heart: the heart can only pump the amount of blood returning to the cardiac chambers which represent the venous return (VR). Focusing on the venous side, the increase in effective compliance during sepsis may create a mismatch between the contained volume and the vascular container.

Since VR is determined by the mean systemic pressure (MSP) and venous resistance, these parameters should be analyzed to theorize VR in septic shock. MSP value is determined by volemia and vascular compliance [12]. Since volemia does not change during the early phase of sepsis because capillary leak is not yet predominant, MSP can be changed only by modifications of vascular compliance, i.e. venous compliance.

Active venodilation has been described as part of septic shock [12]. In the venous capacitance vessels, a loss of normal constrictor tone leads to pool the blood toward the venous circulation. As a consequence, an important fraction of stress volume becomes an unstress volume allowing to shift MSP to the left, and to reduce VR. Using an endotoxin model, Pinsky et al. [13] have shown a depressed venous return as a consequence of splanchnic pooling despite a normal blood volume, assessed by an elevation of hepatic blood volume [14].

However, the presence of venous resistance increase cannot be excluded. It can result from passive increase secondary to vein collapsus or to reflexly mediated venoconstriction. Although the venous resistance component has not received much attention in sepsis, it has been shown in septic patients that forearm venous capacity was decreased in association with an increase in forearm venous tone [15]. At the level of this human circulation, before any treatment, progressive vasodilation was not associated with severe sepsis. It can be concluded that several factors including hypotension might increase local venous resistance, amplifying the decrease in VR.

From the physiological point of view, little is known about the components of the left ventricle afterload. In other words, the impact of severe sepsis on conductive and resistive arterial vessels is not well established from *in vivo* data. Future studies on aortic impedance during sepsis are required to evaluate the modifications of arterial mechanics in term of resistance, compliance and reflective waves [16]. This concept outlines the difficulty to interpret *in vitro* results obtained from different types of isolated arteries and to integrate these results in the *in vivo* patterns.

Moreover, systemic hemodynamic data should be analyzed in the light of the possible intrication between the direct and the indirect mechanisms of vasomotor tone during septic shock, as recently stated by Schumacker [17]. Direct mechanisms may involve a complex network of mediators released in response to endotoxin as cytokines, eicosanoids, nitric oxide, etc. ... Indirect mechanism may result from reflex activation of vasoconstrictive substances as catecholamines, angiotensin, neuropeptides, or from metabolic vasomotion especially during hypoperfusion [18]. The observed effect on vasomotor tone is then the resultant of these components and is difficult to assess clinically, since the calculation of peripheral resistances includes cardiac function and peripheral vasomotion.

In accordance with the above discussion, cardiac output in the pretreatment phase of septic shock should solely be either unchanged or decreased as a result of VR impairment (Fig. 1). The acute treatment of septic shock should depend on which abnormal determinant(s) of venous return is (are) altered. Administration of vasoactive drugs might be confusing because of

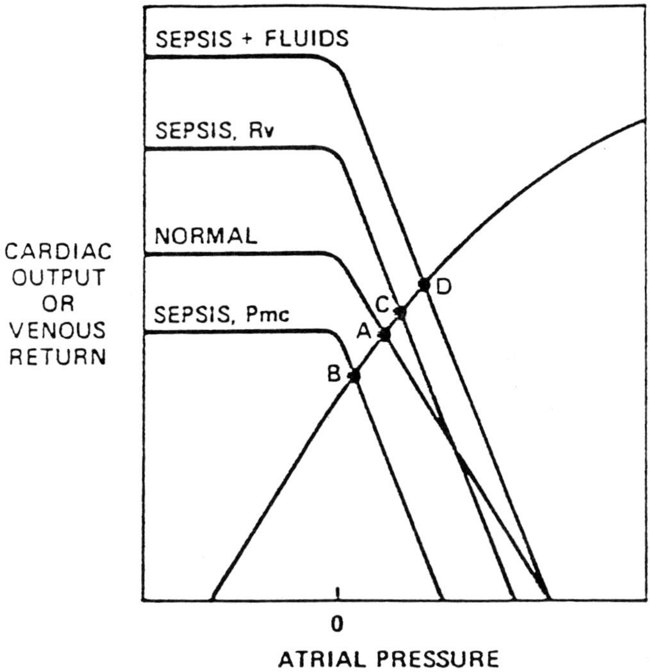

Fig. 1. Sepsis with venodilatation causing a decreased resistance to venous return (Rv) and mean circulatory pressure (Pmc) with no change in cardiac function. Cardiac output (venous return) and atrial pressure may be decreased if Pmc dominates (point A to B), or increased if Rv dominates (point A to C). With fluid therapy, cardiac output and atrial pressure are increased by normalizing Pmc (point D). (From [12] with permission)

their non-specific activity on the vasculature. Fluid therapy remains of primary importance in septic shock according to the venous approach. When septic shock involves venodilation, it is crucial to maintain MSP; when septic shock involves venoconstriction, elevation of MSP is required to overcome the increase in venous resistance.

Finally, vascular failure also concerns microvasculature. *In vivo* studies using intravital microscopy have demonstrated different microcirculatory responses to sepsis induced by *E. Coli.* Vasoconstriction was observed in the gut [19] whereas vasodilation was noted in the hepatic circulation [20]. The response in squeletal muscle seems more complex, as small arterioles dilated, and large arterioles constricted [21]. According to these observations, Vicaut et al. [22] have demonstrated a vasodilation induced by topical TNF application on cremaster muscle of rat, partially mediated by prostaglandins. This model provide the opportunity to study the direct effect of substances involved in the pathogenesis of sepsis, since the substances are locally administered in normal animals. Because of the greater contribution of small arteriolar dilation to the calculated systemic resistance, it is proposed that the differential arteriolar response was sufficient to explain the depressed systemic vascular resistance in sepsis [21].

Regional Aspects

Compared to extensive data on systemic circulatory changes in sepsis, the knowledge on concurrent changes in organ pressure and flow remains limited.

The decrease in systemic vascular resistance does not exclude regional constriction. This has led some authors to propose the concept of distributive shock to describe septic shock [21]. For example, Sibbald et al. [23] found that animals in which sepsis induced by cecal perforation did not manifest an adaptative redistribution in flow from the splanchnic organs to the myocardium. In a rat septic model, Lang et al. [6] found an elevation of cardiac output and flow to myocardium, liver, spleen, small intestine, whereas gastric, pancreatic, portal, renal and squeletal muscle flows were diminished. The use of α-adrenergic blockers could preserve from the depression of regional blood flows, suggesting that adrenergic mechanisms contribute to the regional flow modifications [6]. Moreover, within the organ, excessive blood flow to some territorial units may occur, depriving other units with high metabolic activity, resulting in a "vascular steal phenomenon" [24].

It can be then concluded that this abnormalities are not necessarily shared by all vascular beds, both *between* different organs and *within* different organs.

Vasoplegia

Two types of altered vascular responsiveness need to be described: an impaired vascular smooth muscle response to vasoconstrictive agents; and an impaired endothelium-dependent regulation of the vascular tone.

A depressed vascular responsiveness to exogenous catecholamines has been demonstrated in clinical studies and animal models of sepsis [25,26]. Moreover, this impairment concerns also other vasoconstrictive substances and non-hormonal responses. Some authors have also demonstrated a depressed regional vasodilatory response to ischemia, i.e. an altered reactive hyperemia [15]. Schematically, vasodilation results from an imbalance between vasoconstricting and vasodilating factors acting on vascular smooth muscle cell.

Vasoconstriction/Vasodilation Mechanisms

Vasoconstriction Pathways: In vascular smooth muscle cells, surface receptors respond to neurotransmitters and circulating vasoconstrictor hormones by activating the enzyme phospholipase C via a coupling to guanosine triphosphate binding protein (G protein) located in the plasma membrane. Phospholipase-C-hydrolysates-phosphatidylinositol-4,5-biphosphate to generate two second messengers, diacylglycerol (DAG) and inositol-1,4,5-triphosphate (IP3). DAG activates protein kinase C which phosphorylates several target proteins, while IP3 mobilizes cytosolic calcium from the endoplasmic reticulum. The entry of external calcium through receptor operated channels is facilitated by inositol-1,3,4,5-tetraphosphate (IP4) formed by the phosphorylation of IP3.

Vasodilation Pathways: In addition to an impairment of the vasoconstrictive pathway, vascular hyporesponsiveness might be caused by a stimulation of the vasodilation pathways.

The vasodilation pathways include endothelium-dependent and -independent mechanisms. cAMP and cGMP are the two important mediators of smooth muscle relaxation. Increase in smooth muscle cGMP levels occurs in response to atrial natriuretic factor (ANF) and agents containing the unstable free radical nitric oxide (NO), such as nitrovasodilators or endothelium-derived relaxing factor (EDRF). NO interacts with the iron atom in heme to activate soluble guanylate cyclase, whereas ANF activates a particulate form of guanylate cyclase. These two enzymes stimulate the synthesis of cGMP from GTP. Increase in cAMP is caused by β-adrenergic agonists as well as other activators of adenylate cyclase. Increase in cyclic nucleotides seems to induce vasodilation through the inhibition of constrictive pathways at different molecular levels: phosphoinositide turnover, Ca^{++} disponibility, myosin light chain kinase, via the activity of cGMP and cAMP-dependent protein kinases. However, the specific substrate proteins for these kinases are not well characterized in vascular smooth muscle cells; one predominant mechanism may be the Ca-ATPase activation by phosphorylation of phospholamban by the cGMP-kinase. In addition, the presence of cGMP-dependent protein kinase in vascular smooth muscle cells is required for the reduction of calcium by both cGMP and cAMP, suggesting that the same enzyme mediates the relaxing effects of both cyclic nucleotides.

Hypocontractility

Depression of Contractile Responses: The hypocontractility of vessels has been extensively described using either arteries excised from septic animals or arteries incubated in the presence of LPS. The vascular response to contractile agonists are depressed *in vitro* with a decrease in maximal contraction and an elevation of EC (Fig. 2) [27-29].

A hallmark of hypocontractility is the time-dependency, since contractility diminishes gradually after an endotoxic challenge. Wakabayashi et al. [30] reported in endotoxin-treated rats that aortic hypocontractility precluded the decrease in blood pressure.

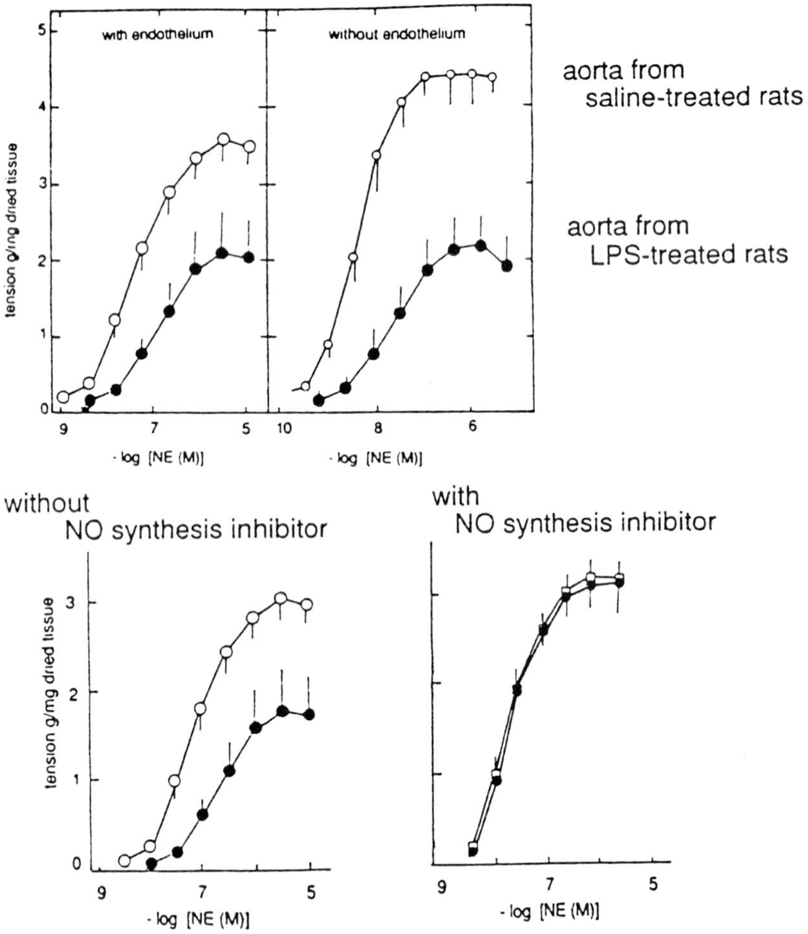

Fig. 2 Upper part: norepinephrine concentration-response curves in aortic rings from saline *(open circle)* and lipopolysaccharide (LPS) treated rats *(filled circle)*. Lower part: norepinephrine concentration-responses curves in aortic rings from saline *(open symbols)* and LPS-treated rats *(filled symbols)*. (From [27] with permission)

Hypocontractility is not mediated by the Endothelium: After LPS treatment, endothelium removal seems not to modify the vascular sensitivity. Julou-Schaeffer et al. [27] showed in aorta from rats treated with LPS that the response to norepinephrine was futher decreased after endothelium removal (Fig. 2). Conversely, McKenna [31] found that vascular endothelium partially contributed to aortic hypocontractility in septic rats.

Hypoconctractility Variability: If hypocontractility concerns the different components of vasculature, its magnitude may vary between vessels. Stoclet et al. [32] showed that unlike the aorta, contractile responses were only slightly reduced in resistance arterioles (mesenteric, femoral) from endotoxin-treated rats. Seaman et al. [14] reported an impaired contractility of hepatic vein to nerve stimulation or to infusion of norepinephrine or angiotensin II in cats. Baker et al. [33] found an alteration of adrenergic response of microcirculation exposed to endotoxin.

Molecular Mechanisms: Many stages of the receptor-mediated contraction seem to be altered and concern several agonists as norepinephrine, phenylephrine, angiotensin II, thromboxane analog U-46619, serotonin and endothelin.

Alterations of membrane signal transduction: Changes in the number of receptors without change in affinity have been described. Indeed, α1-receptor number is reduced in aorta isolated from septic rats [34] but this does not reflect a generalized down-regulation of receptors in sepsis. Numerous other receptors (opioid, β-adrenoreceptor, 5-hydroxytryptamine) are unaltered, and the down-regulation seems to be selective to certain tissues (vascular and hepatic) [34]. Both basal and stimulated phosphatidyl inositol (PI) hydrolysis are suppressed in arteries from endotoxemic animals. Alteration in PI hydrolysis is thus not a receptor specific event. It seems to be mainly due to a decrease in the synthesis of PI since the basal level of inositol monophosphate accumulation is markedly reduced in aorta taken from septic rats [35].

Alterations of intracellular signal transduction: The non-receptor-mediated contractile responses are also depressed such as those induced by Ca, membrane depolarization with KCl and phorbolesters activating proteine kinase C. KCl-induced contractions are markedly reduced in endotoxemic aortas although the corresponding Ca influx via the opening of the voltage-dependent calcium channels is not affected. In addition, intracellular alkalinization-induced contraction was also significantly inhibited in endotoxemic rat aortas [35]. An alteration in intracellular Ca handling or in calcium sensitivity have been proposed to explain hypocontractility. ATP-dependent calcium uptake in vascular smooth muscle at subcellular fractions level, is damaged by endotoxin.

The contractile apparatus seems to be intact: The vascular contraction induced by okadaik acid (inhibitor of myosin-light-chain phosphatase) is normal [35], and Stoclet et al. [32] reported that hypocontractility could be overcome by high calcium concentrations.

It can be concluded that both transmembrane and intracellular signallings are altered by endotoxin whereas the contractile apparatus is intact, indicating that LPS does not operate as a direct toxic cellular agent and that hypocontractility might be reversible.

Role of the L-arginine/Nitric Oxide (NO) Pathway or cGMP as an Effector of Endotoxin-Induced Hyporeactivity

Modifications of the vascular reactivity by NO result from an increase in the cGMP content in smooth muscle, produced by direct stimulation of the soluble guanylate cyclase. Many recent studies evidence that an increase in cGMP by activation of the L-arginine/NO pathway is involved in the vascular hyporeactivity produced by endotoxemia.

L-arginine/Nitric Oxide Pathway: NO has been shown to be released from the L-arginine oxydation pathway in various mammalian cells, including endothelial cells, brain cells, macrophages, neutrophils, platelets, Kupffer cells, and vascular smooth muscle cells [36]. Different enzymes (NO-synthases) are involved in the NO biosynthesis; schematically, one type of NO synthases being Ca^{++}-calmodulin-dependent, constitutive isoform and rapidly activated; the other type being tetrahydrobiopterin-dependent, inducible isoform and requiring time to be activated. The former appears to operate in endothelial and brain cells, while the other has been identified in macrophages [36].

The particulate Ca/calmodulin-dependent enzyme is responsible for over 90% of the EDRF/NO synthesis in endothelial cells. There is, in the vasculature, a continuous utilization of L-arginine for the generation of NO which plays a role in the maintenance of pressure and flow. Vascular smooth muscle cells seem to express only the cytosolic Ca^{++}-independent isoform of NO synthase [32,37], which induction is inhibited by cycloheximide and dexamethasone [38]. A class of L-arginine analogues inhibit both constitutive and inducible forms of NO-synthase.

Involvement of the L-arginine/NO Pathway in Hypocontractility: The activation of the L-arginine/NO pathway appears to be involved in the vascular hyporeactivity induced by endotoxin. First evidence for the possible role of the L-arginine/NO pathway has been given by results of high nitrate and nitrite levels found in urines of septic patients [39]. The *in vivo* response to norepinephrine in rats infused with *E. Coli* LPS can be restored by inhibitors of NO synthesis [40]. In endotoxic pithed rats, a model in which NO is greatly overproduced, arginase pretreatment increases the pressor response to phenylephrine by plasma arginine decrease.

In addition, *in vitro* experiments gave support to the involvement of the L-arginine/NO pathway as the major effector mechanism of vascular hypocontractility. McKenna [28] reported that inhibition of endogenous cGMP production by methylene blue, improved responses of aorta from septic rats to both norepinephrine and KCl. cGMP contents are elevated in aortic rings from LPS treated rats and are associated with hyporeactivity [27,41].

Inflammatory Induction of the L-arginine/NO Pathway in Smooth Muscle: A recent important discovery has demonstrated that L-arginine/NO pathway is activated in smooth muscle itself. The first evidence suggesting an extra-endothelial production of NO-like relaxing factor induced by endotoxin, came from the use of specific inhibitors of NO synthesis. These inhibitors fully reversed the hyporeactivity of endothelium-denuded aorta from endotoxemic rats (Fig. 2) [27]. The same observation was found in conductive and resistive arteries [42]. In addition, the arteries from endotoxemic rats were relaxed by the addition of exogenous L-arginine to the organ bath, whereas those from control rats were not [42]. On isolated medial smooth muscle layer, endotoxin increased cGMP content by the induction of NO synthase [43]. The L-arginine/NO pathway in vascular smooth muscle involves the expression of NO synthase only inducible by immunological mediators, i.e. LPS and cytokines IL-1 and TNFα.

Is L-arginine-derived NO Beneficial or Deleterious? The L-arginine pathway, activated in response to LPS and cytokines, has been evidenced in the arterial wall with seemingly deleterious effects. However, this pathway has also been described in other organs and might play a protective role. L-arginine-derived NO is induced within hepatocytes following production of multiple cytokines by LPS activated Kupffer cells [44]. *In vivo* NO-inhibitor increases liver injury induced by LPS administration. It thus appears that in endotoxemia, hepatocyte-derived NO may protect hepatocytes, either through a direct NO-induced modification in hepatic metabolism, or through a maintained adequate liver blood flow.

In addition, NO produced by vascular cells participates in the cooperation between vascular and blood cells, with an antiaggregant property towards platelets and an antichemotactic activity on leukocytes [45]. Lefer et al. [46] showed that NO provides significant myocardial protection after ischemia and reperfusion. Moreover, an endogenous production of NO may help to maintain vascular integrity after acute endotoxin-induced intestinal damage in rats. Inhaled NO acts as a selective pulmonary vasodilator reversing hypoxic pulmonary vasoconstriction, further supporting the concept of beneficial aspects of NO on regional circulations [47].

In fact, studies on short-term effects of NO-inhibitors in animal models of endotoxin shock become more documented and provide conflicting results. Administration of NO-inhibitors to rats and dogs treated with endotoxin or tumor necrosis factor has been found to increase blood pressure but also to reduce cardiac output [48]. Moreover, administration of NO-inhibitors in LPS-treated rabbits precipitates the fall in blood pressure and the death of the animals [49].

Role of the Cytokines

Cytokines: A Complex Network Involved in the Hemodynamics of Septic Shock: Even though LPS administered to animals is able to produce septic shock, the lethal effect of bacterial LPS is conferred by cells of hematopoietic origin. The transplantation of bone marrow from mice sensitive to LPS (C3H/HeN) to genetically similar mice resistant to LPS (C3H/HeJ) made the latter sensitive to LPS [50]. The macrophage is implicated as a source of septic shock mediators. Among the cytokines released by macrophages in response to LPS, tumor necrosis factor (TNF) produces physiological disturbances which closely mimic those observed upon endotoxin administration [51]. Pretreatment by TNF-specific antibodies prevents death after subsequent administration of lethal doses of endotoxin [52]. In rabbits, anti-TNF antibody infusion, 30-45 min before LPS injection, provides significant protection from hypotension and lethality, and results in inhibition of the LPS-induced serum TNF activity [53]. Even though TNF plays a pivotal role acting as a proximal mediator, it may not be the only mediator in sepsis. Interleukin-1 (IL-1) *per se* is also able to induce a shock-like state in rabbits with hypotension and decreased SVR which can be reversed by IL-1 receptor antagonist treatment [54]. IL-1β synergistically enhances the effects of TNF. While low doses of IL-1β and TNF separately are unable to cause shock, simultaneous administration of these cytokines produces shock [54].

Cytokines Network and the Vascular Wall: Cytokines interact in a network with three essential features. The biological redundancy: individual cytokines have multiple overlapping synergistic activities. The biological amplification: cytokines induce each others as well as their own production in a cytokine cascade. And finally, targets are often sources, adding in complexity of the concurrent messages. TNF, IL-1 and IL-6 are cytokines mainly produced by macrophages, but various other types of cells are found to be sources, especially vascular cells. The vessel has now to be considered as a critical partner in immune and endocrine system. Vascular cells in culture are able to secrete copious amounts of cytokines (TNF, IL-1 and IL-6) with different secretory abilities between endothelial and smooth muscle cells [55]. Recently, LPS has been shown to activate aortic tissue in culture to produce cytokines [28], and IL-1 is able to induce its own expression in an autocrine secretory action [56]. Finally, as a cooperation between blood cells and vascular cells, an amplification of cytokine release is found when rabbit carotids are exposed *in vitro* to LPS-activated macrophages [57].

Contractile Depressive Effect of Cytokines: In vitro, cytokines have been identified as potent inhibitors of vascular contraction via an endothelium-independent mechanism. IL-1 has been reported to inhibit the phenylephrine-induced contraction of rat aorta after a previous exposure to cytokine [58], an effect which was not prevented by indomethacin. TNF had similar depressive effect on the phenylephrine-induced contraction of rabbit carotid [59] and rat aorta [56]. Since KCl-induced contraction is also depressed, the effects of cytokines concern both receptor-dependent and voltage-dependent vasoconstriction.

The depressive effect of cytokines on vascular contractility requires protein synthesis, since their effects are prevented by a cycloheximide pretreatment. It has been then suggested that cytokines effects may represent a novel mechanism for prolonged alterations in vascular responsiveness [58].

In cardiac myocytes, cytokines can produce a marked inhibition both of β-adrenergic agonist stimulated cAMP production, and of contractility. This inhibition concerns the signal transduction across the membrane and may involve changes in the coupling of the stimulatory/inhibitory G proteins to adenylate cyclase [60,61].

Vasodilating Effect of Cytokines: Vasodilating effects of IL-1 and TNFα have been reported in rat pial and cremaster arterioles, partly via prostanoids [22,62]. TNF, in addition to its depressive effect, seems to evoke relaxation of the phenylephrine-contracted rabbit carotid, which is inhibited by methylene blue, suggesting a potential role of cGMP-mediated vasodilation [63]. To support this hypothesis, it was found after stimulation by IL-1 and TNF an increase in cGMP levels in cultured rat smooth muscle cells [58], in bovine mesangial cells, and in renal artery vascular smooth muscle cells via L-arginine pathway activation [64].

LPS induced Cytokines in Vascular Cells: Vascular cells are able to synthesize cytokines. The effect of LPS seems then to be mediated by cytokines produced by the stimulated vascular tissue and furthermore, anti-IL-1 antibodies significantly protect from LPS-induced hypocontractility [28].

Interaction NO/Cytokines in Smooth Muscle Cells: Cytokines induce expression of NO-synthase in smooth muscle cells, from *in vitro* studies. Wood et al. [65] reported in bovine and rat aortic smooth cells formation of NO synthase induced by a 6 h-exposure to LPS, IL-1 and INFγ. In addition, in incubated smooth muscle cells from rat aorta, IL-1β induces a continuous release of a L-arginine-related stable compound, different from NO but vasodilating via guanylate cyclase. *In vivo* inhibition of NO synthesis has been found to prevent TNF-induced shock-like state [66]. It thus appears that besides the well-documented L-arginine pathway in endothelial cells, such a pathway also exists in smooth muscle cells, and cytokines might be the elective agonist.

Role of Other Mediators

Molecular Evidence of other Mechanisms. Wakabayashi et al. [35] argued for other mechanisms for LPS-induced hypocontractility. The LPS-induced impairment of basal and stimulated hydrolysis of phosphoinositides does not seem to be mediated by cytokines. cGMP inhibits inositol monophosphate (IP) accumulation induced by norepinephrine in rat aorta without affecting its basal level. Thus, septic attenuation of both basal and stimulated IP accumulation implicates effector pathways different from cGMP and cytokines.

Role of Bioactive Lipids [67]

Phospholipase A 2 (PLA2) is known to play an important intracellular role in inflammatory processes such as endotoxic shock. In rabbits challenged with IV *E. Coli* endotoxin, plasma PLA2 activity rose 11-fold and correlated with the fall in mean arterial blood pressure. Pretreatment with dexamethasone abrogated both the rise in PLA2 activity and the fall in blood pressure. In human septic shock, serum PLA2 activity rises up to 200-fold above the normal value in relation with the acute hypotensive phase.

Cytokines and PLA2 interact together since IL1- and TNF are potent signals for PLA2 synthesis and secretion. Initial studies reported activation of membrane-bound PLA2 by these cytokines in bovine endothelial cells. IL-1 and TNF also induce the release of soluble PLA2 in vascular smooth muscle cells requiring *de novo* protein synthesis. In septic shock, peak levels of PLA2 correlates with peak TNF levels. The important increase in serum PLA2 after infusions of recombinant human TNF in cancer patients further support this linkage.

The activation of PLA2 metabolic pathway induces a numerous variety of mediators such as proteolytic enzymes, reactive oxygen species, platelet activating factor (PAF), lysophospholipides and eicosanoids.

Prostanoids, including the vasodilator prostacyclin, have been proposed to mediate the vascular hyporesponsiveness by activation of the adenylate cyclase, increasing cAMP levels. Cyclo oxygenase inhibitors have been found to be useful in short-term survival from sepsis, and to be protective against oxydative injuries. However, *in vitro* studies on isolated septic arteries failed to demonstrate a reversion of depressed contractility by indomethacin. Nevertheless, vasodilating effects of IL-1 and TNF in rat pial and cremaster arterioles involve prostanoids [22,62], and IL-1 induces a rapid relaxation of the rabbit isolated mesenteric artery reversed by indomethacin and independent of the L-arginine NO pathway [68].

A Role for Other Mediators?

Many other inflammatory mediators are implied in septic shock. They are organized in cascade systems and act in concert with the cytokine network: especially, the complement system and the contact system [69]. Their direct involvement in septic hypocontractility is not clear and need further studies. However, some different findings can be evoked.

Role of the Complement System in Septic Shock: Levels of the complement products are found either decreased or increased in sepsis, suggesting either activation or consumption. C3a is found significantly higher in patients with shock compared with septic normotensive patients. C5a is the most powerful anaphylatoxin, and intravenous administration of purified C5a into animals can induce a fall in mean arterial blood pressure. Nevertheless, there is no general agreement with respect to the mechanism underlying the hypotensive reactions observed during complement activation. The effects of complement products may be mediated since C5a is able to induce production of cytokines as TNF, IL-1, IL-6 by macrophages.

Role of the Contact System: Both LPS and vascular basement membrane/matrix can activate the contact system. Hageman factor is a permeability factor, and bradykinin is known to be an endothelium-dependent vasodilating factor. Kinins and cytokines interact in a complex way since bradykinin is known to stimulate the release of TNF and IL-1 from macrophages, and in turn cytokines enhance responsiveness of bradykinin-sensitive tissues including vascular tissue.

Dysfunction of the Endothelium

The endothelium is the interface between the blood and the vascular smooth muscle cells and thus occupies a strategic position in the local control of hemodynamics. It can modulate the reactivity of the underlying smooth muscle through several pathways. Moreover, it modulates functions of blood cells, being an active participant of the different phases of inflammation and thrombosis.

It seems that the endothelium is not the mediator of LPS-induced hypocontractility. However, the functions of the endothelium are modified in sepsis and this might be a piece of explanation for the disturbances observed in regional circulations.

The Regulatory Tone Dysfunction: The Role of the Endothelium

The endothelium can release vasoactive factors in response to hormonal substances and physical stimuli.

In vitro studies on cultured endothelial cells show that cytokines stimulate endothelial cells to produce vasodilator as well as vasoconstrictive factors. IL-1 induces the production of prostaglandins (PGI_2, PGE_2) and PAF. IL-1 and TNF induce the production of platelet-derived growth factor (PDGF) which is known to have vasoconstrictive activity, and IL-1 stimulates endothelial cells in culture to secrete endothelin-1. Endothelin-3 plasma concentrations are increased in TNF- or LPS-injected rats [70].

When the ability of the endothelium to produce EDRF is tested by stimulation with acetylcholine, EDRF-release is decreased in LPS-treated vessels, whereas relaxing endothelial-independent responses are not affected [27,71]. Recent *in vivo* studies in human septic shock confirm the occurrence of altered reactive hyperhemia [15]. The impairment of endothelium-mediated vasodilation induced by septic shock is quite similar to that observed in ischemia reperfusion injury. Cytokines, as well, seem to impair the EDRF release. IL-1 inhibits the acetylcholine-induced vasodilation of pre-contracted rabbit aorta [72]. TNF impairs coronary responses to receptor-mediated and endothelium-dependent vasodilators such as acetylcholine and ADP.Conversely, relaxant responses to A-23187 (that releases EDRF independently of endothelial cells receptor), and thoses induced by endothelium-independent vasodilators ($NaNO_2$) are not affected [73]. Similar results have been obtained in isolated cat carotids where inhibition of endothelium-dependent vasodilation induced by TNF was blocked by cycloheximide [74]. Mechanisms underlying this impairment is not known; cytokines may induce free oxygen radicals release from endothelial cells which inactivate EDRF-NO. TGFβ preserves endothelium-dependent relaxation and may be an intrinsic cytoprotective cytokine, since it can antagonize the effects of TNF, inhibit free radical generation and adhesion of neutrophils to the endothelium [73].

The ability of the endothelium from septic vessels to produce vasoconstrictive factors is not known.

The inhibition of endothelium-dependent vasodilation has pathological implications: inferference with compensatory vasodilation and loss of vasodilator reserve may favor local vasoconstriction within organs and subsequent tissue injury.

Activation State of Endothelium [75-77]

LPS and cytokines interact with endothelial cells in multiple ways and induce a phenotype change of the endothelium: the activation state. This state interfers markedly with blood cells functions. Although blood and endothelial cells are interacting in a dynamic way, biomechanical obstructions of vessels can occur in sepsis.

The Pro-coagulant Activity. IL-1 and TNF increase tissue-factor, decrease the endothelial surface thrombomodulin, which markedly inhibit the anticoagulant effects of protein S and protein C, increase the secretion of the inhibitor of tissue plasminogen activator and decrease the secretion of tissue plasminogen activator itself. All these effects tend to tip the balance of the coagulant/anticoagulant molecules on the surface of the endothelium towards fibrin deposition and intravascular coagulation. In addition, depression of EDRF-NO release induced by cytokines favor aggregation of platelets. The formation of microaggregates might favor the development of focal ischemia in sepsis.

The Pro-inflammatory Activity. The second major effect of LPS, IL-1 and TNF on endothelium is the stimulation of increased surface adhesivity for leukocytes. They activate the endothelial cells to stimulate the synthesis of "intercellular adhesion molecule-1" (ICAM-1) and induce the expression of "endothelial-leukocyte adhesion molecule-1" (ELAM-1) causing neutrophils, monocytes and lymphocytes to adhere. Two groups of leukocyte surface receptors are involved as ligands in this leukocyte-endothelium interaction: the integrin receptor family/ICAMs and the selectins/ELAMs.The adherent neutrophils are stimulated by cytokines to release superoxide anions and other secondary inflammatory mediators, which participate in the tissue injury and destruction of host tissue, as it occurs for example in the adult respiratory distress syndrome (ARDS). Another endothelial surface adhesion molecule (called INCAM-110 or VCAM-1) has been identified as a 110 kD IL-1 or TNF-inducible protein. This molecule mediates the adhesion of lymphocytes and monocytes, through a β1 integrin leukocyte ligand (VLA-4). The kinetics of expression of these adhesion molecules suggests that earlier induced ELAM 1 participates in neutrophils adhesion at the early phase of inflammation, IL-8 (neutrophil activating factor) secreted by cytokine activated endothelial cells promoting neutrophils diapedesis through the endothelium. Maximal expression of ICAM-1 occurs after that of ELAM-1, while INCAM-110/VCAM-1 begins to be induced. At a later time, IL-1 and TNF cause endothelial cells to secrete MCP-1 (monocyte chemotactic protein-1, JE gene product) to recruite monocytes to inflammatory sites. These time-dependent modifications of adhesive molecules correlate with changes in leukocyte subtype population involved in the inflammatory response.

The implication in terms of flow may be a microvascular plugging: leukocytes can actively adhere to the endothelium and to each other to finally occlude the larger postcapillary veinules, and allowing ultimately to a no-reflow phenomenon. Moreover, activated leukocytes adhering to the endothelium might release vasoactive products, cytokines with an amplified process, and toxic radicals.

In support of the implication of adhesive molecules in shock, antibodies anti-integrin CD18 protect animals from hemorragic shock injury [78]. Such a protection is in trial in septic shock.

Interactions between Blood Cells and Vascular Wall: The procoagulant and proinflammatory aspects of endothelial activation state occurring in sepsis outline the major role of cellular interactions between blood cells and vascular cells, in terms of both immunomodulation of vasoreactivity and vasomodulation of immune function. LPS-activated polymorphonuclear cells and LPS-activated macrophages release NO and vasodilate when exposed *in vitro* to vessels. LPS-activated macrophages depress contractility of rabbit carotid via induction of the L-arginine/NO pathway of the smooth muscle cells [57].

The Vascular Leakage and Endothelial Injury: Clinical trials of human recombinant cytokines showed a severe side effect of fluid leak from the microvasculature. The cause of vascular leak is unclear.

Endothelial morphological changes occur in cytokines-treated endothelial cells. TNF increases the permeability to macromolecules of endothelial cells monolayers, via an action on membrane-G-proteins.

Endothelial injury can also account for this leakiness. *In vivo* endothelial activation and endothelial injury often coexist. Harlan et al. [79] showed a direct morphological effect of LPS on bovine endothelial cells, including dilation of the intercellular junctions, cell contraction and ruffling of the surface membrane. Young et al. [71] described, using electron microscopy, endothelial injury in vessels isolated from septic animals, with separation of the endothelium from the internal elastic lamina media and increase in inter-endothelial gaps. Many factors may favor the cytotoxicity of LPS: complement system, cytokines, free radicals and leukocyte products. Indeed, cytokine-treated endothelial cells are more susceptible to injury. Oxygen free radicals released by both endothelial and blood cells are known to be cytotoxic, and interaction between oxygen and nitrogen free radicals might lead to the formation of peroxynitrite which is a higher toxic radical. In addition, adhesive leukocytes may mediate LPS endothelium injury through the release of proteases.

Conclusion

If the concept of a septic-induced vasoplegia is generally accepted, the alteration of peripheral vasculature as a specific consequence of septic injury is difficult to assess *in vivo.* Further studies are needed to understand the heterogeneity of vascular alterations occurring in septic shock especially for the left ventricular afterload, the venous return, the resistance and compliance, and the regional circulations. *In vitro* studies give evidence for septic-induced vascular dysfunctions as the depression of vascular contractility and tone. Hypocontractility does not depend from endothelium and is mainly mediated by the cytokine-induced L-argine/nitric oxide pathway in smooth muscle cells. Cytokine activation of the endothelium favors direct interactions between blood and vascular cells. Although the spirit of "the concert of septic mediators" is still not known, except for "chaos" influence, an adequate therapeutic approach in septic shock should integrate these complex pathophysiological events.

References

1. Hess M, Hastillo A, Greenfield L (1981) Spectrum of cardiovascular function during gram-negative sepsis. Prog Cardiovasc Dis 23:279–298
2. Edwards JD, Brown GCS, Nightingale P, et al. (1989) Use of survivors' cardiorespiratory values as therapeutic goals in septic shock. Crit Care Med 17:1098–2002
3. Groeneveld A, Nauta J, Thijs L (1988) Peripheral vascular resistance in septic shock: Its relation to outcome. Intensive Care Med 14:141–147

4. Parker M, Shelhamer J, Natanson C, al. (1987) Serial cardiovascular variables in survivors and nonsurvivors of human septic shock: Heart rate as an early predictor of prognosis. Crit Care Med 15:923–926
5. Parker M, Shelhamer J, Bacharach S (1984) Profound but reversible myocardial depression in patients with septic shock. Ann Intern Med 100:483–490
6. Lang C, Bagby G, Ferguson J, Spitzer J (1984) Cardiac output and redistribution of organ blood flow in hypermetabolic sepsis. Am J Physiol 246:331–337
7. Bernsten A, Gnidec A, Rutledge F, Sibbald W (1990) Hyperdynamic sepsis modifies a PEEP–mediated redistribution in organ blood flow. Am Rev Resp Dis 142:1198–1208
8. Groeneveld A, Bronsveld J, Thijs L (1986) Hemodynamic determinants of mortality in human septic shock. Surgery 99:140–152
9. Tuchschmidt J, Fried J, Swinney R, Sharma O (1989) Early hemodynamic correlates of survival in patients with septic shock. Crit Care Med 17:719–723
10. D'Orio V, Wahlen C, Naldi M, Fossion A, Juchmes J, Marcelle R (1989) Contribution of peripheral blood pooling to central hemodynamic disturbances during endotoxin insult in intact dogs. Crit Care Med 17:1314–1319
11. Guyton A, Jones C, Coleman T (1973) Circulatory physiology: cardiac output and its regulation. WB Saunders
12. Bressack M, Raffin T (1987) Importance of venous return, venous resistance, and mean circulatory pressure in the physiology and management of shock. Chest 92:906–912
13. Pinsky M, Matuschak G (1986) Cardiovascular determinants of the hemodynamic response to acute endotoxemia in the dog. J Crit Care 1:18–31
14. Seaman K, Greenway C (1984) Loss of hepatic venous responsiveness after endotoxin in anesthetized cats. Am J Physiol 246:658–663
15. Astiz M, Tilly E, Rackow E, Weil M (1991) Peripheral vascular tone in sepsis. Chest 99:1072–1075
16. O'Rourke M, Avolio A, Nichols W (1987) Left ventricular–systemic arterial coupling in humans and strategies to improve coupling in disease states. In: E Yin (ed) Ventricular/Arterial Coupling. Springer-Verlag, pp 1–19
17. Schumaker P (1991) Peripheral vascular responses in septic shock. Direct or reflex effects? Chest 99:1057–1058
18. Jones S, Romano F (1989) Dose- and time-dependent changes in plasma catecholamines in response to endotoxin in conscious rats. Circ Shock 28:59–68
19. Withworth P, Cryer H, Garrison R, Baumgarten T, Harris P (1989) Hypoperfusion of the intestinal microcirculation without decreased cardiac output during live Escherichia coli sepsis in rats. Circ Shock 27:111–122
20. Unger L, Cryer H, Garrison R (1989) Differential response of the microvasculature in the liver during bacteremia. Circ Shock 29:335–344
21. Cryer H, Garrison R, Kaebnick H, et al. (1987) Skeletal microcirculatory responses to hyperdynamic Escherichia coli sepsis in unanesthetized rats. Arch Surg 122:86–92
22. Vicaut E, Hou X, Payen D, Bousseau A, Tedgui A (1991) Acute effects of tumor necrosis factor on the microcirculation in cremaster muscle. J Clin Invest 87:1537–1540
23. Sibbald W, Fox G, Martin C (1991) Abnormalities of vascular reactivity in the sepsis syndrome. Chest 100:115–159
24. Groeneveld A, Schneider A, Thijs L (1991) Cardiac alterations in septic shock: Pathophysiology, diagnosis, prognostic, and therapeutic implications. In: Vincent JL (ed) Update in intensive care and emergency medecine Vol 14. Springer-Verlag, pp 126–136
25. Chernow B, Roth B (1986) Pharmacologic manipulation of the peripheral vasculature in shock: Clinical and experimental approaches. Circ Shock 18:141–155
26. Parrat J (1989) Alterations in vascular reactivity in sepsis and endotoxemia. In: Vincent JL (ed) Update in intensive care and emergency medecine. Vol 12, Springer-Verlag, pp 299–308
27. Julou-Schaeffer G, Gray G, Fleming I, Schott C, Parratt J, Stoclet J (1990) Loss of vascular responsiveness induced by endotoxin involves L-arginine pathway. Am J Physiol 259:1038–1043
28. McKenna T (1990) Prolonged exposure of rat aorta to low levels of endotoxin in vitro results in impaired contractility. Association with vascular cytokine release. J Clin Invest 86:160–168

29. Beasley D, Cohen R, Levinsky N (1990) Endotoxin inhibits contraction of vascular smooth muscle in vitro. Am J Physiol. 258:1187–1192
30. Wakabayashi I, Hatake K, Kakishita E, Nagai K (1987) Diminution of contractile response of the aorta from endotoxin injected rats. Eur J Pharmacol 141:117–122
31. McKenna T (1988) Enhanced vascular effects of cyclic GMP in septic rat aorta. Am J Physiol 254:436–442
32. Stoclet J (1991) The L-arginine-NO pathway and cyclic GMP in the vessel wall. Z Kardiol 77:1–4
33. Baker C, Wilmoth F (1984) Microvascular responses to E. Coli endotoxin with altered adrenergic activity. Circ Shock 12:165–172
34. Wakabayashi I, Hatake K, Kakishita E, Hishida S, Nagai K (1989) Desensitization of α-1 adrenergic receptor mediated smooth muscle contraction in aorta from endotoxic rats. Life Science 45:509–515
35. Wakabayashi I, Hatake K, Sakamoto K (1991) Mechanisms of ex vivo aortic hypocontractility in endotoxemic rat. Eur J Pharmacol 199:115–118
36. Moncada S, Higgs E (1991) Endogenous nitric oxide: Physiology, pathology and clinical relevance. Eur J Clin Invest 21:361–374
37. Busse R, Mülsch A (1990) Induction of nitric oxide synthase by cytokines in vascular smooth muscle cells. FEBS (Lett) 275:87–90
38. Rees D, Cellek S, Palmer R, Moncada S (1990) Dexamethasone prevents the induction by endotoxin of nitric oxide synthase and the associated effects on vascular tone: An insight into endotoxic shock. Biochem Biophys Res Commun 173:541–547
39. Wagner D, Young V, Tannenbaum S (1983) Mammalian nitrate biosynthesis: Incorporation 15 NH3 into nitrate is enhanced by endotoxin treatment. Proc Natl Acad Sci USA 80:4518–4521
40. Thiermermann C, Vane J (1990) Inhibition of nitric oxide synthesis reduces the hypotension induced by lipopolysaccharides in the rat in vivo. Eur J Pharmacol 182:591–595
41. Fleming I, Julou–Schaeffer G, Gray G, Parratt JR, Stocklet JC (1991) Evidence that an L-arginine/nitric oxide dependent elevation of tissue cyclic GMP content is involved in depression of vascular reactivity by endotoxin. Br J Phamacol 103:1047–1052
42. Schneider F, Julou-Schaeffer G, Stoclet J (1991) A L-arginine derived relaxing factor is involved in the endotoxin-induced hyporeactivity of resistance vessels to norepinephrine. Circ Shock 34:49–52
43. Gray G, Fleming I, Parratt J, Stoclet J (1991) L-arginine dependent accumulation of cyclic GMP in rat aortic medial smooth muscle layer incubated with LPS. Brit J Pharmacol (Abs)102:123
44. Curran R, Billiar T, Stuehr D, Hofmann K, Simmons R (1989) Hepatocytes produce nitrogen oxides from L-arginine in response to inflammatory products from Kupffer cells. J Exp Med 170:1769–1774
45. Moncada S, Palmer R, Higgs E (1991) Nitric oxide: Physiology, pathophysiology, and pharmacology. Pharm Rev 43:109–142
46. Lefer A (1991) Cytoprotective actions of nitric oxide and NO-donors in ischaemia-reperfusion of coronary and splanchnic circulations. Second International Meeting on the Biology of Nitric Oxide, London (Abs)
47. Frostell C, Fratacci M, Wain J, Jones R, Zapol W (1991) Inhaled nitric oxide: A selective pulmonary vasodilator reversing hypoxic pulmonary vasoconstriction. Circulation 83:2038–2047
48. Klabunde R, Ritger R (1991) Ng-monomethyl-L-arginine restores arterial blood pressure but reduces cardiac output in a canine model of endotoxic shock. Biochem Biophys Res Commun 178:1135–1140
49. Wright C, Rees D, Moncada S (1992) The protective and pathological roles of nitric oxide in endotoxin shock. Cardiovasc Res 26:48–57
50. Manogue K, Cerami A (1988) A macrophage protein that induces a catabolic state and septic shock in infected animals. In: Poste G, Crooke ST (eds) Cellular and molecular aspects of inflammation. Plenum Press, New York, pp 123–150

51. Tracey K, Beutler B, Lowry S (1986) Shock and tissue injury induced by recombinant human cachectin. Science 234:470–474
52. Tracey K, Fong D, Hesse K, et al. (1987) Anti-cachectin antibodies prevent septic shock during lethal bacteremia. Nature 330:662–664
53. Mathison J, Wolfson E, Ulevitch R (1988) Participation of tumor necrosis factor in the mediation of gram-negative bacterial lipopolysaccharide-induced injury in rabbit. J Clin Invest 81:1925–1937
54. Okusawa S, Gelfand J, Ikejima T, Connolly R, Dinarello C (1988) Interleukin-1 induces a shock like state in rabbit. Synergism with tumor necrosis factor and the effect of cyclooxygenase inhibition. J Clin Invest 81:1162–1172
55. Warner S, Libby P (1989) Human vascular smooth muscle cells target for and source of tumor necrosis factor. J Immunol 142:100–109
56. McKenna T, Tituis W (1989) Role of the monokines in altering receptor and non-receptor mediated vascular contracion in sepsis. In: Molecular and cellular mechanisms of septic shock. Alan R Liss Inc, New York, pp 279–303
57. Bernard C, Szekely B, Philip I, Wollman E, Payen D, Tedgui A (1992) Activated macrophages depress the contractility of rabbit carotids via an L-arginine NO dependent effector mechanism. Connection with ampflified cytokine release. J Clin Invest (in press)
58. Beasley D, Brenner B, Schwartz J (1990) Interleukin-1 activates guanylate cyclase in rat vascular smooth muscle cells by inducing nitric oxyde production. FASEB J (Abs) 4: A685
59. Philip I, Bernard C, Payen D, Tedgui A (1989) Depression of contractile response in rabbit carotid artery by tumor necrosis factor. Circulation (Abs) 80:126
60. Gulick T, Chung M, Pieper S, Lange L, Schreiner G (1989) Interleukin-1 and tumor necrosis factor inhibit cardiac myocyte beta adrenergic responsiveness. Proc Natl Acad Sci USA 86:6753–6757
61. Chung M, Gulick T, Rotondo R, Schriener G, Lange S (1990) Mechanism of cytokine inhibition of beta adrenergic agonist stimulation of cyclic AMP in rat cardiac myocyte. Impairment of signal transduction. Circ Res 67:753–763
62. Schibata M, Leffler C, Busija D (1990) Recombinant human interleukin-1 α dilates pial arterioles and increases cerebrospinal fluid prostanoids in piglets. Am J Physiol 259:1486–1491
63. Philip I, Bernard C, Payen D, Bousseau A, Tedgui A (1990) Dual effect of TNF on rabbit carotid reactivity. FASEB J (Abs) 4:A1111
64. Marsden P, Ballermann B (1990) Tumor necrosis factor alpha activates soluble guanylate cyclase in bovine glomerular mesangial cells via a L-Arginine dependent mechanism. J Exp Med 172:1843–1852
65. Wood K, Buga G, Byrns R, Ignarro L (1990) Vascular smooth muscle-derived relaxing factor (MDRF) and its close similarity to nitric oxide. Biochem Biophs Res Commun 173:80–88
66. Kilbourn R, Gross S, Jubran A, et al. (1990) NG-Methyl L-Arginine inhibits tumor necrosis factor hypotension: Implications for the involvement of nitric oxyde. Proc Natl Acad Sci USA 87:3629–3632
67. Pruzanski W, Vadas P (1991) Phospholipase A2: a mediator between proximal and distal effectors of inflammation. Immunol Today 12:143–146
68. Marceau F, Petitclerc E, DeBlois D, Pradelles P, Poubelle P (1991) Human interleukin-1 induces a rapid relaxation of the rabbit isolated mesenteric artery. Br J Pharmacol 103:1367–1372
69. Hack C, Thijs L (1991) The orchestra of mediators in the pathogenesis of septic shock: A review. In: Vincent JL (ed). Update in intensive care and emergency medicine. Vol. 14 Springer-Verlag, pp 232–246
70. Venulappali S, Chiu P, Rivelli M, Cedeno K, Coleman W, Sybertz E (1990) Tumor necrosis factor and hemorrage produce elevation of plasma endothelin in rats. FASEB J (Abs) 4:A456
71. Young J, Headrick J, Berne R (1990) Attenuated responses to endothelium-dependent vasodilators during endotoxic shock. FASEB J 4:A952
72. Robert R, Chapelin B, Neliat G (1990) Effect de I'IL-1 sur la réactivité vasculaire chez le lapin. Réa Med Urg (Abstr)
73. Lefer A, Tsao P, Aoki N, Palladino M (1990) Mediation of cardioprotection by transforming growth factor-beta.Science 249:61–64

74. Aoki N, Siegfried M, Lefrand A (1989) Anti-EDRF effect of tumor necrosis factor in isolated perfused cat carotid arteries. Am J Physiol 256:1509–1512
75. Pober J, Cotran R (1990) The role of endothelial cells in inflammation. Transplantation 50:537–544
76. Pober J, Cotran R (1990) Cytokines and endothelial cell biology. Physiol Rev 70:427–451
77. Cotran R, Pober J (1989) Effects of cytokines on vascular endothelium: Their role in vascular and immune injury. Kidney Int 35:969–975
78. Vedder N, Winn R, Rice C, Chi E, Arfors K, Harlan J (1988) A monoclonal antibody to the adherence-promoting leukocyte glycoprotein, CD18, reduces organ injury and improves survival from hemorragic shock and resuscitation in rabbits. J Clin Invest 81:939–944
79. Harlan JM, Harker LA, Reidy MA, Gajdusek CM, Schartz SM, Striker GE (1983) Lipopolysaccharide -mediated bovine endothelial cell injury in vitro. Lab Invest 48:269–274

New Therapeutic Approaches to Sepsis

Dilemmas in Sepsis Clinical Trials Design and Analysis

R. P. Dellinger and R.C. Straube

Introduction

Analysis of sepsis research studies involving laboratory animal models is straightforward. In such models, all potential prognostic factors such as genetic predisposition, age, sex, infecting organism, inoculum of organisms, time between infection and treatment, environmental conditions, etc... can be specified and standardized between animals in each of the two treatment arms of an experiment. Differences in outcome can, therefore, be ascribed solely to the differences in applied therapy and the relevance of these differences precisely determined by statistics. This experimental purity is rarely achievable in clinical trials. In human trials, the heterogeneity of the patients enrolled in the trial becomes a prominent factor and the complexity, both in design and analysis, increases tremendously.

The clinical entity of sepsis creates particular problems for clinical trial design and analysis. First, the disease is poorly defined. The term "sepsis syndrome" has been used to identify patients for enrollment into sepsis clinical trials. The definitions for sepsis syndrome used in recent large trials vary significantly[1–4]. Inclusion/exclusion criteria are arbitrary and have not been subjected to assessment as to whether they discriminate for patients with the disease or if they are important prognostic factors. Second, the syndrome can have a wide range of etiologic factors varying from gram-negative bacteria to infection with other organisms to non-infectious causes. Third, patients with sepsis frequently have serious underlying diseases which carry their own morbidity, mortality, and may influence the patient's response to therapy targeted at sepsis and its sequelae. Fourth, the natural history of sepsis varies markedly from patient to patient. In some patients, the onset of the disease is clearly defined and rapid resolution occurs within two to three days. In other patients, the onset may be insidious and the patient's course extended. And finally, because of the need to individualize aggressive support and treat for hospital and patient specific organisms, there is no well recognized standard of therapy for such patients. Even within the same institution, physician preferences may create significantly different treatment patterns for patients with similar signs and symptoms.

In its simplest form, the analysis of a clinical trial assumes that patients in each of the treatment arms are identical with the exception of the treatment under study. Such an assumption is warranted in highly homogeneous diseases, however, in heterogeneous diseases such as sepsis, this assumption is violated. To minimize effects of this heterogeneity, clinical trials done in sepsis need to be carefully designed, executed and analyzed. Over the last five to ten years, interest in clinical trial design has mushroomed, and indeed a new area of specialization, clinical epidemiology, has come into existence [5–8]. In the remainder of this chapter, we will highlight a few of the important issues of relevance to the design and analysis of clinical trials in sepsis. We will review phases of drug development and the necessary information to initiate a trial, a few of the key decisions necessary in the design of an efficacy trial, as well as endpoints for efficacy trials, and discuss the organization of large multi-center clinical trials, and finally, the interpretation of clinical trials and their relationship to clinical practice.

Drug Development

The process by which drugs are identified, tested, efficacy determined, and research sponsorship generated has dramatically changed over the course of this century [9]. Prior to the 1940s, the majority of new drug entities were discovered empirically (i.e. penicillin). Increasingly, the chemical structure of potential drugs are being designed by computer analyses. These potential drugs are then tested for biological effect in *in vitro* animal systems. As a result, the number of new, potentially effective drugs has dramatically increased. At the same time, the ethics of clinical trials has undergone similar changes. As a result of Nazi human experimentation during World War II as well as public outcry over several clinical trials in the US during the 1950s, the concept of patient volunteer rights and informed consent have been formalized. In addition, a major force in changing drug development in the US and the world has been the influence of the expansion of the Food and Drug Administration's role from its initial goal of regulation of the quality of food sold interstate, to their role in evaluating the safety, and more recently, the efficacy of new drugs prior to their availability for sales.

Although there is huge variation in precise drug development paths, in general drugs go through six, reasonably distinct phases. Potential new drugs are selected for further research based on *in vitro* studies. Which systems are used for screening is highly dependent upon the type and class of drug being sought. For example, new antibiotics may be screened by their ability to kill specific bacterial strains *in vitro,* monoclonal antibodies may be selected by their ability to bind to specific target antigens, etc. After this initial screening, hopeful candidates are assessed in appropriate animal models. Drugs specifically designed to be used in sepsis are at a disadvantage. The clinical manifestations of sepsis appear to be intricately involved with the host response which includes the cytokine mediator release cascade (such as tumor necrosis factor (TNF) and interleukin-1 (IL-1)) secondary mediators (such as prostacyclins), and end products causing cellular damage (for example, oxygen free radicals). This host response varies markedly from species to spe-

Table 1. Clinical phases of drug testing in sepsis

	Patient Numbers	Toxicity	Efficacy
Phase 1	Small	Yes	No
Phase 2	Moderate	Yes	Not usually
Phase 3	Large	Yes	Yes
Postmarketing	Large	Yes	Consistancy only

cies, and currently, there is no good animal model which accurately reflects all aspects of the human disease. Some models have been shown to accurately reflect specific elements of the human response and are useful in predicting the utility of treatment in patients. These models are however the exception. Some animal models may reproduce one human sepsis response but not others.

In parallel to animal testing, other *in vitro* testings for biological activity are carried out. If the sum of the data suggests that the drug candidate continues to have potential, it undergoes a battery of toxicologic testing. When this data is available, a decision is made as to whether or not the potential benefits of the drug outweigh the observed toxicity.

Once the decision is made to pursue clinical testing, the development process enters into four distinct clinical phases which have been formalized by the FDA (Table 1) [10]. The first of these is Phase I experimentation. These trials are designed to measure the safety and pharmacokinetics of the new compound. Typically, a small number of patients are given increasing doses of the drug. Dosing usually starts significantly below the expected dose used in the clinic and escalation continues to a dose several times that expected to be used. Depending on the compound, the initial subjects receiving the drug may be normal, healthy volunteers. Once the safety and pharmacokinetics profile has been determined in the initial groups, further Phase I testing is done in the population of interest. Thus, in drugs for treatment of sepsis, the initial dosing will occur in normal, healthy volunteers and further Phase I trials will include patients who are diagnosed as having sepsis.

Phase II trials are designed to assess the effectiveness of the drug as well as to determine appropriate clinical doses. Typically, these trials are medium sized, and are conducted in the population in which the efficacy trials are expected to be conducted. Generally, such trials are open-label, however a double-blind design may be employed to decrease selection bias of patient populations. Typically, the sample size for these trials is too small to show statistically conclusive evidence of the efficacy of the drug. They are large enough, however, to allow the identification of significant trends in the data. In addition, many trials will focus on surrogate endpoints and use such information for dose finding. For example, a drug which is expected to lower mortality in sepsis may use, as a dose finding endpoint, the reduction in a particular cytokine level as a measure of biological activity.

Phase III studies are designed to prove the efficacy of a drug. In general, such trials are large, requiring hundreds to thousands of patients. The patient population selected are those patients for which the drug is expected to work and determine the licensed indication for the drug. Because of the requirement for large numbers of patients, such trials usually are multi-center. In sepsis, the usual endpoint for such trials is mortality, specified by either 14 or 28 days. Other parameters of clinical utilities such as days in the hospital, reduction in support needed, and biochemical improvement are included only as secondary endpoints. In general, the FDA requires two Phase III trials to be performed in order for a drug to become licensed.

Providing that the Phase I–III trials have provided compelling evidence of efficacy, a drug will be licensed by the FDA. Post-marketing trials are typically done. Such trials collect further information about safety, especially unusual adverse events, collect data about outcome looking for consistency with data generated from the Phase III trials, and provide information concerning the actual use of the drug in clinical practice.

The logical drug development of testing drugs pre-clinically, then measuring the clinical safety, the clinical effectiveness, and finally the clinical efficacy provides a rational basis by which to judge the utility of a drug in a given condition. Although, the design of clinical trials in all phases of the drug's development are important, Phase III trials, designed to prove efficacy, are the most problematic and will be those on which we will focus in the remainder of our discussion.

Decision to Participate in a Clinical Trial

Physicians who participate in clinical trials are forced into two, sometimes antagonistic positions – that of clinical scientist and that of physician [11, 12]. The scientist demands that every patient in a trial be treated exactly the same and that the trial continues until conclusive evidence of either efficacy or lack of efficacy is available. The physician, on the other hand, is required to provide the optimal care, in the estimation of the physician, for the individual patient. Thus, it is unethical for the physician investigator to participate in the trial if, in his judgment, the available evidence demonstrates one treatment arm is clearly superior (or inferior) to the others. Thus, a physician must critically evaluate all available information on a new drug in order to determine whether participation in a trial is ethical. Some areas for consideration are presented below.

First, the evidence for pre-clinical biological activity needs to be examined. The relevance of the particular *in vitro* assay and/or animal model needs to be examined. The correlation of results from that model system to human experience with other compounds should be evaluated. The internal consistency of the results of the pre-clinical trials needs to be assessed. For example, in septic animal models in which mortality is the outcome, if data on cytokines, blood pressure, organ failure, etc. corroborates the findings of benefit, the findings may be more relevant. In addition, Phase III trials, data concerning effectiveness from Phase I (and sometimes Phase II) trials needs to be examined. The physician investigator must evaluate this likely benefit of the new therapy in light of adverse events predicted both from the animal toxicology and from the safety profile compiled from earlier Phase I and Phase II studies. This benefit/risk ratio must be positive in order for a physician investigator to proceed with a Phase III trial. In addition, the impact of participation in the trial for the individual patient must be examined. For example, the probability of benefit of a new drug must be very high if the drug is to be used instead of a proven lifesaving therapy. If the innovative drug will be given on top of all other forms of standard therapy in settings with very high mortality, the probability of benefit need not be as high. By the same token, it may be unethical for a physician investigator to participate in a double-blind study if he feels that the currently available data shows compelling evidence of efficacy. For example, few physicians would be willing to participate in the new therapy for an invariably fatal disease if the Phase I/II trials had shown that five out of five patients given the new therapy did not succumb.

In addition, patients enrolled in trials are treated differently and these differences may both negatively and positively effect the patients' care. Most studies require laboratory examinations (extra blood work, X-rays, special studies, etc.) which would not normally be performed. All such studies carry some risk. The data obtained may however allow improved patient care. In some settings, the patient may receive improved patient care simply by virtue of being in the clinical trial. Many trials dictate that daily evaluation of the patient be done by the principal investigator, usually a senior attending staff. Their detailed daily review may optimize therapy for that patient in a way that the junior staff who normally review the patients might not be able to provide.

Design of Efficacy Trials

The Clinical Question

Clinical trials are designed to answer specific questions. The more ambiguous the question, the more ambiguous the answer. A surprising large number of clinical trials in sepsis pose nebulous questions. For example: "Will therapy with a new drug improve patient outcome?" Such a study might measure a variety of outcome variables such as death, hospital stay, use of other treatment modalities, development of clinical and laboratory abnormalities, etc. The difficulty in analyzing the results of such trials is one of multiple comparisons, as discussed below. In essence, a positive finding in one outcome variable in such a trial, will generate the hypothesis that the drug positively effects that particular outcome variable rather than proving it. A second trial confirming that finding must be done in order to statistically prove the drug effect. As such, such poorly defined questions should be used primarily for Phase II studies and have no place in Phase III efficacy trials. The more specific the research question, the more compelling the results are in demonstrating efficacy. Inherent in a specific question is a clear definition of the patients who will be examined and the outcome. For example, the question: "Can this new drug reduce all-cause mortality at day 28, using the chi-squared statistics in patients meeting the well defined set of inclusion criteria who have a positive blood culture for gram-positive bacteria", will yield unambiguous "yes" or "no" answer. On the other hand, the question, "Will this new drug benefit very sick patients" may yield conflicting results depending on how "very sick patients" is defined and what parameters are used to assess "make better".

Sample Size

The equation for determining sample size of trial given expected incidence of the endpoint in the placebo group, the expected reduction in incidence in the treated group, the level of statistical significance, and the power of the trial is straight forward [13, 14]. The availability of such calculations via computer programs make the calculations even easier. Despite the ease of calculation, careful attention must be paid to the assumptions underlying sample size determination. The expected incidence of the endpoint in the control group can be surprisingly difficult to ascertain. Relatively trivial differences in the wording of inclusion/exclusion criteria and/or the institutional need for informed consent results in observed mortality in placebo groups in different studies of sepsis to range from 22% to 48%. Similarly, the observed mortality rates at different institutions using identical criteria can vary dramatically from 0 to 100%. Equally important in the calculations of sample size is the percent reduction in the instance of the outcome variable between the treatment and placebo arms which is considered to be important. This reduction must be clinically relevant, and therefore must vary with the outcome parameter being studied. And as the difference between the two treatment arms becomes smaller, the sample size increases. In critically ill patients with sepsis, it may be determined that only dramatic decreases in a biochemical parameter are of clinical significance. Such a trial may require relatively few patients. On the other hand, if the outcome variable is mortality, a much smaller difference of perhaps 10% could be judged to be clinically significant, and therefore the sample size of the trial would need to be increased dramatically.

In sample size calculation, two arbitrary values are assigned. The first of these is the level of "statistical significance". Traditionally, this is set at a probability (p) equal to 0.05. That is to say, if the treatment is ineffective, a statistical significance would still be found 5 out of 100 times the experiment is repeated. Thus, this value gives a measurement of the expected false positive rate of a trial. The second value is that of power calculated by the equation 1-β (the beta error). This is the probability that should the treatment actually be effective, that the clinical trial will fail to show a statistically significance difference between the two arms of the trial, or a measurement of the false negative rate. Traditionally, this value is set at 0.8 or 0.9; however, some investigators use values as low as 0.5. Many studies did not have power to demonstrate anything less than overwhelming treatment effect in their trials because of the small sample size. A sample size large enough to provide a reasonable chance of demonstrating a clinically significant treatment effect is especially important with highly fatal diseases such as sepsis. The risk of discarding potentially life saving new therapies, and in some cases whole classes of therapies, increases as the power of the trial decreases.

Having determined the theoretical number of patients required for the trial, the actual number of patients to be enrolled in the trial then needs to be considered. The majority of large, multi-center trials will enroll some patients who are lost to follow-up, patients who in retrospect fail to meet entrance criteria, and patients who fail to receive a full course of therapy. The overall trial size needs to be increased to account for the estimated number of the unevaluable patients.

Sepsis is a heterogeneous disease process arising from a variety of infectious etiologies and/or simulated by a variety of non-infectious causes. Many of the therapies to be tested in this syndrome would be expected to be efficacious only in that sub-population of patients with a specific etiology [15–18]. Since early therapy is generally accepted to be optimal, the etiologic cause of a patient's septic condition is unlikely to be available at the time the therapy needs to be instituted. For that reason, it is a practical necessity to employ the inefficient trial design of enrolling large number of patients unlikely to benefit from the therapy. Which patients these are, however, can be determined only retrospectively. Thus, the incidence of the sepsis syndrome cause of interest that is expected to exist among all patients enrolled needs to be estimated and the sample size increased accordingly. Thus, in the recent anti-endotoxin monoclonal antibody trials with HA-1A, the target population was patients with endotoxemia. Because of practical difficulties in assaying endotoxin levels in the blood stream, a surrogate target population, those with gram-negative bacteremia, was chosen. Because it was expected that only approximately one-third of the patients with sepsis syndrome would have documented gram-negative bacteremia, the trial size was increased approximately 3 times to guarantee adequate number of patients in the target population. If efficacy is shown in a target population that is a subgroup of the total enrollment, the generalizability of the findings in the subgroup to treatment of the total population is problematic unless the subgroup can be readily identified prospectively.

Homogeneity/Generalizability: In a highly heterogenous disease such as sepsis, the clinical trial must find a balance between a precisely defined homogenous group of patients and clinical relevance of the findings. As the definition of patient characteristics gets tighter, the variability in parameters between patients becomes less and the identity of such patients easier. As inclusion criteria become stricter, the trial more closely approximates that of animal studies. Thus, a trial which enrolled "male patients, aged 26–27 with a preoperative diagnosis of appendicitis who underwent laparotomy at which time a necrotic but non-perforated appendix was found (and who developed sepsis between 24 and 30 hours post-operatively)" will provide a highly homogenous patient population. A physician reading the results of such trials would have no difficulty in determining whether or not the treatment should be used in patients who meet that precise entrance criteria. Difficulty with such homogenous population, however, is that few patients even at large centers will meet such stringent criteria, and there is no internal evidence from the trial to suggest the extent that these findings are representative of what will be seen in other patient populations. For example, in that trial, are those results applicable to patients who have clearly perforated appendices, or conversely, those with significant inflammation but without actual necrosis. Will the results be applicable to females of the same age or to any patient slightly older or slightly younger? A clinical trial with less specific inclusion criteria will provide some information concerning a broader range of patients with the expense of less precision of any one group. From a practical standpoint, the less specific the entrance criteria, the faster the enrollment and the fewer the number of centers required to achieve an appropriate sample size. This in turn will decrease the amount of patient and treatment heterogeneity resulting from enrollment at different centers each with different referral patterns, treatment patterns, and demographic characteristics of their patients. Clearly, there is no accepted standard to guide one in choosing the degree of heterogeneity and generalizability of a trial. Nor is there a template to furnish readers that will allow application of the results of such a trial to their patients.

Similar to the inclusion criteria, the design of the trial as to number of sites can also influence the heterogeneity of patients enrolled. Patients enrolled at one institution from one intensive care unit (ICU) by one physician can be viewed as a baseline low heterogeneity study. Two patients, even in the same unit, or one physician enrolling patients in several ICU in a hospital would be expected to enroll patients slightly more heterogeneously. For example, even though using the same inclusion criteria, two physicians are likely to have slightly different biases as to what patient actually meets inclusion or exclusion criteria. Similarly, patients enrolled in a medical ICU exclusively are more likely to be similar than patients enrolled both in the medical ICU, the surgical ICU, the neurosurgical ICU, or the coronary care unit. Similarly, the involvement of more than one hospital in a clinical trial is likely to dramatically increase the heterogeneity of patients enrolled. Each hospital will have a unique referral pattern which is unlikely to be identical to that of other participating hospitals. Thus, as the number of physicians' units in hospitals increases, so will the heterogeneity of patients enrolled in the trial. With this increased degree of heterogeneity, the exact identity of patients becomes more ambiguous, the amount of variability between patients in outcome parameters is likely to increase.Conversely, the generalizability of the results as well as the ability to detect trends among different patient subgroups is increased with the heterogeneity of trial sites. The uniqueness of one hospital population may make the results irrelevant to another institution. For example, the results of sepsis in patients who have sepsis within the first week of liver transplant, may be totally irrelevant to a physician treating sepsis in a general medical ICU in a community hospital.

One of the concerns of interpreting the results of studies with heterogeneous patient population is whether or not the results can be explained by having sicker patients enrolled in one arm or the other of the trial. As the range of severity of patients increases because of increased heterogeneity, the chances of such mal-distribution occurring is also increased. Three approaches to this problem can be taken. The first of these is to examine whether or not known prognostic factors are maldistributed between the two populations, and if they are, attempt to correct the results to account for these differences using statistical methods (see below). The second method is to identify important prognostic factors and stratify patients at the time of enrollment into the trial by this factor. Thus, if disseminated intervascular coagulation (DIC) is expected to be an overwhelming prognostic factor in the trial, patients with DIC will be randomized to either the control or treatment groups, and patients without DIC will also be randomized thus guaranteeing equal numbers of patients in each arm with DIC and those without DIC. Finally, an adequate randomization scheme should minimize the probability of significant maldistribution. Randomization minimizes the chance for maldistribution of both known prognostic factors and those factors which have not yet been identified and therefore cannot be prospectively corrected (Table 2).

Patient Population Selection: As noted above, the inclusion/exclusion criteria of the study are major determinants in the amount of heterogeneity of patients enrolled in the trial. One of the difficulties associated with attempting to select patients with specific etiologic causes for their sepsis is that few criteria allow discrimination between patients with and without specific etiology. Two general approaches to the selection of patients for septic trials can be employed. The first, which has been the most frequently used method in the past, is to use variations on the "sepsis syndrome" definition first codi-

Table 2. Homogeneity versus heterogeneity in sepsis study population

	Study Length	Generalizability	Precision for Single Group
Homogeneity	Longer	No	Yes
Heterogeneity	Shorter	Yes	No

fied by Bone et al. [19]. This definition has now been used in several large, multi-centered trials, so that the expected mortality as well as other outcome parameters is available in the literature. The problem with this definition is that although the criteria are based on sound theoretical grounds, they are still arbitrary and have not been subjected to analysis for their ability to discriminate between patients with poor and good prognosis, etiologic cause of the sepsis, or the likelihood to respond to the therapy. Another approach to inclusion of patients has recently been entertained by the ACCP/SCCM Consensus Committee on Sepsis Terminology [20]. In this approach, a very general non-specific definition of sepsis is employed, requiring some combination of evidence indicative of infection as well as evidence indicative of a systemic inflammatory response. Once patients are identified, the severity of illness may be assessed using a risk assessment scoring system (i.e. APACHE II) to include those patients with expected mortality above a certain point and below a higher limit.

One of the difficult decisions that needs to be drawn is what patients should be excluded from such a trial. The patient should be excluded if, as a class, they are likely to have a significant different path of physiology to their sepsis, a significantly different prognosis, or significantly different pharmacokinetics. For these reasons, inclusion of patients with HIV infection, neutropenia, burns, bone marrow transplant, etc. needs to be carefully weighted.

Similarly, not only which patient should be enrolled in the trial, but also which patient should be analyzed in a trial must be carefully considered. Should patients who are randomized to receive a drug but never receive it or receive only a partial treatment course be included in the analysis? Patients who do not complete a course of therapy may do so because of severe side effects or even mortality resulting from the drug. Exclusion of such patients from the analysis may mask this downside to the therapy. However, if the intent of the trial is to assess for biological activity of the drug, inclusion of patients with sub-optimal or absent serum concentrations of the medication may dilute the measurement of its actual activity. Likewise, patients who suffer early deaths within the first few minutes or hours after treatment may not represent a drug failure but rather intervention at a stage in the disease at which point the process is irreversible. This arbitrary decision as to appropriate timing is compounded by the fact that a large percent of acute deaths from sepsis will occur within the first 48 h after onset. Therefore, a time period designated as inappropriate to expect an effect may substantially encroach upon the period of maximum mortality and possible efficacy.

As previously discussed, these specific therapies under investigation may be expected to be efficacious only in patients with specific etiologies of their sepsis. In such cases, the precise definition of the target population and the definitions used to classify patients into that population need to be clearly defined. Thus, if the target population is patients with sepsis due to fungal infection, unambiguous definitions for classification of patients having a fungal infection must be given. Should patients with mixed bacterial and fungal infections be included in the population? How will the presence of fungal infection be determined? Will positive cultures be required or are positive stains adequate? Who will determine whether or not specific findings will classify patients as having an infection, the principal investigator or a blinded panel? How should ambiguous findings be judged? For example, is an intubated patient with positive sputum for *Candida* and minimal changes on chest radiograph, infected or colonized.

It should be noted that clinical trials may have one or two different purposes. The first of these is to determine whether or not a new therapy has biological activity, and the second, is whether or not the new therapy has clinical utility. The patient selection process, if the goal is to look for biological activity, is to provide as heterogeneous a patient population as possible. Patients with ambiguous disease or non-standard treatment patterns should be excluded. If, on the other hand, the goal of the clinical trial is to determine clinical utility, how representative the patient enrolled is of all patients with a similar presentation is of paramount importance.

Outcome

A variety of outcome parameters are valid in sepsis syndrome. In a highly fatal disease such as sepsis, mortality provides an unambiguous endpoint. Two types of mortality can be measured. The first of these is all cause mortality. Such an endpoint provides a clean, usually uncontestable result: the patient is either dead or alive. The second mortality endpoint which can be measured is that of cause specific deaths. Patients who develop sepsis often have severe, life threatening disease. In trials with follow-up of several weeks to several months, mortality from the underlying condition can be appreciable. Therapy directed against sepsis is unlikely to affect mortality from patients' underlying condition i.e. severe trauma, or endstage cardiac disease. The difficulty with cause specific mortality is, however, that unlike death itself, the cause of death requires interpretation. Although the extremes of septic death from underlying disease are relatively clear, many patients are in the gray zone in which assignment of death to either underlying disease or sepsis is very arbitrary. Therefore, a majority of trials in sepsis have used all cause mortality as the principal endpoint of the trial. Provided that there is an adequate randomization of patients into the trial, one can expect that non-septic deaths will be evenly distributed between the treatment arms of the trial.

The time period over which mortality will be measured also must be specified. Early work by McCabe et al. [21] suggested that the majority of deaths directly resulting from sepsis occurs within the first 3–5 days after the onslaught of sepsis. With the advent of more aggressive and sophisticated supportive care, many patients with sepsis can be maintained for several weeks but will ultimately succumb [1–4]. A majority of recent studies of sepsis have looked at mortality at either 14 or 28 days. Another decision must be made as to whether deaths at a specific timepoint or actuarial survival curves will be used as the primary determinant of improved survival. The use of Kaplan-Meier survival curves provides important information not only as to the total number of deaths but the pattern of deaths as well [22–25]. A highly potent treatment which interferes directly with the sepsis itself would be expected to have significant impact upon immediate deaths within the first 3 to 5 days, whereas a therapy whose major impact is to protect against sequelae of sepsis without necessarily affecting the course of early deaths may have impact on the survival curve only after several weeks. Such survival curve analyses provide maximal utility for data collected.

One of the more problematic endpoints used for outcome determination is the application of a specific supportive therapy. Such endpoints include intubation, the use of vasopressors, and ICU care. Because such variables rely upon patient judgment as well as local preferences, such endpoints may reflect significantly different physiological states at different institutions. To be completely reliable, such variables can only be reliably used if strict comprehensive treatment protocols are utilized across all centers. When such treatment protocols are not ethically or practically appropriate, the use of underlying physiological measurements at specified time points should be considered.

Bias

The goal of formal clinical trials is to assess the impact of a specific therapy in a well defined population. In order to do so, the outcomes in each of the experimental arms must have as similar an expected outcome as possible.

Table 3. Bias in a sepsis clinical trial

	Occurrence	Defined	Example
Enrollment Bias	Unblinded trial	Difference in severity of illness between experimental arms	Avoiding new therapy in "hopelessly ill" patient because perception is that study drug works
Co-treatment Bias	Unblinded trial	Difference in aggressiveness of treatment between experimental arms	Doing more in patients that received study drug due to a perception that new drug does work
Ascertainment Bias	Unblinded and blinded trial	Increased incidence of morbidities in therapy arm not due to new therapy	New therapy keeps patients alive that would have died but leads to greater incidence of organ failure in these sick patients

Bias is any factor, other than the treatment under study, which would preferentially alter the outcome in one group over the other (Table 3) [7, 26]. Although bias can enter any step of a clinical investigation, formal steps must be taken to minimize bias at three important phases of the trial. Those are at the time of enrollment, in the follow-up period, and at the determination of outcome.

Enrollment bias occurs when patients who are extremely ill are preferentially enrolled in one arm of the trial. Physicians conducting clinic trials may have been convinced from the preclinical data that a new therapy either will or will not work in the patient population in which it is being tested. A physician who believes that new therapy is potentially life saving is more likely to enroll a patient with a high likelihood of dying into the treatment of the trial rather than letting them die. Similarly, a physician may believe that the new therapy is superior and therefore, will enroll the "hopeless" cases into the non-treatment arm to ensure that the drug is not "inappropriately" burdened with non-responding patients. It should be noted that this type of bias can occur either consciously or at a subconscious level. A standard way of minimizing enrollment bias is to randomly allocate patients. It should be noted, however, that most randomization schemes may be circumvented by persistent physicians.

Co-treatment bias is used to describe systematic differences in the aggressiveness of other therapies used depending on whether the patient received active treatment. A physician who believes that a new therapy is lifesaving may categorize such a patient as potentially more salvageable and be more aggressive in supportive care and less likely to recommend discontinuation of therapy than if the patient had received only conventual therapy. To minimize such bias, traditionally, a double-blind study is used. Here the physician is purposely kept uninformed as to which of the possible experimental therapies the patient actually received. In order to be effective, the alternative therapies must be undetectable. The active and placebo therapies must be as indistinguishable as possible. It should be noted that if a new therapy has a consistent side-effect or effect on the disease course, the blinding may be impossible. For example, a physician will have a good idea of whether or not the patient received active therapy if that new drug either dramatically decreases fever within the first hour after treatment or causes unusual side effects as urticaria or flushing in a large number of patients to which it has been given.

Ascertainment bias occurs when the likelihood of documenting an outcome variable is more likely in one treatment arm than the other. For example, patients receiving a new therapy which reduces acute physiological abnormalities, but does nothing for long term morbidity and mortality, may be more rapidly transferred back to the referring hospital making it more difficult to determine that they ultimately died within the follow-up period. Similarly, if a side-effect of a new therapy is severe headaches, the patients receiving the drug may be more likely to undergo CT scanning of the head. Mild to moderate abnormalities may be noted on such scans as a normal part of the sepsis process. Thus even if the true incidence of abnormalities are the same, the fact that more patients underwent the examination leads to the false impression that more patients receiving that therapy have such abnormalities. Again, the standard ways to minimize ascertainment bias is to blind physicians as to what therapy the patient received and specify specific examinations that will be done for all patients at specific timepoints throughout the trial.

In highly fatal illnesses such as sepsis, a unique type of ascertainment bias occurs with efficacious new drugs. Patients who die of sepsis in the immediate 24 to 48 h usually die of intractable hypotension and the resulting cardiovascular problems. If a new therapy keeps such patients alive, these patients are at extremely high risk of developing organ system failure (MOF) as a result of their overwhelming disease. Thus, after enrollment in the trial, three distinct cohorts of patients exist. The first of these are patients who will live regardless of therapy. The second cohort are those who will die regardless of therapy, and the final group are those patients who should have died but are saved by the new drug. This latter group is seen only in the treatment arm of the trial and is expected to have a large number of MOF and are likely to be in the ICU for a prolonged period. Identification of such patients is impossible. Thus, in the treatment group are a mixture of patients destined to live who may have a reduced number of MOF because of the therapy. In addition to this group, however, are those who should have died and have a large number of medical problems resulting from their non-death. If the reduction in mortality is large enough, the incidence of patients with MOF may actually be higher in those receiving the efficacious drug compared to the placebo group. Thus, the ascertainment of non-fatal events is obscured in some patients by the patient's death and this will differentially occur whether or not the patient received or did not receive the efficacious therapy.

Thus, the gold standard for clinical trial design is a randomized prospective double-blind trial [27]. This type of design can minimize the amount of bias involved in the trial. It should be noted, however, that this type of trial may not be appropriate for all diseases. Very rare diseases may not have enough patients available within reasonable amounts of time in order for a double-blind randomized trial to be conducted. Uncommon diseases may require such long patient accrual periods that the introduction of concomitant therapies may make the expected mortality at the beginning and end of the trial significantly different, making the results difficult to interpret. In some diseases, the outcome is so predictable that concurrent controls are not necessary. For example, a new therapy in rabies which prevented death in 90% of afflicted patients would not need concurrent controls to persuade most physicians to use the drug.

Organization of Clinical Trials

It is possible for a single investigator to implement all phases of the clinical trial in a scientifically, rigorous fashion. He/she can randomize drug, administer the drug, determine outcomes and analyze the data. As trials increase in size, and to guarantee to a sceptical readership about the validity of the trial, more formal organizations are usually employed, especially in multicenter trials. Most of the formal organization of large trials are to guarantee that appropriate blinding has been performed, and to decrease the amount of variability in the outcome parameters examined.

A coordinating center is frequently employed to create the randomization code, label the drug, and audit compliance with blinding procedures. In addition, they may be given responsibility such as assuring adequate supplies for the trial are available at each site, track patient enrollment, etc. The use of an independent group not associated with any other aspect of the trial (neither sponsor nor participating institution) minimizes the possibility of intentional bias entering the trial. In most trials, the identity of the study material is available in a coded form to investigators. This can be through a message on the label which is visible after washing with alcohol, opening a sealed envelope, etc. Audits by a coordinating center as to how many cases each at site were unblinded provides an objective assessment of the incidence of unblinding.

For ethical reasons, studies should not be continued once there is clear reasons to believe that one treatment arm of the trial is doing significantly better. This can either be because new therapy is efficacious or because it has significant side effects. Because knowledge of the results of the trial may lead to bias, analysis of the results prior to completion of the trial should be handled by an independent group not associated with the actual conduct of the study. Such a group would be responsible for conducting and analyzing interim results and making the decision whether to continue with the trial or not. Also, the independent group is responsible for monitoring the safety and incidence of unexpected adverse events. Because of their broad responsibilities, such a committee should include statisticians, clinicians, and preferably, an ethicist.

In complex diseases such as sepsis, classification of patients as well as classification of outcomes frequently will involve some degree of physician judgment. Even using standardized classifications for diagnosis of entities such as the adult respiratory distress syndrome (ARDS), two physicians may classify the same patient differently. One way to minimize the amount of heterogeneity in classification is to have one person or group classify all cases in the trial. Such a clinical evaluation committee increases the consistency of classification although not necessarily the accuracy of such a classification. In a similar fashion, different hospital laboratories may use slightly differing assay methods for a test or report the results in different units. If laboratory finding is to be used as a primary outcome variable, the use of a central laboratory will minimize the variability associated with different labs doing that test.

Statistics

The analysis of data generated from most clinical trials in sepsis is a non-trivial exercise. The collaboration of a statistician in the analysis cannot be overemphasized and the involvement of the statistician throughout the trial from the creation of the protocol through the final report of the findings is essential. We will only touch on three critical areas: the need for statistical penalties resulting from multiple looks at the data or from the assessment of multiple endpoints or subgroups, secondary analyses, and the use of statistical adjustment for observed maldistribution.

The standard convention of accepting p=0.05 as the threshold for statistically significance means that there is a one out of twenty chance that a "statistically significant result" is due to chance and not a real difference. This means that if 100 independent endpoints are examined in a trial of an ineffective drug, one would expect about 5 endpoints to have a difference with p=0.05. A number of correction factors to compensate for multiple endpoints have been suggested. The simplest and most conservative is the Bonferroni adjustment in which the threshold for statistical significance is divided by the number of outcomes examined [28]. Using this method, if 10 independent outcomes are analyzed, the level of "statistical significance" would be p=0.005. Outcomes in sepsis trials are likely to be correlated so that this method is likely to be overly conservative. Methods for estimating the adjustment (statistical penalty) required for multiple correlated outcomes have been developed [29, 30] but remain controversial [31]. It can be said, however, that the smaller the number of endpoints examined as a primary analysis, the less problematic the interpretation of the results will be, with a single endpoint being ideal. In a similar fashion, the discussion for multiple endpoints applies as well if multiple subpopulations in the trial are examined separately.

When the data is examined while the trial is still ongoing and a decision to continue or halt the trial is made after examining the results, the probability of potential outcomes is altered since the most extreme results are no longer possible. The level of statistical significance must be adjusted for each of the interim analysis in order to keep the total statistical significance at p=0.05 level (alpha error). A number of well accepted methods are available to calculate the required level of significance for each interim/final analysis [32–35]. All of these methods require that the number of analyses and the resultant effect on a significant p-value be specified prospectively and that no other "peeks" at the data be allowed.

Because the number of primary analyses affect the interpretation of the results, the precise number of subgroups and endpoints must be explicitly stated and the definitions of these analyses unambiguously stated prior to analyzing the data. Because an almost limitless number of subpopulations and endpoints can be created and analyzed retrospectively following completion of the trial (often based on casual observation of apparent differences in the database), analyses of subgroups/endpoints not clearly stated to be a part of the primary analysis cannot be used to prove efficacy. Such secondary analysis results can lead to the creation of new trials specifically targeted to this unexpected subgroup ("hypothesis generating" results) but cannot prove the efficacy ("hypothesis proving" results). This also applies to using slightly different definitions for the subgroup (such as redefining respiratory failure after analyzing the data or altering the PaO_2/FiO_2 ratio definition for ARDS).

Randomization is used to minimize maldistribution both of measured variables as well as unmeasured variables. It is expected that numeric differences will arise in the number of patients with specific demographic, underlying disease(s), and baseline characteristics when comparing the treatment arms of the trial. Few, if any, of the differences in important prognostic factors, are expected to be statistically significant. If important differences arise, there are several methods which allow the analysis to mathematically adjust for this maldistribution [36]. This simplest method is to stratify for that factor. For example, if the incidence of shock is different in the treatment arms, the mortality in patients with shock and the mortality in patients without shock can be compared between the two treatment arms. A summary "p-value" across the shock/no shock groups can be calculated using the Cochran-Haenszel-Mantel method [37, 38]. A more sophisticated approach is to create a statistical model which simultaneously adjusts for several factors. This can be accomplished by modeling the incidence data using logistic regression analyses [39, 40] and survival data using the Cox proportional hazards model [41, 42]. These models make several assumptions about the data and these assumptions must be verified. In general, the most compelling data about efficacy arises from a statistically significant difference in the incidence of the endpoint in the two treatment arms of the trial and the statistical significance remains after correcting for each important prognostic factor singly or in combination. Because of the large number of potential "important prognostic factors", results which are significant only when adjusted must be accepted with caution. Unless the specific method of adjustment and exactly which factors are to be adjusted for are unambiguously stated *a priori*, such analyses must be considered secondary analysis and nonconclusive proof of efficacy.

Conclusion

Clinical trials in sepsis must address the complexity of this heterogeneous syndrome. To extract useful information concerning the efficacy of a new treatment modality, great care must be taken in selecting the patient population of interest (the target population) and the entrance criteria to select for these patients. The question to be answered by the trial must be precise. A limited number (preferably one) of subgroups and endpoints must be prospectively defined and definitions allowing classification of patients precisely and unambiguously stated. A double-blind, randomized clinical trial will provide the most unequivocal results. The conduct of the trial, including standardization of classification (both clinical and laboratory), should be as rigorous as possible. The primary analyses performed should be prospectively defined and clear differentiation between primary ("hypothesis proving") and secondary ("hypothesis generating") analyses clearly made, especially in any report of the trial. Such trials are large and costly but provide the best information concerning the care of the critical ill patients.

References

1. Bone R, Fisher C, Clemmer T, et al. (1987) A controlled clinical trial of high-dose methylprednisolone in the treatment of severe sepsis and septic shock. N Engl J Med 317:653–658
2. The Veterans Administration Systemic Sepsis Cooperative Study Group (1987) Effect of high-dose glucocorticoid therapy on the mortality in patients with clinical signs of systemic sepsis. N Engl J Med 317:659–665
3. Ziegler EJ, Fisher CJ, Sprung CL, et al. (1991) Treatment of gram-negative bacteremia and septic shock with HA-1A human monoclonal antibody against endotoxin. N Engl J Med 324:429–436
4. Greenman RL, Schein RMH, Martin MA, et al. (1991) A controlled clinical trial of E5 murine monoclonal IgM antibody to endotoxin in the treatment of gram-negative sepsis. J Am Med Assoc 266:1097–1102
5. Feinstein AR (1985) Clinical epidemiology. The architecture of clinical research. Little, Brown, and Co, Boston
6. Sackett DL, Haynes RB, Tugwell P (1985) Clinical epidemiology. A basic science for clinical medicine. Little, Brown, and Co, Boston
7. Fletcher RH, Fletcher SW, Wagner EH (1988) Clinical epidemiology. The essentials. 2nd ed, Williams and Wilkins, Baltimore
8. Hulley SB, Cummings SR (1988) Designing clinical research. Williams and Wilkins, Baltimore
9. Iber FL, Riley WA, Murray PJ (1987) Conducting clinical trials. Plenum Medical Book Co, New York, pp 3–17
10. Code of Federal Regulations, Title 21, Part 310
11. Hellman S, Hellman DS (1991) Of mice but not men. Problems of a randomized clinical trial. N Engl J Med 324:1585–1589
12. Passamani E (1991) Clinical trials: Are they ethical? N Engl J Med 324:1589–1592
13. Armitage P (1971) The size of a statistical investigation. In: Statistical methods in medical research. Blackwell Scientific Publications, Oxford, pp 184–188
14. Snedecor GW, Cochran WG (1967) Size of sample. In: Statistical methods. 6th ed. Iowa State University Press, Ames, pp 517–520
15. Simon R (1982) Patient subsets and variation in therapeutic efficacy. Br J Clin Pharmacol 14:473–482
16. Bulpitt CJ (1988) Subgroup analysis. Lancet 2:31–34
17. Yusuf S, Held P, Teo KK, Toresky ER (1990) Selection of patients for randomized controlled trials: Implications of wide or narrow eligibility criteria. Stat Med 9:73–86
18. Yusuf S, Wittes J, Prosbstfield J, Tyroler HA (1991) Analysis and interpretation of treatment effects in subgroups of patients in randomized clinical trials. J Am Med Assoc 266:93–98
19. Bone RC, Fisher CJ, Clemmer TP, et al. (1989) Sepsis syndrome: A valid clinical entity. Crit Care Med 17:389–393
20. ACCP-SCCM Consensus Conference (1992) Definitions for sepsis and organ failure and guidelines for the use of innovative therapies in sepsis. Chest 101:1644–1655
21. Kreger BE, Craven DE, McCabe WR (1980) Gram-negative bacteremia. IV. Re-evaluation of clinical features and treatment in 612 patients. Am J Med 68:344–355
22. Kaplan EL, Meier P (1958) Nonparametric estimation from incomplete observations. J Am Stat Assoc 53:457–481
23. Lee ET (1980) Statistical methods for survival data analysis. Wadsworth, California.
24. Harris EK, Albert A (1991) Survivorship analysis for clinical studies. Marcel Dekker, Inc, New York

25. Miller RG (1981) Survivor analysis. Wiley and Sons, New York
26. Sackett DL (1979) Bias in analytic research. J Chronic Dis 32:51–63
27. Byar DP, Simon RM, Friedewald WT, et al. (1976) Randomized clinical trials. Perspectives on some recent ideas. N Engl J Med 295:74–80
28. Ingelfinger JA, Mosteller F, Thibodeau LA, Ware JH (1987) Problems of multiplicity. In: Biostatistics in clinical medicine, 2nd ed, Macmillian, New York, pp 160–162
29. Pocock SJ (1983) Clinical trials: A practical approach. Wiley and Sons, New York
30. Pocock SJ, Geller NL, Tsiatis AA (1987) The analysis of multiple endpoints in clinical trials. Biometrics 43:487–498
31. Rothman KJ (1990) No adjustments are needed for multiple comparisons. Epidemiol 1:43–46
32. Pocock SJ (1977) Group sequential methods in the design and analysis of clinical trials. Biometrika 64:191–199
33. O'Brien PC, Fleming TR (1979) A multiple testing procedure for clinical trials. Biometrics 35:549–556
34. Lan KKG, DeMets DL (1983) Discrete sequential boundaries for clinical trials. Biometrika 70:659–664
35. Fleming TR, Harrington DP, O'Brien PC (1984) Designs for group sequential tests. Controlled Clinical Trials 5:348–361
36. Breslow NE, Day NE (1980) Initial treatment of the data. In: Statistical methods in cancer research. Vol. 1- The analysis of case-control studies, IARC Scientific Publications, Lyon, pp 90–115
37. Mantel N, Haenszel W (1959) Statistical aspects of the analysis of data from retrospective study of disease. J Natl Cancer Instit 59:799–811
38. Cochran WG (1963) Sampling techniques. 2nd ed, Wiley and Sons, New York
39. Draper N, Smith H (1981) Applied regression analysis. 2nd ed, Wiley and Sons, New York
40. Cornfield J (1962) Joint dependence of the risk of coronary heart disease on serum cholesterol and systolic blood pressure: A discriminant function analysis. Fed Proc 21:58–61
41. Cox DR (1972) Regression models and life tables. J Royal Stat Soc B 34:187–220
42. Armitage P, Gehan EA (1974) Statistical methods for the identification and use of prognostic factors. Internat J Cancer 13:16–36

Experimental Basis of New Therapeutic Approaches to Septic Shock

J. Cohen

Introduction

In 1982, the distinguished scientist, David Tyrrell, wrote a monograph entitled " The Abolition of Infection: Hope or Illusion?" [1]. In it, he drew attention to the fact that the long-expected demise of infection as a "problem" was evidently not going to happen. Issues such as the development of antibiotic resistance in common bacteria, and the contribution of the host to the pathophysiological disease would, he said, require new and innovative approaches to the treatment of infection. The need for these new strategies was particularly apparent in the case of septic shock. Mortality was "stuck", rising to 75% or more in established cases [2], and it was clear that this high mortality was not due simply to the inadequacy of antibiotics.

For these reasons, the last 10 years, and particularly the last 5 years, have seen considerable interest in the pathophysiology of sepsis, and the development of new therapeutic strategies based on modification of the host response, rather than aimed directly at the organism. Such strategies have included monoclonal antibodies to endotoxin and to cytokines, the cloning and expression of circulating receptors or receptor antagonists, and the evaluation of naturally occurring, or pharmaceutically-derived endotoxin binding agents. Not surprisingly, not all of these approaches have equal merit, and before they undergo extensive development they must be tested, screened, and evaluated in a variety of systems. Septic shock has proved to be more difficult than most clinical syndromes to model, and the interpretation of results has led to some controversy.

In this chapter, I shall try and discuss some of these issues, and suggest a general strategy for the evaluation of new agents for septic shock. I shall take as an example tumor necrosis factor-α (TNF), and the several approaches to "anti-TNF".

In Vitro Screening

It is self-evident that most novel therapeutic compounds are first screened for activity *in vitro*. In the case of antibiotics for instance, this is a rather straightforward procedure which generally provides a good general guide to likely efficacy *in vivo*. However in the case of "anti-shock" agents, the situation is less clear. Sepsis is a clinical syndrome caused by many different bacteria. One may take endotoxin as representing gram-negative bacteria, or use the particular target of the intervention – a cytokine, or some other mediator molecule for instance. The difficulty with these approaches is that sepsis is a classical example of a disease greater than the sum of its parts; it is a complex process in which intervention in one area might have only a modest effect on the final outcome. Hence, the successful demonstration of activity *in vitro* against one particular target will not necessarily be reflected in efficacy in *in vivo* models of sepsis. A good example is provided by corticosteroids, which 30 years ago were shown *in vitro* to inhibit some properties of endotoxin [3]. When adequate clinical trials were eventually done, steroid treatment was shown not to be beneficial [4, 5].

Most *in vitro* screening tests depend on the neutralization of a biological property of the target molecule. Hence in the case of an "anti-TNF" (of whatever kind) a standard assay is the ability to neutralize recombinant protein in a cytotoxicity assay, such as the L929 assay. Other, more sophisticated assays are based on TNF-induced expression of class I MHC antigens, or similar properties. While these assays, like all *in vitro* procedures, have their limitations, they do at least provide a general indication of likely *in vivo* activity.

With anti-endotoxin antibodies the picture has been considerably less clear. Although there is no shortage of biological "read-outs" which could serve as an endpoint for a bioassay, it has often been difficult to relate *in vitro* activity with *in vivo* protection. We used two *in vitro* assays to rank a panel of monoclonal antibodies to endotoxin core [6]. First, we measured the binding titre in a standard solid-phase ELISA, and then we determined the dilution of each antibody which would neutralize a fixed concentration of endotoxin in the Limulus assay. When we compared the results of these two *in vitro* tests with the potency of the antibodies in a mouse protection assay, we found no correlation. Similar results have been reported by others [7, 8], thus raising questions about the mode of action of these antibodies.

Initial Tests in Animals

Because of the particular reasons outlined above, experiments in animals are a necessary prerequisite to further clinical development. All such experiments should attempt to limit the numbers of animals to the minimum needed to obtain satisfactory data. Preliminary *in vivo* tests are usually done in small rodents such as mice, rats, or guinea pigs. In the case of sepsis and septic shock however, there are a number of issues that need to be borne in mind (Table 1).

LPS versus Live Infection Challenge. Many of the early studies were done by injecting purified lipopolysaccharide (LPS). Unfortunately, mice and rats are extremely resistant to LPS, and very large doses are necessary to obtain

Table 1. Issuses to be considered in designing animal models of sepsis

1. Use of LPS or bacterial challenge
2. Sensitisation: D – galactosamine; Mucin-hemoglobin, etc...
3. Use of antibiotics
4. Route of infection / challenge
5. Infecting organism: gram-negative vs gram-positive

a response. Furthermore, LPS is just one component (albeit a rather important one) of the organism that is responsible for the syndrome of sepsis, and it could be argued that LPS alone is not the most appropriate challenge. LPS is obtained from bacteria by a number of different chemical procedures, and we do not know if this purified LPS reflects accurately the form in which LPS circulates during sepsis. Finally, the particular method of LPS extraction can alter the biological response. Hence models employing pure LPS can give only limited information, and challenge with live bacteria is preferable.

Many investigators begin their studies with *E. coli,* as a representative gram-negative organism. If the initial studies are encouraging, it is clearly important that the model is extended to include other organisms; *Pseudomonas* and *Klebsiella* are used frequently.

Methods of Increasing Sensitivity to LPS. Because rodents are so resistant to LPS, a number of models have been developed which render the animals more sensitive. These include the use of mucin and hemoglobin [9], lead acetate [10], and D-galactosamine [11]. These maneuvers will certainly reduce the LD_{50} by several orders of magnitude, but the price to be paid is an inevitable alteration of the physiology. Galactosamine, for instance, is a potent hepatotoxin and thus might be expected to modify the hepatic response to sepsis.

The Use of Antibiotics. There are a number of suggestions in the literature indicating that antibiotic-induced bacterial lysis can modify the form in which endotoxin is presented to the host [12]. For this reason, several animal models have been developed in which challenge with live bacteria is followed by the use of antibiotics [13, 14]. Indeed, in some instances, agents have been found to be effective only when antibiotics are added to the protocol [15]. Although there has been a good deal of debate as to whether different classes of antibiotics are more or less potent in this regard [16], in practice this has made little difference. In my view, antibiotic-treated live-challenge models are the most appropriate way to carry out initial *in vivo* screening of new agents for sepsis.

Other Issues in Experimental Design. A number of practical considerations have emerged as being of considerable importance in designing animal models of sepsis. One has been the phenomenon of endotoxin tolerance, whereby minute amounts of endotoxin can tolerise an animal to subsequent, larger doses. In practice, this means that care must be taken to ensure that putative protective antibodies, for example, must be checked for endotoxin contamination since if they are given prophylactically before the bacterial challenge, any apparent protection might be due to the induction of tolerance rather than any specific benefit from the antibody [17]. A similar problem can arise due to the contamination of monoclonal ascitic fluid with cytokines [18].

Most animal models involve the intravenous injection of the challenge, be it LPS or bacteria. However, other routes may yield different answers, and a variety of models should be evaluated. Another variable to consider is timing; agents active prophylactically may not work when given therapeutically, a point of some practical importance. Finally, most of this discussion has assumed that the agent is designed to modify gram-negative sepsis, and indeed this has been the focus of most recent work. However, 40–50% of septicemias are due to gram-positive infections [2], and clinically, gram-negative and gram-positive shocks are indistinguishable. Hence, agents which are designed for the empirical treatment of "sepsis" need to be evaluated in models of gram-positive infection as well, and these are not yet well validated.

TNF as an Example. The first demonstration of the pivotal role of TNF in gram-negative sepsis was an experiment in which a crude rabbit polyclonal antibody protected LPS-challenged mice [19]. The question of whether pure TNF is in fact harmful to mice has been the subject of some debate. Some studies showed that injection of TNF could reproduce many of the pathological features of shock [20], but others presented strong evidence that TNF alone was not injurious [21–23]. The demonstration that monoclonal anti-TNF could protect mice from a live infection challenge was helpful in confirming that anti-TNF might indeed have a clinical role; the same study also demonstrated for the first time that anti-TNF could be protective given *after* the bacterial challenge [13].

TNF also provides a good example of the importance of the route of infection. Most of the early studies (which showed protection) used an intravenous route, but later several investigators evaluated anti-TNF in models of gram-negative peritonitis [24, and Glauser M, personal communication]. Interestingly, anti-TNF was ineffective in these experiments, raising important questions in the design and evaluation of clinical trials.

Theoretically, anti-TNF might be active in both gram-negative and gram-positive infections [25]. Data in gram-positive models are still very preliminary. Anti-TNF appeared to be protective in a baboon model of shock due to *Staph. aureus* [26], but not in a murine model of *Strep. pyogenes* [27]. Further experience with other systems is needed to clarify this situation.

Large Animal Models of Sepsis

The use of large animals offers considerable advantages in the opportunity that it provides to carry out detailed physiological monitoring, and to obtain sequential measurements from the blood or other body fluids. Large animals may also provide initial data on toxicity and pharmacokinetics. The major limitation is the number of animals that can be studied, hence the usual practice of restricting this type of study to molecules that have already demonstrated their potential worth in small animal models.

Dogs [28] and pigs [29] have been widely used for these purposes. Rabbits are not really "large" animals, but because of their extreme sensitivity to LPS and the fact that physiological monitoring is possible, they provide a valuable alternative.

In the case of TNF, the dog, and in particular the rabbit, have been studied widely. Rabbits were used to show that TNF and IL-1 were synergistic [30, 31], and also to characterize the cytokine response to *E. coli* and *Staph. epidermidis* [32]. Natanson et al. [33] showed that in dogs, TNF could reproduce the cardiovascular changes induced by challenge with live *E. coli*.

In addition, a number of investigators have employed primate models of sepsis, primarily because of the limited inter-species cross-reactivity of some agents directed against human TNF. It was in the baboon that Tracey et al. [34] first demonstrated the efficacy of a monoclonal antibody to human TNF, and later studies extended these observations [35–37]. Although these primate studies have been seen as a necessary preliminary to clinical trials of new agents, it should be remembered that there are some drawbacks. The small numbers of animals that can be studied inevitably limits the number of questions that can be asked. Furthermore, primates are in fact rather resistant to endotoxin; in Tracey's experiments, for instance, the dose of bacteria that was injected (approximately 10^{12} organisms) was enormous, and arguably was in effect a pure LPS challenge.

Conclusions

The general approach to the evaluation of new agents for sepsis is summarized in Table 2, but there is no single "gold standard". Numerous studies over the last 15 years have demonstrated that shock is a particularly difficult area to model; fortunately, most of the pitfalls are now well recognized. The development of "anti-TNF" agents illustrates many of the issues that need to be considered when evaluating potential new therapeutic agents for this indication.

Table 2. A Strategy for the evaluation of novel therapeutic agents in sepsis

In Vitro Screening	Large animal model (dogs, pigs, rabbits, primates)
In Vivo tests	– Studies of efficacy
Small animals	– Physiological studies
– LPS challenge	– Toxicology / Pharmacology studies
– Live bacterial challenge	

References

1. Tyrrell DA (1982) The abolition of infection. Hope or illusion? Nuffield Provincial Hospitals Trust, London, pp 1–66
2. Ispahani P, Pearson NJ, Greenwood D (1987) An analysis of community and hospital-acquired bacteraemia in a large teaching hospital in the United Kingdom. Q J Med 63:427–440
3. Flohe L, Giertz H (1987) Endotoxins, arachidonic acid, superoxide formation. Rev Infect Dis 9:553–561
4. Hinshaw LB, Peduzzi P, Young E, et al. (1987) Effect of high-dose glucocorticoid therapy on mortality in patients with clinical signs of systemic sepsis. N Engl J Med 317:659–665
5. Bone RC, Fisher CJ Jr, Clemmer TP, Slotman GJ, Metz CA, Balk RA (1987) A controlled clinical trial of high-dose methylprednisolone in the treatment of severe sepsis and septic shock. N Engl J Med 317:653–658
6. McConnell JS, Appelmelk BJ, Cohen J (1990) Dissociation between Limulus neutralisation and in vivo protection in monoclonal antibodies directed against endotoxin core structures. Microb Pathogen 9:55–59
7. Pollack M, Chia JK, Koles NL, Miller M, Guelde G (1989) Specificity and cross-reactivity of monoclonal antibodies reactive with the core and lipid A regions of bacterial lipopolysaccharide. J Infect Dis 159:168–188
8. Heumann D; Baumgartner JD, Jacot-Guillarmod H, Glauser MP (1991) Antibodies to core lipopolysaccharide determinants: Absence of cross reactivity with heterologous lipopolysaccharides. J Infect Dis 163:762–768
9. Appelmelk BJ, Verweij-Van Vught AM, Maaskant JJ, Schouten WF, Thijs LG, MacLaren DM (1986) Use of mucin and hemoglobin in experimental murine gram-negative bacteremia enhances the immunoprotective action of antibodies reactive with the lipopolysaccharide core region. Antonie van Leeuwenhoek 52:537–542
10. Selye H, Tuchweber B, Bertok L (1966) Effect of lead acetate on the susceptibility of rats to bacterial endotoxins. J Bact 91:884–890
11. Lehmann V, Freudenberg MA, Galanos C (1987) Lethal toxicity of lipopolysaccharide and tumor necrosis factor in normal and D-galactosamine-treated mice. J Exp Med 165:657–663
12. Overbeek BP, Veringa EM (1991) Role of antibodies and antibiotics in aerobic gram-negative septicemia: Possible synergism between antimicrobial treatment and immunotherapy. Rev Infect Dis 13:751–760
13. Silva AT, Bayston KF, Cohen J (1990) Prophylactic and therapeutic effects of a monoclonal antibody to tumor necrosis factor – alpha in experimental gram-negative shock. J Infect Dis 162:421–427
14. Opal SM, Cross AS, Kelly NM, et al. (1990) Efficacy of a monoclonal antibody directed against tumor necrosis factor in protecting neutropenic rats from lethal infection with Pseudomonas aeruginosa. J Infect Dis 161:1148–1152
15. Young LS, Gascon R, Alam S, Bermudez LE (1989) Monoclonal antibodies for treatment of gram-negative infections. Rev Infect Dis 11 (Supp 7):1564–1571
16. Shenep JL (1986) Antibiotic-induced bacterial cell lysis: A therapeutic dilemma. Eur J Clin Microbiol 5:11–12
17. Woods JP, Black JR, Barritt DS, Connell TD, Cannon JG (1987) Resistance to meningococcemia apparently conferred by anti-H.8 monoclonal antibody is due to contaminating endotoxin and not to specific immunoprotection. Infect Immun 55:1927–1928
18. Gearing AJ, Leung H, Bird CR, Thorpe R (1989) Presence of the inflammatory cytokines IL-1, TNF, and IL-6 in preparations of monoclonal antibodies. Hybridoma 8:361–367
19. Beutler B, Milsark IW, Cerami A (1985) Passive immunization against cachectin/tumor necrosis factor protects mice from lethal effect of endotoxin. Science 229:869–871
20. Tracey KJ, Beutler B, Lowry SF, et al. (1986) Shock and tissue injury induced by recombinant human cachectin. Science 234:470–474
21. Rothstein JL, Schreiber H (1988) Synergy between tumor necrosis factor and bacterial products causes hemorrhagic necrosis and lethal shock in normal mice. Proc Natl Acad Sci USA 85:607–611

22. Kiener PA, Marek F, Rodgers G, Lin P-F, Warr G, Desiderio J (1988) Induction of tumor necrosis factor, IFN-gamma, and acute lethality in mice by toxic and non-toxic forms of Lipid A. J Immunol 141:870–874
23. Silva AT, Appelmelk BJ, Buurman WA, Bayston KF, Cohen J (1990) Monoclonal antibody to endotoxin core protects mice from Escherichia coli sepsis by a mechanism independent of tumor necrosis factor and interleukin-6. J Infect Dis 162:454–459
24. Bagby GJ, Plessala KJ, Wilson LA, Thompson JJ, Nelson S (1991) Divergent efficacy of antibody to tumor necrosis factor alpha in intravascular and peritonitis models of sepsis. J Infect Dis 163:83–88
25. Freudenberg MA, Galanos C (1991) Tumor necrosis factor alpha mediates lethal activity of killed gram-negative and gram-positive bacteria in D-galactosamine-treated mice. Infect Immun 59:2110–2115
26. Hinshaw LB, Emerson TE Jr, Taylor FB Jr, et al. (1992) Lethal Staphyococcus aureus-induced shock in primates: Prevention of death with anti-TNF antibody. J Trauma (in press)
27. Wayte J, Silva AT, Cohen J (1991) Role of tumour necrosis factor (TNF) in experimental gram-positive sepsis. Interscience Conference on Antimicrobial Agents and Chemotherapy, Chicago. (Abst) 789
28. Natanson C, Danner RL, Elin RJ, et al. (1989) Role of endotoxemia in cardiovascular dysfunction and mortality. Escherichia coli and Staphylococcus aureus challenges in a canine model of human septic shock. J Clin Invest 83:243–251
29. Rokke O, Revhaug A, Osterud B, Giercksky KE (1988) Increased plasma levels of endotoxin and corresponding changes in circulatory performance in a porcine sepsis model: The effect of antibiotic administration. Prog Clin Biol Res 272:247–262
30. Okusawa S, Gelfand JA, Ikejima T, Connolly RJ, Dinarello CA (1988) Interleukin- 1 induces a shock-like state in rabbits. Synergism with tumor necrosis factor and the effect of cyclooxygenase inhibition. J Clin Invest 81:1162–1172
31. Weinberg JR, Wright DJ, Guz A (1988) Interleukin-1 and tumor necrosis factor cause hypotension in the conscious rabbit. Clin Sci 75:251–255
32. Wakabayashi G, Gelfand JA, Jung WK, Connolly RJ, Burke JF, Dinarello CA (1991) Staphylococcus epidermidis induces complement activation, tumor necrosis factor and interleukin-1, a shockk-like state and tissue injury in rabbits without endotoxemia. Comparison to Escherichia coli. J Clin Invest 87:1925–1935
33. Natanson C, Eichenholz PW, Danner RL, et al. (1989) Endotoxin and tumor necrosis factor challenges in dogs simulate the cardiovascular profile of human septic shock. J Exp Med 169:823–832
34. Tracey KJ, Fong Y, Hesse DG, et al. (1987) Anti-cachectin/TNF monoclonal antibodies prevent septic shock during lethal bacteraemia. Nature 330:662–664
35. Minami A, Fujimoto K, Aozaki Y, Nakamura S (1988) Augmentation of host resistance to microbial infections by recombinant human interleukin-1 alpha. Infect Immun 56:3116–3120
36. Hinshaw LB, Tekamp-Olson P, Chang AC, et al. (1990) Survival of primates in LD100 septic shock following therapy with antibody to tumor necrosis factor (TNF alpha). Circ Shock 30:279–292
37. Exley AR, Buurman WA, Bodmer M, Cohen J (1989) Monoclonal antibody to recombinant human tumor necrosis factor in the prophylaxis and treatment of endotoxic shock in Cynomolgus monkeys. Clin Sci 76:50p

Anti-Endotoxin Antibodies: A Critical Appraisal

J.D. Baumgartner

Introduction

More than 20 years ago, the hypothesis has been made that antibodies to the core region of endotoxin (lipopolysaccharide, LPS) might afford protection against a great variety of gram-negative strains serologically distinct in their O antigen specificities [1, 2]. These antibodies were elicited by immunization with rough mutants of gram-negative bacilli, the LPS of which is devoid of O antigen, thus exposing the core region at the surface of the bacterial membrane. It was postulated that these antibodies could recognize an epitope of the core region shared by endotoxins from pathogenic gram-negative bacteria. The initial studies were performed with antisera or immunoglobulin fractions. Recently, investigations were performed with anti-core LPS monoclonal antibodies, in particular antibodies to the lipid A region of LPS. However, the concept has been the subject of considerable debates [3, 4]. Several points remain unclear:

1) the epitope of core LPS which is responsible for the postulated cross-reactivity of anti-core LPS antibodies has not been precisely characterized;
2) the mode of action of the polyclonal or monoclonal anti-core LPS antibodies that were reported to be protective has not been demonstrated. Although it is postulated that they might neutralize endotoxins, no experimental evidence for such a mode of action has yet been published;
3) the factor responsible for the protection observed in some experimental models and in some clinical studies with polyclonal antisera has not been clarified: that the protection was antibody-mediated was even not demonstrated;
4) the discrepant results of the protective experiments are difficult to understand because opposite results were sometimes obtained using similar animal models;
5) the clinical studies with polyclonal antibody preparations are puzzling because only one was successful, another was possibly successful, whereas four failed;
6) the clinical studies with two monoclonal anti-lipid A antibodies did not allow to solve the problems because the results with both antibodies were discordant and because only subsets of randomized patients appeared to be protected.

Cross-reactive Epitope(s) of Core LPS or of Lipid A

In contrast to the highly variable outer side chains of LPS (O antigens), the inner core and the lipid A region of LPS is structurally conserved among gram-negative bacteria, with only a limited degree of variability. It was therefore postulated that antibody(ies) recognizing epitope(s) of the core LPS could cross-react with a large variety of strains. However, this hypothesis is still unproven because the postulated common epitope of core LPS could not be precisely characterized, and because the actual demonstration of cross-reactivity of core LPS antibody or of anti-lipid A antibody with smooth bacteria or with LPS has been exceedingly difficult, even with the use of monoclonal antibodies. While some groups have reported observations suggesting that various polyclonal or monoclonal core LPS antibodies might be cross-reactive, other attempts have revealed little or no cross-reactivity, or cross-reactivities with only a few strains of gram-negative bacteria [3, 5]. Some of these discrepancies might be explained by the different serologic methods used, because LPS are amphiphilic substances that are difficult to use as antigens, because they form aggregates, they bind poorly to ELISA plates, and they promote non-specific sticking of immunoglobulins to LPS hydrophobic regions. Some sticky immunoglobulins might therefore be misinterpreted as cross-reacting antibodies, especially in ELISA [6, 7].

The advent of monoclonal antibody technology did not solve the problem because discrepant results on cross-reactivities of anti-lipid A monoclonal antibodies with LPS from pathogenic gram-negative bacteria have been published. Some monoclonal antibodies have been reported to specifically bind to the lipid A part of endotoxin and to be cross-reactive with a large variety of gram-negative strains [8–14]. However, the reactivity of these latter monoclonal antibodies was tested in ELISA and, thus, their epitope specificity and their pattern of cross-reactivity deserve confirmation. Two of them, one murine (designated as E5) [12] and one human (subsequently designated as HA-1A or Centoxin[R]) [13], both of the IgM class, have been tested for the treatment of patients with gram-negative infections [15, 16]. We have extensively studied one of these antibodies. *In vitro*, we observed that it bound moderately to lipid A and Re LPS, and poorly to LPS from pathogenic smooth gram-negative bacteria. It bound to a large range of gram-negative bacteria and also to gram-positive bacteria, fungi and to lipids unrelated to lipid A such as cardiolipin and lipoproteins. The apparent affinity for lipid A was lower than 10^4 M^{-1}. This very weak affinity and the broad binding pattern suggested non-specific interactions with hydrophobic substances and questioned the specificity of this antibody for lipid A [3, 17]. This is further suggested by studies performed with this antibody which revealed that it bound to vascular endothelial cells *in vivo*, and to most tissues of all organs after incubation *in vitro* (Protocol Number C41T-003, Centocor, Malvern, PA).

Using bacterial and synthetic lipid A antigens and murine monoclonal antibodies, five different epitopes could be defined in *E. coli* type lipid A

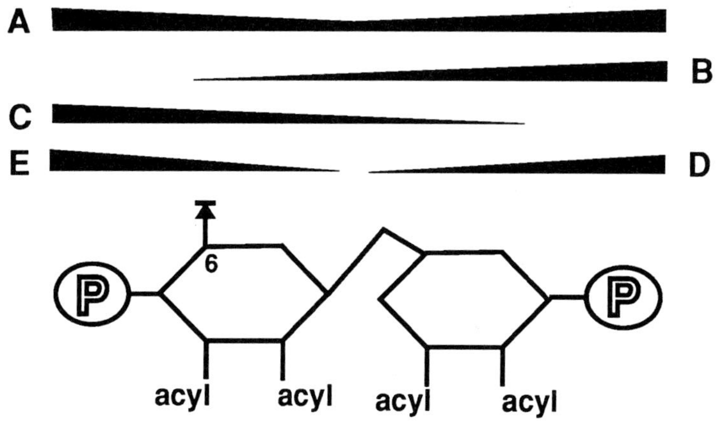

Fig. 1. Schematic diagram of the epitope specificities of anti-lipid A antibodies. Shown are disaccharide (A, B, C) and monosaccharide (D, E) reactive specifities. These antibodies cross react with purified lipid A's of different bacterial origin, but they do not cross react with the lipid A component of LPS when the saccharide portion of LPS has not been chemically removed. The LPS saccharides attach to lipid A in position 6 (arrow). (Adapted from [18] with permission)

(Fig. 1) [18]. All epitopes resided in the hydrophilic lipid A backbone region. Antibodies recognizing these epitopes cross-reacted with a large variety of free lipid A of distinct bacterial origin. However, it was emphasized that these antibodies did not cross-react with LPS, i.e. the attachment of the core region to lipid prevented the binding of anti-lipid A antibodies to the lipid A component of LPS. Furthermore, it is well-known that immunization with complete LPS does not elicit antibodies to the core region, a fact also indirectly supporting the possibility that antibodies to core LPS cannot access the core region of complete LPS. Therefore, at the present time, *in vitro* studies have not allowed to clearly and undoubtfully define an epitope specificity in the inner core of LPS that is shared by a large variety of bacterial strains, and the possibility that the conserved chemical structures in the inner core and in the lipid A regions are not expressed or are cryptic in LPS from pathogenic strains still remains.

Mode of Action of Anti-Core LPS Antibodies

Although antisera or monoclonal antibodies directed against various epitopes of the core LPS or against lipid A were sometimes reported as cross-protective, the effector mechanism of the observed protection was not elucidated. These antibody preparations did not increase the intravascular clearance of bacteria or LPS, were not opsonic *in vitro*, and were not bactericidal in the presence of complement [19–21]. Therefore, it was postulated that they directly neutralized LPS, presumably by steric hindrance of the toxic moiety of the molecule. However, no demonstration of this hypothesis has been reported. Although the monoclonal antibodies E5 and HA-1A were also postulated to neutralize endotoxins, i.e. to protect by blocking the toxic effect of endotoxin thus preventing the release of the mediators of shock, *in vitro* or *in vivo* data supporting this claim are lacking. In fact, the only reported experimental study of this kind showed that HA-1A did not suppress LPS-induced TNF and IL-6 serum levels in mice, in contrast to type-specific antibodies [22]. The knowledge of the mode of action of these antibodies would however appear to be crucial not only to define more precisely the subsets of patients that might benefit from these treatments, but also, owing to the controversial results of experimental and clinical studies, to indirectly confirm that they might be able to afford protection.

Factor Responsible for the Protection Afforded by Anti-Core LPS Antisera

In addition to these difficulties to define *in vitro* the shared epitope and the corresponding hypothetical cross-reactive anti-core LPS antibody, the factor responsible for the protection reported after immunization of rabbits with the J5 mutant of *E. coli* O111 or with the Re mutant of *Salmonella minnesota* S128 has not been clarified. The protection observed in some of the clinical studies with human J5 antiserum [23, 24] remained of unclear origin because outcome could not be convincingly correlated with anti-J5 LPS antibodies [23, and personal unpublished data]. In addition, immunization with an *E. coli* J5 vaccine of 70 volunteers who donated their plasma for one of these studies [24] induced no increase in anti-Re LPS or in anti-lipid A antibodies [25]. Thus, the protection afforded by J5 antiserum was not attributable to anti-J5 LPS, to anti-Re LPS or to anti-lipid A antibodies. Therefore, clinical studies with polyclonal anti-core LPS antisera cannot be considered as evidence that antibodies to lipid A can afford cross-protection against gram-negative bacteremia. In addition, previous experimental studies have failed to establish that anti-lipid A antisera were protective [26–31]. These findings are important when considering the experimental and clinical data gathered with the two antibodies E5 and HA-1A mentioned above.

Protection Experiments in Animal Models

Since the precise specificity and the mode of action of the antibodies responsible for the postulated cross-protection have not been determined despite the availability of monoclonal antibodies, the whole concept relies up to now mainly on the interpretation of protection experiments in animals and in humans. The first studies, suggesting that antisera directed against rough mutants of GNB might protect against unrelated smooth GNB or endotoxins, have been published almost 20 years ago [1, 2, 32], and some subsequent experiments gave similar results. As previously discussed, the factor[s] responsible for protection could not be demonstrated. Moreover, controversies have emerged as to the very existence of the cross-protection afforded by antisera to rough mutants. Indeed, several investigators were not able to reproduce the demonstration of a protective effect of core LPS antisera in animal models of gram-negative sepsis. A striking example of these difficulties to reproduce protective results came from Greisman et al. [33–36]. This group has investigated during several years anti *E. coli* J5 and anti-*S. minnesota* Re rabbit sera and was unable to reproduce the experiments demonstrating that these antisera could protect against smooth LPS or bacteria. Similar contradictory results were also found with core LPS monoclonal antibodies. Some authors found cross-protection with anti-lipid A monoclonal antibodies [8, 12, 13] while others found no protection even when testing many different anti-core LPS antibodies [11, 22, 37, 38, and personal unpublished data].

A puzzling example of divergent observations came from the human IgM monoclonal antibody HA-1A. This antibody, tested as a crude hybridoma supernatant, was reported to protect against LPS in the dermal Shwartzman reaction in rabbits and against lethal gram-negative bacteremia in mice [13]. Based on these promizing data, the cells isolated from the original clone were licenced to two companies: Centocor (Malvern, PA), the organizer of the clinical study [15], and Merieux (Lyon, France). Using the purified antibody produced by Merieux instead of hybridoma fluid, neither Merieux laboratories nor we could reproduce protection against gram-negative bacteria or endotoxin [22] in various models, including models similar to those of Teng et al. [13]. We have recently duplicated these negative results using commercially acquired HA-1A produced by Centocor (Centoxin^R) [personal unpublished data].

The discrepant results of the protective experiments with various anti-core LPS antibodies are difficult to explain because the specificities and the mode of action of the antibodies under investigations are unclear. The animal models that were used, the mode of challenge, as well as the nature of LPS or of bacteria used for challenge, were all parameters which could have an impact on the protective efficacy of these antibodies [4]. These considerations cannot explain all the discrepancies however, since opposite results were sometimes obtained using similar antibodies, similar animal models and similar bacterial or LPS challenges. Therefore, one can postulate that additional, still undiscovered, negative or positive factors might sometimes operate. For instance, a well described artifact can result from the LPS contamination of the antibody preparation. Minute amounts of LPS administered prophylactically induce a state of tolerance to LPS and therefore can protect animals against subsequent bacterial or LPS challenges [39, 40]. Since antibodies tested in protection experiments are almost uniformally administered before bacterial or LPS challenge, such an artifact cannot be ruled out in many published experiments. When testing monoclonal antibodies, the degree of purification is also crucial. Indeed, ascites and hybridoma fluids can contain various proteins and peptides, such as cytokines, some of which might be able to bind to LPS or to induce some tolerance to LPS in experimental animals. In addition, antibiotics are added to culture medium to prevent bacterial contaminations. These antibiotics might provide by themselves some protection when injected to animals together with the monoclonal antibody. Most protective experiments reported, including those by Teng et al. [13], have involved ascites or hybridoma fluids. Therefore, the precise description of the control and of the antibody preparation is crucial for the interpretation of experimental data in animals.

Clinical Studies with Human Anti-*E. coli* J5 Antiserum and with Purified Intravenous Immune Globulins

There have been four clinical studies using whole human serum or plasma from volunteers after immunization with *E. coli* J5 boiled cells, and two stu-

Table 1. Clinical studies with human J5 antiserum, with human J5 immune plasma, or with anti-core LPS intravenous immune globulins (IVIG).

Type of preparation (reference)	Study population	Result
Therapeutic studies		
J5 antiserum [23]	suspicion of gram-negative bacteremia and shock	reduction in mortality
J5 plasma (E. Girardin et al., unpublished data]	fulminant meningococcal purpura	no apparent effect
Anti- *E.coli* J5 IVIG [41]	gram-negative septic shock	no efficacy
Prophylactic studies		
J5 antiserum [42]	neutropenic cancer patients and bone marrow transplant recipients	no prevention of fever and of gram-negative sepsis
J5 plasma [24]	high-risk post-surgical patients	• no prevention of gram-negative infections • prevention of shock and death due to gram-negative infections (statistically significant with one-tailed Fisher's tests)*
Anti-Re LPS IVIG [A.Cometta et al., unpublished data]	high-risk post-surgical patients	no efficacy

*The P values obtained with the Chi-square test are 0.10 for the difference in the incidence of gram-negative shock between J5 plasma (15/136 patients) and normal plasma (6/126) recipients, and 0.08 for the associated mortality (9/136 and 2/126, respectively).

dies with hyperimmune intravenous immunoglobulins G (IVIG) (Table 1). Only two of them were successful or possibly successful. In three studies, the antibodies were administered for the treatment of gram-negative bacteremias or septic shock. In the first and well-known therapeutic study, 304 patients with a septic syndrome received a single intravenous infusion of either *E. coli* J5 antiserum or pre-immune (control) serum, near the onset of illness [23]. Among the 212 patients with gram-negative bacteremia, the mortality rate was significantly reduced in J5 antiserum recipients, especially in patients with shock at entry (from 77% to 44%, respectively). However, this study suffered from the absence of evaluation of the severity of illnesses among the patients at entry other than by listing underlying diseases. Moreover, there was an unusually high mortality in the control group of patients with septic shock (77%). In a second therapeutic study *E. coli* J5 immune plasma was compared to pre-immune plasma for the treatment of fulminant meningococcemia in children. J5 immune plasma was prepared from volunteers immunized with a vaccine provided by E.J. Ziegler, with a schedule similar to that in the previous study [23]. The trial was recently discontinued after 73 children had been enrolled, because the intermediate analysis did not reveal an improved survival in the J5 plasma recipients. Although the objective of randomizing 100 patients was not obtained, this study suggested nevertheless that a major impact of J5 immune plasma on the mortality of meningococcemia was unlikely (E. Girardin et al., unpublished data). The third study investigated the protective efficacy of a purified anti-*E. coli* J5 IgG preparation (J5-IVIG) obtained from volunteers immunized with J5 vaccine. In this multicenter study, 70 patients with established gram-negative septic shock received blindly a single dose of 200 mg/kg body weight of either control IVIG (Sandoglobulin^{R}) or of J5-IVIG [41]. Mortality from gram-negative septic shock was identical in the two groups (49% and 50%). In addition, J5-IVIG did not reduce the number of systemic complications of shock and did not delay the occurrence of death. This study suggested therefore that anti-J5 LPS IgG was not effective in the treatment of gram-negative septic shock.

In three other studies, the antibody preparations were administered for the prophylaxis of systemic gram-negative infections in high-risk patients. In surgical patients at high risk of developing gram-negative infections, repeated doses of J5 immune plasma did not prevent the acquistion of new focal gram-negative infections, but seemed to prevent the development of gram-negative septic shock (15 cases in 136 control patients versus 6 cases in 126 J5 recipients) and its fatal outcome (9 versus 2 deaths, respectively) [24]. However, the study should be analyzed with caution because the results were of borderline statistical significance: the number of patients developing septic shock was small and statistical evaluation was performed with one-tailed tests and was not significant with two-tailed tests (Table 1). In another prophylactic study, 150–200 ml of J5 antiserum was administered at the onset of neutropenia in 100 patients with 109 episodes of prolonged neutropenia (mean 17 days) [42]. When compared to control serum, J5 antiserum did not reduce the number of febrile days, the number of gram-negative bacteremic episodes, or death from these infections. This inability to demonstrate a beneficial effect was attributed to the insufficient amount of antibody administered, because most febrile episodes occurred 1 week or more after the administration of one single plasma unit. The third prophylactic study was performed in surgical patients at high-risk of developing infections. Patients were randomized to receive intravenously either a standard human IVIG preparation (Gammagard^{R}), or an IVIG preparation enriched in anti-Re LPS antibodies (core-LPS IVIG), or albumin as placebo. In the 329 evaluable patients, the number of acquired infections was significantly lower in patients treated with the standard-IVIG than in those receiving core-LPS IVIG or albumin. No difference in the occurrence of focal or systemic gram-negative infections was observed between core-LPS IVIG and albumin. The mortality due to infections was not significantly different between the 3 prophylactic groups. Therefore, anti-Re LPS IgG did not have a detectable impact on the prevention of gram-negative infections and on their systemic complications (A. Cormetta et al., unpublished data).

The two studies with hyperimmune IVIG were performed to duplicate the two possibly successful studies of J5 anti-serum or immune plasma [24, 43]. The study designs were therefore very similar, except that purified IVIG were used instead of serum or plasma. The failure of hyperimmune IVIG cannot be explained by an insufficient amount of anti-J5 LPS IgG or anti-Re LPS IgG (respectively) administered to the patients since this amount was far above the amount that was administered through the infusion of antiserum or plasma in the two successful studies [23, 24]. One possible explanation for the ineffectiveness of core LPS IVIG is that IgM antibodies, which were absent from the IVIG preparations, might be necessary for protection. However, since the mode of action of anti-core LPS antibodies is unknown, there is no solid basis for such a claim. Although some experimental data suggested that IgM-enriched serum fractions were more effective than IgG-enriched fractions [44], other studies had found that IgG antibodies were as effective or even more effective than IgM [45, 46]. Thus, another possible explanation is that anti-J5 LPS and anti-Re LPS antibodies cannot afford cross-protection against heterologous bacteria, and that the protection observed with the immune serum or plasma was attributable to other factors. These disappointing results underscore the need for a more precise knowledge of the immunochemistry of LPS and of the mechanisms of protection of anti-LPS antibodies.

Clinical Studies with Monoclonal Antibodies

As stated previously, two monoclonal antibodies, one murine (designated as E5) and one human (subsequently designated as HA-1A) both of the IgM class, have been tested for the treatment of patients with gram-negative infections in prospective, randomized, double-blind, multicenter trials [15, 16].

E5 has been reported to bind to lipid A and to protect experimentally when administered in association with antibiotics [12], but the precise material and methods have not been published. The discrepant results gathered with HA-1A have been summarized in the previous paragraphs.

In the first clinical study of E5 [16], patients with a suspected gram-negative septic syndrome were randomly assigned to receive intravenously either the antibody (2 mg/kg body weight daily for 2 consecutive days), or an identical volume of saline. No decrease of the mortality was observed among the whole study population (468 evaluable patients) nor among the 316 patients with a documented gram-negative sepsis syndrome. However, when the results in subgroups were analyzed, there was a statistically significant decrease of the mortality in the 137 patients without shock at entry (P=0.03), whereas the 179 patients with shock were not protected. Among the patients without shock, a comparable reduction in mortality occurred in both bacteremic and non-bacteremic patients. Since this study suggested that E5 was effective only in a subgroup of patients without shock, a finding which had not been anticipated, a confirmatory multicenter study has been initiated. This second study was recently completed and included about 835 patients with a sepsis syndrome without shock. Two-third of the cases proved to be due to gram-negative infections. This trial failed to confirm that E5 could reduce the mortality among non-shock patients with gram-negative sepsis [47].

The second antibody, HA-1A, was studied in 543 patients with a presumptive diagnosis of gram-negative sepsis [15]. The patients were randomized to receive intravenously either a single dose of 100 mg of HA-1A, or a similar

Table 2. Mortality due to sepsis and all causes in the HA-1A trial, according to patient subgroup. (Adapted from [49] with permission).

Subgroup	Mortality at 14 days due to sepsis and all causes[1]		P value		
	Placebo	HA-1A	Sepsis over		All causes over
	patients dead/all patients (%)		14 days	28 days	28 days
gram-negative bacteremia	32/95 (34)	25/105 (24)	0.12	0.039	0.014
gram-negative sepsis	47/145 (32)	40/137 (29)	0.56	0.29	0.18
gram-negative infection	61/207 (29)	56/194 (29)	0.89	0.47	0.30

[1]Mortality due to sepsis equaled mortality due to all causes at 14 days.
The group called "gram-negative sepsis" was an aggregate of the groups "gram-negative bacteremia" and "probable gram-negative sepsis"; the group called "gram-negative infection" was an aggregate of the groups "gram-negative sepsis" and "possible gram-negative sepsis".
From these data, it can be calculated that the mortality at 14 days in patients with probable gram-negative sepsis was 15/50 (30%) in the placebo arm and 15/32 (47%) in the HA-1A arm, and the mortality in patients with possible gram-negative sepsis was 14/62 (23%) and 16/57 (28%), respectively.

volume of human albumin. Of the 543 patients, 401 had gram-negative infections, among which 200 had positive blood cultures at randomization. Among the remaining patients with non-bacteremic gram-negative infections, 117 were classified as "probable" gram-negative sepsis and 84 as "possible" gram-negative sepsis. HA-1A did not reduce the mortality in the overall study population, nor in the 201 patients with non-bacteremic gram-negative infections (Table 2). However, there was a significant decrease of the mortality in the subgroup of patients with gram-negative bacteremia (P=0.014).

This result contrasts with the results of the first E5 study because, in the HA-1A study, only bacteremic patients appeared to be protected, and because the difference was the most obvious among the 102 patients who were in shock at study entry, and was marginal in the 98 patients who were not in shock (Table 3). Moreover, in view of the postulated mechanisms of protection (which is that HA-1A neutralized endotoxin [15]), the absence of effectiveness in patients with gram-negative sepsis syndromes without positive blood cultures is unexpected, since endotoxin also plays a crucial role in this population of patients [48]. Furthermore, when analyzing this study in details, it appeared that there might have been imbalances in risk factors at randomization between placebo and HA-1A recipients in the subgroup of 200 patients with gram-negative bacteremia [49]. Indeed, a total of 101 serious complications (disseminated intravascular coagulations, adult respiratory distress syndromes, acute hepatic failures and acute renal failures) (calculated from table 4 of the study [15]) were present at entry among the 95 placebo recipients compared to 85 among the 105 HA-1A recipients. These 16 additional serious complications in the placebo group might account for some of the higher death rate in this group (13 deaths in excess). In addition, more patients in the placebo arm than in the HA-1A arm received inadequate or unknown antibiotic (17% vs 10%) [50]. Inappropriate antimicrobial therapy was strongly associated with death in patients with gram-negative bacteremia (in the placebo group: mortality of 67%, compared with 27% with appropriate therapy). In a recent editorial, R.P. Wenzel pointed out that the monoclonal antibody studies were all analyzed primarily

Table 3. Mortality due to sepsis in patients with gram-negative bacteremia, according to the presence or absence of shock. (Adapted from [50] with permission).

	Mortality at 14 days			Mortality over 28 days
	Placebo	HA-1A	P value	P value
All patients	32/95 (34%)	25/105 (24%)	0.12	0.039
Patients with shock	23/48 (48%)	13/54 (24%)	0.012	0.023
Patients without shock	9/47 (19%)	12/51 (24%)	0.60	--

under corporate direction and not initially by major investigators from academic centers [51]. This fact, in part, generated a second-look analysis based on the informations presented to an open advisory-committee meeting held by the Food and Drug Administration (FDA) on September 4, 1991 [50]. This reassessment suggested that the data analysis presented at the FDA meeting differed from that reported by Ziegler et al. [15], and concluded that the initial report of the HA-1A study by Ziegler et al. was unduly optimistic. They noted that a significant result was found in only one of many overlapping groups; that the statistical result was marginal; that a protective effect was seen only at clinical centers with high mortality and only in patients with shock; that the APACHE II system used to stratify patients might have been inappropriately applied; that patients who received inadequate or unknown antibiotic treatment were included in the analysis; and that the data were not stratified according to the time elapsed before the antibody or placebo was infused [50].

Inasmuch as the clinical studies with anti-lipid A monoclonal antibodies are difficult to assess and the preclinical studies have given inconsistent data, one may take the view at the present time that the treatment of the gram-negative septic syndrome with antibodies directed to lipid A or to other epitopes of the core LPS should still be considered as investigational. In contrast to some European countries which have already licensed HA-1A, the FDA decided recently that the effectiveness of HA-1A was not yet conclusively proven and asked for an additional well-controlled trial (The Wall Street Journal and the New York Time, April 16, 1992).

Conclusions

None of the investigated anti-lipid A antibodies has emerged yet as an established therapeutic modality that can be administered routinely to patients with septic shock. The epitope specificity, the mode of action, and the experimental protective power of these antibodies are subject to caution. Clearly, additional basic experiments are warranted to clarify the efficacy of these antibodies and to establish the fundamental scientific knowledge that would be mandatory before settling new clinical trials.

References

1. Braude AI, Douglas H (1972) Passive immunization against the local Shwartzman reaction. J Immunol 108:505–512
2. McCabe WR (1972) Immunization with R mutants of S. minnesota. I. Protection against challenge with heterologous gram-negative bacilli. J Immunol 108:601–610
3. Baumgartner JD (1991) Immunotherapy with antibodies to core LPS: A critical appraisal. Infect Dis Clin North Am 5:915–927
4. Ziegler EJ (1988) Protective antibody to endotoxin core: The emperor's new clothes? J Infect Dis 158:286–290

5. Baumgartner JD, Eggimann P, Glauser MP (1992) Management of septic shock: new approaches. In: Remington JS, Swartz MN (eds.) Current Clinical Topics in Infectious Diseases, Volume 12. Blackwell Scientific Publications Inc., Cambridge, pp 165–187
6. Heumann D, Baumgartner JD, Jacot-Guillarmod H, Glauser MP (1991) Antibodies to core lipopolysaccharide determinants: Absence of cross-reactivity with heterologous lipopolysaccharides. J Infect Dis 163:762–768
7. Freudenberg MA, Fomsgaard A, Mitov I, Galanos C (1989) ELISA for antibodies to lipid A, lipopolysaccharides and other hydrophobic antigens. Infection 17:322–328
8. Dunn DL, Bogard WC Jr, Cerra FB (1985) Efficacy of type-specific and cross-reactive murine monoclonal antibodies directed against endotoxin during experimental sepsis. Surgery 98:283–289
9. Kirkland TN, Colwell DE, Michalek SM, McGhee JR, Ziegler EJ (1986) Analysis of the fine specificty and cross-reactivitiy of monoclonal anti-lipid A antibodies. J Immunol 137:3614–3619
10. Erich T, Schellekens J, Bouter A, Van Kranen J, Brouwer E, Verhoef J (1989) Binding characteristics and cross-reactivity of three different antilipid A monoclonal antibodies. J Immunol 143:4053–4060
11. Appelmelk BJ, Verweij-van Vught AMJJ, Maaskant JJ, et al. (1988) Production and characterization of mouse monoclonal antibodies reacting with the lipopolysaccharide core region of gram-negative bacilli. J Med Microbiol 26:107–114
12. Young LS, Gascon R, Alam S, Bermudez LE (1989) Monoclonal antibodies for treatment of gram-negative infections. Rev Infect Dis 11 (Suppl. 7):1564–1571
13. Teng NNH, Kaplan HS, Hebert JM (1985) Protection against gram-negative bacteremia and endotoxemia with human monoclonal IgM antibodies. Proc natl Acad Sci USA 82:1790–1794
14. Bogard WC Jr, Dunn DL, Abernethy K, Kilgarriff C, Kung PC (1986) Isolation and characterization of murine monoclonal antibodies specific for gram-negative bacterial lipopolysaccharide: Association of cross-genus reactivity with lipid A specificity. Infect Immun 55:899–908
15. Ziegler EJ, Fisher CJ, Sprung CL, et al. and the HA-1A Sepsis Study Group (1991) Treatment of gram-negative bacteremia and septic shock with HA-1A human monoclonal antibody against endotoxin. A randomized, double-blind, placebo-controlled trial. N Engl J Med 324:429–436
16. Greenman RL, Schein RMH, Martin MA, et al. and the Xoma Sepsis Study Group (1991) A controlled clinical trial of E5 murine monoclonal IgM antidoby to endotoxin in the treatment of gram-negative sepsis. JAMA 266:1097–1102
17. Baumgartner JD, Heumann D, Glauser MP (1991) The HA-1A monoclonal antibody for gram-negative sepsis. N Engl J Med 325:281–282 (Letter)
18. Rietschel ETh, Seydel U, Zähringer U, et al. (1991) Bacterial endotoxin: Molecular relationships between structure and activity. Infect Clin North Am 5:753–779
19. Ziegler EJ, Douglas H, Sherman JE, Davis CE, Braude AI (1973) Treatment of E. coli and Klebsiella bacteremia in agranulocytic animals with antiserum to a UDP-Gal epimerase-deficient mutant. J Immunol 111:433–438
20. Young LS, Stevens P, Ingram J (1975) Functional role of antibody against "core" glycolipid of Entereobacteriaceae. J Clin Invest 56:850–861
21. Young LS, Stevens P (1977) Cross-protective immunity to gram-negative bacilli: Studies with core glycolipid of Salmonella minnesota and antigens of Streptococcus pneumoniae. J Infect Dis 136:174–180
22. Baumgartner JD, Heumann D, Gerain J, Weinbreck P, Grau GE, Glauser MP (1990) Association between protective efficacy of anti-lipopolysaccharide (LPS) antibodies and suppression of LPS-induced tumor necrosis factor α and interleukin-6. Comparison of O side chain-specific antibodies with core LPS antibodies. J Exp Med 171:889–896
23. Ziegler EJ, McCutchan JA, Fierer J, et al. (1982) Treatment of gram-negative bacteremia and shock with human antiserum to a mutant Escherichia coli. N Engl J Med 307:1225–1230
24. Baumgartner JD, Glauser MP, McCutchan JA, et al. (1985) Prevention of gram-negative shock and death in surgicall patients by prophylactic antibody to endotoxin core glycolipid. Lancet 2:59–63

25. Baumgartner JD, Heumann D, Calandra T, Glauser MP (1991) Antibodies to lipopolysaccharides after immunization of humans with the rough mutant Escherichia coli J5. J Infect Dis 163:769–772
26. Galanos C, Luederitz O, Westphal O (1971) Preparation and properties of antisera against the lipid-A component of bacterial lipopolysaccharides. Eur J Biochem 24:116–122
27. Mullan NA, Newsome PM, Cunnington PG, Palmer GH, Wilson ME (1974) Protection against gram-negative infections with antiserum to lipid A from Salmonella minnesota R595. Infect Immun 10:1195–1201
28. Hodgin LA, Drews J (1976) Effect of active and passive immunizations with lipid A and Salmonella minnesota Re 595 on gram-negative infections in mice. Infection 4:5–10
29. Johns MA, Bruins SC, McCabe WR (1977) Immunization with R mutants of Salmonella minnesota. II. Serological response to lipid A and the lipopolysaccharide of Re mutants. Infect Immun 17:9–15
30. Bruins SC, Stumacher R, Johns MA, McCabe WR (1977) Immunization with R mutants of Salmonella minnesota. III. Comparison of the protective effect of immunization with lipid A and the Re mutant. Infect Immun 17:16–20
31. Mattsby-Baltzer I, Kaijser B (1979) Lipid A and anti-lipid A. Infect Immun 23:758–763
32. Chedid L, Parant M, Parant F, Boyer F (1968) A proposed mechanism for natural immunity to enterobacterial pathogens. J Immunol 100:292–301
33. Greisman SE, DuBuy JB, Woodward CL (1978) Experimental gram-negative bacterial sepsis: Reevaluation of the ability of rough mutant antisera to protect mice. Proc Soc Biol Med 158:482–490
34. Greisman SE, DuBuy JB, Woodward CL (1979) Eperimental gram-negative bacterial sepsis. Prevention of mortality not preventable by antibiotics alone. Infect Immun 25:538–557
35. Greisman SE (1982) Experimental gram-negative bacterial sepsis: Optimal methylprednisolone requirements for prevention of mortality not preventable by antibiotics alone. Proc Soc Biol Med 170:436–442
36. Greisman SE, Johnston CA (1987) Failure of antisera to J5 and R595 rough mutants to reduce endotoxemic lethality. J Infect Dis 157:54–64
37. Miner KM, Manyak CL, Williams E (1986) Characterization of murine monoclonal antibodies to Escherichia coli J5. Infect Immun 52:56–62
38. Pollack M, Chia JKS, Koles NL, Miller M, Guelde G (1989) Specificity and cross-reactivity of monoclonal antibodies reactive with the core and lipid A regions of bacterial lipopolysaccharide. J Infect Dis 159:168–188
39. Woods JP, Black JR, Barrittt DS, Connell TD, Cannon JG (1987) Resistance to meningococcemia apparently conferred by anti-H.8 monoclonal antibody is due to contaminating endotoxin and not to specific immunoprotection. Infect Immun 55:1927–1928
40. Chong KT, Huston M (1987) Implications of endotoxin contamination in the evaluation of antibodies to lipopolysaccharides in a murine model of gram-negative sepsis. J Infect Dis 156:713–719
41. Calandra T, Glauser MP, Schellekens J, Verhoef J, the Swiss-Dutch J5 Immunoglobulin Study Group (1988) Treatment of gram-negative septic shock with human IgG antibody to Escherichia coli J5: A prospective, double-blind, randomized study. J Infect Dis 158:312–319
42. McCutchan JA, Wolf JL, Ziegler EJ, Braude AI (1983) Ineffectiveness of single-dose human antiserum to core glycolipid (E. coli J5) for prophylaxis of bacteremic, gram-negative infection in patients with prolonged neutropenia. Schweiz Med Wschr 113 (Suppl. 14):40–45
43. Just HM, Vogel W, Metzger M, Pelka RD, Daschner FD (1986) Treatment of intensive care unit patients with severe nosocomial infections. Intensive Care Med 345–352
44. McCabe WR, DeMaria A Jr, Berberich H, Johns MA (1988) Immunization with rough mutants of Salmonella minnesota: Protective activity of IgM and IgG antibody to the R595 (Re chemotype) mutant. J Infect Dis 158:291–300
45. Davis CE, Ziegler EJ, Arnold K (1978) Neutralization of meningococcal endotoxin by antibody to core glycolipid. J Exp Med 147:1007–1017
46. Zinner SH, McCabe WR (1976) Effects of IgM and IgG antibody in patients with bacteremia due to gram-negative bacilli. J Infect Dis 133:37–45

47. Wenzel R, Bone R, Fein A, et al. (1991) Results of a second double-blind, randomized, controlled trial of anti-endotoxin antibody E5 in gram-negative sepsis. In: 31st Interscience Conference of Antimicrobial Agents and Chemotherapy. Am Soc Microbiology (Abst 1170):294
48. Danner RL, Elin RJ, Hosseini JM, Wesley RA, Reilly JM, Parillo JE (1991) Endotoxemia in human septic shock. Chest 99:169–175
49. Carlet J, Offenstadt G, Chastang C, et al. (1991) The HA-1A monoclonal antibody for gram-negative sepsis. N Engl J Med (Letter) 325:280
51. Warren HS, Danner RL, Munford RS (1992) Anti-endotoxin monoclonal antibodies. N Engl J Med 326:1153–1157
51. Wenzel RP (1992) Anti-endotoxin monoclonal antibodies – A second look. N Engl J Med (Editorial) 326:1151–1153

The Case for Immunotherapy Against Endotoxin in Sepsis and Septicemia

H.R. Michie

Introduction

Conventionally treated severe gram-negative infection has an unpredictable outcome. Institution of appropriate antibiotic therapy, drainage of septic foci and adequate ventilatory, fluid and inotropic support where needed will result in survival of roughly half of the septic individuals [1,2]. The remainder will develop a variety of potentially lethal sequelae including profound hypotension, coagulopathy and progressive organ failure and most of these patients will die. Mortality in this latter group has not improved significantly in the last two decades and the enormous cost of caring for such patients is associated with a poor reward. Furthermore a "cure" for septicemia progressing to multiple organ failure might have a greater impact on total patient survival than a cure for breast cancer according to some calculations. It might be considered that following publication of a Phase III clinical trial in a premier journal that demonstrated a 39% reduction in mortality in those with gram-negative sepsis when treated with a human moncolonal antibody against the Lipid A (a component of the endotoxin of all gram-negative strains of bacteria) this approach might be adopted with considerable enthusiasm and a desire to make such therapy available to all appropriate patients as rapidly as possible [3]. The reality is that this therapy has attracted an almost unprecedented degree of controversy [4-7]. In this chapter, only the human monoclonal anti-endotoxin antibody HA-1A (Centoxin^R) will be considered in depth. The other anti-endotoxin antibody E5 (a murine antibody) has been evaluated in two Phase III clinical trials. In neither study taken individually has it been shown to increase survival in the group of patients with gram-negative sepsis and hypotension, the clinical scenario most likely to be attributable to circulating endotoxin and where an IgM antibody against endotoxin would, on theoretical grounds, be most likely to be effective [8]. For this reason, the author cannot find any compelling case for further evaluation of this agent.

The controversy concerning HA-1A can be summarized in terms of three broad themes which will considered in turn:

1. Is the pivotal trial suggesting efficacy of HA-1A flawed?
2. If HA-1A works, how does it work?
3. Cost-effectiveness.

Is the Pivotal HA-1A Trial Flawed?

Trials of new agents for the treatment of severe sepsis and septic shock are notoriously difficult to perform for the following reasons:

a) Severe sepsis is not so much a disease in itself as a most unwelcome complication occurring following trauma, instrumentation of an infected viscus or surgery. Much less commonly does *de novo* infection lead to septic shock (e.g. meningococcal septicemia). Patients cannot be recruited in advance but rather must be identified rapidly and with insufficient characterization at the time that clinical deterioration occurs. In retrospect the deterioration of many patients will be found to be due to non-gram-negative infection, cardiovascular/cerebrovascular events, other complications of surgery or metabolic abnormalities unrelated to endotoxin. For this reason, many patients recruited will with hindsight be found to have been inappropriately entered into the study. Additionally, in the absence of post-mortem data, other causes of death will remain unrecognized.
b) Gram-negative septicemia is a condition *par excellence* where therapeutic intervention must be rapid. Although irreversible detioration may occur over minutes, hours or days the time course from suspected infection to potentially lethal and irreversible alterations is often a matter of a few hours. In a clinical trial permission of the sponsors must be sought, the drug must be made available, full pre-treatment parameters must be documented and permission of relatives obtained. These requirements necessarily entail significant delay and the "window of opportunity" may be missed in many patients.
c) Even if clinical deterioration is originally attributable to severe endotoxemia, secondary phenomena may accelerate the deterioration which could not possibly be reversed by anti-endotoxin therapy. These include myocardial infarction, cerebrovascular events, ischemia/reperfusion injury and profound acidemia. These events are very commonly observed in the intensive therapy unit and are a major source of mortality.
d) Enrolment of a patient in a Phase III trial provides considerable financial gain for the unit concerned and the temptation may exist to enrol a patient who fulfils the entry requirements for a particular protocol but who would never be seriously considered for receipt of an expensive treatment outside of a clinical trial. In the pivotal trial [3] mortality in those receiving placebo in centers recruiting more than twenty patients ranged from 40-100% (Table 1).
e) A reduction in mortality from a new agent in septic shock cannot occur in the absence of adequate surgery, correct use of antibiotics and a generally extremely high standard of care, standards which are known to vary widely between centers. Additionally, it may be found in retrospect when cultures and sensitivities become available that the antibiotics used were ineffective. In the pivotal trial in patients with gram-negative bacteremia

Table 1. A comparison of HA-1A and placebo in the highest enrolling centers

Center no	N	28 day mortality rate (%) Placebo	HA-1A	Reduction
10	21	40	18	55
13	25	67	19*	72
28	33	46	40	13
89	22	100	43*	57

* = $P < 0.05$

Table 2. The effect of adequacy of antibiotics on survival during gram-negative bacteremia with and without HA-1A

	28 day mortality rate (%) Placebo	HA-1A	Reduction
Adequate	42% (32/76)	28% (27/95)	33%
Inadequate	75% (9/12)	57% (4/12)	24%

12/88 patients in the placebo group were found to have received inappropriate antibiotics and this was associated with a much higher mortality than those receiving suitable antibiotics (Table 2).

f) Gram-negative sepsis may occur in the terminal phase of other conditions associated with significant immunosuppression. An anti-endotoxin therapy may prevent death in patients dying *of* sepsis but not in those dying *with* sepsis. Conditions where death is highly likely even if endotoxin is neutralized include recurrent aortic graft infection, multiple hepatic abscesses, >80% burns, and necrotizing pancreatitits with superimposed infection.

For these reasons, it has reasonably been estimated that the "perfect" anti-endotoxin agent would only reduce mortality by about 50% in appropriate cases, the remainder beings victims of delay in treatment, incorrect supportive and other therapy or lethal comorbidities. Table 1 summarizes the results of the pivotal trial and it can be seen that intervention with HA-1A produces an increase in survival very close to the 50% figure which suggests that the agent is highly effective. Nevertheless the efficacy of the agent has been attacked on the following grounds.

HA-1A was only Effective in Patients with Gram-negative Bacteremia

The protocol for the pivotal trial was designed to determine whether HA-1A was effective in gram-negative bacteremia, not in all patients recruited. Ba-

1. binding is determined by the amount of antibody and antigen present;
2. binding of antibody is saturable with limited antigen of antibody;
3. binding of antibody is inhibitible by excess antigen of antibody;
4. binding of antibody is competitively inhibited by other antibodies with similar antigen specificities [12].

This exhaustive work leaves no doubt that HA-1A is highly specific in its binding to lipopolysaccharide.

Nevertheless, when human monocytes in tissue culture are incubated with the endotoxins of a wide variety of gram-negative organisms they are stimulated to release the various cytokines which are believed to mediate the deleterious effects on the host, particularly the cytokine tumor necrosis factor (TNF). The addition of HA-1A in such tissue culture experiments does not prevent elaboration of such cytokines. This suggests that HA-1A does not directly neutralize endotoxin, at least in tissue culture. However, when the he-

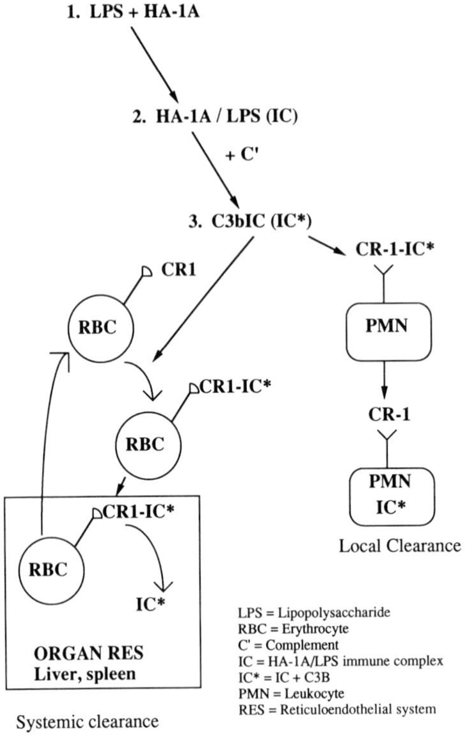

Fig. 1. A proposed mechanism of action of HA-1A. HA-1A binds to lipopolysaccharide and the immune complex so formed activates complement. The C3B component of complement binds to the immune complex and this conjugate binds either to an erythrocyte or to a neutrophil through the CR-1 receptor. When the conjugate is bound to an erythrocyte it is not internalized but is broken down in the reticuloendothelial system with neutralization of lipopolysaccharide. If bound to a neutrophil then the conjugate is internalized in that cell. Neither pathway results in the induction of cytokines. This mechanism has been clearly demonstrated *in vitro* but awaits verification *in vivo*. Animals other than primates lack CR-1 receptors on erythrocytes so that the mechanism cannot be validated in such species

althy host is exposed to endotoxin in low dosage the normal binding of endotoxin is not through the CD-14 mechanisms that triggers cytokine release but to another polypeptide BPI following which it is transferred to the liver for detoxification without the triggering of cytokine release (Dr Fisher describes such mechanisms in detail pp 339-344). It is clear that in sepsis natural stores of polypeptides such as BPI become depleted and more endotoxin becomes available for binding to CD-14 receptors and subsequent cytokine release. Recent work by Dadonna et al. (P Dadonna, personal communication) has shown that HA-1A, *in vitro,* fulfils all the characteristics required of an agent that will take endotoxin out of the cytokine-activating pathway and into the non-cytokine activating pathway (Fig. 1). This mechanism is complement-dependent, erythrocyte dependent and CR-1 dependent. Dadonna et al. have shown that HA-1A binding of endotoxins of various strains is dependent on all such cells and other moieties being present . Feldman has further shown that in tissue culture in leukapheresis packs when all such moieties are present that HA-1A prevents endotoxin-induced cytokine release from monocytes (Marc Feldman, personal communication). If these *in vitro* findings are substantiated in human models, then much of the existing controversy concerning mode of action of HA-1A should be resolved.

Cost-effectiveness of HA-1A

There can be little doubt, if the cost of HA-1A were comparable to that of most conventional antibiotics that, based on existing evidence, it would now be widely used on both sides of the Atlantic. However, at somewhat less than $4000 for a single infusion (the total recommended dose) it is clearly an agent that cannot be used indescriminantly and yet the crafting of suitable guidelines is difficult. One suggestion is that the selection criteria used in the Phase III trial should be employed [4]. The difficulty with this approach is that some of these criteria were present for medico-legal rather than clinical reasons (pregnancy, age < 18 years). Others were present to lessen the heterogeneity of the population studied (burned patients and recipients of transplants). Although such criteria were quite appropriate in the context of a clinical trial they would seem less appropriate for an approved drug being used in a clinical setting where the mortality rate is high. The author would propose the following algorithm for the use of agents such as HA-1A.

Step 1. The mortality and morbidity of the underlying condition should be assessed. If sepsis has ensued following surgery for all but the earliest upper gastrointestinal or biliary malignancies, then costly life saving therapy would seem inappropriate when the five year survival is negligible and the quality of life prior to death is poor.

Step 2. The likelihood that the acute deterioration the patient's condition can be attributed to gram-negative bacteremia must be assessed. This involves the evaluation of all available bacteriological cultures and the clinical assessment of the patient. Nevertheless in acute bacteremia the chances of obtaining confirmatory bacteriological evidence before irreversible changes have occurred is small so that for the forseeable future the diagnosis of gram-negative bacteremia will remain a clinical one.

Step 3. Use a scoring system such as the APACHE II system to estimate the likelihood of death [11]. It remains a political, financial and ethical issue whether an expensive agent should be used when the risk of death is 1%, 5%, 10% or 50%. The data suggest that HA-1A saved more lives than placebo at all stratifications of risk but that the efficacy was greatest when the risk of death was highest (Table 1).

Step 4. Ensure that all available conventional therapies are in insututed. It cannot be too strongly stressed that anti-endotoxin immunotherapy is no substitute for drainage of septic foci and adequate antibiotics. Table 2 contains data derived from the pivotal trial and showed that irrespective of the presence of HA-1A mortality was much higher when the antibiotics employed were inappropriate.

Step 5. If the case for immunotherapy is equivocal then it seem reasonable to observe the patient closely and decide over the ensuing minutes or hours whether deterioration or improvement is occurring. If deterioration is present and it seems likely that endotoxemia is the cause then the case for immunotherapy is strong.

A particularly difficult situation occurs when laparotomy is performed and gross peritoneal contamination with faeces or pus is present. Many such patients will have an uneventful recovery following conventional therapy but 20-30% will proceed to hypotension, multiple organ failure and disseminated intravascular coagulation. In an ideal world all such patients should probably receive immunotherapy since clinical deterioration often does not begin until several hours after surgery but once it commences it proceeds with devastating speed. If immunotherapy is withheld provisionally then it is clear that re-evalation on an hourly basis at least is necessary.

During the transition of immunotherapy from a laboratory tool to clinical practice the issue of cost has received prominence. Table 3 shows the calculated cost of immunotherapy with HA-1A in terms of life-years saved (calculated from the results of the pivotal trial) and demonstrates that in comparison with other accepted clinical modalities the cost is in no way exorbitant. The whole problem has been confounded by the rapid arrival of a costly agent into countries whose clinical budgets have not yet taken into account the new technology and there is understandable concern that the indiscriminant use of such agents would prove financially crippling. Particularly in the USA there are concerns that if agents such as HA-1A were licensed for the treatment of serious gram-negative infections but were withheld from particular patients considered inappropriate for its use then this could form the basis of claims of malpractice. There can be no question that there should be nationally or internationally agreed guidelines for the use of such

Table 3. A comparison of the cost effectiveness of immunotherapy with the antiendotoxin antibody HA-1A compared with accepted therapeutic interventions

Therapeutic intervention	Cost per life-year saved ($)
Hemodialysis	34,750
Hypertension	32,000
Heparin for DVT prophylaxis	81,143
HA-1A	5,515

agents. Even if definitions are inadequate and the guidelines were considered flawed by some individuals it is clear that some agreement over indications is better than no consensus at all.

Conclusion

It seems a reasonable estimate that between 30-50% of patients who die from gram-negative sepsis could be salvaged if there were an effective agent which neutralized endotoxin available for clinical use. Two double blinded randomized trials and one openlabel cohort study have suggested that antibodies against endotoxin can reduce the death rate from gram-negative bacteremia by this extent. The case for the use of such antibodies in clinical practice now seems a very strong one. There is a compelling need for new methods to identify rapidly the individuals most likely to benefit from such an approach while excluding those who are either likely to survive with conventional therapy or who are dying from causes other than gram-negative sepsis.

References

1. Ledingham I McA, McArdle CS (1978) Prospective study of the treatment of septic shock. Lancet, 1:1194–1197
2. Kreger BE, Craven DE, McCabe WR (1980) Gram-negative bacteremia IV. Re-evaluation and treatment in 612 patients. Am J Med 68:344–355
3. Zeigler EJ, Fisher CJ, Sprung CL, et al. (1991) Treatment of Gram-negative bacteremia and septic shock with HA-1A human monoclonal antibody against endotoxin. N Eng J Med 324:429–436
4. Bone RC (1991) Monoclonal antibodies to endotoxin. New allies against sepsis? JAMA 266:1125–1126
5. Baumgartner JD, Heuman D, Glauser MP (1991) The HA-1A monoclonal antibody for Gram-negative sepsis. N Eng J Med (letter) 325:281–282
6. Taylor D (1991) Centoxin – birth of a budgetbuster. BMJ 302:1229
7. Schmidt GA (1991) The HA-1A monoclonal antibody for Gram-negative sepsis. N Eng J Med (letter) 325:280–281

8. Greenman RL, Schein RMH, Martin MA, et al. (1991) A controlled clinical trial of E5 murine monoclonal IgM antibody to endotoxin in the treatment of gram-negative sepsis. JAMA 266:1097–1102
9. Smith CR (1992) HA-1A - additional clinical data. Presented at the 12th International Symposium on Intensive Care and Emergency Medicine, Brussels
10. Ziegler EJ, McCutchan JA, Fierer J, et al. (1982) Treatment of Gram-negative bacteremia and shock with human antiserum to a mutant Escherichia coli. N Eng J Med 307:1225–1230
11. Knaus WA, Draper EA, Wagner DP, Zimmerman JE (1985) APACHE II: a severity of disease classification system. Crit Care Med 13:818–829
12. Morrison D (1992) HA-1A – mode of action. Presented at the 12th International Symposium on Intensive Care and Emergency Medicine, Brussels

Bactericidal Permeability Increasing Protein: A Potent Naturally Occurring Anti-Endotoxin Protein

C.J. Fisher, S.M. Opal, and M.N. Marra

Introduction

Sepsis syndrome is the systemic inflammatory response associated with severe infection, bacteremia, and/or endotoxemia and is a leading cause of morbidity and mortality among hospitalized patients despite the use of potent antibiotics and intensive support procedures. Approximately 400,000 to 500,000 cases are reported each year in the United States, and the incidence is increasing. In the ten year period ending 1987, the discharge diagnosis of sepsis syndrome had increased by 139% with an average mortality of 40 to 45% [1-5]. The systemic inflammatory response is generally initiated by an exogenous challenge from bacterial toxins stimulating release of endogenous mediators such as tumor necrosis factor (TNF), interleukin-1 (IL-1), IL-6, bradykinin, and other important pro-inflammatory mediators [5-11]. Both gram-positive and gram-negative bacteria produce sepsis syndrome [1]. In approximately 60% of cases with a known etiology, sepsis is associated with gram-negative bacteria.

Endotoxin is the lipopolysaccharide (LPS) component of gram-negative bacterial cell walls, which by stimulating release of pro-inflammatory mediators, can lead to shock, disseminated intravascular coagulation, multiorgan dysfunction, and ultimately death in patients with sepsis syndrome [5-7,11]. Lipid-A is the biologically active component of endotoxin and is highly conserved among different gram-negative species. Antibodies directed against endotoxin core determinants reduce the lethal effects of gram-negative bacteremia and endotoxemia in animal models [12,13]. Immunotherapy with human polyclonal J5 antiserum directed against core determinants prevents death in animal models of gram-negative bacteremia, reduces mortality in patients with gram-negative bacteremia [14], and protects high-risk surgical patients from developing septic shock [15]. Recently, two clinical trials using monoclonal antibodies directed against endotoxin core determinants observed up to a 40% reduction in mortality in patients with gram-negative sepsis or gram-negative bacteremia, when combined with conventional intensive care support [3,16]. It should be noted that neither monoclonal antibody clinical trial demonstrated an intent-to-treat reduction in mortality [3,16]. While the results of these monoclonal antibody clinical trials are interesting, other more potent approaches to neutralizing endotoxin appear to have greater promise.

Neutrophil Host Defense Responses

Human neutrophil granules contain proteins which are important in host defense against bacterial pathogens. Granule proteins released from activated neutrophils facilitate opsonization, phagocytosis, tissue digestion, and antimicrobial activity. Human neutrophils respond to endotoxin stimulation, both *in vitro* and *in vivo*, with a dramatic increase in cell surface expression for CR-1 and CR-3 [17-20]. This increase for CR-1 and CR-3 expression facilitates cell binding to soluble complexes or particles bearing C-derived peptides before phagocytosis [17]. Once phagocytosis has occurred, the nascent phagolysosome is fused with azurophil granules. Azurophil granules contain potent non-oxidative antimicrobial proteins which are involved in the killing and degradation of bacteria [21-25].

Bactericidal Permeability Increasing Protein (BPI)

Bactericidal permeability increasing protein (BPI) was first described in 1978 by Weiss, et al. [26] as one of several naturally occurring cationic antimicrobial proteins found in the azurophil granules of the human neutrophil. BPI is a 55,000 M.W. protein which binds to the surface of susceptible gram-negative bacteria *in vitro* and alters membrane permeability resulting in cell death [26,27]. The bactericidal activity of BPI *in vitro* has been shown to be completely inhibited by serum albumin suggesting that the function of BPI *in vivo* may not be direct killing of bacteria as previously described by Manion et al. [28]. Since BPI demonstrated specificity for LPS containing bacteria, Marra et al. [29] investigated the possibility that BPI may inhibit the activity of LPS. Using flow microfluorimetry, these authors analyzed the surface expression for CR-1 and CR-3 as a measure of neutrophil stimulation response to LPS. Purified BPI completely inhibited CR up-regulation on neutrophils stimulated with both rough and smooth LPS chemotypes at 1.8 to 3.6 nM. In comparison, complete inhibition of LPS stimulated neutrophils was observed with 0.4 nM of polymixin-B. Since polymixin-B binds stoichiometrically to the lipid A moiety of LPS, this would suggest that on a molar basis it requires five-fold greater BPI to bind to the lipid-A moiety than the amount required for polymyxin B [29]. Monocytes stimulated with LPS secrete TNF. Pre-incubating neutrophils with BPI prevents LPS stimulation of TNF expression and LPS mediated CR up-regulation. Further, BPI inhibits LPS in the LAL assay and neutralizes LPS from both smooth and rough chemotypes as well as lipid A. [29].

Animal Experiments with BPI

BPI appears to have a very potent anti-LPS effect *in vitro,* and therefore, we evaluated its role in a series of animal models to determine its potential therapeutic benefit. We isolated and purified human BPI, and cloned and expressed recombinant BPI (r-BPI), and found both BPI and r-BPI to possess potent endotoxin neutralizing activity *in vitro*. Both purified and recombinant BPI bind LPS and inhibit LPS mediated neutrophil and monocyte stimulation. Since the protein has endotoxin neutralizing activity, and most probably functions naturally to regulate the inflammatory response to endotoxin, BPI was studied in experimental models of endotoxin injury.

The Dermal-Shwartzman reaction is used to assess anti-endotoxin activity *in vivo*. New Zealand white female rabbits were initially inoculated intradermally with *E. coli* 0111:B4 endotoxin, and 18 h later were given an intravenous challenge of the 0111:B4 endotoxin. Immediately following the intravenous endotoxin challenge, the animals received either normal saline for the control group or recombinant BPI. The animals were then monitored for seven days for the degree of induration or the presence or absence of dermal necrosis at the initial site of inoculation. Intravenous administration of BPI remarkably improved the tolerance of the rabbits to endotoxin. Induration was significantly reduced from 336.6 ± 23.1 mm^2 to 223.8 ± 17.6 mm^2 ($P=0.0013$). Further, significant dermal necrosis was observed in nine of the ten normal saline treated animals, whereas none of the nine BPI treated animals developed any dermal necrosis following intravenous endotoxin challenge ($p<0.001$).

Since some proteins from the azurophil granules, such as defensin, are quite potent [21,22], BPI was evaluated for any evidence of potential toxicity. Both rats and mice tolerated up to 10 mg/kg BPI without any evidence of toxicity. The animals continued to feed and gain weight normally. Evaluation of blood counts, serum electrolytes, and standard biochemical determinations revealed no abnormalities over seven days of study. Necropsy examination revealed no gross abnormalities on inspection of the major organs of the test animals and histological examination revealed no pathological changes.

Once BPI was demonstrated to be non-toxic and to possess potent LPS neutralizing capabilities, it was then studied in endotoxin challenged animals for both protection and salvage. Intravenous injection of *E. coli* 0111:B4 endotoxin (50.0 mg/kg) into CD-1 mice was 100% lethal in all control animals within 24 h, whereas, 15 of 16 mice treated with 10 mg/kg of BPI immediately following the endotoxin challenge survived ($p = 0.0001$). Further studies revealed dose dependent protection following the simultaneous administration of BPI in escalating doses compared to the endotoxin challenge required to produce 50% lethality (LD_{50}). Compared to saline controls, the LD_{50} of mice treated with 10 mg/kg of BPI was 32-fold greater. Additionally, the ability of BPI to provide protection against a wide variety of heterologous intravenously administred endotoxins was assessed. In addition to the 0111:B4 at 50 mg/kg, the Rc mutant at 25 mg/kg, lipid-A at 25 mg/kg, and 055 LPS at 50 mg/kg, were tested. All the endotoxin challenge control groups had 100% mortality. The BPI treated 0111:B4 endotoxin challenged mice had 19 out of 20 survivors ($p<0.0001$). Further, no deaths were observed in any of the BPI treated groups which received the other endotoxin challenges ($p<0.05$) [30]. In addition to providing significant protection against lethal endotoxin challenge, BPI also is capable of significant rescue following both lethal endotoxin and gram-negative bacteremia challenges.

Proposed Mechanism of Action for BPI

BPI has a high affinity binding domain for the lipid A component of endotoxin. Further, BPI shares considerable sequence homology with LPS binding protein (LBP) [31]. LBP appears to play a significant role in mediating the LPS inflammatory signal by binding to the lipid A portion of LPS and then binding to CD-14 receptors and thus transmitting the LPS inflammatory signal [32]. Conversely, it appears BPI binds to lipid A but does not bind to CD-14 and therefore blocks the LPS signal.

Conclusions

Bactericidal permeability increasing protein is a naturally occurring biologic response blocking protein with potent anti-endotoxin properties. BPI provides significant protection in the Dermal Shwartzman LPS model and is non-toxic. BPI inhibits LPS mediated CR-1 and CR-3 up regulation and prevents LPS stimulation of TNF expression. Further, BPI provides significant protection and rescue salvage in lethal animal models of endotoxin and gram-negative bacteremia challenges. We believe that BPI is a very potent naturally occurring anti-endotoxin protein which shows considerable promise as a potential therapeutic agent in patients with endotoxin mediated illness. The exciting possibility that BPI may be a specific therapeutic agent to enhance the natural negative feedback mechanisms for regulating endotoxic shock in humans is worth investigation.

References

1. Bone RC, Fisher CJ Jr, Clemmer TP, et al. (1989) Sepsis Syndrome: A valid clinical entity. Crit Care Med 17:389–393
2. Bone RC, Fisher CJ Jr, Clemmer TP, et al. (1987) A controlled clinical trial of high-dose methylprednisolone in the treatment of severe sepsis and septic shock. N Engl J Med 317:653–658
3. Ziegler EJ, Fisher CJ Jr, Sprung CL, et al. (1991) Treatment of gram-negative bacteremia and septic shock with HA-1A human monoclonal antibody against endotoxin. N Eng J Med 324:429–436
4. Incrase in national hospital discharge survey rates for septicemia - United States, 1979-1987 (1990) MMWR 39:31–34
5. Kreger BE, Craven DE, McCabe WR (1980) Gram-negative bacteremia IV. Re-evaluation of clinical features and treatment in 612 patients. Am J Med 68:344–355
6. Michie HR, Manogue KR, Spriggs DR, et al. (1988) Detection of circulating tumor necrosis factor after endotoxin administration. N Engl J Med 318:1481–1486

7. Calandra T, Glauser MP (1990) Cytokines and septic shock. Diagn Microbiol Infect Dis 13:377–381
8. Calandra T, Gerain J, Heumann D, et al. (1991) High circulating levels of interleukin-6 in patients with septic shock: Evolution during sepsis, prognostic value, and interplay with other cytokines. Am J Med 91:23–29
9. Calandra T, Baumgartner JD, Grau GE, et al. (1990) Prognostic values of tumor necrosis factor/cachectin, interleukin-1, interferon-α and interferon-γ in the serum of patients with septic shock. J Infec Dis 161:982–987
10. Okusawa S, Gelfand JA, Ikejima T, et al. (1988) Interleukin-1 induces a shock-like state in rabbits synergism with tumor necrosis factor and the effect of cyclooxygenase inhibition. Clin Invest 81:1162–1172
11. Morrison DC (1987) Endotoxin and desease mechanism. Ann Rev Med 38:417
12. McCabe WR, DeMaria A Jr, Berberich H, et al. (1988) Immunization with rough mutants of Salmonella Minnesota: Protective activity of IgM and IgG antibody to the R 595 (Re chemotype) mutant. J Infect Dis 158:291–300
13. Ziegler EJ, Teng NNH, Douglas H, et al. (1987) Treatment of Pseudomonas bacteremia in neutropenic rabbits with human monoclonal IgM antibody against E. coli, lipid-A. Clin Res 35:619A
14. Ziegler EJ, McCutchan JA, Fierer J, et al. (1982) Treatment of gram-negative bacteremia and shock with human antiserum to a mutant E. coli. N Engl J Med 307:1225–1230
15. Baumgartner JD, Glauser MP, Mc Cutchan JA, et al. (1985) Prevention of gram-negative shock and death in surgical patients by antibody to endotoxin core glycolipid. Lancet 2:59–63
16. Greenman RL, Schein RMH, Martin, et al. (1991) A controlled clinical trial of E5 murine monoclonal IgM antibody to endotoxin in the treatment of gram-negative sepsis. JAMA 266:1097–1102
17. Fearon DT, Wong WW (1983) Complement ligand-receptor interactions that mediate biological responses. Ann Rev Immunol 1:243
18. Berger J, O'Shea JO, Cross NS, et al. (1984) Human neutrophils increase expression of C3bi as well as C3b receptors upon activation. J Clin Invest 74:1566
19. Davis CF, Moore FD, Rodrick ML, Fearon DT (1987) Neutrophil activation after burn injury: Contributions of the classic complement pathway and of endotoxin. Surgery 102:477
20. Moore FD, Moss NA, Revhaug D, et al. (1987) A single dose of endotoxin activated neutrophils without activating complement. Surgery 102:200
21. Ganz T, Selsted ME, Szklarek D, et al. (1985) Defensins: Natural peptide antibiotics of human neutrophils. J Clin Invest 76:1427
22. Wilde CG, Griffith JE, Marra MN, et al. (1989) Purification and characterization of HPN-4. A novel member of the Defensin family. J Biol Chem 264:11200
23. Biondin J, Janoff A (1976) The role of lysosomal elastase in the digestion of E. coli proteins by human polymorphonuclear leukocytes. J Clin Invest 58:971
24. Gabay JE, Scott RW, Campanelli S, et al. (1989) Antibiotic proteins of human polymorphonuclear leukocytes. Proc Natl Acad Sci USA 86:5610
25. Houde CJ, Gray BH (1986) Physiologic effects of a bactericidal protein from human polymorphonuclear leukocytes on pseudomonas aeruginosa. Infect Immun 52:90
26. Weiss J, Elsbach P, Olsson I, Odegerg H (1978) Purification and characterization of a potent bactericidal and membrane active protein from the granules of human polymorphonuclear leukocytes. J Biol Chem 253:2664
27. Weiss J, Muello K, Victor M, Elsbach P (1984) The role of lipopolysaccharide in the action of the bactericidal/permeability-increasing neutrophil protein on the bacterial envelope. J Immunol 132:3109
28. Manion BA, Weiss J, Elsbach P (1990) Separation of sublethal and lethal effects of polymorphonuclear leukocytes on E. coli. J Clin Invest 85:853
29. Marra MN, Wilde CG, Griffith JE, et al. (1990) Bactericidal/permeability-increasing protein has endotoxin-neutralizing activity. J Immunol 144:662–666
30. Opal SM, Fisher CJ, Marra MN, Scott RW, Palardy JE (1991) Bactericidal/permeability-increasing protein is a novel therapeutic modality in the treatment of endotoxic shock. Clin Res 39:351

31. Tobias PS, Matison JC, Ulevitch RJ (1988) A family of lipopolysaccharide binding proteins involved in responses to gram-negative sepsis. J Biol Chem 263:13479
32. Schuman RR, Leong SR, Flaggs GW, et al. (1990) Structure and function of lipopolysaccharide binding protein. Science 249:1429

Strategies for Modulation of Systemic and Tissue Cytokine Responses to Sepsis

S.F. Lowry, K.J. VanZee, and L.L. Moldawer

Introduction

The morbidity and mortality attending episodes of sepsis remain high despite widespread advances in technologies directed at support of systemic hemodynamic performance and organ function [1]. The sequelae of sepsis are particularly challenging in the setting of prolonged stressful injury, wherein repeated or sustained endotoxinemic or bacteremic events often eventuate in a progressive deterioration of immunological competence and solid organ function.

While it is now evident that several definable pathways can, in varying degree, initiate and sustain the clinical responses characteristic of sepsis and septic shock, it currently appears that the cytokine class of mediators are nearly uniformly operative within the context of sepsis induced shock and tissue destruction. The cytokines, especially those of a more proximal and pro-inflammatory nature such as tumor necrosis factor (TNF) and interleukin-1 (IL-1) species, have received much attention as pathophysiological determinants of septic shock and the sepsis syndrome [2]. Those antigenic events initiating the appearance of TNF and IL-1 also promote the production of other cytokines, such as interleukin-6 (IL-6) or interleukin-8 (IL-8), which are less globally inflammatory in nature and serve more highly specialized immunological and metabolic functions. Although a description of this classical cytokine cascade remains difficult to document except under the most extreme of clinical conditions [3], our previous studies in gram-negative bacteremic primates have defined both the temporal nature of this cascade and the relative maximal magnitudes of acute cytokine responses during bacteremia (Fig. 1) [4].

Cytokine Activity in Experimental Sepsis

Tumor Necrosis Factor

An immense body of evidence now supports the concept of TNF as a major early determinant of cytokine induced shock.The origins of such data arose from early work identifying TNF as a macrophage product responsible for endotoxin induced mortality in LPS sensitive murine models [5-8]. Sub-

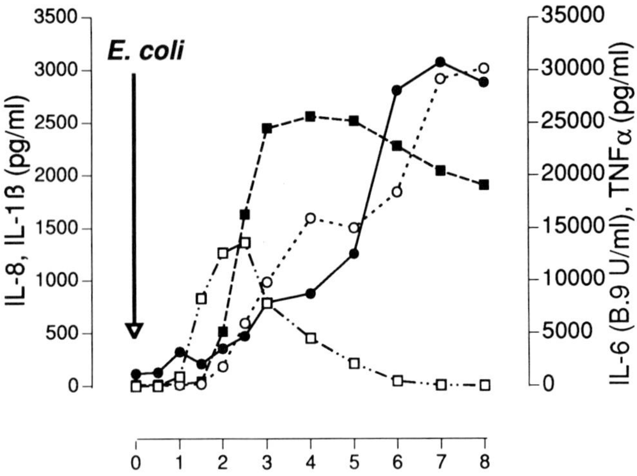

Fig. 1. Circulating cytokine levels in septic shock. Blood samples were obtained every 30 to 60 min from baboons that had received a lethal dose of live *E. coli*. Mean cytokine levels for each timepoint are shown for TNFα (❑), IL-1β (■, IL-6 (○), and IL-8 (●) and were determined by ELISA (TNFα, IL1β, and IL-8) and by B.9 hybridoma proliferation assay (IL-6).

sequent investigators outlined the specificity and essentiality of TNF to endotoxin mortality by demonstrating the protective capacity of neutralizing antibodies against TNF. It was also evident from other experimental studies that the administration of exogenous TNF reproduced many of the systemic and tissue-specific pathological sequelae of clinical sepsis [9,10]. The clinical relevance of TNF related events in the evolution of infectious shock was emphasized by studies wherein monoclonal antibodies directed against a human TNF epitope fully prevented the early deterioration of hemodynamic function as well as the late tissue injury components of *E. coli* bacteremia [11]. These initial studies also suggested that other mediators, such as more distal cytokines, might also be essential to the evolution of septic shock, or as is more likely, to the full expression of systemic and tissue responses which characterize the sepsis and multiorgan system failure (MOF) syndromes. For example, the co-administration of IL-1 or interferon-γ appear to enhance the lethality of sublethal TNF doses [12].

Recent surveys have enumerated the *in vitro* biological characteristics of TNF [13,14]. Unfortunately, efforts to translate the known properties of this cytokine to specific clinical events remain elusive. The *in vivo* appearance of TNF elicits not only a cascade of further cytokine mediators, several of which share similar functions, but also a counter-regulatory neuro-endocrine response which serves to variably amplify or attenuate the activities of TNF and other cytokines [15,16]. Hence, it is clinically impractical to attribute

Table 1. Cytokine levels during sepsis and critical illnes correlation with outcome

		TNF[a]		IL-1[a]		IL-6[a]		IL-8[a]	
Reference	Disease	Survivors	Non Survivors	Survivors	Non Survivors	Survivors	Non Survivors	Survivors	Non Survivors
Waage et al. [20]	meningitis +/- shock	8/68 (WEHL: 10μ/ml)	10/11						
Marone et al. [21]	burns/sepsis	8/26 (ELISA: 34pg/ml)	12/17						
Girardin et al. [22]	purpural sepsis	410±50 pg/ml) (RIA)	830±240						
Waage et al. [23]	meningococcal sepsis	5/5 (WEHI:2-3 pg/ml)	5/5	0/4 (LBRM:0.02μ/ml)	3/4	<3 (B9:15-20pg/ml)	>750		
de Groote et al. [24]	gram-negative sepsis	___ (ELISA)	___						
Debets et al. [25]	sepsis	3/24 (ELISA:5-10pg/ml)	8/19						
Damas et al. [26]	septic shock	139±21 (RIA:2pg/tube)	614±281	447±60 (RIA:10pg/tube)	496±34				
Cannon et al. [27]	septic shock			153±30 (RIA:20-80pg/ml)	93±9				
Calandra et al. [28]	septic shock	180 (RIA:100pg/ml)	330	300 (RIA:150pg/ml)	480				
Munoz et al. [29]	sepsis	143±25 (RIA:70pg/ml)	217±41	275±112 (RIA:70pg/ml)	121±59	638±158 (μ/ml) (7TDI)	15,205±6430		
Danner et al. [30]	shock					3.06±1.14 (ELISA)	3.98±1.50	3.77±0.49 (ELISA)	1.48±0.39

[a] number of patients with detectable levels/total number of patients, or mean level ( ) = (specific assay: reported level of assay sensitivity)

any sepsis induced event, perhaps other than acute hemodynamic collapse, specifically to TNF. The problem inherent in defining a specific *in vivo* role for TNF likewise extends to most other members of this mediator class.

It is evident from those studies in which TNF has been exogenously administered to experimental animals and humans, that excessive activity of this cytokine initiates many components of the inflammatory stress response [17-19]. In addition to acute alterations of cardiovascular performance, increased release of neuro-endocrine stress hormones, activation of coagulation pathways, as well as significant stimulation of immune function and metabolic regulation all occur within minutes to hours after the administration of TNF. Such studies demonstrate that many clinical events predicted by the known *in vitro* activities of this cytokine are evoked by pharmacological influences of TNF. However, circulatory TNF levels of similar magnitude in sepsis and critically ill patients is much less frequent, or predictable, than would be anticipated by the incidence of associated responses (Table 1) [20-30].

The capacity to document such *in vivo* TNF activity clinically may be influenced by a variety of factors including sample timing and assay sensitivity. However, the frequent discordance between clinical events suggestive of a TNF influence and a lack of detectable protein raises other issues regarding the direct role of TNF to post-infection or injury responses. TNF, like several other cytokines, exhibits polymorphism which, in the form of a cell associated species, may exert influences at the tissue level without release of soluble protein [31-33]. Although neither the molecular regulation nor clinical significance of such cell associated species have been fully elucidated, such mechanisms may permit a broader temporal range of TNF activity than would be predicted by detectability of the circulating ligand.

Interleukin-1

Species of this cytokine, like TNF, are only sporadically detected in the circulation of patients with severe injury or infection. While it was previously held that IL-1 shared many pro-inflammatory characteristics with TNF, the capacity for this protein to induce conditions of shock were believed to be limited. Recent studies have questioned these assumptions as IL-1, either singly [34] or in combination with TNF [35] or other proximal components of the cytokine cascade, has been demonstrated to produce some degree of hemodynamic compromise and tissue injury. In fact, IL-1 when administered in sufficient doses, appears capable of initiating many of the cardiovascular and metabolic sequelae associated with sepsis and severe tissue injury.

The production of IL-1 is promoted by a variety of inciting antigenic stimulae, as well as other members of the cytokine family [2,36]. While this protein is detected with less frequency during experimental and clinical conditions of sepsis, it nevertheless maintains a significant proximal role in the cytokine cascade which attends overwhelming infection (Fig. 1) and appears to be necessary for the full expression of subsequent cytokine appearance and activity. Recent data would suggest that a significant degree of immune cell activation or of tissue injury is necessary for the appearance of the circulating form of IL-1, which is predominantly the beta species [37]. Although the circulating as well as the predominant cellular form (alpha) share only 26% amino-acid homology, both bind with equal affinity to the same cell surface receptors and induce similar biological responses [38]. In a manner similar to TNF, these IL-1 species are capable of exerting significant biological responses within the local tissue environment, and likely do so at low levels of receptor occupancy [39].

The ability to identify *in vivo* host toxicities specific to IL-1 are also limited. Many of the tissue responses attributable to IL-1 are similar to those exhibited by TNF, or may arise from frank synergy between these or other cytokines. Recent experimental studies have served to clarify these issues, as the exogenous administration of IL-1 α reproduces many of the acute hematological and metabolic perturbations reminiscent of severe bacterial infection in the absence of a detectable TNF response [34]. Such studies also suggest that the TNF component is necessary for induction of severe shock, whereas IL-1 is equally, if not more potent on a molar basis, for the further induction of subsequent cytokine responses.

Interleukin-6

The appearance of cirulating forms of other cytokines, especially those subserving more specialized functions, such as IL-6, is also inducible by the activity of TNF and IL-1. While a clear precursor requirement for these proximal cytokines to the *in vivo* production of IL-6 is not defined, the temporal relationship of IL-6 appearance within the cytokine cascade suggests a strong relationship to antecedent TNF or IL-1 stimulation during severe infection. Further evidence to support such a relationship arises from studies in which either TNF or IL-1 activity is attenuated during infection, with a resultant diminution in the IL-6 response [40,41].

In contrast to the readily demonstrable toxicities of TNF and IL-1, neither the range of biological functions attributable to IL-6 nor studies of exogenous administration of this cytokine suggest significant inherent toxicity of this protein alone [42]. Some evidence does attest to a potential adverse role for IL-6 during endotoxinemic states or those associated with prior activation hy pro-inflammatory cytokines, as anti-IL-6 monoclonal antibodies provide protection from lethal *E. coli* infection as well as TNF administration in mice [43]. While the mechanism for such protection remains poorly defined, recent data suggest that TNF or IL-1 enhanced expression of GP130, a cell associated glycoprotein that binds to the IL-6/IL-6 receptor complex, may contribute to enhanced IL-6 signal transduction [44]. As this complex is not induced by IL-6 alone, such amplification of the IL-6 signal pathway via antecedent TNF and IL-1 activity may serve to promote the toxicity of IL-6.

Interleukin-8

Paralleling the circulating appearance of IL-6 is that of IL-8, a 6-10kD cytokine with potent *in vitro* chemoattractant and activation properties. The production of IL-8 by a diverse array of cell types is responsive to numerous stimulae, including LPS, TNF, and IL-1, but not of IL-6 [45]. Whereas the defined *in vitro* activities of this cytokine, in association with its appearance during experimental and clinical sepsis [46] conditions make IL-8 an additional candidate for promoting adverse host responses to sepsis, the exogenous administration of this single cytokine to primates does not provoke either systemic or tissue insult nor the appearance of other inflammatory cytokines [47]. The available evidence would suggest that IL-8, like other distal cytokines of a specialized functional nature may contribute to the progressive tissue destruction attending severe infection largely in the context of antecedent or continuing stimulation of the pro-inflammatory cytokines, TNF and IL-1.

Clinical Studies of Cytokine Activity

Endotoxemia

Efforts to characterize both the temporal nature of cytokine appearance and the clinically relevant magnitude of such responses have been aided by the administration of sublethal endotoxin (LPS) doses to normal subjects [4,49]. Under these circumstances, a cytokine cascade is likewise evident, although the magnitude of circulating levels are far less than those observed during endotoxemia or bacteremia in animals [16,48,49]. Further, evidence of a circulating IL-1 response to LPS has been inconsistent. The temporal relationship between cytokine appearance and systemic symptomatology is remarkably consistent, with the evolution of chills/myalgias and pyrogenic responses being superimposable upon the peak TNF and IL-6 responses, respectively. By contrast, the initial neutropenia attending LPS administration precedes the detection of any cytokines within the circulation and the later (3-6 h) neutrophilia more closely parallels the development of hypercortisolemia [50].

Several approaches to the control of LPS induced symptomatology have sought to interrupt the normal production of cytokines or that of the purported cellular signal pathways activated by cytokines. Among the agents readily affecting the normal production of TNF are glucocorticoids and oxypentifylline. When subjects are treated with such agents prior to LPS administration, the appearance of circulating TNF is markedly attenuated and much of the symptomatology, including febrile responses, are abrogated. While such studies suggest that a pro-inflammatory cytokine response is necessary for such LPS induced manifestations, agents which block the generation of prostanoid mediators also produce similar influences [16].

Tumor Necrosis Factor

An extensive clinical experience with the administration of TNF as an antitumor therapy attests to the *in vivo* activities of this protein in humans [54,55]. Such studies have likewise defined distinct toxicities associated with TNF therapy, with evidence of hemodynamic compromise following dosages in excess of 250-300 ug/m2. Additional hematological and metabolic effects are observed at much lower doses of TNF. It has been observed that increases in resting energy expenditure as well as systemic and regional tissue metabolic changes may evolve with the administration of a single 10 ug/m2 or greater [19]. The striking similarities between host sequelae attending LPS administration and those of TNF exposure have been noted [56].

Recent studies have systematically evaluated the responses to TNF administration in normal humans. Diverse hematologic, coagulation, hormonal, and metabolic alterations reminiscent of those arising from severe infection and tissue injury are evoked by intravenous TNF administration [17,18]. These studies, like those performed in clinical trials with TNF therapy, noted the onset of these events within minutes after administration of the protein, suggesting a direct linkage of TNF to such sequelae.

Interleukin-1

Far less definitive data referable to the direct contribution of IL-1 species in the post-infectious or injury states is available. Although limited trials of IL-1 administration as a biological response modifier are underway, the observed systemic and regional responses have not been fully characterized [57]. It would appear, however, that similar systemic toxicities and metabolic events to those observed with TNF administration are induced by IL-1. Whether IL-1 will exhibit the same degree of hemodynamic compromise attributable to equimolar doses of TNF has yet to be established in clinical trials. As the exogenous administration of IL-1 has not been proven to induce a significant TNF response in primates [34], it may be suggested that both cytokines are necessary for full expression of the cardiovascular collapse associated with activation of this pathway.

Pre-Clinical Studies with Antagonist Therapies

Recent experimental studies investigating the potential therapeutic utility of direct cytokine antagonism serve to both illuminate the complexity of the cytokine system during sepsis and critical illness as well as suggest the potential benefits and limitations of these strategies. These interventional studies have been performed in a variety of species with similar results being obtai-

Table 2. Cytokine responses to endotoxin and *E. coli* in primates: the influence of anti-cytokine therapies

Reference		Peak TNF (pg/ml)	Peak IL-1β (pg/ml)	Peak IL-6 (B.9u/ml)	Survival
Fischer et al. [34]	LPS (500 μg/Kg bolus)	1,000 - 1,700	ND	3500 - 4200	7/7
VanZee et al. [46]	Bacteremia (10^{10}-10^{11} cfu/Kg *E. coli*)	32,000 - 42,000	300 - 800	26,000 - 34,000	3/7 (@24hr)
Fischer et al. [41]	Bacteremia + IL-1ra	28,000 - 35,000	300 - 800	10,000 - 18,000	7/7 (@24hr)
Tracey et al. [40]	Bacteremia (10^{11} cfu/Kg *E. coli*)	17,000 - 24,000	1,700 - 2,500	10,000 - 27,000	0/6 (@24hr)
Fong et al. [40]	Bacteremia + TNF mAB	<1,000	200 - 500	500 - 1,500	3/3 (>48hr)

ND - not detectable by ELISA

ned in several models of gram-negative bacteremia. The current discussion will focus upon our own evaluations of such therapies in a primate model of overwhelming bacteremia.

TNF Blockade

The administration of anti-TNF monoclonal antibodies prior to challenge with an otherwise LD100 dose of live *E. coli* provided essentially complete protection against the stress hormone response, shock and death in baboons (Table 2) [11]. Such therapy, when provided 2 h prior to bacterial challenge, also significantly attenuated the appearance of IL-1 and IL-6, suggesting the importance of TNF in initiating the cytokine cascade [40]. Further, such anti-TNF therapy prevents both histological and functional deterioration of critical organs, as these parameters remained normal in all organs examined, with the exception of the adrenal gland for up to 7 days after treatment. The hematological and metabolic responses of primates treated with anti-TNF antibodies also exhibited a significant attenuation compared with untreated cohorts [40], although these influences may, in part, be related to a less severe stress hormone background [58].

We [60] have recently investigated the efficacy of other antagonist strategies directed against TNF activity in this model. Naturally occurring soluble inhibitors of TNF in the circulation of endotoxinemic and critically ill subjects have recently been defined as the extracellular domains of the type I and II TNF receptors. These soluble receptors bind to circulating TNFα and prevent detection of the protein by standard immunoassays and bioassays. Although the functional significance of such soluble TNF antagonists remains unclear [59], recombinant species of soluble TNF receptors is appealing as a therapeutic modality. We have performed preliminary studies evaluating the efficacy of this therapeutic stratagem in our primate bacteremia model. These studies have demonstrated a lack of toxicity associated with a 3 h infusion of the type I recombinant soluble TNF receptor. More importantly, such treatment acutely neutralizes the immunological detection and bioactivity of TNF induced by severe bacteremia and maintains hemodynamic performance and organ function in a manner similar to that provided by anti-TNF monoclonal antibodies [60].

Interleukin-1 Antagonism

Circulating levels of IL-1β in the range of 300-2500 pg/ml are achieved during gram-negative bacteremia in primates (Table 2) [40]. However, the extent to which this cytokine precipitates, or perhaps more importantly serves to propagate, the deterioration of systemic and tissue function during sepsis has been an issue of considerable debate. Our previous studies in primates suggested that doses of exogenous IL-1α of 10-100 μg/kg could also produce a state of diminished cardiac output as well as produce lactacidemia and adrenal injury similar to equimolar doses of TNF [34]. Although such treatment did not evoke the full spectrum of sequelae observed with TNF, such responses were observed in the absence of any detectable TNF levels. Such findings, in addition to those noted in other animal species with IL-1 administration, suggested that this cytokine may also be of principal importance in the evolution of septic syndromes.

Several groups have utilized the naturally occurring IL-1 receptor antagonist as a means of modulating the influences of IL-1 during sepsis and bacteremia [41,61,62]. This protein, when present in quantities of 500-1000 molar excess to IL-1, effectively prevents the binding of IL-1 to its receptor and does so without any known toxicity or inherent agonist activity. We have recently utilized a recombinant species of this IL-1 receptor antagonist in our primate model of bacteremia and demonstrated improved survival to gram-negative bacteremia [41]. This improvement in outcome was achieved despite a fully intact circulating TNF response and only partial abrogation of other inducible cytokines, such as IL-6 (Table 2). These results are suggestive of an important role for endogenous IL-1 activity as contributory to the acute sequelae of sepsis.

Identification of Cytokine Activity in Clinical Sepsis

As noted above, circulating cytokines, particularly the pro-inflammatory proteins TNF and IL-1, are not consistently detected during conditions of clinical shock, infection or severe tissue injury. An examination of the levels of these cytokines, measured either at study entry or serially during the critical illness phase, reveals a wide variability with respect to the incidence of detection and of the absolute values obtained. The reasons for these discrepancies have been widely discussed [2,63]. Except under the most extreme of conditions, such as meningococcemia, there is little evidence to suggest that levels of circulating TNF and IL-1 above those achieved with lesser degrees of infection are consistently detected.

A number of prospective studies have evaluated the presence of two or more cytokines during conditions of sepsis and critical illness (Table 1). Given the implications of the above discussion regarding the potential for synergy between TNF and IL-1 or other cytokine mediators, it would not be surprising that documentation of more global cytokine activation is associated with increased morbidity and mortality. An examination of these reported series tends to confirm this impression, wherein patients not surviving their septic insult frequently exhibit not only simultaneous detection of TNF and IL-1 but also greater levels of these cytokines than do surviving patients. Additionally, these patients usually display greater levels of IL-6 than do surviving subjects.

An additional confounding problem in the interpretation of cytokine levels and their correlation with clinical course and outcome is the probability that non-circulating forms may contribute substantially to activity at the tissue level. Indeed, local or compartmentalized production of cytokines, particularly of TNF and IL-1, are well documented [31-33]. A variety of cell types are capable of producing cell associated forms of these cytokines and may exert localized agonist activity even in the absence of circulating species. Such organ specific TNF and IL-1 bioactivity is inducible by a diverse array of antigenic stimulae in the experimental setting. Although the relevance of such observations to prolonged cytokine influences during human sepsis has yet to be fully defined, it is speculated that these species contribute to the progressive organ dysfunction of injured and infected patients [64].

The problems inherent to assay sensitivity, sporadic production of many cytokines, and of influences exerted by cell associated species, all serve to confound any current interpretations of cytokine contribution during clinical sepsis and injury. Further, the ability to translate *in vitro* functions attributable to any single cytokine to observed clinical events is hampered by the breadth of functional overlap exhibited by many members of this mediator class. As a consequence, much of the *in vivo* biological activity currently attributed to cytokines remains largely speculative. Further definition of these events will require the utilization of specific antagonist therapies to dissect the individual and synergistic influences exerted by cytokines in the clinical responses to sepsis and injury.

It is also increasingly evident that the host capacity for cytokine production and responsiveness is modulated by a number of biological variables and countervailing clinical influences. Such influences include endogenous mechanisms for the regulation of cytokine production and activity. As evidence of this teleologic function, the appearance of natural cytokine antagonists, such as soluble TNF receptors or of the IL-1 receptor antagonist discussed above, are emblematic of the host efforts, albeit limited, to limit the destructive activity of excessive cytokine production. Although the mechanisms regulating the production of these natural antagonists remain unclear, preliminary data would suggest that their appearance is, at least partially, independent of prior cytokine activity [36]. These findings suggest a complex interplay of other mediator signals serving to attenuate cytokine activities.

Perhaps most readily identifiable among the mediators influencing activation of the cytokine system is the neuro-endocrine hormone system. Activation of the stress hormonal response follows to a variable degree upon all infectious or injurious stimulae. While the immunological and metabolic functional consequences arising from such enhanced hypothalamic-pituitary-adrenal activity are well described, the *in vivo* relationship between these signal pathways and those of micromediator systems, such as cytokines, has only recently been appreciated. It is well established that *in vitro* cytokine responses to LPS antigen exposure can be transiently attenuated by glucocorticoids [8], and that this response can be restored by interferon-gamma [65]. We have recently demonstrated that antecedent hypercortisolemia for periods up to 12 h prior to LPS administration in humans essentially abrogates the appearance of circulating TNF [51]. This attenuation of the cytokine cascade also diminishes the systemic symptomatology and pyrogenic response to LPS.These observations may partially explain the lack of cytokine detection both during the early phases of host counter-regulatory hormonal responses to endotoxinemia as well as during later periods of sustained endocrine stress. This also underscores the necessity of broadly defining the antecedent as well as concurrent hormonal background in evaluation of cytokine activity in patients.

Cytokine production and activity in the critically ill patient may also be influenced by a large number of therapeutic agents [1]. Additionally, the potential for enhanced antigenic stimulation for cytokine production may arise from antimicrobial agents which cause bacterial lysis. Other clinical circumstances may also predispose to amplification, especially under circumstances where prolonged periods of bowel rest or total parenteral nutrition may be necessary. We have recently documented the influence of such nutritional therapies in normal subjects who were challenged with LPS after a one week period of oral nutrition or a similar period of parenteral feeding. The sytemic

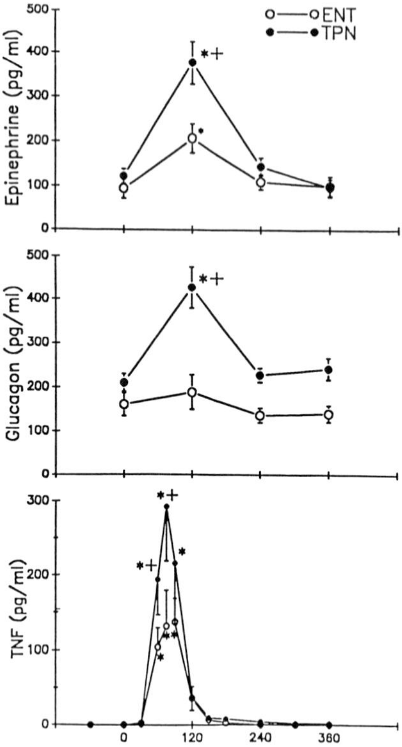

Fig. 2. Hormonal and tumor necrosis factor (TNF) levels in response to endotoxin in normal subjects. Epinephrine, glucagon, and TNF levels in arterial blood before (t=0) and after intravenous endotoxin administration. Subjects were studied 12 h after the cessation of 7 days of enteral feedings (ENT) or total parenteral nutrition (TPN).

as well as splanchnic tissue production of TNF was significantly enhanced by such a lack of antecedent intestinal feeding (Fig. 2) [66]. The potential impact of this variable needs to be considered in the interpretation of cytokine data as well as in the clinical management of injured or septic patients.

It is suspected that excessive cytokine activity adversely influences critical organ function. A limited number of studies [21,28] also suggest that increased circulating cytokine levels are more readily evident during states of MOF. Although the functional significance of these observations remains to be clarified, the available evidence suggests that a failure to effectively clear excessive cytokines may represent a fundamental host defect leading to MOF. This may also be true at the regional tissue level where, despite the inability to detect a circulating cytokine response, progressive tissue destruction is associated with enhanced cytokine bioactivity [67]. Given the evidence to suggest that some tissue fixed immune cell populations do not effectively produce cytokine antagonists, such as IL-1ra [36], organs relatively enriched with such cell populations may be predisposed to excessive cytokine influences. Recent studies have documented the dramatic local production of TNF and IL-1 within tissues such as the pulmonary vasculature and hepatic bed [15]. Whether such tissues exhibit defective generation of cytokine antagonists, or alternatively an enhanced sensitivity to such cytokines, remains to be determined in man.

Clinical Strategies for Modulating Cytokine Influences

It is evident that therapeutic regimens directed against excessive cytokine activity hold promise for enhancing the successful management of septic and injured patients. The current wealth of pre-clinical data impugns cytokines, particularly the pro-inflammatory cytokines TNF and IL-1, as significant mediators of sepsis induced morbidity and mortality. Unlike current therapies directed against a single antigenic determinant [68], it is apparent that cytokine activity is inducible by a wide variety of ligands of both microbial and endogenous origin. Hence, therapies directed against such a broader range of stimulae are appealing under conditions where the offending stimulus is not well defined.

Some concerns must arise from the use of agents directed against any endogenously derived mediator, few, if any, of which have been conserved for the sole purpose of host destruction. A growing body of literature attests to the beneficial influences of cytokines, ranging from preservation of immunological competence, to interorgan and tissue substrate utilization, and wound healing [2,69]. We are currently far from a comprehensive understanding of the integrative biology of cytokine functions nor of their relationship with other signal pathways. Further, we have yet, at either the experimental or clinical levels, to assess the potential consequences of selective blockade of individual components of these teleologically integrated response mechanisms.

Despite these theoretical concerns, there is little pre-clinical evidence to suggest that anti-cytokine therapies produce acutely adverse consequences. When administered prior to activation of the cytokine cascade, their capacity to attenuate the hemodynamic consequences of bacterial infection are impressive. However, similarly impressive protective effects may not be observed when these agents are utilized during therapeutic modes. Under such circumstances, the risk/benefit relationships may be more difficult to assess and the potential for untoward adverse consequences exaggerated.

The era of cytokine response modification in the critically ill patient has evolved with such rapidity and intensity that current interventional capacity outstrips our comprehension of the salient clinical mechanisms. Such therapies will be broadly applied if they prove effective in the numerous clinical trials assessing efficacy in the septic patient. One cannot help but wonder, however, if such trials may not overlook some of the finer details regarding patient selection and the timing of therapeutic interventions in the critically ill. Many current trials are designed to utilize dosing regimens derived from limited pre-clinical assessment of circulating cytokine levels. The possible existence of ongoing or recurring tissue cytokine production and the necessity to attenuate such influence over a longer treatment period will need to be addressed in future trials. More prolonged or repeated dosing schedules may ultimately prove superior to an abbreviated period of intervention. This is particularly true of patients with evidence of progressive MOF in whom, as noted above, neither effective endogenous systemic nor regional protective measures are evoked.

Several current trials have sought to evaluate anti-cytokine strategies as single agent therapy. To date, only that utilizing the 72-hour infusion of IL-1 ra has been reported, with the results of a recently completed Phase II clinical trial suggesting a dose-dependent relationship to 28 day survival. Although the achievement in survival of the 99 patients accrued to this trial were not statistically significant, the mortality of placebo treated patients was similar to that observed in previously reported trials of anti-endotoxin antibodies [68,70].

Conclusion

The next several years will provide exciting additional insights into the biological application of anti-cytokine therapies. While it can be anticipated that some patient populations will benefit from these therapies, the dilemmas accruing to clinicians from these new biological agents are potentially enormous. The need to define these populations carefully and the likelihood that potentially costly combination therapies may prove more efficacious than single agent regimens will also serve to heighten the conflict between appropriate patient care and societal cost/benefit pressures. These sometimes opposing pressures may be further amplified if anti-cytokine therapies prove effective not only in gram-negative sepsis but also against a broader range of microbes.

References

1. Bone RC (1991) A critical evaluation of new agents for the treatment of sepsis. JAMA 266:1686–1691
2. Fong Y, Moldawer LL, Shires GT, Lowry S (1990) The biological characteristics of cytokines and their implication in surgical injury. Surg Gynecol Obstet 170:363–378
3. Waage A, Brandtzaeg P, Halstensen A, Kierulf P, Espevik T (1989) The complex pattern of cytokines in serum from patients with meningococcal septic shock: Association between interleukin-6, interleukin-1, and fatal outcome. J Exp Med 169:333–338
4. VanZee KJ, Lowry SF (1992) Identification and effects of cytokines during experimental and clinical sepsis. In: Dunn DL (ed) Humoral Immunity and Antibody Therapy During Septic Shock (in press)
5. Beutler B, Milsark IW, Cerami AC (1985) Passive immunization against cachectin/tumor necrosis factor protects mice from lethal effect of endotoxin.Science 229:869–871
6. Beutler B, Milsark IW, Cerami A (1985) Cachectin/tumor necrosis factor: Production, distribution, and metabolic fate in vivo. J Immunol 135:3972–3977
7. Beutler B, Greenwald D, Hulmes JD, et al. (1985) Identity of tumour necrosis factor and the macrophage-secreted factor cachectin. Nature 316:552–554
8. Beutler B, Krochnin N, Milsark IW, Luedke C, Cerami A (1986) Control of cachectin (tumor necrosis factor) synthesis: Mechanisms for endotoxin resistance. Science 232:977–980
9. Tracey KJ, Beutler B, Lowry SF, et al. (1986) Shock and tissue injury induced by recombinant human cachectin.Science 234:470–474
10. Tracey KJ, Lowry SF, Fahey TJ, et al. (1987) Cachectin/tumor necrosis factor induces lethal septic shock and stress hormone responses in the dog. Surg Gynecol Obstet 164:415–442
11. Tracey KJ, Fong Y, Hesse DG, et al. (1987) Anti-cachectin/TNF monoclonal antibodies prevent septic shock during lethal bacteremia. Nature 330:662–664
12. Philip R, Epstein LB (1986) Tumor necrosis factor as immunomodulator and mediator of monocyte cytotoxicity induced by itself, γ-interferon and interleukin-1. Nature 323:86–89
13. Larrick JW, Wright SC (1990) Cytotoxic mechanism of tumor necrosis factor α. FASEB J 4:3215–3223
14. Beutler B, Cerami A (1989) The biology of cachectin /TNF - a primary mediator of the host response. Ann Rev Immunol 7:625–655
15. Fong Y, Marano MA, Moldawer LL, et al. (1990) The acute splanchnic and peripheral tissue metabolic response to endotoxin in man. J Clin Invest 85:1896–1904
16. Michie HR, Manogue KR, Spriggs DR, et al. (1988) Detection of circulating tumor necrosis factor after endotoxin administration. N Engl J Med 318:1481–1486
17. van der Poll T, Büller HR, ten Cate H, et al. (1990) Activation of coagulation after administration of tumor necrosis factor to normal subjects. New Engl J Med 322:1622–1627
18. van der Poll T, Romijn JA, Endert E, Borm JJJ, Büller HR, Sauerwein HP (1991) Tumor necrosis factor mimics the metabolic response to acute infection in healthy humans. Am J Physiol 261:457–465
19. Starnes Jr HF, Warren RA, Jeevanandam M, et al. (1988) Tumor necrosis factor and the acute metabolic response to tissue injury in man. J Clin Invest 82:1321–1325
20. Waage A, Halstensen A, Espevik T (1987) Association between tumour necrosis factor in serum and fatal outcome in patients with meningococcal disease. Lancet1:355–357
21. Marano MA, Fong Y, Moldawer LL, et al. (1990) Serum cachectin/tumor necrosis factor in critically ill patients with burns correlates with infection and mortality. Surg Gynecol Obstet 170:32–38
22. Girardin E, Grau GW, Dayer JM (1988) Tumor necrosis factor and interleukin-1 in the serum of children with severe infectious purpura. N Engl J Med 319:397–400
23. Waage A, Brandtzaeg P, Halstensen A, Kierulf P, Espevik T (1989) The complex pattern of cytokines in serum from patients with meningococcal septic shock: Association between interleukin-6, interleukin-1, and fatal outcome. J Exp Med 169:333–338

24. de Groote MA, Martin MA, Densen P, Pfaller MA, Wenzel RP (1989) Plasma tumor necrosis factor levels in patients with presumed sepsis: Results in those treated with antilipid A antibody vs placebo. JAMA 262:249–251
25. Debets JMH, Kampmeijer R, van der Linden MPMH, Buurman WA, van der Linden CJ (1989) Plasma tumor necrosis factor and mortality in critically ill septic patients.Crit Care Med 17:489–494
26. Damas P, Reuter A, Gysen P, Demonty J, Lamy M, Franchimont P (1989) Tumor necrosis factor and interleukin-1 serum levels during severe sepsis in humans. Crit Care Med 17:975–978
27. Cannon JG, Tompkins RG, Gelfand JA, et al. (1990) Circulating interleukin-1 and tumor necrosis factor in septic shock and experimental endotoxin fever. J Infect Dis 161:79–84
28. Calandra T, Baumgartner JD, Grau GE, et al. and the Swiss-Dutch J5 Immunoglobulin Study Group (1990) Prognostic values of tumor necrosis factor/cachectin, interleukin-1, interferon-α, and interferon-γ in the serum of patients with septic shock. J Infect Dis 161:982–987
29. Munoz C, Misset B, Fitting C, Blériot JP, Carlet J, Cavaillon JM (1991) Dissociation between plasma and monocyte-associated cytokines during sepsis. Eur J Immunol 21:2177–2184
30. Danner RL, Suffredini AF, Van Dervort AL, et al. (1990) Detection of interleukin 6 (IL-6) and interleukin 8 (IL-8) during septic shock in humans. Clin Res 38:352
31. Kriegler M, Perez C, DeFay K, Albert I, Lu SD (1988) A novel form of TNF/cachectin is a cell surface cytotoxic transmembrane protein: Ramifications for the complex physiology of TNF. Cell 53:45–53
32. Keogh CV, Fong Y, Barber A, et al. (1990) Identification of a novel cell-associated murine tumor necrosis factor. Arch Surg 125:79–85
33. Munoz C, Carlet J, Fitting C, Misset B, Blériot JP, Cavaillon JM (1991) Dysregulation of in vitro cytokine production by monocytes during sepsis. J Clin Invest 88:1747–1754
34. Fischer E, Marano MA, Barber A, et al. (1991) Interleukin-1α administration can replicate the hemodynamic and metabolic responses to sublethal endotoxemia. Am J Physiol 261:442–452
35. Dinarello CA (1991) The proinflammatory cytokines interleukin-1 and tumor necrosis factor and treatment of the septic shock syndrome. J. Infect Dis 163:1177–1184
36. Dinarello CA (1991) Interleukin-1 and interleukin-1 antagonism. Blood 77:1627–1652
37. Hogquist KA, Unanue ER, Chaplin DD (1991) Release of IL-1 from mononuclear phagocytes. J Immunol 147:2181–2186
38. Dinarello CA (1988) Biology of interleukin-1. FASEB J 2:108–115
39. McIntyre KW, Stepan GJ, Kolinsky KD, et al. (1991) Inhibition of interleukin-1 (IL-1) binding and bioactivity in vitro and modulation of acute inflammation in vivo by IL-1 receptor antagonist and anti-IL-1 receptor monoclonal antibody. J Exp Med 173:931
40. Fong Y, Tracy KJ, Moldawer LL, et al. (1989) Antibodies to cachectin/TNF reduce interleukin-1β and interleukin-6 appearance during lethal bacteremia. J Exp Med 170:1627–1633
41. Fischer E, Marano MA, Van Zee KJ, et al. (1992) Interleukin-1 receptor blockade improves survival and hemodynamic performance in E. coli septic shock, but fails to alter host responses to sublethal endotoxemia. J Clin Invest (in press)
42. Preiser JC, Schmartz D, Van der Linden P, et al. (1991) Interleukin-6 administration has no acute hemodynamic or hematologic effect in the dog. Cytokine 3:1–4
43. Starnes HF, Pearce MK, Tewari A, Yim JH, Zou JC, Abrams JS (1990) Anti-IL-6 monoclonal antibodies protect against lethal Escherichia coli infection and lethal tumor necrosis factor-α challenge in mice. J Immunol 145:4185–4191
44. Klein CE, Ozer HL, Traganos F, Atzpodien J, Oettgen HF, Old LJ (1988) A transformation-associated 130-kD cell surface glycoprotein is growth controlled in normal human cells. J Exp Med 167:1684–1696
45. Hannum CH, Wilcox CJ, Arend WP, et al. (1990) Interleukin-1 receptor antagonist activity of a human interleukin-1 inhibitor. Nature 343:336–340
46. VanZee KJ, DeForge LE, Fischer E (1991) Interleukin-8 circulates during septic shock, endotoxemia, and following interleukin-1 administration. J Immunol 146:3478–3482
47. VanZee KJ, Fischer E, Hawes AS, et al. (1992) The sequelae of IL-8 administration in nonhuman primates. J Immunol (in press)

48. Hesse DG, Tracey KJ, Fong Y, et al. (1988) Cytokine appearance in human endotoxemia and primate bacteremia. Surg Gynecol Obstet 166:147–153
49. van Deventer SJH, Büller HR, ten Cate JW, Aarden LA, Hack CE, Sturk A (1990) Experimental endotoxemia in humans: Analysis of cytokine release and coagulation, fibrinolytic, and complement pathways. Blood 76:2520–2526
50. Richardson RP, Rhyne CD, Fong Y, et al. (1989) Peripheral blood leukocyte kinetics following in vivo lipopolysaccharide (LPS) administration to normal human subjects: Influence of elicited hormones and cytokines. Ann Surg 210:239–245
51. Barber AE, Coyle SM, Fong Y, et al. (1990) Impact of hypercortiosolemia on the metabolic and hormonal responses to endotoxin in man. Surg Forum 41:74–77
52. Waage A, Sorensen M, Stordal B (1990) Differential effect of oxypentifylline on tumour necrosis factor and interleukin-6 production. Lancet1:543–545
53. Zabel P, Schönharting M, Wolter DT, Schade UF (1989) Oxypentifylline in endotoxemia. Lancet 2:1474–1477
54. Schiller JH, Storer BE, Witt PL, et al. (1991) Biological and clinical effects of intravenous tumor necrosis factor-α administered three times weekly. Cancer Res 51:1651–1658
55. Warren RS,Starnes HF Jr, Gabrilove JL, Oettgen HF, Brennan MF (1987) The acute metabolic effects of tumor necrosis factor administration in humans. Arch Surg 122:1396–1400
56. Michie HR, Spriggs DR, Manogue KR, et al. (1988) Tumor necrosis factor and endotoxin induce similar metabolic responses in human beings. Surgery 104:280–286
57. Tewari A, Buhles WC, Starnes HF (1990) Preliminary report: Effects of interleukin-1 on platelet counts. Lancet1:712–714
58. Fong Y, Albert JD, Tracey KJ, et al. (1991) The influence of substrate background on the acute metabolic response to epinephrine and cortisol. J Trauma 31:1467–1476
59. Aderka D, Engelmann H, Maor Y, Brakebusch C, Wallach D (1992) Stabilization of the bioactivity of tumor necrosis factor by its soluble receptors. J Exp Med 175:323–329
60. VanZee KJ, Kohno T, Fischer E, Rock CS, Moldawer LL, Lowry SF (1992) Tumor necrosis factor (TNF) soluble receptors circulate during experimental and clinical inflammation and can protect against excessive TNFα in vitro and in vivo. Proc Natl Acad Sci USA (in press)
61. Ohlsson K, Björk P, Bergenfeldt M, Hageman R, Thompson RC (1990) Interleukin-1 receptor antagonist reduces mortality from endotoxin shock. Nature 348:550–552
62. Wakabayashi G, Gelfand JA, Burke JF, Thompson RC, Dinarello CA (1991) A specific receptor antagonist for interleukin-1 prevents Escherichia coli-induced shock in rabbits. FASEB J 5:338–343
63. Cohen J (1991) Clinical role of tumor necrosis factor in septic shock. In: Vincent JL (ed) Update in Intensive Care and Emergency Medicine Vol 14, Springer-Verlag, New York, pp 262–268
64. Lowry SF (1990) The route of feeding influences injury responses. J Trauma 30:510–515
65. Luedke CE,Cerami A (1990) Interferon-gamma overcomes glucocorticoid suppression of cachectin/tumor necrosis factor biosynthesis by murine macrophages. J Clin Invest 86:1234–1240
66. Fong Y, Marano MA,Barber A, et al. (1989) Total parenteral nutrition and bowel rest modify the metabolic response to endotoxin in man. Ann Surg 210:449–457
67. Gisberg HS, Moldawer LL, Sehgal PB, et al. (1991) A mouse model for investigating the molecular pathogenesis of adenovirus pneumonia. Proc Natl Acad Sci USA 88:1651–1655
68. Ziegler EJ, Fisher CJ Jr, Sprung CL, et al. (1991) Treatment of gram-negative bacteremia and septic shock with HA-1A monoclonal antibody against endotoxin: A randomized, double-blind, placebo-controlled trial. N Engl J Med 324:429–436
69. Luger A, Graf H, Schwarz HP, Stummvoll HK, Luger TA (1986) Decreased serum interleukin-1 activity and monocyte interleukin-1 production in patients with fatal sepsis. Crit Care Med 14:458–461
70. Greenman RL, Schein RM, Martin MA, et al. (1991) A controlled clinical trial of E5 murine monoclonal IgM antibody to endotoxin in the treatment of gram-negative sepsis. JAMA 226:1097

Blocking Cytokines in Infectious Diseases

C. A. Dinarello

Introduction

Cytokines possessing biological properties primarily which are inflammatory in nature are important to the outcome of infectious diseases. To begin this overview, a distinction is to be made between the local effects of some cytokines and the consequences of high, systemic blood levels. The ultimate function of the host defense system is the elimination of the invading organism whether by phagocytosis and antibody formation as is the case in most bacterial infections, or the induction of cytotoxic T-cells for elimination of virus infected cells. Inflammation is the price the host pays for an efficient and effective defense system. In the extreme, death is the price paid. Some degree of this inflammation is, in part, due to the biological effects and balance of cytokines, notably IL-1, TNF, INFγ, TNFβ, FGF, IL-6 and the family of neutrophil and monocyte chemotactic cytokines. Some of these cytokines, for example the chemotactic and neutrophil activating cytokines, have particular importance for the local events in the lungs. Cytokines, particularly interferons and TNF, are important in the pathogenesis and defense against viral infections. Whether local or systemic, infections induce the liver to synthesize a variety of proteins collectively called acute phase proteins. The importance of IL-6 and the interactions of this cytokine with IL-1, TNF and TGFβ in the acute phase response of the liver are of fundamental importance because the acute phase proteins are likely down-regulating the inflammation of cytokines. However, the role of IL-1 and TNF in systemic and life-threatening bacterial infections is the focus of this chapter.

The local effects of some cytokines involve the recruitment of phagocytic cells essential for the elimination of the microorganisms. Twenty years ago, it was clearly shown that despite high titers of specific antibodies and bactericidal blood levels of antibiotics, neutropenic humans with bacterial infection could not clear the organism unless an infusion of these cells was administered. However, phagocytosis of microorganisms results in the release of a variety of substances which are themselves detrimental to the host.

These phagocytic cells are also activated by the same cytokines which are responsible for inducing their emigration from the blood into the infected tissue. For example, GM-CSF acts to recruit cells from the bone marrow and also primes neutrophils for subsequent enzyme release. There is ample evidence that products of this activation cause host damage. Another example is the family of neutrophil chemotactic peptides of which IL-8 is most cited. The effect of IL-8 on neutrophils is to induce degranulation and the release of enzymes such as elastase which cause tissue destruction. Superoxide radicals produced by activated neutrophils cause significant damage. Local infection and local inflammation are well tolerated but when the organism is particularly virulent, no local measures can contain the infection and systemic infection (sepsis) becomes a life-threatening event. In some cases, death is the consequence of an efficient host response to massive sepsis. How do we know this?

For many years, the general assumption was that microorganisms produced lethal toxins which, upon entrance into the circulation, caused hypotension, decreased perfusion of vital organs, acidosis and death. It made no difference whether these were endotoxins from gram-negative bacteria or enterotoxins from gram-positive *Staphylococci.* The breakthrough came when antibodies to TNF blocked death in mice to a lethal endotoxin challenge. This experiment clearly established that blocking TNF would prevent a host-medicated self-destructive process. The conclusion made from this experiment is that the infectious organism (or its toxins) induces the host to made a lethal amount of TNF. Blocking TNF with monoclonal antibodies has reduced deaths in baboons and humans.

The other cytokine which is important to the systemic response to sepsis is IL-1. Blocking IL-1 using the IL-1 receptor antagonist (IL-1ra) prevents letal shock in mice, rabbits and humans. Both anti-TNF and IL-1ra have been effective in reducing deaths in humans with sepsis in Phase II trials, and these "cytokine antagonists" are presently in separate Phase III trials for sepsis. Therefore, the role of these two cytokines in the consequences of infection is hardly a matter of speculation.

IL-1 and TNF

IL-1 and TNF affect nearly every tissue and organ system. Most studies on the biology of IL-1 and TNF have been carried out by injecting either cytokine into animals, but in the last 5 years, human subjects have also been injected with recombinant IL-1 or TNF. The results of those studies confirm that either cytokine can mimic a disease state, particularly acute infection or inflammation. However, in either situation, the biological responses of humans or animals to infection can also result in the synthesis of counter regulatory cytokines, which could modulate the host response. A good example of this is the cytokines TGFβ which reduces gene expression and synthesis of IL-1 and TNF induced by LPS. Another cytokine is IL-4 which also reduces IL-1 and TNF production following LPS.

How much of the response to infection or injury is, in fact, due to either IL-1 or TNF? The recent cloning of a naturally occurring IL-1 receptor antagonist (IL-1ra) and the isolation from the urine of the two soluble receptors (extracellular domains) for TNF have allowed one to examine how much of the biological responses to disease are due to IL-1 or TNF by specific blockade of either cytokine. The ability of the IL-1ra to block IL-1 receptors in animals or humans without agonist activities has reduced the severity of infectious diseases, such as *E. coli* shock, lethal bacterial sepsis, endotoxemia and *staphylococcal* sepsis. Similarly, blocking TNF with anti-TNF antibodies or soluble TNF receptors have reduced lethality to *E. coli* infection or LPS in mice and baboons. These results demonstrate that both IL-1 and TNF play essential roles in mediating the responses to infection and inflammation.

In healthy subjects, northern hybridization, *in situ* hybridization or polymerase chain reaction in peripheral blood mononuclear cells (PBMC) do not show evidence of TNF and IL-1 mRNA. However, adherence of PBMC to glass or polystyrene triggers TNFα and IL-1β gene expression, but, in the strict absence of LPS, gene expression for either cytokine occurs without translation into their respective proteins [1]. Circulating human blood in plastic tubing at 200 ml/min for 4 h at 37° C under strict LPS-free conditions does not trigger the transcription of these cytokines [2]. In the presence of complement activation however, only transcription but not translation of IL-1 and TNF takes place [2,3]. Thus, these cytokines are under both transcriptional as well as translational control. However, as few as 5 LPS molecules per human monocyte is sufficient to trigger the synthesis of IL-1 and TNF for several hours. Numerous reports of "spontaneous" IL-1 production in various disease states such as AIDS, or in the laboratory by infection of mononuclear cells with the HIV, can be artifactual because of the LPS contamination of culture media [4-6].

Recombinant human TNFα has been injected into human subjects and many of its systemic effects, such as fever, leukopenia, and hypotension, which were studied in animals, have been observed in humans [7]. When humans are injected intravenously with LPS, the leukopenia which develops rapidly correlates directly with the circulating level of TNF [8]. When TNF (1 μg/kg) is injected as a bolus intravenously into healthy human subjects, there is an immediate fall in circulating neutrophils followed by a leukocytosis. Lymphopenia remains for a more prolonged time [9]. The levels of lactoferrin were elevated in the circulation during the time of neutropenia suggesting neutrophil activation [9]. There was also a 40-fold increase in circulating IL-6 levels. Of course, fever and headache accompanied the response. Of note, at this dose of TNF, there was no significant fall in systemic blood pressure [10]. There is also evidence that following TNF, there is activation of several clotting parameters, including an increase in plasminogen activator inhibitor levels [10]. These are other aspects of the human response to TNF, similar to the changes observed in acute infection and inflammation.

Since TNF induces the synthesis and release of IL-1, IL-8 and IL-6 from monocytes, fibroblasts, and endothelial cells, it is possible that these cytokines augment the action of TNF. Nearly every biological property of IL-1 has also been observed with TNF. These include fever [11], the induction of PGE_2 and collagenase synthesis in a variety of tissues [12], bone and cartilage resorption, inhibition of lipoprotein lipase [13], increases in hepatic acute-phase proteins and complement components, and a decrease in albumin synthesis [14]. Slow-wave sleep and appetite suppression are also observed following the injection of TNF [15]. Both molecules induce fibroblast proliferation and collagen synthesis. IL-1 can function as a cofactor for stem cell activation (hemopoietin-1 activity) [16], whereas TNF suppresses bone marrow colony formation [17]. Both IL-1 and TNF induce the synthesis of colony-stimulating factors [18,19].

In experimental animals, TNF produces hypotension, leukopenia, and local tissue necrosis. On a weight basis in rabbits, TNF is more potent than IL-1 in producing a shock [20]. However, in humans, IL-1β or IL-1α, when given intravenously [21], appears to be more potent in producing hypotension than TNF [10]. Administration of anti-TNF antibodies to baboons [22] or rabbits prevents the shock induced by endotoxin [23]. The shock-like responses to TNF likely reflect the effects on the vascular endothelium. TNF stimulates PGI_2, PGE_2, and PAF production by cultured endothelium. In addition, like IL-1, TNF stimulates procoagulant activity, leukocyte adherence, and plasminogen activator inhibitor on these cells. TNF also induces a capillary-leak syndrome.

Despite the similarities, receptors for TNF and IL-1 are distinct and specific, and receptor binding to the respective ligand is only displaced by the specific cytokine. Furthermore, IL-1 down regulates the receptor for TNF [24].

IL-1α and IL-1β have been administered to humans in Phase I trials. Systemic administration of intravenous IL-1 from 10-100 ng/kg has produced fever, sleepiness, anorexia, generalized myalgias, arthralgias, headache, some gastrointestinal disturbances; at higher doses, hypotension has been observed [21,25]. The subcutaneous route is associated with less side effects. Laboratory data confirm the neutrophila-inducing property of IL-1 but increased circulating platelets have also been observed [25]. In general, the early experience in humans are consistent with previous observations in the rabbit and other animals.

Comparison of IL-1, TNF, and IL-6

The biological properties of TNF share remarkable similarities to those of IL-1 (Table 1). When the two cytokines are used together in experimental studies, the net effect often exceeds the additive effect of each cytokine. Potentiation or frank synergism between these two molecules has been demonstrated in studies on fibroblast production of PGE_2, the cytotoxic effect on certain tumor cells, and when administered to tumor-bearing mice. IL-1 acts synergistically with TNF to protect rats exposed to lethal hyperoxia or radiation. IL-1 cytotoxic effects on the insulin-producing beta cells of the islets of Langerhans is dramatically augmented by TNF. Rats receiving intravenous infusions of IL-1 or TNF manifest metabolic changes reflected in plas-

Table 1. Comparison of IL-1, TNF, and IL-6

Biological property	IL-1	TNF	IL-6
Endogenous pyrogen fever	+	+	+
Slow wave sleep	+	+	-
Hepatic acute-phase proteins	+	+	+
T cell activation	+	+	+
B cell activation	+	+	+
B cell Ig synthesis	-	-	+
Fibroblast proliferation	+	+	-
Stem cell activation (hemopoietin-1)	+	-	+
Nonspecific resistance to infection	+	+	+
Radioprotection	+	+	-
Cyclooxygenase, PLA_2 gene expression	+	+	-
Synovial cell activation	+	+	-
Endothelial cell activation	+	+	-
Shock syndrome	+	+	-
Induction of IL-1, TNF, and IL-8	+	+	-
Induction of IL-6	+	+	-

ma amino-acid levels, but, when given together, negative nitrogen balance and muscle proteolysis can be demonstrated. Although high doses (10-20 μg/kg) of TNF produce a shock-like state with tissue damage, IL-1 and TNF act synergistically to produce hemodynamic shock and pulmonary hemorrhage at doses of only 1 μg/kg when given together [20]. The synergism between these two cytokines seems to be due to second message molecules rather than up regulation of cell receptors; in fact, IL-1 reduces TNF receptors [24,26].

In some models, the production of IL-6 appears to be under the control of IL-1; for example, mice subjected to an inflammatory event induced by intramuscular turpentine fail to produce IL-6 when pretreated with anti-IL-1 receptor antibodies [27]. In baboons injected with *E. coli*, anti-TNF antibodies prevent the appearance of IL-6 in the circulation [28]. Like IL-1 and TNF, IL-6 is an endogenous pyrogen and an inducer of acute-phase responses. Since IL-1 and TNF induce IL-6 levels, IL-6 often correlate with the amount of fever and disease in patients. Many studies demonstrate that IL-6 levels are elevated in patients with a variety of infectious diseases. In fact, the best correlations of the severity of an infectious disease with any cytokine is clearly with the levels of IL-6, not IL-1 or TNF. However, it is important to note that unlike IL-1 and TNF, there is no evidence except for one study [29], that IL-6 is a lethal cytokine. In that study, antibodies to IL-6 reduced mortality of mice to LPS. However, IL-6 does not cause shock in mice or primates regardless of the amount given either alone or withTNF.

IL-6 does not induce endothelial cell adhesion molecules and does not stimulate the genes for cyclooxygenase [30], phospholipase A_2, nor nitric oxide synthase. Finally, unlike soluble receptors for TNF and IL-1 which bind and

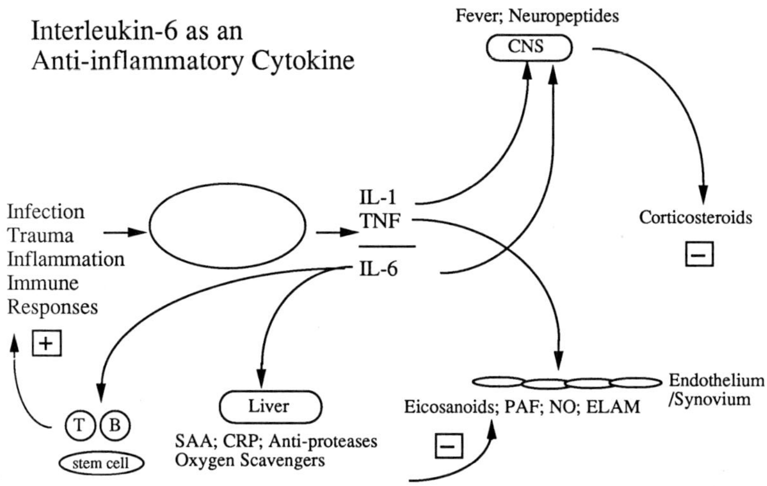

Fig. 1. IL-6 as an anti-inflammatory cytokine. Infection, trauma, inflammation and immune responses stimulate a variety of cells to produce IL-6. IL-6, like IL-1 and TNF, triggers the CNS to increase the hypothalamic set-point which results in fever. IL-6, similar to IL-1 and TNF, also stimulates neuropeptide release. The effect of ACTH is to stimulate corticosteroids which can have an endogenous anti-inflammatory effect (negative sign in box). IL-6, unlike IL-1 and TNF, does not stimulate endothelial or synovial lining cells. IL-6 is a potent inducer of several hepatic acute phase proteins which function as oxygen scavengers and anti-proteases. These acute phase proteins exert a negative influence on inflammatory processes. IL-6 has positive effect (as noted by the positive sign in the box) on resolution of infection by stimulating bone marrow stem cells and T and B lymphocytes which help remove the invading organism

reduce their respective biological activities, soluble p80 receptors for IL-6 *enhance* the activity of this cytokine [31,32]. IL-6 suppresses LPS- and TNF-induced IL-1 production [33]. In general, IL-6 appears to be an anti-inflammatory peptide. Of considerable importance is the observation that IL-6 acts as hemopoietin-1 on bone marrow cultures [16]. The spectrum of acute phase proteins induced by IL-6 includes many anti-proteases and one interpretation of the biological significance of IL-6 is the anti-inflammatory property of these anti-proteases. Figure 1 illustrates the proposed anti-inflammatory effects of IL-6.

IL-1 Antagonism

It appears that nature developed several mechanisms for blocking the activity of IL-1. Naturally occurring substances which specifically inhibit IL-1 have been detected in the serum of human volunteers injected with bacterial LPS [34], urine of febrile patients [35], plasma following hemodialysis [36], supernatants of human monocytes adhering to IgG coated surfaces [37], and urine of patients with monocytic leukemia [38]. An IL-1 specific inhibitory molecule of 52-66 kDa secreted from a human myelomonocytic cell line [39], and the mouse macrophage cell line P388D [40] have also been reported. Another inhibitory material isolated from the urine of pregnant women had been identified as uromodulin, which is a glycosylated form of the Tamm-Horsfall protein.The carbohydrate portion of uromodulin binds IL-1 as well as TNF and other cytokines, and this IL-1 inhibitor is non-specific. IL-1 inhibitory activities have also been reported from virus infected monocytes, blood neutrophils, UV-exposed keratinocytes, Epstein-Barr infected B-cell lines, and from normal submandibular glands.

The IL-1 receptor antagonist (IL-1ra) was originally called the "IL-1 inhibitor" [37,38,41,42]; it was a 23-25 kDa protein purified from the urine of patients with monocytic leukemia [38,42,43]. Natural IL-1 inhibitor blocked the ability of IL-1 to stimulate synovial cell PGE_2 production, thymocyte proliferation, and decreased insulin release from isolated pancreatic islets [38,42,44,45]. It appears that the IL-1-specific inhibitory activities found in the serum during endotoxemia [34] is likely the IL-1ra [46], but the IL-1 specific inhibitor for the M20 myelomonocytic cell line [39] does not share identity with the IL-1ra [47]. In each case, the IL-1 inhibitory activity was shown to prevent IL-1 but not IL-2 or mitogen-induced T-cell proliferation. The "IL-1 inhibitor" blocked the binding of IL-1 to receptors on T-cells and fibroblasts but did not affect the binding of TNF or IL-2 to their receptors [42,45]. The IL-1 inhibitor also did not bind to IL-1 itself.

Using the IL-1 inhibitor purified from adherent monocytes [37,48], N-terminal sequence was obtained and the molecule was cloned [49]. The cDNA sequence codes for a polypeptide of approximately 17 kDa, whereas the 25 kDa molecular weight is due to glycosylation. The amino-acid sequence deduced from the cDNA revealed a 26% amino-acid homology to IL-1β, and a 19% homology to IL-1α. Conserved amino-acids as defined by Dayoff [50] revealed a 41% homology of the IL-1ra to IL-1β, and 30% to IL-1α. The IL-1ra was also cloned from U937 cells and reported as the IL-1 receptor antagonist protein (IRAP) [51].

Similar to the purified naturally occurring IL-1 urinary inhibitor [42], the recombinant IL-1 inhibitor competes with the binding of IL-1 to its cell surface receptors. Because of its sequence homology and mode of activity, the IL-1 inhibitor was re-named as IL-1 receptor antagonist. Recombinant human IL-1ra expressed by *E. coli* is not glycosylated but blocks binding of IL-1 equally as well as the glycosylated natural form. Antibodies produced to the recombinant human IL-1ra recognize the purified urinary IL-1 inhibitor of Seckinger and Dayer establishing that the IL-1 inhibitor and IL-1ra are the same molecule [52].

The IL-1ra blocks IL-1 activity *in vitro* and *in vivo. In vivo,* the IL-1ra competes with IL-1 for occupancy of the IL-1 receptor type I (IL-1RtI) on T-cells and fibroblasts with nearly the same affinity as that for *bone fide* IL-1, but without demonstrable agonist activity [48]. To date, attempts to show agonist activity of IL-1ra on a variety of cells *in vitro* have failed. Humans have been injected with large amounts of IL-1ra, and symptoms or signs of agonist properties have not been observed. In a Phase I trial of the IL-1ra, blood levels were in excess of 20 μg/ml and there were no indications of altered homeostatic parameters [53].

When IL-1ra occupies the type I receptor, there is no evidence of internalization nor of protein kinase activity [54]. Early reports showed that in murine pre-B-cell lines which expresses only the p68 IL-1R (IL-1RtII), there was no blockade of IL-1 binding by the IL-1ra [48,51,55]. However, the human IL-1ra blocks the binding of IL-1 to human cells bearing the IL-1RtII such as neutrophils and B-cells [56], as well as human peripheral myelomonocytic leukemia cells [57]. In addition, IL-1ra blocks the binding of IL-1β to human blood monocytes, a type II receptor bearing cell [58]. Using murine T-cells (IL-1RtI), the human IL-1ra blocks the binding of IL-1 at nearly equimolar concentrations; however, a 10-50-fold molar excess of the IL-1ra is required to block the binding of human IL-1 to human type II receptor bearing cells [56].

It is not surprizing that recombinant IL-1ra will block the activity of IL-1 in various animal models of disease. Rabbits [59] or baboons [60] injected with IL-1 develop hypotension which is reversed by prior administration of the IL-1ra. However, a larger question remains: during acute or chronic disease, several cytokines are produced but what is the effect of specific blockade of IL-1? The results of several studies have now been published and demonstrate that IL-1 receptor blockade significantly reduces the severi-

Table 2 . Reduction in severity by human IL-1ra in animal models of various diseases

Death in rabbits from endotoxin (LPS)	[59,80]
Death in mice from endotoxin (LPS)	[81]
Death in newborn rats from *Klebsiella pneumoniae*	[82]
Hemodynamic shock and tissue damage in rabbits from *E. coli*	[80]
Hemodynamic shock in rabbits fram *Staphylococcus epidermidis*	[83]
Hemodynamic shock and death in baboons from *E. coli*	[60]
Cerebral malaria in mice	[84]
Streptococcal wall-induced arthritis in rats	[85]
Collagen-induced arthritis in mice	[86]
Inflammatory bowel disease in rabbits	[87]
Onset of spontaneous diabetes in BB rats	[88]
Hypoglycemia and CSF production in mice following endotoxin	[89]
Proliferation and CSF production of acute myeloblastic leukemia cells	[57]
Proliferation of chronic myelogenous leukemia cells	[90]
Neutrophil accumulation in inflammatory peritonitis	[91]
Sciatic nerve regeneration in mice	[92]
Graft *versus* host disease in mice	[93]
Experimental enterocolitis in rats	[94]
Indomethacin-induced intestinal ulceration in rats	[94]
LPS-induced pulmonary inflammation in rats	[95]

ty of several inflammatory disease (reviewed in [61]). Table 2 lists these data.

The balance of IL-1 and IL-1ra production may be critical to the outcome of disease. IL-1ra is synthesized in septic animals and humans with a variety of infectious or inflammatory diseases. The balance between the amount and secretion of IL-1 and its receptor antagonist may be critical in some diseases. IL-1 and IL-1ra gene expression and protein synthesis are differently regulated [37,62,63]. For example, IL-1β is transcribed and synthesized in cells before IL-1ra. The dysregulation in production of the agonist and antagonist in human disease has recently been studied by Rambaldi et al. [57] who examined spontaneous gene expression for IL-1β and IL-1ra in fresh cells from patients with acute myelogenous leukemia. Cells from each of 11 patients studied spontaneously expressed the gene for IL-1β whereas the leukemic cells from only 1 of 11 patients expressed IL-1ra following stimulation.

During experimental endotoxemia in humans [46], in sepsis [64], or in systemic juvenile rheumatoid arthritis [65], large amounts of circulating IL-1ra has been found. In several studies on circulating IL-1β during infection in humans, levels rarely exceed 500 pg/ml [66,67]. During experimental endotoxemia in humans, levels of IL-1β reach a maximal concentration of 150-200 pg/ml after 3-4 h, and then fall rapidly; in these same individuals, the peak levels of IL-1ra occur after 4 h, exceed the molar concentration of IL-1β by 100-fold and are sustained for 12 h [46]. During *E. coli* sepsis in baboons, peak IL-1ra levels occur 8-10 h later [64]. Thus, production of a small amount of IL-1, but a large amount of the IL-1ra, appears to be a natural response in some clinical situations. Endogenously produced IL-1ra probably contributes to limiting the severity of disease, but may be inadequate in overwhelming infection or acute inflammation. Providing exogenous IL-1ra in some of these latter situations may have beneficial effects as observed in animal models. In humans with various forms of sepsis (either gram-negative, gram-positive or fungal), significantly reduced mortality from 45% to 16% ($p<0.015$) was observed using 133 mg/h constant infusion of IL-1ra for 72 h (Charles Fisher Jr. et al, presented at Society of American Thoracic Surgeons, San Francisco, November, 1991).

Unlike IL-1, IL-1ra with a classical signal peptide is readily secreted into the extracellular compartment whereas in the same cell culture, only 50% of the IL-1β and less than 10% of IL-1α is secreted. An intracellular form of IL-1ra without a signal peptide has been described in keratinocytes [68], and it is speculated that intracellular IL-1ra in these cells acts to counter the biological activity of IL-1α which remains in the cytosolic compartment of keratinocytes. However, this is not the case in human monocytes stimulated with endotoxin where nearly all of the IL-1α is intracellular, but less than 10% of IL-1ra remains in these cells. Nevertheless, the concept that intracellular IL-1α is biologically active has received recent experimental support [69], and the balance of IL-1 to IL-1ra should be considered for both intra-cellular and extracellular compartments.

The extracellular domain of the IL-1RtI has been expressed and shown to bind both forms of IL-1. Unlike soluble TNF, IL-6 and INFγ receptors which occur naturally in the urine [32,70], soluble IL-1R have yet to be found naturally. When the recombinant soluble IL-1RtI was given to mice undergoing heart transplantation, survival of the heterotopic allografts was increased. Lymph nodes directly injected with allogeneic cells have reduced hyperplasia with the use of the soluble IL-1RtI [71]. However, it is unclear from these experiments how much of the effects of the soluble type I receptor is due to decreased inflammation rather than to decreased immuno-res-ponsiveness. There are no data suggesting that the type I IL-1R is naturally shed; however, conditioned media from the IL-1RtII-bearing Raji cells contain the soluble form (35-45 kDa) of the IL-1RtII [72]. Recently, an IL-1 binding protein (soluble form of an IL-1R) was found circulating in humans with inflammatory disease and appears to be related to the type II receptor [73].

TNF Antagonism

The effects of monoclonal antibodies to TNF have been discussed above. However, antibody therapies in humans have their limitations and hence attention has been focused on the use of soluble receptors for TNF which act as antibodies but have the distinct advantage of being natural products and unlikely to induce an antibody response to a foreign protein. Soluble TNFRs which represent the extracellular domains of the two TNFR (TNFRtI and TNFRtII) were initially discovered in the urine of healthy humans [70,74,75], and hence the presence of these molecules in a normal body fluid suggests that they are constantly being produced.The soluble TNFRs are proteolytic cleavage products, not separate products of alternate mRNA splicing as is the case with other receptors such as IL-4. Circulating levels of soluble TNFRtI and TNFRtII in the serum or plasma of healthy humans are in the 1-2 ng/ml range [76], and are elevated in patients during infection and with metastatic disease [77]. Like IL-1ra, the host response to infection includes a brisk production of TNF antagonistic molecules.

The effects of blocking TNF using the soluble forms of the TNFRtI have yielded the same data as that of the antibodies. *E. coli* induced shock in baboons [78], and death in mice from LPS [79] have been observed when animals are treated with soluble TNFR. Clinically, the amounts of soluble TNFR required to block these events are high, but the use of chimeric molecules, in which the soluble TNFR is linked covalently to the Fc portion of Ig, results in a prolonged circulating half-life and greater effectiveness that the native form.

Contrary to antibodies to the IL-1RtI which block IL-1 responses, antibodies to the TNF are not blocking but rather induce a TNF response [74]. The mechanism of action of TNF appears to be cross-linking of two receptors, and the cross-linked receptors are responsible for triggering signal transduction. Thus, it appears that antagonism to IL-1 has 4 possibilities (IL-1ra, anti-IL-1, anti-IL-1R and soluble IL-1R) whereas for TNF antagonism, there are at present, anti-TNF and soluble TNFR. Regardless of the approach taken,the data consistently show that blocking either IL-1 or TNF (using any of the available antagonistic molecules) reduces the severity, sometimes completely, of the consequences to infectious and inflammatory disease processes. What does this mean in terms of the role of either IL-1 or TNF alone? The current interpretations that *both* IL-1 and TNF orchestrate the deleterious effects of infection and injury, and that blocking the activity of either one of these cytokines prevents the full consequences of the disease. This interpretation is consistent with the known synergistic effects of IL-1 and TNF in that blocking one cytokine prevents the synergism.

Conclusion

Although antibiotics and support systems have reduced the mortality due to bacterial infections, 40-50% mortality is still an unacceptable statistic. Anti-LPS (anti-lipid A) passive immunotherapy has reduced this mortality but only in patients with documented gram-negative bacteremia. However, anti-cytokine therapy such as monoclonal antibodies to TNF and the IL-1ra have reduced mortality to all infectious causes. IL-1ra is presently in Phase III trials as is monoclonal anti-TNF. Two other strategies are soluble (extracellular domains) receptors to TNF and IL-1. These are now entering Phase I trials but animal data strongly support that similar to antibodies to TNF and IL-1ra, these anti-cytokine therapies will also be effective.

Acknowlegements. These studies are supported by NIH Grant AI 15614.

References

1. Schindler R, Clark BD, Dinarello CA (1990) Dissociation between interleukin-1β mRNA and protein synthesis in human peripheral blood mononuclear cells. J Biol Chem 265:10232–10237
2. Schindler R, Lonnemann G, Shaldon S, Koch KM, Dinarello CA (1990) Transcription, not synthesis, of interleukin-1 and tumor necrosis factor by complement. Kidney Int 37:85–93
3. Schindler R, Gelfand JA, Dinarello CA (1990) Recombinant C5a stimulates transcription rather than translation of IL-1 and TNF; cytokine synthesis induced by LPS, IL-1 or PMA. Blood 76:1631–1638
4. Molina JM, Scadden DT, Amirault C, et al. (1990) Human immunodeficiency virus does not induce interleukin-1, interleukin-6, or tumor necrosis factor in mononuclear cells. J Virology 64:2901–2906
5. Molina JM, Scadden DT, Byrn R, Dinarello CA, Groopman JE (1989) Production of tumor necrosis factor alpha and interleukin-1 beta by monocytic cells infected with human immunodeficiency virus. J Clin Invest 84:733–737
6. Molina JM, Schindler R, Ferriani R, et al. (1990) Production of cytokines by peripheral blood monocytes/macrophages infected with human immunodeficiency virus type 1 (HIV-1). J Inf Dis 161:888–893

7. Chapman PB, Lester TJ, Casper ES, et al. (1987) Clinical pharmacology of recombinant human tumor necrosis factor in patients with advanced cancer. J Clin Oncol 6:1942–1951
8. Michie HR, Manogue KR, Spriggs DR, et al. (1988) Detection of circulating tumor necrosis factor after endotoxin administration. N Engl J Med 318:1481–1486
9. van der Poll T, van Deventer SJH, Hack CE, et al. (1992) Effects of leukocytes following injection of tumor necrosis factor into healthy humans. Blood (in press)
10. van der Poll T, Bueller HR, ten Cate H, et al. (1990) Activation of coagulation after administration of tumor necrosis factor to normal subjects. N Engl J Med 322:1622–1627
11. Dinarello CA, Cannon JG, Wolff SM, et al. (1986) Tumor necrosis factor (cachectin) is an endogenous pyrogen and induces production of interleukin-1. J Exp Med 163:1433–1450
12. Dayer JM, Beutler B, Cerami A (1985) Cachectin/tumor necrosis factor stimulates collagenase and prostaglandin E2 production by human synovial cells and dermal fibroblasts. J Exp Med 162:2163–2168
13. Beutler B, Cerami A (1987) Cachectin: More than a tumor necrosis factor. N Engl J Med 316:379–385
14. Perlmutter DH, Dinarello CA, Punsal PI, Colten HR (1986) Cachectin/tumor necrosis factor regulates hepatic acute-phase gene expression. J Clin Invest 78:1349–1354
15. Shoham S, Davenne D, Cady AB,Dinarello CA, Krueger JM (1987) Recombinant tumor necrosis factor and interleukin-1 enhance slow-wave sleep.Am J Physiol 253:142–149
16. Moore MA, Warren DJ (1987) Synergy of interleukin-1 and granulocyte colony-stimulating factor: In vivo stimulation of stem-cell recovery and hematopoietic regeneration following 5-fluorouracil treatment of mice. Proc Natl Acad Sci USA 84:7134–7138
17. Zucali JR, Broxmeyer HE, Gross MA, Dinarello CA (1988) Recombinant human tumor necrosis factors alpha and beta stimulate fibroblasts to produce hemopoietic growth factors in vitro. J Immunol 140:840–844
18. Zucali JR, Dinarello CA, Oblon DJ, Gross MA, Anderson L, Weiner RS (1986) Interleukin-1 stimulates fibroblasts to produce granulocyte-macrophage colony-stimulating activity and prostaglandin E2. J Clin Invest 77:1857–1863
19. Bagby GCJ, Dinarello CA, Wallace P, Wagner C, Hefeneider S, McCall E (1986) Interleukin-1 stimulates granulocyte macrophage colony-stimulating activity release by vascular endothelial cells. J Clin Invest 78:1316–1323
20. Okusawa S, Gelfand JA, Ikejima T, Connolly RJ, Dinarello CA (1988) Interleukin-1 induces a shock-like state in rabbits. Synergism with tumor necrosis factor and the effect of cyclooxygenase inhibition. J Clin Invest 81:1162–1172
21. Smith J, Urba W, Steis R, et al. (1990) Interleukin-1 alpha: Results of a phase I toxicity and immunomodulatory trial. Am Soc Clin Oncol 9:717
22. Tracey K, Fong Y, Hesse DG, et al. (1987) Anti-cachectin/TNF monoclonal antibodies prevent septic shock during lethal bacteremia. Nature 330:662–664
23. Mathison JC, Wolfson E, Ulevitch RJ (1988) Participation of tumor necrosis factor in the mediation of gram-negative bacterial lipopolysaccharide-induced injury in rabbits. J Clin Invest 81:1925–1937
24. Holtmann H, Wallach D (1987) Down regulation of the receptors for tumor necrosis factor by interleukin-1 and 4-beta-phorbol-12-myristate-13-acetate. J Immunol 139:1161–1167
25. Tewari A, Buhles WC Jr, Starnes HF Jr (1990) Preliminary report: Effects of interleukin-1 on platelet counts. Lancet 336:712–714
26. Wallach D, Holtmann H, Aderka D, et al. (1989) Mechanisms which take part in regulation of the response to tumor necrosis factor. Lymphokine Res 8:359–363
27. Gershenwald JE, Fong YM, Fahey TJ, et al. (1990) Interleukin-1 receptor blockade attenuates the host inflammatory response. Proc Natl Acad Sci USA 87:4966–4970
28. Fong Y, Tracey KJ, Moldawer LL, et al. (1989) Antibodies to cachectin/tumor necrosis factor reduce interleukin-1b and interleukin-6 appearance during lethal bacteremia. J Exp Med 170:1627–1633
29. Starnes HF, Pearce MK, Twari A, Yim JM, Zou JC,Abrams JS (1990) Anti-monoclonal antibodies protect against lethal Escherichia coli infection and lethal tumor necrosis factor-α challenge in mice. J Immunol 145:4185–4191

30. Dinarello CA, Cannon JG, Mancilla J, Bishai I, Lees J, Coceani F (1991) Interleukin-6 as an endogenous pyrogen: Induction of prostaglandin E2 in brain but not in peripheal blood mononuclear cells. Brain Res 562:199–206
31. Novick D, Engelmann H, Wallach D, Leitner O, Revel M, Rubinstein M (1990) Purification of soluble cytokine receptors from normal human urine by ligand-affinity and immunoaffinity chromatography. J Chromat 510:331–337
32. Novick D, Engelmann H, Wallach D, Rubinstein M (1989) Soluble cytokine receptors are present in normal human urine. J Exp Med 170:1409–1414
33. Schindler R, Mancilla J, Endres S, Ghorbani R, Clark SC, Dinarello CA (1990) Correlations and interactions in the production of interleukin-6 (IL-6), IL-1, and tumor necrosis factor (TNF) in human blood mononuclear cells: IL-6 suppresses IL-1 and TNF. Blood 75:40–47
34. Dinarello CA, Rosenwasser LJ, Wolff SM (1981) Demonstration of a circulating suppressor factor of thymocyte proliferation during endotoxin fever in humans. J Immunol 127:2517–2519
35. Liao Z, Grimshaw RS, Rosenstreich DL (1984) Identification of a specific interleukin-1 inhibitor in the urine of febrile patients. J Exp Med 159:125–136
36. Shaldon S, Koch KM, Bingel M, Granolleras C, Deschodt G, Dinarello CA (1987) Modulation of plasma interleukin-1 and its circulating protein inhibitor (CPI) by hemodialysis and hemofiltration. Kidney Int (Abs) 31:245
37. Arend WP, Joslin FG, Thompson RC, Hannum CH (1989) An IL-1 inhibitor from human monocytes: Production and characterization of biologic properties. J Immunol 143:1851–1858
38. Seckinger P, Dayer JM (1987) Interleukin-1 inhibitors. Ann Inst Pasteur/Immunol 138:461–516
39. Barak V, Treves AJ, Yanai P, et al. (1986) Interleukin-1 inhibitory activity secreted by a human myelomonocytic cell line (M20). Eur J Immunol 16:1449–1452
40. Isono N, Kumagai K (1989) Production of interleukin-1 inhibitors by the murine macrophage cell line P388D which produces interleukin-1. Microbiol Immunol 33:43–57
41. Arend WP, Joslin FG, Massoni RJ (1985) Effects of immune complexes on production by human monocytes of interleukin-1 or an interleukin-1 inhibitor. J Immunol 134:3868–3875
42. Seckinger P, Lowenthal JW, Williamson K, Dayer JM, MacDonald HR (1987) A urine inhibitor of interleukin-1 activity that blocks ligand binding. J Immunol 139:1546–1549
43. Mazzei GJ, Seckinger PL, Dayer JM, Shaw AR (1990) Purification and characterization of a 26-kDa competitive inhibitor of interleukin-1. Eur J Immunol 20:683–689
44. Dayer-Metroz MD, Wollheim CB, Seckinger P, Dayer JM (1989) A natural interleukin-1 (IL-1) inhibitor counteracts the inhibitory effect of IL-1 on insulin production in cultured rat pancreatic islets. J Autoimmun 2:163–171
45. Balavoine JF, de Rochemonteix B, Williamson K, Seckinger P, Cruchaud A, Dayer JM (1986) Prostaglandin E2 and collagenase production by fibroblasts and synovial cells is regulated by urine-derived human interleukin-1 and inhibitor(s). J Clin Invest 78:1120–1124
46. Granowitz EV, Santos A, Poutsiaka DD, et al. (1991) Circulating interleukin-1 receptor antagonist levels during experimental endotoxemia in humans. Lancet 1:1423–1424
47. Barak V, Peritt D, Flechner I, et al. (1991) The IL-1 specific inhibitor from the M20 cell line is distinct from the IL-1 receptor antagonist. Lymphokine Cytokine Res 10:437–442
48. Hannum CH, Wilcox CJ, Arend WP, et al. (1990) Interleukin-1 receptor antagonist activity of a human interleukin-1 inhibitor. Nature 343:336–340
49. Eisenberg SP, Evans RJ, Arend WP, et al. (1990) Primary structure and functional expression from complementary DNA of a human interleukin-1 receptor antagonist. Nature 343:341–346
50. Dayoff MO, Barker WC, Hunt LT (1983) Establishing homologies in protein sequences. Meth Enzymol 91:524–545
51. Carter DB, Deibel MRJ, Dunn CJ, et al. (1990) Purification, cloning, expression and biological characterization of an interleukin-1 receptor antagonist protein. Nature 344:633–638
52. Seckinger P, Klein-Nulend J, Alander C, Thompson RC, Dayer JM, Raisz LG (1990) Natural and recombinant human IL-1 receptor antagonists block the effects of IL-1 on bone resorp-

tion and prostaglandin production. J Immunol 145:4181–4184
53. Granowitz EV, Porat R, Gelfand JA, et al. (1991) Effects of intravenous interleukin-1 receptor antagonist in healthy humans subjects. Cytokine (Abs) 3:501
54. Dripps DJ, Brandhuber BJ, Thompson RC, Eisenberg SP (1991) Effect of IL-1ra on IL-1 signal transduction. J Biol Chem 266:10331–10336
55. Young P, Kumar V, Lillquist J, et al. (1990) A site-specific mutant of IL-1 beta with reduced activity but wild type binding. Lymphokine Res 9:599
56. Granowitz EV, Mancilla J, Clark BD, Dinarello CA (1991) The IL-1 receptor antagonist inhibits IL-1 binding to the type II IL-1 receptor. J Biol Chem 266:14147–14150
57. Rambaldi A, Torcia M, Bettoni S, et al. (1991) Modulation of cell proliferation and cytokine production in acute myeloblastic leukemia by interleukin-1 receptor antagonist and lack of its expression by leukemic cells. Blood 78:3248–3253
58. Granowitz EV, Clark BD, Vannier E, Callahan MV, Dinarello CA (1992) Effect of IL-1 blockade on cytokine synthesis. I. IL-1 receptor antagonist inhibits IL-1-induced cytokine synthesis and blocks the binding of IL-1 and its type II receptor on human monocytes. Blood (in press)
59. Ohlsson K, Bjork P, Bergenfeldt M, Hageman R, Thompson RC (1990) Interleukin-1 receptor antagonist reduces mortality from endotoxin shock. Nature 348:550–552
60. Fischer E, Marano MA, VanZee KJ, et al. (1992) IL-1 receptor blockade attenuates the hemodynamic and metabolic consequences of lethal E. coli septic shock. J Clin Invest (in press)
61. Dinarello CA, Thompson RC (1991) Blocking IL-1: Effects of IL-1 receptor antagonist in vitro and in vivo. Immunol Today 12:404–410
62. Poutsiaka D, Clark BD, Vannier E, Dinarello CA (1991) Production of interleukin-1 receptor antagonist and interleukin-1β by peripheral blood mononuclear cells is differentially regulated. Blood 78:1275–1281
63. Arend WP, Smith MFJ, Janson RW, Joslin FG (1992) IL-1 receptor antagonist and IL-1b production in human monocytes are regulated differently. J Immunol (in press)
64. Fischer E, Poutsiaka DD, VanZee KJ, et al. (1992) Levels of interleukin-1 receptor antagonist circulates in experimental inflammation and in human disease. Blood (in press)
65. Prieur AM, Kaufmann MT, Girscelli C, Dayer JM (1987) Specific interleukin-1 inhibitor in serum and urine of children with systemic juvenile chronic arthritis. Lancet 2:1240–1242
66. Cannon JG, Gelfand JA, Tompkins RG, Hegarty MT, Burke JF, Dinarello CA (1992) Plasma IL-1β and TNFα levels in humans following cutaneous injury. Critcal Care Med (in press)
67. Cannon JG, Tompkins RG, Gelfand JA, et al. (1990) Circulating interleukin-1 and tumor necrosis factor in septic shock and experimental endotoxin fever. J Inf Dis 161:79–84
68. Haskill S, Martin M, VanLe L, et al. (1991) cDNA cloning of a novel form of the interleukin-1 receptor antagonist associated with epithelium. Proc Natl Acad Sci USA 88:3681-3685
69. Maier JAM, Voulalas P, Roeder D, Masiag T (1990) Extension of the life span of human endothelial cells by an interleukin-1α antisense oligomer. Science 249:1570-1574
70. Engelmann H, Aderka D, Rubinstein M, Rotman D, Wallach D (1989) A tumor necrosis factor-binding protein purified to homogeneity from human urine protects cells from tumor necrosis factor toxicity. J Biol Chem 264:11974-11980
71. Fanslow WC, Sims JE, Sassenfeld H, et al. (1990) Regulation of alloreactivity in vivo by a soluble form of the interleukin-1 receptor. Science 248:739-742
72. Giri J, Newton RC, Horuk R (1990) Identification of soluble interleukin-1 binding protein in cell-free supernatants. J Biol Chem 265:17416-17419
73. Symons JA, Eastgate JA, Duff GW (1991) Purification and characterization of a novel soluble receptor for interleukin-1. J Exp Med 174:1251-1254
74. Engelmann H, Holtmann, H, Brakebusch C, et al. (1990) Antibodies to a soluble form of a tumor necrosis factor (TNF) receptor have TNF-like activity. J Biol Chem 265:14497-14504
75. Engelmann H, Novick D, Wallach D (1990) Two tumor necrosis factor-binding proteins purified from human urine. Evidence for immunological cross-reactivity with cell surface tumor necrosis factor receptors. J Biol Chem 265:1531-1536
76. Liabakk NB, Sundan A,Waage A, et al. (1991) Development of immunoassays for the detection of soluble tumor necrosis factor receptors. J Immunol Methods 141:237-243

77. Aederka D, Engelmann H, Wallach D (1991) Serum levels of TNF receptors in patients with metastatic disease. J Cancer Res 51:5602-5607
78. Fischer E, Marano MA, VanZee KJ, et al. (1992) Soluble TNF receptors blocks E. coli shock in baboons. Proc Natl Acid Sci USA (in press)
79. Lesslauer W, Tabuchi H, Gentz M, et al. (1991) Recombinant soluble TNF receptor proteins inhibit LPS-induced lethality in mice. Cytokine (Abs) 3:497
80. Wakabayashi G, Gelfand JA, Burke JF, Thompson RC, Dinarello CA (1991) A specific receptor antagonist for interleukin-1 prevents Escherichia coli-induced shock. FASEB J 5:338-343
81. Alexander HR, Doherty GM, Buresh CM, Venzon DJ, Norton JA (1991) A recombinant human receptor antagonist to interleukin-1 improves survival after lethal endotoxemia in mice. J Exp Med 173:1029-1032
82. Mancilla J, Garcia P, Dinarello CA (1991) IL-1 receptor antagonist can either protect or enhance the lethality of Klebsiella pneumoniae sepsis in newborn rats. Cytokine (Abs) 3:502
83. Aiura K, Gelfand JA, Wakabayashi G, et al. (1991) Interleukin-1 receptor antagonist blocks Staphylococcal induced shock in rabbits. Cytokine (Abs) 3:498
84. van der Meer JWM, Curfs JHAJ, Thompson RC, Eling WMC (1991) The effect of IL-1ra in murine cerebral malaria. Cytokine (Abs) 3:497
85. Schwab JH, Anderle SK, Brown RR, Dalldorf FG, Thompson RC (1992) Pro- and anti-inflammatory roles of IL-1 in recurrence of bacterial cell wall-induced arthritis in rats. Inf Immun (in press)
86. Wooley PH, Whalen JD, Chapman DL, et al. (1990) The effect of an interleukin-1 receptor antagonist protein on type II collagen and antigen-induced arthritis in mice. Arthritis and Rheumat (Abs) 33:S20
87. Cominelli F, Nast CC, Clark BD, et al. (1990) Interleukin-1 gene expression, synthesis and effect of specific IL-1 receptor blockade in rabbit immune complex colitis. J Clin Invest 86:972-980
88. Dayer-Metroz MD, Duhamel D, Rufer N, et al. (1992) IL-1ra delays the spontaenous autoimmune diabetes in the BB rat. Eur J Clin Invest (Abs) (in press)
89. HenricsonBE, Neta R, Vogel SN (1991) An interleukin-1 receptor antagonist blocks lipopolysaccharide-induced colony-stimulating factor production and early endotoxin tolerance. Infect Immun 59:1188-1191
90. Estrov Z, Kurzrock R, Wetzler M, et al. (1992) Suppression of CML colony growth by IL-1 receptor antagonist and soluble IL-1 receptors: A novel application for inhibitors of IL-1 activity. Blood (in press)
91. McIntyre KW, Sepan GJ, Kolinsky DK, et al. (1991) Interleukin-1 receptor antagonist blocks acute inflammatory responses to IL-1 and other agents in vivo. J Exp Med 173:931-939
92. Guenard V, Dinarello CA, Weston PJ, Aebischer P (1991) Peripheral nerve regeneration is impeded by interleukin-1 receptor antagonist released from a polymeric guidance channel. J Neurosci Res 29:396-400
93. McCarthy PL, Abhyankar S, Neben S, et al. (1992) Inhibition of interleukin-1 by interleukin-1 receptor antagonist prevents graft versus host desease. Blood (in press)
94. Sartor RB, Holt LC, Bender DE, Murphy ME, McCall RD, Thompson RC (1991) Prevention and treatment of experimental enterocolitis with a recombinant interleukin-1 receptor antagonist. Gastroenterology (Abs) 100:A613
95. UlichTR, Yin SM, Guo KZ, Del CJ, Eisenberg SP, Thompson RC (1991) The intratracheal administration of endotoxin and cytokines. III. The interleukin-1 (IL-1) receptor antagonist inhibits endotoxin- and IL-1-induced acute inflammation. Am J Pathol 138:521-524

Platelet Activating Factor: Rationale for the Use of PAF-Antagonists in Sepsis

J.P. Mira, J.F. Dhainaut, and F. Brunet

Introduction

Septic shock, especially due to gram-negative infection, continues to be an increasingly serious clinical problem carrying high mortality rate despite significant advances in antimicrobial therapeutics [1]. Moreover, this treatment has little effect on endotoxin (LPS), and may even promote the release of LPS from bacteria [2]. Release of LPS or other bacterial debris activate various humoral and cellular cascades which result in an effective defense against infection [3]. In many cases, however, this response becomes exaggerated causing tissue damage [4,5]. These host defense systems include complement, kinin and clotting cascades with activation of macrophages and various leukocytes [3]. These cells, in turn, release several potent mediators.

Recently, vasoactive mediators such as opioids, serotonin, histamine... have been implicated in this response. Among them, a labile factor released from platelets in the presence of antigen and leukocytes, has been described by Benveniste et al. [6,7] who first coined the term platelet activating factor (PAF). Hensen and Pinckard [8,9] gave PAF a potentiel role in pathology when they described it as the mediator of IgE anaphylaxis in the rabbit. This ether lipid has also been suggested as an important mediator in septic and endotoxic shock [10,11]. This suggestion is based on the following evidence:

(1) Infusion of exogenous PAF into animals and humans mimics many of the effects of sepsis and endotoxin [11,13]. The administration of picomolecular concentrations of PAF is associated with systemic hypotension and increased vascular permeability [11-13];
(2) PAF is produced during endotoxemia in animals and severe sepsis in humans [11-13]; and
(3) Several structurally different PAF antagonists have been reported to inhibit endotoxin-induced hypotension, lung injury and mortality [11,13].

This chapter summarizes the evidence which implicates PAF as a key mediator in inflammatory response to sepsis, and proves PAF antagonists are able to protect or reverse pathophysiological derangements in various forms of endotoxemia and septic shock.

PAF as a Key Mediator in Sepsis

Systemic Effects of PAF Administration

The administration of picomolecular concentrations of PAF produces the two most prominent and species-universal effects, i.e. **enhanced vascular permeability** [14-17] and **systemic hypotension** [14,15,18,19]. PAF can increase systemic [17,20], microvascular [21,22], and pulmonary permeabilities [23,24]. The increased permeability is suggested to occur at postcapillary venules [21], and plasma molecules as large as very low density proteins extravasate from the vascular system [17]. At low doses, the effect of PAF is direct, and the concentration required to induce extravasation in the guinea pig is several-fold less than that needed for the extravasation induced by leukotrienes or histamine [25,26]. The hypotensive effect of PAF is also a non-platelet-mediated occurrence [27]. Permeability and hypotension are independent events, since hypotension occurs at lower doses, and is immediate and reversible [28]. Conversely, the extravasation response needs 4-10 min to peak and several hours to reverse [26,29].

The major effects of PAF are accompanied by a variety of autonomic responses such as **respiratory distress** and **hematologic abnormalities** [14,15]. In contrast, these last changes depend on the platelet's sensitivity to PAF and are largely species-specific. The infusion of PAF into the sensitive species: guinea pig [30] and rabbit [31] (baboon and man are intermediate sensitivity [32]), results in rapid and pronounced thrombocytopenia and leukopenia associated with severe hypoxemia due to bronchoconstriction. Conversely, in those species with reduced platelet sensitivity (rat, rhesus primate), PAF lacks such effects [33].

Vascular Effects of PAF. The hypotensive response may be the result of vasodilatation, but the effect of PAF on blood vessels is difficult to examine in *in vivo* preparations since systemic hypotension elicits sympathetic mediated vasoconstriction [34]. However, at constant perfusion pressure, low doses of PAF produce a direct vasodilatory response of mesenteric, hindquarter and renal vessels [35]. Furthermore, intracoronary injections produce coronary vasodilation in the dog [36] and pig [37]. The vascular endothelium has been suggested to be required for the hypotensive activity of PAF in the rat [38], but not in the rabbit [39]. Other possible vasoactive mechanisms have been hypothesized: renin inhibition, central action, alpha-adrenergic antagonism [40]...

However, systemic administration of PAF is also shown to constrict rat pulmonary vessels *in vitro* [41], pig pulmonary vessels *in vivo* [42], and dog coronary vessels [43]. The constrictor responses are usually observed when large doses of PAF are utilized, and might be mediated by arachidonate metabolites such as thromboxane A2 (TXA2) [18,35] or leukotrienes [44]. Recently, Salari et al. [45] have examined the effects of PAF on isolated rat arteries. PAF did not cause contraction or relaxation. It must be mentioned, however, that, when endothelial cells were removed, 60% of the tissue slightly (10%) relaxed in response to PAF. These findings are in agreement with those of Baranes et al. [46] who reported that PAF did not contract or relax arteries but relaxed the venous tissue, in contrast to the Santamaria et al.'s report [47]. Conversely, PAF, in the presence of platelets, caused profound contraction of the aortic strips, implying that PAF was inducing the release of secondary mediator from platelets. TXA2 is probably responsible for the observed contraction, since this effect was entirely blocked by TXA2 antagonists.

Cardiac Effects of PAF. Systemic administration of PAF in doses which induce hypotension is accompanied by a low cardiac output. This alteration of cardiac output may be, especially when using large doses of PAF, the result of the decreased venous return due to peripheral vasodilatation, reduction plasma volume secondary to enhanced vascular permeability [14,17], and, in the most sensitive species, right ventricular failure due to severe pulmonary hypertension [35]. Studies conducted in isolated heart preparations have also found to produce direct myocardial depression [48,49]. Moreover, if PAF-induced severe arrhythmias [18] contributing to cardiac failure, the role of the coronary hypoperfusion remains controversial [37], but seems to be dose dependent [45]. Indeed, in isolated heart preparation, PAF at low concentration (~2 nmol) caused an initial increase in ventricular pressure and coronary flow, followed by a more prolonged decrease while coronary perfusion pressure increased (~30%). Higher concentrations of PAF (>50 nmol) immediately produced a sharp decrease in ventricular pressure and coronary flow since coronary perfusion pressure continued to increase. Interestingly, only the second phase of PAF action (decreased contractile force), was mediated through the generation of eicosanoids. This suggests that PAF might have a direct action on the cardiac cell action potential or contractile proteins independently of arachidonic acid products.

Lung Effects of PAF

Lungs taken from PAF-treated animals reveal edematous changes by increased vascular permeability [24]. In isolated perfused lungs, edema formation can be induced by PAF in the absence of circulating blood elements, although, at least in the rabbit, the addition of platelets to the perfusate increased both the pulmonary pressure and the extent of edema formation [50].

Finally PAF was shown to act on all the components of the cardiopulmonary system not only directly but also by a variety of mediators such as amines (histamine, serotonin, catecholamines), arachidonate metabolites (TXA2, leukotrienes), and other humoral and cellular products of activated cells (oxygen radicals, lysomal enzymes) [14].

Evidence for PAF Release in Sepsis

Variety of Cell Types Responsible for Synthesizing PAF

Release of large quantities of PAF is believed to result from activation of leukocytes, mast cells and macrophages during stimulation by immune complexes [14]. Salari et al. [45] found that PAF was essentially synthesized by macrophages in response to endotoxin. Endotoxin required at least 30 min to cause generation of PAF by these cells. Its most striking action was found to be its priming of the macrophages to respond to another inflammatory agent, such as zymosan. This effect was also observed for the neutrophils. However, the neutrophils were less responsive to endotoxin. These findings support the previous reports, showing that macrophages are the principle target cells of endotoxin action [51]. Enhanced release of PAF from spleen lymphocytes taken from rats exposed to bacterial peritonitis was also reported [52].

Recently, Leaver et al. [12] reported that human mononuclear cells responded to endotoxin by releasing PAF during short-term (60 min) incubations in a dose-dependent response. A paracrine action of PAF released from monocytes is supported by the elegant experiments of Salari and Walker [53], in which the perfusion medium from endotoxin-challenged monocytes produced greater cardiac effects than the addition of endotoxin-stimulated monocytes into the heart. These experiments suggest that the monocyte may contribute substantially to the PAF released during human endotoxemia.

Blood PAF Levels in Endotoxic and Septic States

Although PAF was shown to be produced and released by many cellular elements of immune and non-immune origin, and by immune and nonimmune stimuli, there is only little information on PAF production *in vivo* during pathophysiological processes [14]. The instability of PAF in the circulation, together with problems in the development of specific and sensitive assays for the measurement of PAF, has limited our knowledge about the effect of endotoxin in PAF release. Salari et al. [45] have recently resolved this issue. Using HPLC analysis, they studied the murine metabolism of PAF *in vivo*. Fig. 1 (left panel) shows the HPLC profile after 10 min of tritiated PAF intravenous administration, and the time course of PAF metabolism is shown in the right panel. Tritiated PAF was metabolized over 60 min into lyso-PAF (~30%), acyl-PAF (~10%), and some degraded products (~10%), and the remainder was found in the form of PAF. This study showed that most of the administered PAF remained in the circulation as PAF and not lyso-PAF, suggesting that, if PAF is generated after administration of endotoxin, it should be possible to detect it using bioassay techniques.

The first description of the presence of PAF in the blood was made by Pinckard et al. [54] in rabbits with systemic anaphylaxis. A PAF-like substance, that preceded the blood volume reduction due to plasma extravasa-

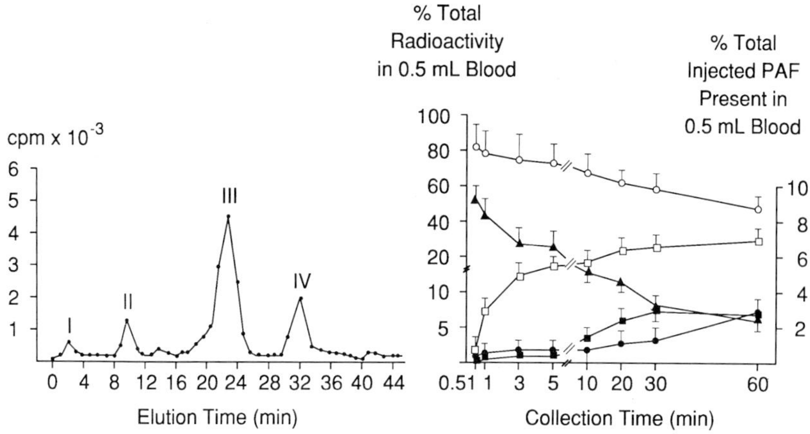

Fig. 1. Biosynthesis and metabolism of PAF in vivo. Left panel: HPLC profile of 0.5 ml blood sample injected with ^{3}H-PAF, obtained 10 min after PAF administration. Degraded products (I), acyl-PAF (II), PAF (III), and Lyso-PAF (IV). Right panel: Time course of ^{3}H-PAF metabolism in vivo. PAF (o), lyso-PAF (‡), acyl-PAF (·), and degraded products (•). Total radioactivity present in 0.5 ml blood (Δ). Mean ± SD (n = 9). (Redrawn from [45] with permission)

tion, appeared in the liver and the spleen of mice after challenge with IgG [52]. Therefore, PAF is considered to play a major role in the anaphylaxis or other forms of allergic reactions.

More interestingly, strong evidence also suggests that PAF is produced in septic conditions since elevated plasma levels of PAF were found during *E. coli* [55] and *S. enteritidis* [11,56] endotoxemia. Intravenous administration [45,55] was accompanied by a rapid increase (three times the baseline value) in PAF level in blood; this level began to decrease after 5 min and reached the initial value about 20 min (Fig. 2). After intraperitoneal injection of *S. enteritidis* in rats [11], the increase in blood PAF was quantitatively similar, but delayed to 20 min. Moreover, the high level of PAF persisted throughout the 2-h period of observation (Fig. 3, upper panel), suggesting either a high level of continued production or a marked depression in the activity of the plasma acethylhydrolase that normally degrades PAF [57].

An increase in the concentration of circulating PAF has also been reported in patients with sepsis [13,52]. Furthermore, Diez et al. [13] have shown that the high concentrations of PAF in patients with septicemia were accompanied with a reduced number of free accessible PAF receptors on platelets. This study may indicate that platelets from these septic patients had reacted with endogenous PAF and this had caused downregulation of the receptors and an enhanced internalization of PAF, or even trapping of PAF, into another compartment.

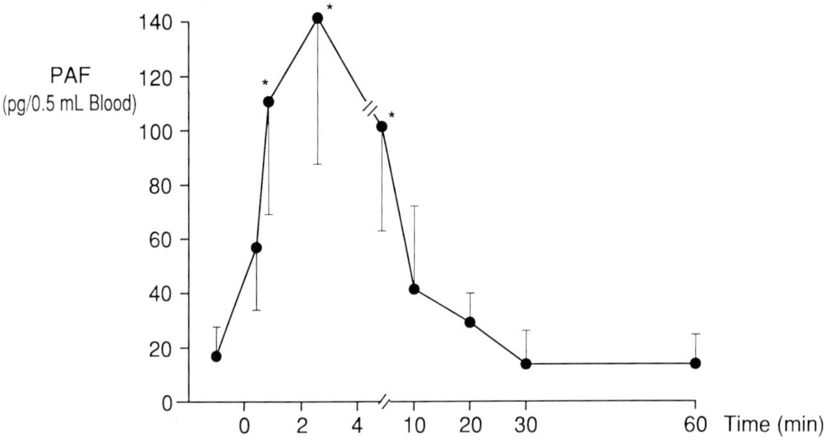

Fig. 2. Effect of endotoxin (10 ml/kg) on the synthesis and release of PAF in blood. PAF detected in 0.5 ml of blood taken at various time intervals. Mean ± SD (n = 8). (Redrawn from [45] with permission)

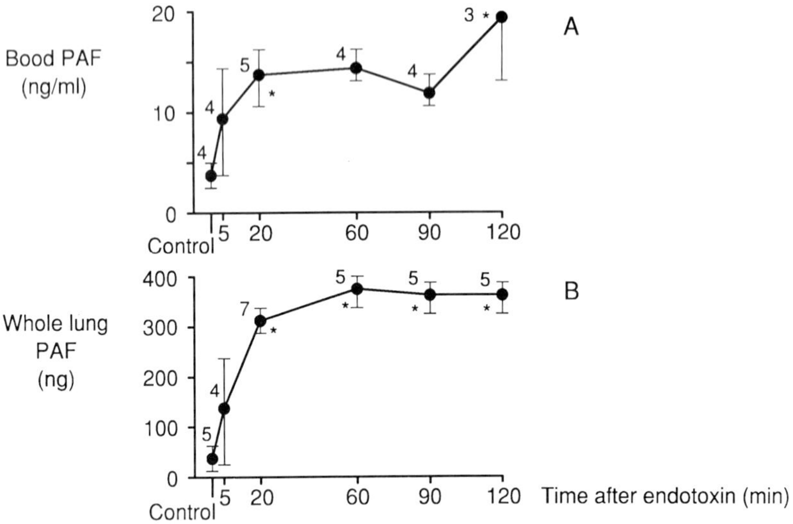

Fig. 3. (**A**) Blood PAF levels after endotoxin treatment in rats. Shown are the means (and standard errors) of blood PAF values in different groups of rats after intraperitoneal injection of 20 mg/kg S Enteritidis endotoxin. The numbers indicate the number of animals in each group. *P <0.05 from control values. (**B**) Lung PAF levels after endotoxin treatment. (Redrawn from [11] with permission)

PAF-mediated Organ Dysfunction in Endotoxin-treated Animals

Chang et al. [11] have shown that endotoxemia in rats was followed by a more impressive increase of the PAF levels in the **lung** than in the blood (Fig. 3). This might suggest either that the primary source of PAF production is in the lung or that the cells that produce PAF are sequestred in the lung after endotoxemia. Although neutrophils are sequestrated in the lung after endotoxin administration [58], neutropenia did not reduce the endotoxin-stimulated in the PAF concentrations in the lung, suggesting that neutrophils were not necessary for lung PAF synthesis. The pulmonary endothelial cells appear to be probable sources of PAF, since Camussi et al. [59,60] have recently reported both *in vitro* and *in vivo* release of PAF from injured pulmonary endothelial cells, and since pulmonary endothelial injury is a prominent finding in endotoxemia. Furthermore, the recovery of PAF in the pulmonary lavage fluid has been reported [61,62], but an inflammatory alveolitis seems not detectable until 24 h after endotoxin injection [63,64], and the lung lavage concentrations did not reflect lung tissue concentrations [11].

The **kidney** may also synthesize PAF [65]. However, in the Chang et al.'s study [11], both the baseline and post-endotoxin values of renal PAF were markedly lower than those found in the lung, although the degree of enhancement by endotoxin was similar in the two organs. Tolins et al. [66] have shown that, even in the absence of systemic hypotension in the rat, both intrarenal PAF infusion and intravenous administration of LPS produced a significant decrease in renal blood flow and glomerular filtration rate by marked afferent arteriolar vasoconstriction. Endotoxin administration in rats results in a rapid increase in phospholipase A2 activity in plasma, liver, renal and intestinal tissues. Activation of this enzyme would be expected to result in increased release of lyso-PAF and arachidonic acid from membrane phospholipids [56]. Then, PAF and vasoactive arachidonic acid metabolites are cogenerated and coparticipate in the endotoxin-induced acute renal failure.

Intraperitoneal administration of PAF or endotoxin to fasted rats disrupts the cyclic occurrence of migrating myoelectronic complexes which are replaced by an irregular spiking activity at both duodenal and jejunal levels [67]. Endogenous release of PAF is partially responsible for the intestinal motor alterations induced by endotoxin, but the release of prostaglandins also participates in this dysfunction.

Identified PAF antagonists

The activity of many PAF antagonists discussed in this section is summarized in Table 1.

Protection of PAF Antagonists in Endotoxin and Septic Shock

In endotoxin shock, PAF antagonists provide significant protection, especially against the hemodynamic derangements. The PAF antagonist CV-3988 has been shown to inhibit endotoxin-induced hypotension when given as pretreatment or after hypotension already developed following endotoxin administration in the rat [11,45,68], and also to block endotoxin-induced gastrointestinal damage [94]. Of primary importance is the finding that this PAF antagonist improves the survival rate of rats exposed to a highly lethal endotoxin shock [68]. These earlier findings are substantiated by several studies using a variety of PAF antagonists. For example, the PAF antagonists ONO-6240 and SRI 63-072 inhibit endotoxin-induced hemodynamic and hematologic derangements, but have little effect on pulmonary hypertension and hypoxemia in the sheep [95]. SRI 63-441 blocks all major endotoxin responses in several animals [11,45,73], especially inhibiting the endotoxin-induced lung vascular leak and improving the impaired hypoxic pulmonary vasoconstriction after endotoxin, as well as CV-3988 [11]. These last two PAF antagonists do not protect against leukopenia and only SRI 63-441 affected the metabolic acidosis in the endotoxin-treated rats [11].

Treatment with WEB-2086, a synthetic derivative of triazolodiazepine, 90 min to 2 h after endotoxin injection, significantly reduced lung injury and lethality in the rat (Fig. 5) [96]. The protective effect of WEB-2086 was the result of neither cyclooxygenase blockade, because the release of TXB2 by endotoxin-treated lungs was not affected by WEB-2086, nor oxidative stress reduction [96].

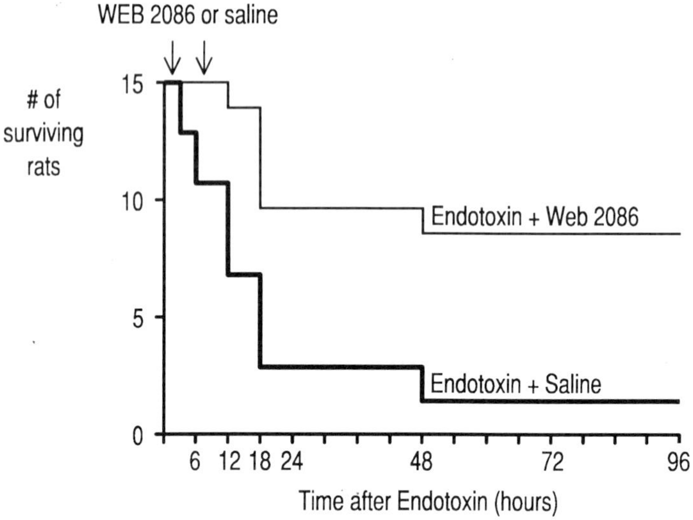

Fig. 5. Effect of WEB-2086 posttreatment of endotoxin-induced lethality. Shown are number of surviving rats at various time points after intraperitoneal injection of 20 mg/kg endotoxin.WEB-2086 (10 mg/kg) or saline was injected at 2 h (intravenous) and 6 h (intraperitoneal) after endotoxin. All deaths occurred during the first 48 h after endotoxin injection. The two survival curves are significantly different ($P < 0.005$) by the method of Mantel and Haenszel. (Redrawn from [96] with permission)

Other antagonists, kadsurenone and L-652731, were also shown to reverse the systemic hypotension produced by endotoxin administration in the rat [97], while a different PAF antagonist FR-900452 was shown to block endotoxin-induced thrombocytopenia and leukopenia in the rabbit [87,88].

The role of PAF in endotoxin shock has also been substantiated by the beneficial effects of the highly selective and potent PAF antagonist BN-52021 which was shown to markedly reduce the hypotensive response as well as the thrombocytopenia produced by *S. typhimurium* endotoxin in guinea pigs [97], and a significant dose-dependent inhibition of the lethality was observed [18,84]. This effect was associated with a lower increase in the rectal temperature of animals, suggesting that this antagonist has an effect on the release of IL-1. Indeed, when added at 10^{-12} M to adherent rat monocytes stimulated with endotoxin, PAF induced a significant increase in IL-1 synthesis and release [18]. In platelet-depleted animals, BN-52021 afforded total protection against the drop in arterial pressure, suggesting that platelets contribute to hypotension by releasing an unknown factor, not inhibited by this PAF antagonist [98]. Administered curately in the late phase of shock (90 min), BN-52021 was yet able to restore the systemic blood pressure. Furthermore, endotoxin-induced pulmonary hypertension, renal functional abnormalities, and ulcerations of the gastrointestinal tract were also partially abolished by BN-52021 [18]. Indeed, vasoactive arachidonic acid metabolites may also play a role in the multiple organ dysfunction.

Conclusion

Over the past decade, PAF has achieved the status of an important inflammatory mediator. The potential for the presence and involvement in human disease is easily concluded from the reports described in this chapter. Their findings provide a rationale for the use of PAF antagonists in patients with severe sepsis. A multicenter, randomized, double blind, clinical trial, studying the efficacy of BN-52021 in patients with sepsis syndrome, is in progress in France.

References

1. Luce JM (1987) Pathogenis and management of septic shock. Chest 91:883–888
2. Shenep JL, Morgan KA (1984) Kinetics of endotoxin release during antibiotic therapy for experimental gram-negative bacteria sepsis. J Infect Dis 150:380–388
3. Dhainaut JF, Hamy I, Schremmer B (1990) Manipulation of the immuno-inflammatory cascade in sepsis: facts and perspectives. In: Vincent JL (ed). Update in Intensive Care and Emergency Medicine Vol 10, Springer-Verlag, Berlin, pp 100–108
4. Larrick JW (1989) Antibody inhibition of the immuno-inflammatory cascade. J Crit Care 4:211–224
5. Warren HS, Chedid LA (1987) Strategies for treatment of endotoxemia: Significance of the acute-phase response. Rev Infect Dis 9:630–638

6. Benveniste J, Henson PM, Cochrane CG (1972) Leukocyte-dependent histamine release from rabbit platelets: The role of IgE-basophils and platelet-activating factor. J Exp Med 136:1356–1368
7. Benveniste J (1974) Platelet-activating factor, a new mediator of anaphylaxis and immune complex deposition from rabbit and human basophils. Nature 249:581–583
8. Henson PM, Pinckard RN (1976) Platelet-activating factor (PAF) as a mediator in IgE anaphylaxis. Fed Proc (Abs) 35:516
9. Henson PM, Pinckard RN (1977) Platelet-activating factor (PAF): A possible mediator of anaphylaxis in the rabbit and a trigger for the vascular deposition of circulating immune complexes. Monogr Allergy 12:13–26
10. Feuerstein G, Hallenbeck JM (1987) Prostaglandins, leukotrienes and platelet activating factor in shock. Ann Rev Pharmacol Toxicol 27:301–313
11. Chang SW, Feddersen CO, Henson PM, Voelkel NF (1987) Platelet activating factor mediates hemodynamic changes and lung injury in endotoxin-treated rats. J Clin Invest 79:1498–1509
12. Leaver HA, Qu JM, Smith G, Howie A, Ross WB, Yap PL (1990) Endotoxin releases platelet-activating factor from human monocytes in vitro. Immunopharmacology 20:105–113
13. Diez FL, Nieto M, Fernandez-Gallardo S, Gijon MA,Sanchez-Crespo M (1989) Occupancy of platelet receptors for platelet-activating factor in patients with septicemia. J Clin Invest 83:1733–1740
14. Feuerstein G, Stren AL (1988) Platelet-activating factor and shock. Prog Biochem Pharmacol 22:181–190
15. Saunders RN, Handley DA (1987) Platelet activating factor antagonists. Ann Rev Pharmacol Toxicol 27:237–255
16. Wendmore CV, Williams TJ (1981) Platelet-activating factor (PAF), a secretory product of polymorphonuclear leukocytes, increases vascular permeability in rabbit skin. Br J Pharmacol 74:916–918
17. Handley DA, Arbeeny CM, Lee ML, Van Valen RG, Saunders RN (1984) Effect of platelet-activating factor on endothelial permeability to plasma macromolecules. Immunopharmacology 8:137–142
18. Braquet P, Touqui L, Shen T, Vargaftig B (1987) Perspectives in platelet-activating factor. Pharmacol Rev 39:97–145
19. Blank ML, Snyder F, Byers LW, Brooks B, Muirhead EE (1979) Antihypertensive activity of an alkyl ether analog of phosphatidylcholine. Biochem Biophys Res Commun 90:1194–1200
20. Handley DA, Van Valen RG, Melden MK, Saunders RN (1984) Evaluation of dose and route effects of platelet-activating factor-induced extravasation in the guinea pig. Thromb Haemostatis 52:34–36
21. Björk J, Smedegard G (1983) Acute microvascular effects of PAF-acether, as studied by intravital microscopy. Eur J Pharmacol 96:87–94
22. Björk J, Lindbom L, Gerdin B, Smedegard G, Arfors KE, Benveniste J (1983) PAF-acether (platelet-activating factor) increases microvascular permeability and effects endothelium-granulocyte interaction in microvascular beds. Acta Physiol Scand 119:305–308
23. Bessin P, Bonnet J, Apffel D, et al. (1983) Acute circulatory collapse caused by platelet activating factor (PAF-acether) in dogs. Eur J Pharmacol 86:403–413
24. Mojarad M, Hamasaki Y, Said SI (1983) Platelet-activating factor increases pulmonary microvascular permeability and induced pulmonary edema. A preliminary report. Bull Eur Physiopathol Respir 19:253–256
25. Hwang SB, Li CH, Lam MH, Shen TY (1985) Characterization of cutaneous vascular permeability induced by platelet-activating factor in guinea pigs and rats and its inhibition by a platelet-activating factor receptor antagonist. Lab Invest 52:617–630
26. Handley DA, Farley C, Deacon R, Saunders RN (1986) Evidence for distinct systemic extravasation effects of platelet-activating factor, leukotrienes B4, C4, D4 and histamine in the guinea pigs. Prostaglandins Leukotrienes Med 21:269–277

27. Sanchez-Crespo M, Alonso F, Inarrea P, Egido J (1981) Non platelet-mediated vascular actions of 1-O-alkyl-2-acetyl-sn-3-glycerol phosphorylcholine (a synthetic PAF). Agents Actions 11:566–567
28. Handley DA, Van Valen RG, Melden MK, Flury S, Lee ML, Saunders RN (1986) Inhibition and reversal of endotoxin, aggregated IgG and PAF-induced hypotension in the rat by SRI 63072, a PAF receptor antagonist. Immunopharmacology 12:11–17
29. McManus LM, Pinckard RN, Fitzpatrick FA, O'Rourke RA, Crawford MH, Hanahan DJ (1981) Acetyl glyceryl ether phosphorylcholine (AGEPC): Intravascular alterations following intravenous infusion in the baboon. Lab Invest 45:303–307
30. Vargaftig BB, Lefort J, Chignard M, Benveniste J (1980) Platelet-activating factor induces a platelet-dependent bronchoconstriction unrelated to the formation of prostaglandin derivatives. Eur J Pharmacol 65:185–192
31. Mc Manus LM, Hanahan DJ, Demopoulos CA, Pinkard RN (1980) Pathobiology of the intravenous infusion of acetylglycerylether-phosphorylcholine (AGEPC), a synthetic platelet activating factor (PAF) in the rabbit. J Immunol 124:2919–2924
32. Winslow CM, Andersson RC, D'Aries FJ, et al. (1987) Toward understanding the mechanism of action of PAF receptor antgonists. In Winslow CM, Lee ML (ed) New Horizons in Platelet Activating Factor Research, Wiley, New York, pp. 153–164
33. Sanchez-Crespo M, Alonso F, Inarrea P, Vlvares V, Egido J (1982) Vascular actions of synthetic PAF-acether (a synthetic platelet activating factor) in the rat: Evidence for a platelet independent mechanism. Immunopharmacology 4:173–185
34. Zukowska GZ, Blank M, Snyder F, Feuerstein G (1985) The adrenergic system and the cardiovascular effects of PAF platelet activating factor (1-0-hexadecyl-2-acethyl-sn-glycero-3-phosphorylcholine) in SHR and WKY rats. Clin Exp Hyperten A7:1015–1031
35. Feuerstein G, Goldstein R (1987) Effect of PAF on the cardiovascular system. In: Snyder (ed) Platelet Activating Factor, Plenum Press, New York, pp 403–424
36. Jackson CV, Schumacher WA, Kunkel SL, Driscoll EM, Lucchesi BR (1986) Platelet-activating factor and the release of a platelet-derived coronary artery vasodilatator substance in the canine. Circ Res 58:218–229
37. Feuerstein G, Boyd LM, Erza D, Goldstein RE (1983) Effect of platelet activating factor on coronary circulation of the domestic pig. Am J Physiol 246:466–471
38. Kasuya Y, Masuda Y, Shigenobu K (1984) Possible role of endothelium in the vasodilatator response of rat thoracic aorta to platelet-activating factor (PAF). J Pharmacol Dyn 7:138–142
39. Lefer DJ, Lefer AM (1986) Failure of endothelium to mediate potential vasocactive action of platelet activating factor. Int Res Commun Syst Med Sci 14:356–357
40. Kamitani T, Katamoto M, Tatsumi M, et al. (1984) Mechanism(s) of the hypotensive effect of synthetic 1-0-octadecyl-2-0-acetyl-glycero-3-phosphorylcholine. Eur J Pharmacol 98:357–366
41. Gillespie M, Bowdy P (1986) Impact of platelet-activating factor on vascular responsiveness in isolated rat lungs. J Pharmac Exp Ther 236:396–402
42. Goldstein R, Erz D, Laurindo F, Feuerstein G (1986) Coronary and pulmonary vascular effects of leukotrienes and PAF-acether. Pharmacol Res Commun 18:151–162
43. Sybertz EJ, Watkins RW, Baum T, Pula K, Rivelli M (1985) Cardiac, coronary and vascular effects of acethyl-glyceryl-ether-phosphorylcholine in the anesthetized dogs. J Pharmacol Exp Ther 232:156–162
44. Voelkel N, Worthen S, Reeves J, Henson P, Murphy R (1982) Non-immunologic production of leukotrienes induced by platelet-activating factor. Science 218:286–288
45. Salari H, Demos M, Wong A (1990) Comparative hemodynamics and cardiovascular effects of endotoxin and platelet-activating factor in rat. Circ Shock 32:189–207
46. Baranes J, Hellegouarch A, Lettegarat M, et al. (1986) The effect of PAF-acether on the cardiovascular system and their inhibition by a new specific PAF–acether receptor antagonist BN 52021. Pharmacol Res Commun 18:717–737
47. Santamaria R, Pourrias B, Benveniste B (1983) First PAF-acether Symposium. J Pharmacol S1:14

48. Camussi G, Alloatti G, Montrucchio G, Meda M, Emanulli G (1984) Effect of platelet-activating factor on guinea pig papillary muscle. Experientia 40:697–699
49. Saeki S, Masugi F, Ogihara T, et al. (1985) Effect of 1-0-alkyl-2-acethyl-sn-glycero-3-phosphorylcholine (platelet-activating factor) on cardiac function in perfused guinea pig heart. Life Sci 37:325–329
50. Heffner JE, Shoemacker SA, Canham EM, et al. (1983) Platelet-induced pulmonary hypertension and edema. A mechanism involving acethyl-glyceryl-ether-phosphorylcholine and thromboxane A2. Chest 83:78–85
51. Miller CL (1982) Endotoxin action on macrophages. In: Collins JA, Murawski K, Schafer AW (eds) Massive transfusion in surgery and trauma. Alan R. Liss, New York, pp. 91–97
52. Inarrea P, Gomes-Cambronero J, Pascual J, Carmen-Ponte M, Hernando L, Sanchez-Crespo M (1985) Synthesis of PAF-acether and blood volume changes in gram-negative sepsis. Immunopharmacology 9:45–52
53. Salari H, Walker MJA (1989) Cardiac dysfunction caused by factors released from endotoxin-activated macrophages. Circ Shock 27:263–272
54. Pinckard RN, Farr RS, Hanahan DJ (1979) Physicochemical and functional identity of platelet-activating factor (PAF) release in vivo during IgE anaphylaxis with PAF released in vitro from IgE sensitized basophils. J Immunol 123:1847–1856
55. Doebber T, Wu MS, Robbins J, Choy B, Chang M, Shen T (1985) Platelet activating factor (PAF) involvement in endotoxin induced hypotension in rats; Studies with PAF receptor antagonist kadsurenone. Biochem Biophys Res Commun 127:799–808
56. Braquet P, Paubert-Braquet M, Bessin P, Vargaftig BB (1987) Platelet-activating factor: A potential mediator of shock. In: Samuelsson B, Paoletti R, Ramwell PW (eds) Adv Prostglandins, Thromb Leukotriene Res Vol. 17 Raven Press, New York, pp. 822–827
57. Grandel KE, Farr RS, Wanderer AA, Eisenstadt TC, Wasserman SJ (1985) Association of platelet-activating factor with primary acquired cold urticaria. N Engl J Med 313:405–409
58. Meyrick B, Brigham KL (1983) Acute effects of Escherichia coli endotoxin on the pulmonary microvascularization of anesthetized sheep: Structure, function relationship. Lab Invest 48:458–470
59. Camussi G, Pawlowski I, Bussolino F, Caldwell PRB, Brentjens J, Andres G (1983) Release of platelet-activating factor in rabbits with antibody-mediated injury of the lung: The role of leukocytes and of pulmonary endothelial cells. J Immunol 131:1802–1807
60. Camussi G, Aglietta M, Malavasi F, et al. (1983) The release of platelet activating factor from human endothelial cells in culture. J Immunol 131:2397–2403
61. Prevost MC, Cariven C, Simon MF, Chap H, Douste-Blazy L (1984) Platelet-activating factor (PAF) is released into rat pulmonary alveolar fluids as a consequence of hypoxia. Biochem Biophys Res Commun 119:58–63
62. Fasules J, Stenmark KR, Henson PM, Voelkel NF, Tucker A, Reeves JT (1985) Platelet-activating factor in lung lavage of chronically hypoxic neonatal calves. Am Rev Respir Dis (Abs) 133:A227
63. Rinaldo JE, Dauber JH, Christman J, Rogers RM (1984) Neutrophils alveolitis following endotoxemia: Enhancement by previous exposure to hyperoxia. Am Rev Respir Dis 130:1065–1071
64. Chang JC, Lesser M (1984) Quantitation of leukocytes in bronchoalveolar lavage samples from rats after intravascular injection of endotoxin. Am Rev Respir Dis 129:72–75
65. Pirotsky E, Bidault J, Burtin C, Gubler MC, Benveniste J (1984) Release of platelet-activating factor, slow-reacting substance, and vasoactive amines from isolated rat kidneys. Kidney Int 25:404–410
66. Tolins JP, Vercelloti GM, Wilkowske MHaB, Jacob HS, Raij L (1989) Role of platelet activating factor in endotoxemic acute renal failure in the male rat. J Lab Clin Med 113:316–324
67. Pons L, Droy-Lefaix MT, Braquet P, Buéno L (1989) Involvement of platelet activating factor (PAF) in endotoxin induced intestinal motor disturbances in rats. Life Sci 45:533–541
68. Terashita Z, Taushima S, Yoshioka Y, Nomura H, Inada Y, Nishikawa K (1983) CV-3988 - A specific antagonist of platelet-activating factor (PAF). Life Sci 32:1975–1981
69. Terashita Z, Imura Y, Nishikawa K, Sumida S (1985) Is platelet activating factor (PAF) a mediator of endotoxin shock? Eur J Pharmacol 109:257–263

70. Handley DA, Lee ML, Saunders RN (1985) Evidence for the direct effect on vascular permeability of platelet-activating factor induced hemoconcentration in the guinea pig. Thromb Haemostasis 54:756–759
71. Handley DA, Deacon RW, Farley C, Saunders RN, Van Valen RG (1985) Biological effects of PAF in the non-human primate Cebus apella. Fed Proc (Abs) 44:1268
72. Miyamoto T, Ohno H, Yano T, Okada T, Hamabaka N, Kawasaki A (1985) ONO-6240: A new potent antagonist of platelet activating factor. Adv Prostaglandins Thromb Leukotriene Res 15:719–720
73. Handley DA, Tomesch JC, Saunders RN (1986) Inhibition of PAF-induced responses in the rat, guinea pig, dog and primate by the receptor antagonist SRI 63-441. Thromb Haemostasis 56:40-44
74. Berri K, Barner R, Cassal JM, Hadvary P, Hirth G, Muller, K (1985) PAF: From agonists to antagonists by synthesis. Prostaglandins (Abs) 30:691
75. Hadvary P, Baumgartner HR (1985) Interference of PAF-acether antagonists with platelet aggregation and with the formation of platelet thrombi. Prostaglandins (Abs) 30:694
76. Sediry P, Caillard CG, Floch A, et al. (1985) 48740 RP: A specific PAF-acether antagonist. Prostaglandins (Abs) 30:688
77. Coeffier E, Borrel MC, Lefort J, et al. (1985) Effect of PAF-acether antagonists RP 48740 and BN 52021, on platelet activating and bronchoconstriction induced by PAF-acether and structural analogous in guinea pig. Prostaglandins (Abs) 30:699
78. ShenTY, Hwang SB, Chang MN, et al. (1985) Characterization of a platelet-activating factor receptor antagonist isolated from haifenteng (Piper futokadsura): Specific inhibition of in vitro and in vivo platelet-activating factor-induced effects. Proc Natl Acad Sci USA 82:672–676
79. Hwang SB, Lam MH, Li CH, Shen TY (1986) Release of platelet-activating factor and its involvement in the first phase of carrageening-induced rat foot edema. Eur J Pharmacol 120:33–41
80. Doebber T, Wu M, Biftu T (1986) Platelet activating factor (PAF) mediation on rat anaphylactic responses to soluble immune complexes.Studies with PAF receptor antagonist L-652 731. J Immunol 136:4659–4668
81. Handley DA, Farley C, Melden MK, Deacon RW, VanValen RG, Saunders RN (1986) Comparative oral and parenteral activities of several PAF antagonists in the rat and guinea pig. Presented at Platelet Activating Factor, 2nd Int. Conf. Gatlingburg, Tenn.
82. Braquet P, Godfroid JJ (1986) PAF-acether specific binding sites: 2. Design of specific antagonists. Trend Pharmacol Sci 7:397–403
83. Sanchez-Crespo M, Fernandez-Gallardo S, Nieto ML, Baranes J, Braquet P (1985) Inhibition of the vascular actions of IgG aggregates by BN 52021, a highly specific antagonist of PAF-acether. Immunopharmacology 15:69–75
84. Etienne A, Hecquet F, Souland F, Spinnewyn B, Clostre F, Braquet P (1985) In vivo inhibition of plama protein leakage and salmonella enteritidis-induced mortality in the rat by a specific PAF acether antagonist BN 52021. Agents Actions 17:368–370
85. Touvay C, Etienne A, Braquet P (1985) Inhibition of antigen-induced lung anaphylaxis in the guinea pig by BN 52021 a new specific PAF-acether antagonist isolated from Ginko biloba. Agents Actions 17:371–372
86. Foegh ML, Khirabadi BS, Braquet P, Ramwell PW (1985). Platelet-activating factor antagonist BN 52021 prolongs experimental cardiac allograft survival. Prostaglandins (Abs) 30:718
87. Okamoto M, Yoshida K, Nishikiwa M, et al. (1986) FR-900452 a specific inhibitor of platelet-activating factor (PAF) produced by Streptomyces phalofaciens. J Antibiot 39:198–204
88. Okamoto M, Yoshida K, Uchida I, Kohsada M, Aoki H (1986) Studies of platelet-activating factor (PAF) antagonists from microbial products. II Pharmacological studies of FR-49175 in animal models. Chem Pharm Bull 34:345–348
89. Kornecki E, Ehrlich YM, Lemox RW (1984) Platelet-activating factor induced aggregation of human platelets specifically inhibited by triazolobenzodiazepines. Science 226:1954–1957
90. Camussi G,Tetta C, Bussolino F (1983) Inhibitory effect of prostacyclin (PGI 2) on neutropenia induced by intravenous injection of platelet-activating factor (PAF) in the rabbit. Prostaglandins 25:343–349

91. Myers AK, Ramey E, Ranwell P (1983) Glucocorticoid protection against PAF-acether toxicity in mice. Br J Pharmacol 79:595–598
92. Feuerstein G, Lux WE, Snyder F, Erza D, Faden AI (1984) Hypotension produced by platelet-activating factor is reversed by thyrotropin-releasing hormone.Circ Shock 13:255–260
93. Westwick J, Marks G, Powling MJ, Kakkar VV (1983) Diltiazem, the cardiac channel calcium antagonist, is a potent, selective and competitive inhibitor of platelet-activating factor on human platelets. J Pharmacol 14:62–68
94. Wallace JL, Whittle BJR (1986) Prevention of endotoxin-induced gastrointestinal damage by CV-3988, an antagonist of platelet-activating factor. Eur J Pharmacol 124:209–210
95. Toyofuku T, Kubo K, Kobayashi T, Kusama S (1986) Effects of ONO-6240, a platelet activating factor antagonist, on endotoxin shock in unanesthetized sheep. Prostaglandins 31:271–280
96. Chang SW, Fernyak S, Voelkel NF (1990) Beneficial effect of a platelet activating factor antagonist, WEB 2086, on endotoxin-induced lung injury. Am J Physiol 257:153–158
97. Wu M, Biftu T, Doebber T (1986) Inhibition of the platelet-activating factor (PAF) induced in vivo responses in rats by trans-2,5-(3,4,5-trimethoxyphenyl) tetrahydrofuran(L-652,731), a PAF receptor antagonist. J Pharmac Exp Ther 239:841–845
98. Adnot S, Lefort J, Lagente V, Braquet P, Vargaftig BB (1986) Interference of BN 52021, a PAF-acether antagonist, with endotoxin-induced hypotension in the guinea-pig. Pharmacol Res Commun 18:197–200

Mediator Gene Expression in Sepsis: Implications for Therapy

K.L. Brigham, A.E. Canonico, and J.T. Conary

Introduction

Diffuse lung injury resulting in the clinical entity commonly called the adult respiratory distress sydrome (ARDS), remains highly lethal. Since the clinical description of the syndrome about 20 years ago, mortality in published series of patients has changed very little. This is true in spite of major advances in the technology of critical care medicine. Although a large amount of research has dramatically enhanced the understanding of mechanisms of lung injury and respiratory failure in ARDS, this has, so far, not translated into demonstrably effective pharmacological interventions.

However, there are several pharmacological interventions currently being studied which hold promise. For example, a large multi-center prospective placebo controlled trial of the efficacy of the non-steroidal anti-inflammatory agent ibuprofen in patients with sepsis is currently underway and promises important new information about this class of drugs in this clinical setting. Preliminary clinical studies with the anti-oxidant n-acetylcysteine in patients with established ARDS and respiratory failure also appear promising. Conclusions about efficacy for this class of glutathione repleting drugs must await completion of definitive large studies. Other promising pharmacological interventions include a whole range of antioxidant substances, airway installation of surfactant, and manipulation of the generation or effects of various lipid mediators including platelet activating factor and eicosanoids. Recognition that diffuse lung injury resulting in ARDS is, at its root, an inflammatory condition has heavily influenced the development of therapeutic rationales.

The rapid development of techniques of molecular biology permitting manipulation of DNA has provided new opportunities for understanding the pathogenesis of diffuse lung injury and for developing novel therapies. Information describing the inflammatory process at the molecular level is directly applicable to many forms of diffuse lung injury. As alteration in expression of genes encoding important proteins in the process of injury is understood more thoroughly, new therapeutic rationales will emerge. For example, pharmacological interventions which have their effect as a result of altering gene expression may become useful. In addition, the new field of gene therapy may also be expanded to apply to acute diseases like ARDS.

This chapter will summarize some of the information relevant to alterations in gene expression which occur in the process of lung injury and how the techniques of molecular biology might be used in developing rationales for therapy and strategies for preventing or treating patients with diffuse lung injury. The chapter is not meant to be encyclopedic, but simply to illustrate the current advantages and potential for molecular biological methods in understanding and treating diffuse lung injury.

Experimental Endotoxemia as a Model of ARDS

Although ARDS occurs in humans in a number of clinical settings, in many reported series the predominant risk factor is sepsis [1,2,3]. As a result of that fact and of the fact that the pathophysiology of responses to endotoxemia in some experimental animals resembles the pathophysiology of ARDS, animal models of endotoxemia have been studied by numerous investigators interested in the clinical syndrome. For the past twenty years, we have used a chronically instrumented unanesthetized sheep endotoxemia model to study alterations in lung structure and function which we infer are relevant to the clinical syndrome of ARDS [4-7].

Fig. 1 schematically summarizes some of the pathophysiological responses to endotoxemia in chronically instrumented sheep. The response includes changes in function of both airways and the lung circulation. Alterations in lung mechanics include decreases in lung compliance and increases in resistance to airflow across the lungs. In addition to those acute changes in airway function, airway reactivity is also increased during the first few hours

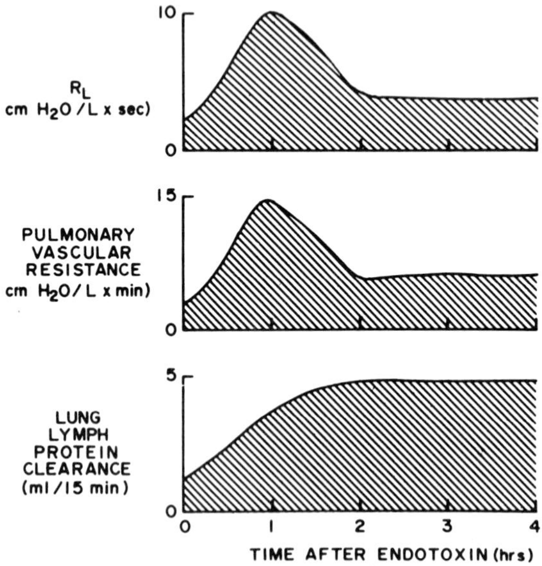

Fig. 1. Schematic representation of some changes in lung function caused by endotoxemia in sheep

following endotoxemia [8]. Pulmonary hypertension is a uniform and characteristic response to endotoxemia and is also common in patients with ARDS. In the sheep model, there is a marked early increase in pulmonary artery pressure and a more modest elevation in pulmonary vascular resistance which persists for several hours. The normal hypoxic vasoconstrictor response is lost following endotoxemia [9]. If sufficient doses of endotoxin are given to unanesthetized sheep, there evolves over 7 to 9 h a syndrome indistinguishable from the clinical syndrome of ARDS [10]. Animals develop severe respiratory failure, refractory hypoxemia, and diffuse pulmonary edema, and die of respiratory failure [10].

Bovine pulmonary artery endothelial cells in culture also are susceptible to toxic injury by low concentrations of endotoxin [11]. Since, in the whole animal, endothelial injury is an early and conspicuous event in the evolution of respiratory failure [12], endotoxin induced injury in cultured endothelial cells may have relevance to endotoxin induced injury of the whole lung.

Both the whole animal endotoxin preparation and cultured endothelial cell responses to endotoxin have been useful in deciphering pathogenetic mechanisms involved in acute lung injury. Information derived from a large body of research in these preparations now provides rationales for selection of pharmacological interventions which may be useful in humans.

Alterations in Gene Expression in Acute Lung Injury

Acute lung injury examplified by experimental responses to endotoxemia is a complexity of events. Release of numerous mediators, cytokines and other

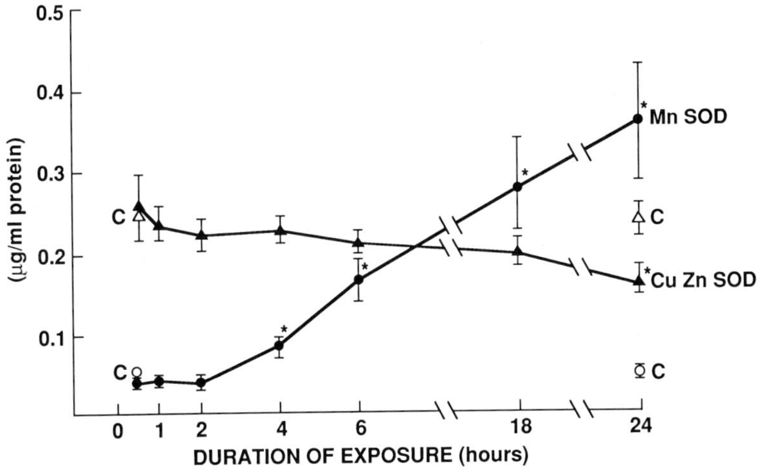

Fig. 2. Effects of endotoxin exposure on lung endothelial cell content of superoxide dismutase (SOD). (From [16] with permission)

chemicals which may participate in functional and structural derangements of the lung can be demonstrated. In addition, there is recent evidence that synthesis of several proteins which may directly or indirectly affect lung function is affected by endotoxin at a molecular level.

Several different kinds of data suggest that endotoxin induced injury of the lung involves, either directly or indirectly, oxidant stress [13-15]. Since oxidant stress might be thought to increase endogenous synthesis of antioxidant substances, we looked at the effects of endotoxin exposure of cultured bovine endothelial cells on endothelial cell content of several antioxidant enzymes. We found that endotoxin increased the amount of manganese superoxide dismutase (MnSOD) in a time course shown in Fig. 2 [16]. This increase in mitochondrial associated SOD was not accompanied by an increase in copper zinc SOD (the cytosolic form). In addition, as shown in Table 1, endotoxin exposure did not cause increases in lung endothelial cell content of catalase or of mitochondrial enzymes other than MnSOD [16]. In more recent studies, we have measured messenger RNA specific for MnSOD in the same endothelial cell cultured preparation, and have found that endotoxin exposure increases expression of the MnSOD gene (Meyrick, unpublished).

Numerous studies have demonstrated in both whole animals and in cultured cell preparations that endotoxin exposure causes release of several prostanoids [17-19]. In endothelial cells in culture, the increase in release of endothelial derived prostanoids (prostacyclin and PGE_2) appears to result, at least in part, from increased expression of the gene encoding the protein prostaglandin synthase. In our preliminary studies in both cultured endothelial cells and in the sheep endotoxin model, it appears that PGH synthase is induced as a consequence of endotoxin exposure, and that this molecular level event is important in the generation of prostanoids [20,21].

Table 1. Protein and enzyme concentrations in endothelial cells exposed to endotoxin. (From [16] with permission).

Time after endotoxin exposure, h	Protein	Glutathione Peroxidase	Catalase	Cyto-chrome-*c* oxidase	Fumarase
Control					
1	8.42±0.52	34±7	12±1	19±5	123±13
24	8.87±0.54	29±5	12±1	15±1	126±8
Endotoxin					
0.5	9.01±0.76	33±7	12±2	21±2	129±15
1	8.98±0.66	32±5	11±1	19±4	125±11
2	8.93±0.63	32±8	10±1	23±8	119±14
4	9.15±0.49	33±8	11±1	17±5	113±11
6	8.73±0.53	32±6	12±1	18±5	117±13
18	7.99±0.56	25±5	11±1	16±2	118±12
24	7.56±0.60	15±2	10±2	17±4	104±12

The endothelins are a family of peptides with potent biological properties. Endothelin 1 is a pulmonary vasoconstrictor which appears to be generated during inflammatory responses and, therefore, could participate in the pulmonary vasoconstriction typical of the endotoxin response. We looked at the time course of endothelial generation by the lung in sheep following endotoxin infusion and found increased production and release of endothelin in a manner consistent with increased expression of the gene encoding this peptide [22].

The macrophage derived cytokine, tumor necrosis factor (TNF), has been proposed as an important mediator of the physiological events of sepsis. We found that when TNF was infused into sheep, it was possible to reproduce many of the structural and functional features of the endotoxin response [23,24]. Endotoxin is the classic stimulus for generation of TNF by macrophages. The generation of TNF by macrophages following endotoxin exposure appears to involve increase in expression of the gene encoding the cytokine.

All of these data, and others, are consistent with the notion that endotoxin, a principal stimulus for acute lung injury resulting in ARDS in humans, induces increased expression of genes encoding a number of peptides which could be important either in the pathophysiology of respiratory failure, or in protecting the lung against extensive injury.

It is possible that a category of pharmacological interventions could be identified which would either exaggerate induction of genes encoding protective proteins, or repress induction of genes encoding destructive proteins. For example, in macrophages in culture, endotoxin induced increases in messenger RNA for TNF can be suppressed by the addition of prostaglandin E_2 to the cultures [25]. Since macrophages also generate prostaglandin E_2, it has been suggested that this may reflect a control system within the macrophage. In the sheep endotoxin model, we found that infusion of large amounts of prostaglandin E_2 significantly attenuated pulmonary responses to endotoxemia [26]. It is possible that this effect of prostaglandin E_2 is mediated via an effect on gene expression characteristic of the inflammatory response.

The Conventional View of Gene Therapy

As the techniques for analyzing and manipulating DNA have developed, a number of specific genetic abnormalities associated with specific clinical diseases have been identified. Classic examples related to the lungs would include alpha-1 antitrypsin deficiency and cystic fibrosis. Since in these cases, the disease appears to be a consequence of the lack of generation of a single normal protein, and the specific genetic abnormality is identified, it is presumed that the disease could be cured by introducing into the host genome a gene encoding the deficient protein which functions normally. A substantial body of work is now in progress in experimental preparations, and some preliminary work in humans is designed to test the notion that this is a safe and effective rationale for treating diseases which are a consequence of a genetic abnormality.

Several strategies for delivering genes into intact organisms have been used. The most common strategy is to engineer cells in culture using retroviral vectors which assure insertion of the DNA into the genome of the cultured cells, and reimplanting these transformed cells into the intact organism. Such cells might correct the disease if engineered to hyperexpress a gene encoding a secreted protein deficient in the host. An example here in the lungs would be alpha-1 antitrypsin deficiency. Both genetically engineered fibroblasts and genetically engineered lymphocytes have been used in this manner.

For deficiencies of proteins which are either intracellular or integral to the cell, the problem is somewhat different. For example, the cystic fibrosis transmembrane regulator (CFTR) gene, the expression of which is abnormal in patients with cystic fibrosis, encodes a transmembrane protein which must be present in respiratory epithelium for ion transport to function normally. To effectively treat patients with cystic fibrosis, the CFTR gene would have to be expressed in a sufficient number of respiratory epithelial cells to correct the physiological abnormalities.

The goal for most of conventional gene therapy is to permanently alter host cells in a manner which assures that they will express the deficient gene, and will confer the ability to express the deficient gene to subsequent generations of cells. The goal here is a permanent alteration in the host genome.

Transient Gene Therapy (Gene Therapeutics)

Most diseases of the lungs, and other organs for that matter, are not, so far as we know, a consequence of a genetic abnormality. In the current context, ARDS is a transient disease. Patients are at risk, they either develop the syndrome or they do not, and they either live or die. As far as the pathogenesis of ARDS is understood, it is not a direct consequence of a genetic abnormality. However, if it were possible to transiently alter gene expression for proteins which were either protective or deleterious, then this might represent a novel therapeutic rationale.

Such approaches are at least theoretically possible. DNA which functions can be introduced into cells in a form in which it does not readily incorporate into the host genome. This is known in cultured cells as transient transfection. DNA in the form of plasmids which do not replicate in eukaryotic cells can be introduced by a variety of techniques into cultured cells and the encoding portions of the introduced DNA expressed in the host cells transiently. The potential for using this approach as a therapeutic modality, that is using DNA as a drug, has been termed transient gene therapy, or gene therapeutics.

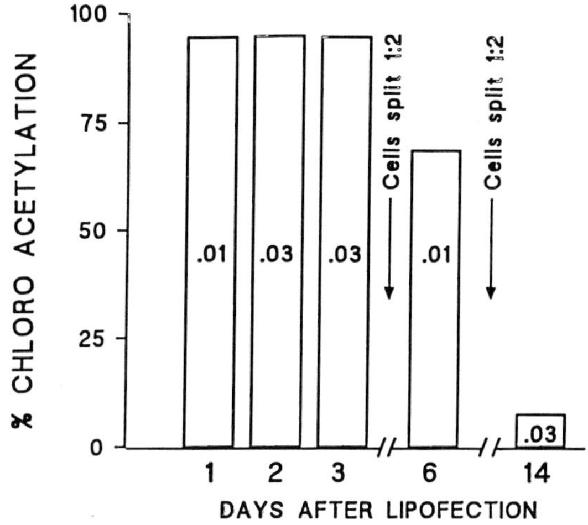

Fig. 3. Time course of expression of CAT activity in endothelial cells transfected with 10 μg DNA per 60-mm dish. All samples were incubated for 4 h in the CAT assays, and the numbers in the bars are milligrams of cell protein in the assay. The cells were split 1/2 on day 3 and day 6 after lipofection. CAT activity began to decline slightly after the first split of the cells and by 14 days after lipofection (8 days after the last split of the cells), was markedly reduced although still detectable. (From [29] with permission)

ARDS should be vulnerable to this approach. A principal focus of work in this area, presently, is the development of strategies for delivering genes into the cells of lungs of intact organisms.

Delivery of Genes to the Lungs

To date, two methods have been published for delivering genes directly into the lungs. Rosenfeld et al. [27] have used an adeno-virus vector delivered through the airways to express the human alpha-1 antitrypsin gene or the human CFTR gene in the lungs of cotton rats. It appears possible to obtain functioning cDNA in the lungs using this technique, although the quantitative generation of gene product may not yet have been demonstrated to reach therapeutic levels.

We have used small cationic unilamellar liposomes, originally described for use of transfection of cells in culture, and DNA in the form of plasmids to transiently express genes in the lungs of mice, rats, rabbits, and sheep [20,30,32].

Felgner et al. [28] originally described the synthesis of cationic liposomes which associated by charge with DNA and escorted DNA into cells in culture. Since that original description, several commercial preparations of these liposomes have become available. We initially tested whether lung endothe-

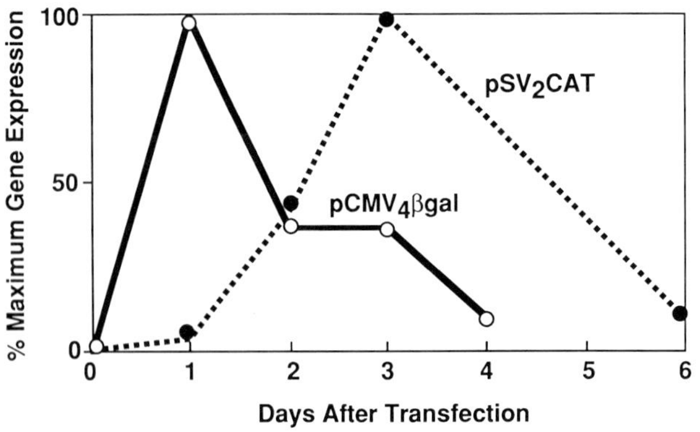

Fig. 4. Time course of expression of two different DNA constructs in transfected lung endothelial cells in culture

lial cells in culture would be vulnerable to transfection using this technique called lipofection [29]. As shown in Fig. 3, expression of the prokaryotic gene chloramphenicol acetyl transferase was achieved in lung endothelial cells in culture when a plasmid containing the cDNA for that gene driven by an RSV promote was introduced into the cells by lipofection. Expression of the gene was exuberant and lasted for days, even following splitting of the cells. Fig. 4 shows the time course of expression of the beta-glactosidase gene in a construct which the gene was driven by a CMV promoter, and the CAT gene driven by an RSV promoter. In both cases the cDNA for the reporter gene was contained in a plasmid and was introduced by lipofection in the cultured bovine lung endothelial cells. It is obvious that the method of lipofection works in lung endothelial cells in culture. The data suggests that the time course of expression may be manipulable by choosing the DNA construct. We tested whether the technique of lipofection could be used to transfect the lungs *in vivo* with foreign DNA. We reasoned that, since the lungs were the first microvascular bed seen by intravenously injected substances, intravenous injection of DNA liposome complexes might transfect endothelial cells in the lung. In addition, the lung is uniquely available by administering DNA liposome complexes through the airways. In the initial studies in mice reported in 1989 [30], we injected DNA liposome complexes either intravenously or intratracheally into mice. The DNA construct contained chloramphenicol acetyl transferase gene as a reporter driver by an SV-40 early promoter. The time course of expression of the CAT gene in the lungs of mice is shown in Fig. 5. The time course was similar to that which we saw in cultured endothelial cells. Expression of the foreign gene began at about day 1, peaked at about day 3, and persisted for several days thereafter. Table 2 summarizes the data using the CAT reporter gene in mice. From those data it

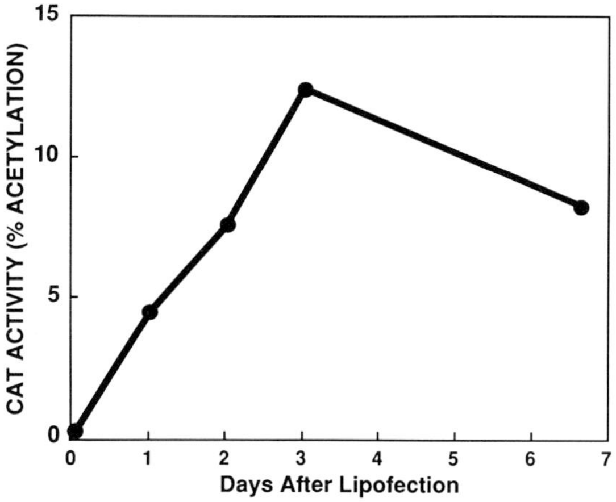

Fig. 5. Time course of expression of CAT gene in lungs of mice following intravenous lipofection

appeared that there was a dose related expression of DNA delivered by lipofection intravenously in the lungs. When material was injected via the airway, greater expression in the lung was seen for a similar dose of DNA. Intraperineal injection of the DNA liposome complexes resulted in no expression of the foreign gene. In those studies, we found expression of the gene limited to the lungs, that is we saw no detectable chloramphenicol acetyl transferase activity in either liver or kidneys regardless of the dose or route of DNA liposome injection.

We have now constructed additional vectors containing the cNDA for human alpha-1 antitrypsin driven by a CMV promoter. When this DNA construct complexed to small cationic liposomes is injected intravenously or delivered by aerosol to rabbits, expression of the gene can clearly be demon-

Table 2. CAT activity in lungs, liver and kidneys 72 hours following DNA-liposome injection into mice (from [30] with permission).

Route	% Chloramphenicol Acetylation per h per µg Protein X 10^{-2}		
	Lungs	Liver	Kidneys
Intravenous			
30 µg DNA per mouse	24.5	0	0
15 µg DNA per mouse	10.1	0	0
Intratracheal			
30 µg DNA per mouse	35.7	0	0
Intraperitoneal			
30 µg DNA per mouse	0	0	0

strated in the lungs. It appears that the alpha-1 antitrypsin gene product localizes to the epithelium in the airways regardless of the route by which the foreign DNA is delivered. Using a similar construct with the ovine PGH synthase gene in rabbits, we also have been able to show expression of the introduced CDNA in the lungs [31,32]. Recently, we have completed studies in sheep in which we have instilled the alpha-1 antitrypsin construct via bronchoscope into a lung sub-segment and subsequently demonstrated generation of human alpha-1 antitrypsin by the transfected segment removed from the animal (Canonico et al., unpublished).

All of these data clearly demonstrate the phenomenon that it is possible to deliver functioning foreign DNA into the lungs of intact animals. Using liposomes, the delivery procedure appears to be safe, at least acutely. Quantitative questions remain. It is not clear yet that sufficient generation of protein is achieved via this route to effect a therapeutic outcome.

What Genes Should be Manipulated to Treat ARDS?

As the delivery technologies are developed sufficiently to make this approach to gene therapy feasible clinically, further development of therapy will depend on the development of effective rationales for selecting genes, the expression of which should be altered to prevent or treat acute lung injury. In theory, it would be possible either to increase amounts of gene product or decrease them by introducing sense cDNA driven by a strong promoter, or anti-sense DNA driven by a strong promoter. There is good reason to think that expression of several genes could be altered in a way that could be beneficial to the lungs.

For example, as discussed above, oxidant stress appears to be an important common denominator for many types of acute lung injury. The endogenous proteins superoxide dismutase and catalase and other proteins are intimately involved in redox regulation in the lungs as in other organs. There is evidence that hyperexpression of manganese superoxide dismutase inside lung cells might protect them from oxidant stress. The human manganese SOD cDNA is available, and in theory could be delivered by the strategies discussed above in a manner which would enhance the resistance of the lungs to oxidant stress. Similar rationale could be used for a variety of other proteins including antiproteases (proteolytic injury may also be important in acute lung injury).

If foreign genes could be selectively introduced into sub-populations of lung cells, this might pave the way for gene therapeutics used in a manner to protect against pathological changes in lung function. For example, the endothelial derived prostanoids, prostaglandin E_2 and prostacyclin, have many effects which might be protective of the lung. Prostaglandin E_2 is generally anti-inflammatory, and prostacyclin is a pulmonary vasodilator. If the intravenous delivery of cDNA selectively transfected endothelial cells in the lungs, then the principal product of hyperexpression of prostaglandin synthase would be expected to be prostaglandin E_2 and prostacyclin. Our early experimental data suggest this to be true [20].

If the generation of cytokines is principally a consequence of increases in gene expression, then it might be possible to manipulate production of cytokines using gene therapeutics. If TNF is a mediator of the pathology of endotoxemia for example, and anti-sense DNA for TNF were hyperexpressed in the cells which generate TNF, then it might be possible to diminish production of this toxic mediator over a transient period of time during which the lungs were at risk for injury.

It is obvious from this discussion that a large list of potential genes, either the hyperexpression or diminished expression of which might be beneficial to the lungs, could be generated.

Potential Problems

The principal problems currently in developing this technology for clinical application are the demonstration of safety and efficacy. It seems intuitively likely that the introduction of DNA in forms which do not readily incorporate into the host genome should be safer than altering the host genome with foreign DNA. However, introducing foreign DNA in any form into the cells of humans has long term consequences which remain unknown.

Most of the studies to date have failed to demonstrate high concentrations of gene product in the lungs regardless of the manner or route by which it is introduced. Obviously, efficacy will depend upon the quantitative generation of the protein encoded by the introduced gene. It is likely that this problem will be overcome, by the development of more efficient vectors and more efficient delivery systems for the lungs. However, it will be important to demonstrate efficacy in animal models prior to applying such technology in the clinical setting.

Conclusion

Current understanding of the pathogenesis of acute lung injury resulting in the clinical syndrome of ARDS provides a basis for multiple rationales for both pharmacological and other interventions. The development of the techniques of molecular biology now allows those investigating acute lung injury to understand the pathogenesis of the injury at a molecular level.This understanding will allow the design of pharmacological interventions which may affect gene expression as their principal mode of action.In addition, the development of strategies for delivering functioning DNA to the lungs in a form in which the DNA does not alter the host genome and is expressed only transiently, may allow gene therapy to be applied in this acute self-limited clinical situation. Initial studies in that regard appear promising.

It seems likely that the tools of molecular biology, over the years, will have a major impact on both the understanding and therapy of the processes involved in acute lung injury and the clinical syndrome of ARDS.

References

1. Harris TR, Bernard GR, Brigham KL, et al. (1990) Lung microvascular transport properties measured by multiple indicator dilution methods in ARDS patients: A comparison between patients reversing respiratory failure and those failing to reverse. Am Rev Respir Dis 141:272–280
2. Bernard GR, Brigham KL (1989) Increased lung vascular permeability: Mediators and therapies. In: Shoemaker WC (ed) Textbook of Critical Care, 2nd edn. Saunders Co, Philadelphia, PA, pp. 1049–1054
3. Brigham KL (1991) Corticosteroids in ARDS. In: Zapol WM, Lemaire F (eds) The lung. A series of monographs and textbooks. Marcel Dekker Inc, New York, NY, pp 285–304
4. Brigham KL, Bowers RE, Haynes J (1979) Increased sheep lung vascular permeability caused by E. coli endotoxin.Circ Res 45:292–297
5. Brigham KL, Padove SJ, Bryant DM, McKeen CR, Bowers RE (1980) Diphenhydramine reduces endotoxin effects on lung vascular permeability in sheep. J Appl Physiol (Respirat Environ Exercise Physiol) 49:516–520
6. Brigham KL, Bowers RE, KcKeen CR (1981) Methylprednisolone prevention of increased lung vascular permeability following endotoxemia in sheep. J Clin Invest 67:1103–1110
7. Brigham KL, Begley CJ, Bernard GR, et al. (1983) Septicemia and lung injury. Clin Lab Med 3:719–744
8. Hutchison AA, Hinson JM Jr, Brigham KL, Snapper JR (1983) The effects of endotoxin on airway responsiveness in sheep. J Appl Physiol (Respirat Environ Exercise Physiol) 54:1463–1468
9. Hutchison AA, Ogletree ML, Snapper JR, Brigham KL (1985) Effect of endotoxemia on hypoxic pulmonary vasoconstriction in unanesthetized sheep. J Appl Physiol (Respirat Environ Exercise Physiol) 58:1463–1468
10. Esbenshade AM, Newman JH, Lams PM, Jolles H, Brigham KL (1982) Respiratory failure after endotoxin infusion in sheep: Lung mechanics and lung fluid balance. J Appl Physiol (Respirat Environ Exercise Physiol) 53:967–976
11. Meyrick B, Hoover R, Jones MR, Berry LC Jr, Brigham KL (1989) In vitro effects of endotoxin on bovine and sheep lung microvascular and pulmonary artery endothelial cells. J Cell Physiol 138:165–174
12. Meyrick B, Brigham KL (1983) Acute effects of Escherichia coli endotoxin on the pulmonary microcirculation of anesthetized sheep: Structure function relationships. Lab Invest 48:458–470
13. Birgham KL, Meyrick BO, Berry LC, Repine JE (1987) Antioxidants protect cultured bovine lung endothelial cells from injury by endotoxin. J Appl Physiol 63:840–850
14. Brigham KL (1987) Mechanisms of lung endothelial injury. In: Will JA, Dawson CA,Weir EK,Buckner EK (eds) Pulmonary circulation in health and disease, Academic Press Inc, Florida, pp 363–369
15. Brigham KL (1987) Mechanisms of endothelial injury. In: Ryan US (ed) Pulmonary endothelium in health and disease. Marcel Dekker Inc, pp 207–236
16. Shiki Y, Meyrick BO,Brigham KL, Burr IM (1987) Endotoxin increases superoxide dismutase in cultured bovine pulmonary endothelial cells. Am J Physiol 252:436–440
17. Brigham KL (1989) Mediators of the inflammatory process. In: Henson P, Murphy R (eds) Prostanoids: Handbook of inflammation, vol 6: Mediators of the inflammatory process. Elsevier Science Publishers, pp 1–14

18. Ogletree ML, Begley CJ, King GA, Brigham KL (1986) Influence of steroidal and non-steroidal anti-inflammatory agents on accumulation of arachidonic acid metabolites in plasma and lung lymph after endotoxemia in awake sheep: Measurements of prostacyclin and thromboxane metabolites and I2-HETE. Am Rev Respir Dis 133:55–61
19. Meyrick BO, Ryan US, Brigham KL (1986) Direct effects of E. coli endotoxin on structure and permeability of pulmonary endothelial monolayers and the endothelial layer of intimal explants. Am J Pathol 122:140–151
20. Conary JT, Canonico AE, Parker RE, Christman BW, King G, Brigham KL (1992) Expression of a CMV promoter driven ovine prostaglandin G/H synthase gene in the lungs of rabbits. Am Rev Respir Dis 145:A850
21. Conary JT, Brown DL, Shepherd VE, Christman BW, King G, Brigham KL (1992) Expression of a CMV promoter driven ovine prostaglandin G/H synthase gene in cultured lung endothelial cells. Am Rev Respir Dis, 145:A839
22. Rummel TS, Parker RE, Conary JT, Brigham KL (1992) Time course of endotoxin-induced lung endothelin-1 production in sheep. Am Rev Respir Dis 145:A850
23. Johnson J, Brigham KL, Meyrick B (1991) Morphological changes in lungs of anesthetized sheep following intravenous infusion of recombinant human tumor necrosis factor alpha. Am Rev Respir Dis 144:179–186
24. Wheeler AP, Jesmok G, Brigham KL (1990) Tumor necrosis factor's effects on lung mechanics, gas exchange, and airway reactivity in sheep. J Appl Physiol 68:2542–2549
25. Kunkel SL, Spengler M, May AM, Spengler R, Larrick I, Remick D (1988) Prostaglandin E_2 regulated macrophage-derived tumor necrosis factor gene expression. J Biol Chem 263:5380–5384
26. Brigham KL, Serafin W, Zadoff A, Blair I, Meyrick B, Oates J (1988) Prostaglandin E_2 attenuation of sheep lung responses to endotoxin. J Appl Physiol 64:2568–2574
27. Rosenfeld MA, Siegfried W, Yoshimurc K, et al. (1991) Adeno-virus-mediated transfer of a recombinant α1-antitrypsin gene to the lung epithelium in vivo. Science 252:431–434
28. Felgner PL, Gadek TR, Holm M, et al. (1987) Lipofection: A highly efficient, lipid-mediated DNA-transfection procedure. Proc Natl Acad Sci 84:7413–7417
29. Brigham KL, Meyrick B, Christman B, Berry LC Jr, King G (1989) Expression of a prokaryotic gene in cultured lung endothelial cells following lipofection with a plasmid vector. Am J Resp Cell Molec Biol 1:95–100
30. Brigham KL, Meyrick B, Christman B, Magnuson M, King G, Berry LC Jr (1989) In vivo transfection of murine lungs with a functioning prokaryotic gene using a liposome vehicle. Am J Med Sci 298:278–281
31. Canonico AE, Conary JT, Christman BW, Meyrick BO, Brigham KL (1991) Expression of a CMV promoter driven human α-1 antitrypsin gene in cultured lung endothelial cells and in the lungs of rabbits. Clin Res 39:219
32. Canonico AE, Conary JT, Meyrick BO, Brigham KL (1992) In vivo expression of a CMV promoter driven human alpha-1 antitrypsin (alpha-1AT) gene after intravenous or airway administration of DNA/liposome complex. Am Rev Respir Dis 145:A200

Subject Index